AMERICA'S
TOP
DOCTORS
FOR
CANCER

Text by John J. Connolly, Ed.D.

&

Jean Morgan, M.D.

A CASTLE CONNOLLY GUIDE

CASTLE
CONNOLLY
MEDICAL LTD.

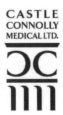

The selection of medical providers for inclusion in this book was based in part on opinions solicited from physicians, nurses, and other health care professionals. The author and publishers cannot assure the accuracy of information provided to them by third parties, since such opinions are necessarily subjective and may be incomplete. The omission from this book of particular health care providers does not mean that such providers are not competent or reputable.

The purpose of this book is educational and informational. It is not intended to replace the advice of your physician or to assist the layman in diagnosing or treating illness, disease, or injury. Following the advice or recommendations set forth in this book is entirely at the reader's own risk. The author and publishers cannot ensure accuracy of, or assume responsibility for, the information in the book as such information is affected by constant change. Liability to any person or organization for any loss or damage caused by errors or omissions in this book is hereby disclaimed. Whenever possible, readers should consult their own primary care physician when selecting health care providers, including any selection based upon information contained in this book. In order to protect patient privacy the names of patients cited in anecdotes throughout the book have been omitted.

Reproduction in whole or part, or storage in any data retrieval system and reproduction therefrom, is strictly prohibited and violates Federal copyright and trademark laws.

The confidence of our readers in our editorial integrity is crucial to the success of the Castle Connolly Guides. Any use of the Castle Connolly name, or of any list or listing (or portion of either) from any Castle Connolly Guide, for advertising or for any commercial purpose, without prior written consent, is strictly prohibited and may result in legal action.

For more information, please contact:

Castle Connolly Medical Ltd., 42 West 24th St, New York, New York 10010

212-367-8400x10

E-mail: info@castleconnolly.com

Web site: http://www.castleconnolly.com.

Library of Congress Catalog Card Number 2005927293

ISBN 1-883769-24-8 (paperback)

ISBN 1-883769-64-7 (hardcover)

Printed in the United States of America

ABOUT THE PUBLISHERS

John K. Castle has spent much of the last three decades involved with healthcare institutions and issues. Mr. Castle served as Chairman of the Board of New York Medical College for eleven years, an institution where he served on the Board of Trustees for twenty-two years.

Mr. Castle has been extensively involved in other healthcare and voluntary activities as well. He served for five years as a public commissioner on the Joint Commission on Accredition of Healthcare Organizations (JCAHO), the body which accredits most public and private hospitals throughout the United States. Mr. Castle has also served as a trustee of five different hospitals in the metropolitan New York region, including New York Presbyterian Hospital, where he continues to serve.

Mr. Castle is also the Chairman of the Columbia Presbyterian Science Advisory Council and a Director of the Whitehead Institute for Biomedical Research. He is a Fellow of New York Academy of Medicine and has served as a Trustee of the Academy. He is Chairman of the United Hospital Fund of New York's Capital Campaign. He continues as Director Emeritus of the United Hospital Fund. He is a Life Member of the MIT Corporation, the governing body of the Massachusetts Institute of Technology.

Mr. Castle is the Chairman and Co-Publisher of Castle Connolly Medical Ltd. and affiliated companies which publish *America's Top Doctors*; *Top Doctors: New York Metro Area* and other books to help people find the best healthcare. Castle Connolly Graduate Medical Publishing Ltd. publishes more than a dozen guides to assist resident physicians in preparing for their medical specialty boards.

ABOUT THE PUBLISHERS

John J. Connolly, Ed.D. is the President & CEO of Castle Connolly Medical Ltd., and is the nation's foremost authority on identifying top physicians. Dr. Connolly's experience in healthcare is extensive.

For over a decade he served as President of New York Medical College, the nation's second largest private medical college. He is a Fellow of the New York Academy of Medicine, a Fellow of the New York Academy of Sciences, a Director of the New York Business Group on Health, a member of the President's Council of the United States Hospital Fund, and a member of the Board of Advisors of Funding First, a Lasker Foundation initiative. Dr. Connolly has served as a trustee of two hospitals and as Chairman of the Board of one. He is extensively involved in healthcare and community activities and has served on a number of voluntary and corporate boards including the Board of the American Lyme Disease Foundation, of which he is a founder and past chairman, and the Board of Advisors of the Whitehead Institute for Biomedical Research. He is also a Director and Vice Chairman of the Professional Examination Service. He holds a Bachelor of Science degree from Worcester State College, a Master's degree from the University of Connecticut, and a Doctor of Education degree in College and University Administration from Teacher's College, Columbia University.

Dr. Connolly has authored or edited nine books and has been interviewed by more than 100 television and radio stations nationwide including "Good Morning America," "20/20," "48 Hours," Fox Cable News, CNN, and "Weekend Today in New York," and he and Castle Connolly have been featured in major newspapers and magazines including *The New York Times*, the *Chicago Tribune*, the *Daily News* and the *Boston Herald, Redbook, Town & Country, Good Housekeeping, Boardroom Reports* and regional magazines including *New York, Chicago, Philadelphia, St Louis, San Francisco* and *Atlanta* magazines.

MEDICAL ADVISORY BOARD

FOREWORD

Vincent T. DeVita, Jr., M.D.
Director, National Cancer Institute
(1980-1988)

As a physician, I've spent my professional career valuing the ability to find the right information and resources I need - quickly, efficiently and with the confidence that my sources are reliable. Similarly, healthcare consumers need to be able to find reliable information about the very best medical and healthcare services is critical, especially when confronting a diagnosis of cancer. That's why I like Castle Connolly's newest consumer guide, *America's Top Doctors for Cancer*.

In creating this guide to more than 2,000 of the nation's leading medical specialists involved in the prevention, diagnosis and treatment of various cancer in both adults and children, Castle Connolly has invested a tremendous amount of time, energy and money in its research, screening and evaluation processes. To illustrate some of the complexity of doing this kind work, let me share a story with you. In my capacity as Director of the NCI from 1980 to 1988, I was often deluged with phone call requests, frequently from members of Congress or other well-placed individuals, to help them with their own personal problem with cancer or that of a friend or relative - and "pretty damn quick". They were not satisfied with just going to any doctor when their life, or the life of a friend or loved one was at stake - they wanted to know "who was doing what and where" and they wanted suggestions about the top doctors for their particular type of cancer. I often felt guilty that only a privileged few had access to this type of information. (This lack of fundamental information for the average patient is exactly what motivated Castle Connolly to start their "Top Doctors" series in 1991.)

FOREWORD

The National Cancer Act had been established in 1971 by an Act of the U.S. Congress as part of a national "War on Cancer." Among its mandates for NCI was the creation of a cancer information service to get relevant information rapidly to cancer patients. Two unique individuals deserve credit and recognition for the role that they played in creating this information service. This part of the Cancer Act mandate was actually the brainchild of the philanthropist Mary Lasker, who was also one of the main architects of the passage of the Cancer Act itself. She had her finger on the pulse of the American public and was concerned, and correctly so in my view, that researchers and organizations that supported them, like the NIH, had a tendency to ignore the practical applications of their work for the public, despite the fact that their research was paid for by tax dollars. From the time of the passage of the act, Mary Lasker pursued each subsequent National Cancer Institute (NCI) Director to build this information service. In 1981, Mr. Richard Bloch, of H&R Block, then a member of the National Cancer Advisory Board, and himself a successfully treated lung cancer patient, approached the NCI Director about his dream that a patient could use computerized information services to enter their personal information and get, in return, the most up-to-date management recommendations, and names of doctors using them. He was motivated by his own experience. He had had to fight his way through the system, being told by several doctors that he was incurable before he found where to go, and the physicians to provide the treatment that ultimately cured him. It was his goal, a goal to which he dedicated the rest of his life; to see that cancer patients like him got the information they needed.

With the strong advocacy of Mary Lasker and Richard Bloch, in 1984 NCI launched the PDQ system at the National Library of Medicine.

It was the first computerized database in the world, aimed at the general public, devoted to a single disease, cancer. PDQ included lists of institutions, treatment protocols, and physicians devoted to managing cancer patients, all geographically matrixed, to allow patients, regardless of their status, to find the most appropriate doctor, treatment, and or clinical trial for them anywhere in the country and in their locale as well. Ironically, this aspect of PDQ - a list of specialists that seemed so logical and necessary - was controversial. From cancer specialists themselves, we heard that since not all cancer specialists (for example Cancer Surgeons) are "certified" by boards that test their qualifications for the cancer part of their work, the PDQ lists did not include " board certification" as a selection criteria. The PDQ physician list was also constructed primarily by using input and lists from specialty organizations. By building our list with assistance from specialty organizations, we were told, we had abrogated peer review and would be including doctors who might be only marginally qualified as specialists. To identify all doctors who were capable of providing modern care for cancer patients, on an individual basis, was not within the capability of the NCI or any government or private institution at the time. And to identify who were among the most qualified to diagnosis and treat specific types of cancers was simply not within our purview. And yet we knew that finding the right doctor at the right time could be a matter of life and death.

Fast-forward to 2005 - PDQ and the Cancer Information Service have played a big part in the decline in national mortality rates from cancer in the US that began in 1990 and has continued since then. PDQ has now become a more complex information system about cancer and

FOREWORD

NCI cancer programs. But regrettably, the one thing that patients appreciated the most - the list of cancer doctors - is no longer a part of the PDQ system.

Castle Connolly's *America's Top Doctors for Cancer* represents the much-needed and long-overdue answer for consumers – and physicians - seeking the top cancer specialists. Their physician-led Research Team has tackled some of the tough issues and developed criteria for selection, built on the foundation of Castle Connolly's well-respected national survey process that has enabled them to identify the leading physicians in more than twenty medical specialties associated with the prevention, diagnosis and treatment of cancers. The breadth and depth of the information they offer on each profiled physician will enable readers to be empowered consumers, to make informed decisions about the right doctor for their particular type of cancer. The guide also includes valuable information on some of the nation's most outstanding medical centers and specialty hospitals that are involved in the treatment of cancers.

America's Top Doctors for Cancer will be an invaluable resource – a user-friendly, trusted source of information from an independent nationally renowned healthcare research and information company. I believe that using Castle Connolly's *America's Top Doctors for Cancer* as a key source of information will help cancer patients and their loved ones navigate the complexities of the American healthcare system to find – and receive – the highest quality medical care.

Vincent T. DeVita, Jr., M.D.
Amy and Joseph Perella Professor of Medicine
Yale Cancer Center, Yale School of Medicine
(New Haven, Connecticut) January, 2005
Director, National Cancer Institute (1980-1988)

TABLE OF CONTENTS

SECTION I: INTRODUCTION & GENERAL INFORMATION

SECTION II: USING THIS GUIDE TO FIND A DOCTOR

SECTION III: PHYSICIAN LISTINGS AND PARTICIPATING HOSPITALS

SECTION IV: APPENDICES

SECTION V: INDICES

SECTION I

INTRODUCTION

• 1 •

CANCER IN THE U.S. TODAY

If you or someone you love has been diagnosed with cancer, this book is for you. Although one in four Americans will be told they have cancer at some point during their lives, it is important to emphasize this no longer automatically carries a grim prognosis. Due to advances in treatment and, more importantly, early detection, people with cancer are living longer as well as healthier and more productive lives. While the overall quality of medical care throughout the United States is generally of very high quality, and in many places is superb, there are still those rare, complex or extremely difficult problems that demand resources beyond the ordinary or that require talents that are exceptional.

Many cancers are potentially curable, provided they are detected in the early stages.

There is no denying fear is the most common reaction to the word "cancer," at least initially. Cancer has recently emerged as the leading cause of death of Americans under age 85. Bernadine Healy, M.D., former Director of the National Institute of Health, wrote in *U.S. News and World Report* that cancer is both "sneaky and inexplicably virulent in many of its forms." These characteristics go a long way toward making cancer even more formidable than heart disease, another major killer.

1

INTRODUCTION

However, Dr. Healy also described how advances in identification and prevention have restrained cancer from "galloping" through our population. We are all familiar with PAP smears which can identify early forms of cervical cancer in women, or the Prostate-Specific Antigen (PSA) test for prostate cancer in men, as well as colonoscopies that permit doctors to remove potentially cancerous polyps from the colon.

Today, many people are completely cured or are able to cope with their cancer as a chronic disease. There are nearly ten million cancer survivors in the U.S. alone

Many cancers are potentially curable, provided they are detected in the early stages. Growing awareness of early warning signs and symptoms, together with advances in screening, have resulted in major improvements in cancer survival.

Prevention is even more important. Jane E. Brody, one of the nation's leading health columnists, recently wrote in *The New York Times* about life-enhancing changes involving diet and exercise we can make that may enable us to live cancer-free beyond the age of 85.

At the same time that methods of diagnosis and prevention have advanced, so too has our ability to treat cancer. In fact, today, many people are completely cured or are able to cope with their cancer as a chronic disease. There are nearly 10 million cancer survivors in the U.S. alone.

Americans' risk of getting cancer and dying from cancer continues to decline and survival rates for many cancers continue to improve. The *Annual Report to the Nation on the Status of Cancer, 1975-2001*, which is a collaboration among the American Cancer Society (ACS), the Centers for Disease Control and Prevention (CDC), the National Cancer Institute (NCI), and the North American Association of Central Cancer Registries (NAACCR), provides updated information on cancer rates and trends in the United States, found that overall observed cancer incidence rates dropped 0.5 percent per year from 1991 to 2001, while death rates from all types of cancer combined dropped 1.1 percent per year from 1993 to 2001.

In keeping with the current hopeful climate for cancer patients, the purpose of this book is to help you approach your diagnosis and treatment in the most effective way possible.

Cancer can occur in any cell in the body when the mechanisms that regulate normal cell growth fail. As a result, the cell experiences uncontrolled and excessive growth. These rapidly multiplying cells may go on to invade local tissues or spread (metastasize) to other parts of the body.

The field of cancer research is growing in leaps and bounds. Research is essential, not only to improve current methods of treatment, but also to develop new ways of treating what had previously been considered intractable types of cancer. As medical research and technology advances, more treatments and drugs are being introduced to combat cancer. In fact, every day we can read of new developments which may give renewed hope to many cancer patients.

Research is essential, not only to improve on current methods of treatment, but also to develop new ways of treating what had previously been considered intractable types of cancer.

The huge amount of information now available about all aspects of cancer can be quite daunting. New tests, new drugs, new technology, all may present a bewildering choice for many patients. You need guidance, and also psychological support, as you navigate through this strange new world. That's why it's vital for you to consult and be treated by a physician highly experienced in and knowledgeable about your particular type of cancer.

In certain types of cancer, different specialists may combine their efforts to work together as a team. For example, in successful skull base tumor surgery, the otolaryngologist and neurological surgeon operate together.

INTRODUCTION

Different major medical centers may concentrate on different types of cancer treatments, their physicians working together to provide the "team approach" as needed. In other words, you're not just selecting a single doctor, but an entire hospital for your treatment.

• 2 •

WHY TOP DOCTORS AND TOP HOSPITALS

Finding the best physicians and best hospitals for your care is a major factor in achieving the best possible outcome. The average person may not be familiar with the various medical specialties, or know what constitutes medical education and the specifics of doctor "training" that period of residencies and fellowships that follows medical school. As a result, it is difficult for most Americans to choose physicians or hospitals in a well-informed fashion. Most people still find a doctor by asking a friend for a recommendation, or picking a name from a health plan directory or even a phone book.

In addition to listing excellent physicians identified by the Castle Connolly research team through our surveys, this book will describe the process you can use to find a "top doctor" for any medical problem or need. It will also provide up-to-date information on leading hospitals, and list valuable resources for cancer patients and their families. These resources are found in the appendices.

At times, our healthcare system, while good, may seem less than consumer friendly. The United States (and Canada) has many thousands of exceptionally well-trained and dedicated professionals involved in providing the best healthcare possible. Managed care, despite its shortcomings, has brought some much-needed structure to the healthcare delivery system. Most plans require that you have a primary care physician as well as specify referrals

INTRODUCTION

to selected specialists and hospitals. The health plans have the ability to monitor and assess the care delivered to you at all times, regardless of provider or location, because the plan has all your medical records in order to affect appropriate payment.

Unfortunately, the advantages offered by managed care plans have too frequently been directed toward controlling costs rather than enhancing quality. The hospitals and doctors to which patients are referred for more services or complex care are often selected on the basis of cost rather than other, more medically relevant, criteria. Therefore, even though a health plan directory may list a number of "centers of excellence" and several specialists for a given problem, they may not be the best for your particular needs.

> *Even the best doctors and the best hospitals are not perfect. Cancer treatment is a combination of art and science*

Asking your primary care physician for a referral to a specialist can be a good place to start. However, too many of us don't have a close relationship with that all important "quarterback" of our healthcare, and this type of referral also has its limitations. Is the recommendation being made on the basis of a personal or professional relationship? Is the specialist to whom you are being referred truly the best, or is he or she simply in your primary care physician's group or in the network of your health plan? Even if your primary care physician is making a referral free from outside considerations, how broad is his or her knowledge of this particular specialty? Most primary care physicians have a limited number of referral channels. They are busy caring for their own patients and rarely have the time to devote hours of research to identifying top doctors for referrals. Typically, their referral network is local rather than regional or national

If you are already under the care of an excellent specialist, and he or she refers you to another specialist or sub-specialist for a particular problem, you can be confident of a more "meaningful" referral. When physicians are continually dealing with a specific disease, such as cancer, they are usually more aware of advances in the field, as well as the names of the top practitioners.

As the patient, finding the best physicians and best hospitals for your care is your responsibility. "Get a second opinion" is a common refrain. Everyone has heard stories of patients who were told by one physician (even at a top hospital) that their case was hopeless and yet, when they continued their search, they found another doctor or hospital that provided a different plan of treatment and perhaps even a cure.

Even the best doctors and the best hospitals are not perfect. Cancer treatment, like other medical care, is a combination of art and science. Frequently, opinions on diagnosis and treatment may differ - even among top doctors. That's why it's so important for you to seek second or even third opinions when a diagnosis, even one not involving cancer, is serious or may necessitate major surgery.

As the patient, finding the best physicians and best hospitals for your care is your responsibility.

One of the best known and inspirational stories of a patient undertaking this kind of search is that of Lance Armstrong, the six time Tour de France champion cyclist. When Armstrong was first diagnosed with testicular cancer he received a grim prognosis from a number of excellent physicians at some of the nation's leading cancer centers. The recommended courses of treatment would have destroyed his ability to continue competing professionally. Refusing to accept that limitation, he continued his search until he found a physician and institution that offered different treatment options. As most people know, the treatment was successful. Four of Armstrong's cycling championships have come since his recovery from cancer.

Of course, there is a difference between seeking additional medical opinions and simply bouncing around from doctor to doctor until you find one that tells you what you want to hear. You need to find a doctor, hospital and treatment plan in which you have confidence, and which you honestly believe, based on extensive research, will work for you. Depending on the circumstances, it may be possible to find another physician or hospital that can offer a superior plan, or it may be that no better treatment options currently exist.

"Hope springs eternal" is not just a trite saying. It is something that should drive every patient and every doctor, simply because there are always unexpected and sometimes unexplainable remissions or cures occurring with cancer, and new breakthroughs in treatment could be just around the corner.

There is a significant amount of evidence that patients who are optimistic and fight, rather than surrender to their disease, have generally better outcomes. A positive attitude and the support of family and friends, as well as physicians and nurses, can be an important factor in your recovery. Knowing as much as possible about your diagnosis and your treatment options is another.

> *There is a significant amount of evidence that patients who are optimistic and fight, rather than surrender to their disease, have generally better outcomes*

Reaching an initial diagnosis usually involves a number of medical tests including x-rays, MRIs and analysis of tissue samples obtained by a biopsy. It may be necessary to repeat these tests, or perform more specialized ones, in order to gain more thorough information or firmly establish a questionable diagnosis.

In the case of breast cancer, the disease is first likely to be identified either through a mammogram or else the discovery of a lump during a routine self or physician exam. Any breast lumps need to be biopsied for confirmation of cancer. Once that occurs, you will be referred to a surgeon who has special expertise in this field. He or she will recommend one or more possible treatments, including a total mastectomy, a lumpectomy, radiation therapy and chemotherapy.

A suspicion of prostate cancer usually occurs following evidence of an enlarged prostate or an elevated PSA test. A urologist will make a definitive diagnosis based on a biopsy and examination of that tissue by a pathologist. Once cancer is found, the urologist can treat it by removing the prostate.

Both the breast cancer and prostate cancer patient face the same basic questions: Is the surgeon treating you the most qualified and, more importantly, is surgery the only or best solution to deal with your disease?

Just like a number of additional options exist for breast cancer, surgery is not the only way to deal with prostate cancer, and may have unwanted side effects. Other alternative treatments include radiation therapy. In addition, since prostate cancer usually develops very slowly, some patients, especially older ones, may choose "watchful waiting." However, because most patients initially see a surgeon at the time of their diagnosis, they may end up having surgery without fully exploring the other alternatives.

Knowledge is not just power; in some instances it can make all the difference in not only your long-term survival, but also the quality of your life. This is why it is essential for you to be an informed consumer and find the best possible healthcare for yourself. This book will help you find the very best doctors and hospitals to treat cancer.

FACTORS TO CONSIDER WHEN IDENTIFYING A TOP DOCTOR

1. Medical Education

2. Residency & Fellowships

3. Board Certification

4. Hospital Appointment

5. Academic and Other Professional titles

6. Insurance Accepted

7. Personality

• 3 •

HOW CASTLE CONNOLLY IDENTIFIED THE TOP DOCTORS FOR CANCER

C astle Connolly is best known for its series of consumer guides including *America's Top Doctors, Top Doctors: New York Metro Area* and *Top Doctors: Chicago Metro Area*. These books list "top doctors" in their respective regions. Both the New York and Chicago editions list primary care physicians as well as other specialists and sub-specialists. *America's Top Doctors* does not include any primary care physicians, but it lists the nation's top referral specialists. The Castle Connolly Guides are trusted by consumers and physicians alike. In fact, over 50% of the physicians listed in the Guides use them to make referrals.

Doctors *do not* and *cannot* pay to be listed in any Castle Connolly Guides. They are selected based on their nomination by peers solicited through mail and

The physcians we have identified and listed are clearly among the best as nominated by their peers and screened by our research team

11

phone surveys, and on an extensive review of their credentials by the Castle Connolly physician-led research team.

For *America's Top Doctors for Cancer*, Castle Connolly sent nomination forms to all 4,765 physicians listed in *America's Top Doctors*. In addition, nominations were solicited from the presidents and vice presidents of over 250 of the nation's leading medical centers and specialty hospitals as well as over 1,300 physicians in the Society of Surgical Oncology and over 500 physicians on the editorial boards of leading journals in the cancer field, as well as those involved in related conferences, foundations, working groups and societies.

> *The goal in creating this list was to select physicians viewed by their peers as the best in preventing, diagnosing and treating cancer and its related ramifications*

Over five thousand different physicians were nominated by their peers for inclusion in this guide. Of course, many of them received multiple nominations. In addition to the thousands of mail surveys, the Castle Connolly research team made hundreds of phone calls to leading specialists and sought additional nominations as well as using these conversations to reinforce the nominations received through the mail nomination process.

The Castle Connolly physician-led research team reviewed and analyzed the nominations and narrowed the field to those being considered for inclusion in *America's Top Doctors for Cancer.* They contacted these physicians and asked them to complete an extensive biographical form describing their medical education, residencies, fellowships, hospital appointments and more. Particularly, we were interested in the physicians' area of special expertise; that is, the particular type of cancer (e.g. lung, breast, brain tumors, etc.,) or procedures (e.g. radical prostatectomy) in which the physician had particular experience, interest and expertise.

Finally, the research team checked on the disciplinary histories of the physicians by screening those that may have been disciplined by a medical board or state agency. After this intensive review, the final list was created.

The goal in creating this list was to select physicians viewed by their peers as the best in preventing, diagnosing and treating cancer and its related ramifications. Castle Connolly does not claim these are the only excellent doctors treating cancer in this country. Our nation is fortunate in having a generally excellent cadre of well-trained, dedicated physicians. The physicians we have identified and listed, however, are clearly among the very best as nominated by their peers and screened by our research team. In addition, they practice, for the most part, at major medical centers and leading specialty hospitals where they, and their patients, can receive the support of other highly skilled doctors, nurses and technicians as well as having access to the sophisticated and expensive equipment, laboratories and other resources that advance the level of cancer treatment and care from good to excellent. Furthermore, many of these physicians are engaged in teaching or research, or both. While the academic nature of their practice can limit the amount of time available to see patients, it keeps them, their colleagues and their institutions on the "cutting edge" of cancer treatment.

The laboratories, technicians, intensive care beds, research fellows, scientists and specially trained nursing staff, equipment and, especially, the volume of patients and research subjects so necessary to enable these professional teams to continually develop and hone their skills, typically exist only in metropolitan areas or at university-based medical centers.

One important factor in our selection was geographic coverage. Some patients may be unable to travel long distances to a major medical center or specialty hospital due to financial resources, overall health status or some other reason. For them, a hospital in the immediate region is the only possible alternative. Since this is a guide for consumers and as many physicians

INTRODUCTION

use our guide to make referrals we felt it was important to have broad geographic coverage and attempted to identify the top doctors for cancer in every state.

The reality is that the critical resources, the very best doctors and hospitals, are not dispersed evenly throughout the nation. For good reason they are clustered in large metropolitan areas or at academic medical centers that are part of major universities. It is only in these settings where it is possible to gather the combination of resources necessary to mount and maintain a superior medical program. The laboratories, technicians, intensive care beds, research fellows, scientists, specially trained nursing staff, equipment and, especially, the volume of patients and research subjects so necessary to enable these professional teams to continually develop and hone their skills, typically exist only in metropolitan areas or at university-based medical centers.

> *Since this is a guide for consumers and as many physicians use our guide to make referrals we felt it was important to have broad geographical coverage and attempted to identify the top doctors for cancer in every state*

Therefore, it may be necessary for many Americans, if they are motivated to seek out the very best doctors and hospitals, to travel many miles, if possible, to obtain their care. It is also this reality that has motivated many outstanding medical centers and specialty hospitals to reach out and establish relationships with community hospitals throughout the nation. While it is not always possible to bring the labs, scientists, equipment and leading physicians to these communities, it is possible to raise the overall level of cancer care through these relationships.

14

• 4 •

JUDGING THE QUALIFICATIONS OF A PHYSICIAN

The National Cancer Institute has declared its intention to "eliminate suffering and death due to cancer by the year 2015." While that is clearly an ambitious goal, and one many may feel is unrealistic, it nonetheless demonstrates the optimism physicians and scientists are beginning to feel about the battle against cancer. As Ellen V. Sigal, Ph.D, founder and chairperson of Friends of Cancer Research in Washington, D.C. and a member of the National Cancer Institutes Board of Scientific Advisors, stated: "The consensus among the science community is that for the first time we understand the genetic underpinnings of this disease."

"How do you identify a top doctor?" is an important question for all Americans, not just those diagnosed with cancer. As we mentioned earlier, too many Americans are incredibly casual in selecting physicians and hospitals. They may pick a name from their health plan directory, or even from a phone book, with the location of the doctor's office being the primary factor in their selection. Others may simply ask a friend or relative and the recommendation they receive may be based on how well the person "likes" the doctor rather than on any particular medical expertise or skill.

The specialists listed in *America's Top Doctors for Cancer* are clearly among the best in the nation and have been identified through a rigorous

15

research process and thorough screening by the Castle Connolly physician-led research team. Through our extensive surveys and research we have done much of the work in finding a top referral specialist, but they are not the only excellent physicians in the nation.

"How do you identify a top doctor?" is an important question for all Americans, not just those diagnosed with cancer

So, how does one judge the qualifications of a physician who may not be listed in this Guide? If someone was trying to find a specialist on their own, how should they go about it? How can someone tell when a physician has the appropriate training in a specialty and how does one distinguish what is meaningful and what is not from among all those plaques and certificates on a doctor's wall?

The reality is that few of us see only one doctor in our lifetime. Each of us may be cared for by a primary care physician, an ophthalmologist, an orthopaedist, a dermatologist, a surgeon or a number of other specialists. The choices can be many and they can be among the most important choices we make.

The following pages will outline the process for selecting a well-qualified physician. In fact, what is written here reflects much of the logic that underlies the selection of physicians for this book. This section will help not only in finding a top specialist in this Guide, but it also should be helpful in choosing among the many specialists, primary care doctors and other physicians, that a person will need to consult throughout his/her life.

EDUCATION

The review of a prospective doctor's education and training should begin with medical school. While some may feel that the institution at which a physician earned a bachelor's degree could be an indication of the doctor's quality, most people in the medical field do not believe it plays a major role. A degree from a highly selective undergraduate college or university will help an aspiring doctor gain admission to a medical school, but once there, all students are peers. Furthermore, where a doctor trains (i.e. completes residency) is more important than medical school in judging quality. American medical schools are highly standardized, at least in terms of basic quality standards.

A group known as the Liaison Committee for Medical Education (LCME) accredits all U.S. medical schools that grant medical degrees (MDs) and osteopathic degrees (DOs). Most also are accredited by the appropriate state agency, if one exists, and by regional agencies that accredit colleges and universities of all kinds.

Where a doctor trains (i.e. completes residency) is more important than medical school in judging quality. American medical schools are highly standardized, at least in terms of minimal quality

Fortunately, U.S. medical schools have universally high standards for admission, including success on the undergraduate level and on the Medical College Admissions Tests (MCATs). Although frequently criticized for being slow to change and for training too many specialists, the system of medical education in the United States has assured consistent high quality in medical practice. One recent positive change is a strong effort in most medical schools to diversify the composition of the student body. While these schools have been less successful in enrolling racial minorities, the number of women in U.S. medical schools has increased to the point that women now make up about 50 percent of most classes. In certain specialties preferred by women medical graduates (pediatrics, for example), it is possible that in coming years the majority of specialists will be female.

Most doctors practicing in the United States are graduates of U.S. medical schools, but there are two other groups of doctors who make up a significant portion (25%) of the total physician population. They are (1) foreign nationals who graduated from foreign schools and (2) U.S. nationals who graduated from foreign schools. (Canadian medical schools are not considered foreign.)

INTRODUCTION

FOREIGN MEDICAL GRADUATES

Foreign medical schools vary greatly in quality. Even some of the oldest and finest European schools have become virtually "open door," with huge numbers of unscreened students making teaching and learning difficult. Others are excellent and provided the model for our system of medical education.

The fact that someone graduated from a foreign school does not mean that he or she is a poor doctor. Foreign schools, like those in the U.S., produce both good and poor doctors. Foreign medical graduates who wish to practice here must pass the same exam taken by U.S. graduates for licensure. It is true the failure rate for foreign graduates is significantly higher. In the first year of using the new United States Medical Licensing Exam (USMLE), 93 percent of U.S. medical school graduates passed Step II, the clinical exam, as compared with only 39 percent of the foreign graduates. It is clear that the quality of many foreign schools, if not individual doctors, is not the same as U.S. medical schools, at least as measured by our standards. Nonetheless, many communities and patients have been well served by foreign medical graduates practicing in this country—often in areas where it has been difficult to attract graduates of American schools. About 25% of practicing physicians in the U.S. today are graduates of foreign medical schools.

> *If in doubt about a doctor's training, ask the doctor if the residency program he or she completed was in the specialty of the practice; if not, ask why not*

In addition, many foreign medical schools and their teaching hospitals are world renowned for their leadership in medical care, research and teaching, and many of the technologies and techniques we utilize in the U.S. today have been developed and perfected in foreign countries.

RESIDENCY

Most doctors practicing today have at least three years of postgraduate training (following the MD or DO) in an approved residency program. This not only is an important step in the process of becoming a competent doctor, but it is also a requirement for board (specialty) certification. Most people assume that a prospective doctor needs to complete a three-year residency program to obtain a medical license. That is not an accurate assumption! New York State, for example, requires only one postgraduate year. However, since all approved residencies last at least three years and some, such as those in neurosurgery, general surgery, orthopaedic surgery and urology, may extend for five or more years, it is important to know the details of a doctor's training. Licensure alone is not enough of a basis on which to choose a physician.

Without undertaking extensive and detailed research on every residency program, the best assessment you can make of a doctor's residency program is to see if it took place in a large medical center whose name you recognize. The more prestigious institutions tend to attract the best medical students, sometimes regardless of the quality of the individual residency program. If in doubt about a doctor's training, ask the doctor if the residency he or she completed was in the specialty of the practice; if not, ask why not.

It is important to know the details of a doctor's training. Licensure alone is not enough of a basis on which to choose a physician

It is also important to be certain that a doctor completed a residency that has been approved by the appropriate governing board of the specialty, such as the American Board of Surgery, the American Board of Radiology, or the American Osteopathic Board of Pediatrics. These board groups are listed in Appendices A and B. If you are really concerned about a doctor's training, you should call the hospital that offered the residency and ask if the residency program was approved by the appropriate specialty group. If still in doubt, consult the publication Directory of Graduate Medical

INTRODUCTION

Education Programs, often called the "green book," found in medical school or hospital libraries, which lists all approved residencies.

BOARD CERTIFICATION

With an MD or DO degree and a license, an individual may practice in any medical specialty with or without additional specialized training. For example, doctors with a license, but no special training, may call themselves a surgeon, oncologist or radiologist. This is why board certification is such an important factor. It assures the physician has had specific training in that specialty and has passed the board exam. The American Board of Medical Specialties (ABMS) recognizes 25 specialties and more than 90 subspecialties. Visit www.abms.org or call 866-275-2267 for more information. Eighteen boards certify in 20 specialties under the aegis of the American Osteopathic Association (AOA). Visit www.osteopathic.org or call 800-621-1773 for more information. Doctors who have qualified for such specialization are called board certified; they have completed an approved residency and passed the board's exam.

You can be confident that doctors who are board certified have, at a minimum, the proper training in their specialty and have demonstrated their proficiency through supervision and testing.

(See Appendix A for an approved ABMS list; see Appendix B for the AOA list). While many doctors who are not board certified call themselves "specialists," board certification is the best standard by which to measure competence and training.

You can be confident that doctors who are board certified have, at a minimum, the proper training in their specialty and have demonstrated their proficiency through supervision and testing. While there are many non-board certified doctors who are highly competent, it is more difficult to assess the level of their training. While board certification alone does not guarantee competence, it is a standard that reflects successful completion of an appropriate training program. If it is impossible to find a doctor in your area who is board certified in a particular subspecialty, for example, Medical Oncology or Radiation Oncology, at least be certain the physician is board certified in a related specialty such as Internal Medicine or Radiology.

Board certified doctors are referred to as Diplomates of the Board. Some of the colleges of medical specialties (e.g., the American College of Radiology, the American College of Surgeons) have multiple levels of recognition. The first is basic membership and the second, more prestigious and difficult to obtain, is status as a Fellow. Fellowship status in the colleges is meaningful and is based on experience, professional achievement and recognition by one's peers, including extensive experience in patient care. It should be viewed as a significant professional qualification.

BOARD ELIGIBILITY

Many doctors who have been more recently trained are waiting to take the boards. They are sometimes described as "board eligible," a common term that the ABMS advocates abandoning because of its ambiguity. Board eligible means that the doctor has completed an approved residency and is qualified to sit for the related board's exam. Another term that is used is "board qualified." Once again, the term has no official standing, but could mean the doctor has completed residency and is awaiting the board exam. It could also mean the doctor took and failed to pass the exam to become board certified.

Each member board of the ABMS has its own policy regarding the use and recognition of the board eligible term. Therefore, the description "board eligible" should not be viewed as a genuine qualification, especially if a doctor has been out of medical school long enough to have taken the certification exam. To the boards, a doctor is either board certified or not. Furthermore, most of the specialty boards permit unlimited attempts to pass the exam and, in some cases, doctors who have failed the exam twice or even ten times, continue to call themselves board eligible. In Osteopathic Medicine, the board eligible status is recognized only for the first six years after completion of a residency.

INTRODUCTION

In addition to the approved lists of specialties and subspecialties of the ABMS and AOA, there are a wide variety of other doctors and groups of doctors who call themselves specialists. At present there are at least 100 such groups called "self-designated medical specialties." They range from doctors who are working to create a recognized body of knowledge and subspecialty training to less formal groups interested in a particular approach to the practice of medicine. These groups may or may not have standards for membership. There is no way to determine the true extent of their members' training, and neither the ABMS or the AOA recognizes them. While you should be cautious of doctors who claim they are specialists in these areas, many do have advanced training and the groups at least offer a listing of people interested in a particular approach to medical care. Rely on board certification to assure yourself of basic competence, and use membership in one of these groups to indicate strong interest and possible additional training in a particular aspect of medicine.

RECERTIFICATION

A relatively new focus of the specialty boards is the area of recertification. Until recently, board certification lasted for an unlimited time. Now, almost all the boards have put time limits on the certification period. For example, in Internal Medicine and Radiology, the time limit is ten years. These more stringent standards reflect an increasing emphasis on recertification by both the medical boards and state agencies responsible for licensing doctors.

Since the policies of the boards vary widely, it is a good procedure to check a doctor's background to see when certification was awarded. If the date was seven to ten years ago, see if he or she has been recertified. Unfortunately, many boards permit "grandfathering," whereby already certified doctors do not have to be recertified, and recertification requirements apply only to newly certified doctors. Even if recertification is not required, it is good professional practice for doctors to undertake the process. It assures you, the patient, that they are attempting to stay current.

Many states have a continuing medical education requirement for doctors. These states typically require a minimum number of continuing medical education (CME) credits for a doctor to maintain a medical license.

Seven states require 150 CME credits over a three-year period. Osteopathic doctors are required to take 120 hours of CME credits within three years to maintain certification.

FELLOWSHIPS

The purpose of a fellowship is to provide advanced training in the clinical techniques and research of a particular specialty. Fellowships usually, but not always, are designed to lead to board certification in a subspecialty such as medical oncology which is a subspecialty of internal medicine. Many physicians listed in this Guide have had fellowship training. In the U.S. there are a variety of fellowship programs available to doctors, which fall into two broad categories: approved and unapproved. Approved fellowships are those that are approved by the appropriate medical specialty board (e.g., the American Board of Radiology) and lead to subspecialty certificates. Fellowship programs that are unapproved are often in the same areas of training as those that are approved, but they do not lead to subspecialty certificates.

The purpose of a fellowship is to provide advanced training in the clinical techniques and research of a particular specialty

Unfortunately, all too often, unapproved fellowships exist only to provide relatively inexpensive labor for the research and/or patient care activities of a clinical department in a medical school or hospital. In such cases, the learning that takes place is secondary and may be a good deal less than in an approved fellowship. On the other hand, any fellowship is better than none at all and some unapproved fellowships have status for a valid reason that should not reflect negatively on the program. For example, the fellowship may have been recently created, with approval being sought. There are also some areas of medicine not yet recognized for sub-specialty certification, such as Transplant Surgery.

INTRODUCTION

Some physicians may have completed more than one fellowship and may be boarded in two or more subspecialties. In addition, some physicians may pursue fellowship training and subspecialty certification but then choose to practice in their primary field of certification. For example, a doctor who is board certified in internal medicine also may have obtained board certification in oncology, but may choose to practice primarily internal medicine. For the most part, the physicians in this guide practice in their sub-specialties.

PROFESSIONAL REPUTATION

There are practitioners who meet every professional standard on paper, but who are simply not good doctors. In all probability, the medical community has ascertained this and, while the individual may still practice medicine, his or her reputation will reflect that collective assessment. There are also doctors who are outstanding leaders in their fields because of research or professional activities but who are not particularly strong, or perhaps even active, in patient care. It is important to distinguish that kind of professional reputation from a reputation as a competent, caring doctor in delivering patient care or, in the case of this guide, as an outstanding practitioner in a given specialty.

HOSPITAL APPOINTMENT

Most doctors are on the medical staff of one or more hospitals and are known as "attendings;" some, however, are not. If a doctor does not have admitting privileges or is not on the attending staff of a hospital, you may wish to consider choosing a different doctor. It can be very difficult to ascertain whether or not the lack of hospital appointment is for a good reason. For example, it is understandable that some doctors who are raising families or heading toward retirement choose not to meet the demands (meetings, committees, etc.) of being an attending.

The best doctors usually practice at the best hospitals

However, if you need care in a hospital, the lack of such an appointment means that another doctor will have to oversee that care. In some specialties, such as dermatology and psychiatry, doctors may conduct their entire practice in the

24

office and a hospital appointment is not as essential, or as good a criterion for assessment, as in other specialties.

While mistakes are made, most hospitals are quite careful about admissions to their medical staffs. The best hospitals are highly selective, so a degree of screening (or "credentialing") has been done for you. In other words, the best doctors usually practice at the best hospitals. Since caring for a patient in a hospital is often a team effort involving a number of specialists, the reputation of the hospital to which the doctor admits patients carries special weight. Hospital medical staffs review their colleagues' credentials and authorize performance of specific procedures. In addition, they typically review and reappoint their medical staff every two or three years. In effect, this is an additional screening to protect patients. It is especially true of hospitals that have what are known as closed staffs, where it is impossible to obtain admitting privileges unless there is a vacancy that the administration and medical staff deem necessary to fill. If you are having a surgical procedure and are concerned about the doctor's skill or experience, it may be worthwhile to call the Medical Affairs Office at the doctor's hospital to see if he or she is authorized to perform that procedure in that hospital.

> *Physicians listed in this guide are primarily on the staffs of major medical centers, university teaching hospitals and leading specialty hospitals.*

The reasons for a hospital's selectivity are easy to understand: no hospital wishes to expose itself to liability and every hospital wants to have the best reputation possible in order to attract patients. Obviously, the quality of the medical staff is immensely important in creating that reputation.

Physicians listed in this guide are primarily on the staffs of major medical centers, university teaching hospitals and leading specialty hospitals. Occasionally, some may be on staff at a community hospital for one or two days a week and spend the majority of their time at the teaching hospital. There are many excellent physicians on the staffs of community hospitals that call themselves "medical centers," but they are typically not physicians who attract complex cases and referrals regionally, nationally and even internationally.

To learn about a hospital, visit its website. It is also useful to review a hospital's accreditation status under the Joint Commission on the Accreditation of Healthcare Organizations at www.JCAHO.com.

A last and very important reason why a hospital appointment is an essential requirement in your choice of doctor is that some states permit doctors to practice without malpractice insurance. If you are injured as a result of a doctor's poor care, you could be without recourse. However, few hospitals permit doctors to practice in them unless they carry malpractice insurance. This not only protects the hospital, but the patient as well.

MEDICAL SCHOOL FACULTY APPOINTMENT

> *Doctors who are full-time academicians are more likely to be in the forefront of new techniques and research, especially when it comes to a disease like cancer.*

Many doctors have appointments on the faculties of medical schools. There is a range of categories from "straight" appointments, meaning full-time appointment as professor, associate professor, assistant professor or instructor, to clinical ranks that may reflect lesser degrees of involvement in teaching or research. If someone carries what is known as a straight academic rank (e.g. "professor of surgery," without "clinical" in the title), this usually means that the individual is engaged full-time in medical school research, teaching activities and patient care. The title "clinical professor of surgery" usually identifies a part-time or adjunct appointment and less direct involvement in medical school activities such as teaching and research.

Doctors who are full-time academicians are more likely to be in the forefront of new techniques and research, especially when it comes to a disease like cancer. They also have the advantage of the support of other faculty, residents and medical students.

When you are seeking a subspecialist, a doctor's relationship to a medical school becomes more meaningful since medical school faculties tend to be made up of sub-specialists. You are less likely to find large numbers of general or primary care practitioners engaged full-time on a medical school faculty. The newest approaches and techniques in medicine, for the most part, are explored and developed by medical school faculties in their laboratories and clinical practice settings. This is where they practice their sub-specialties, as well as teach and conduct research.

MEDICAL SOCIETY MEMBERSHIP

Most medical society memberships sound very prestigious and some are; however, there are many societies that are not selective and virtually any doctor can join. In addition, membership in many of the more prestigious societies is based on research and publication or on leadership in the field and may have little to do with direct patient care. While it is clearly an honor to be invited to join these groups, membership may be less than helpful in discerning whether a doctor can meet your needs.

There is a good deal of evidence that there is a positive relationship between quantity of experience and quality of care

EXPERIENCE

Experience is difficult to assess. Obviously, in most cases, an older doctor has more experience; on the other hand, a younger doctor has been more recently immersed in the challenge of medical school, residency, or even a fellowship, and may be the more up-to-date. If a doctor is board certified, you may assume that assures at least a minimal amount of experience, but since it could be as little as a year, check the date of graduation from medical school or completion of residency to know precisely how long a doctor has been in practice.

INTRODUCTION

There is a good deal of evidence that there is a positive relationship between quantity of experience and quality of care. That is, the more a doctor performs a procedure, the better he or she becomes at it. That is why it is important to ask a doctor about his or her experience with the procedure that you need. Does the doctor see and treat similar cases every day, every week or only rarely? Of course, with some rare diseases, "rarely" is the only possible answer, but it is the relative frequency that is critical. In some states, data is available on volume or numbers of certain procedures performed at hospitals. For volume and outcome information in other states, visit the web site of Health Care Choices at www.healthcarechoices.org. There is a good deal of controversy, however, on the validity and usefulness of such data. Opponents cite the fact that some of the data is produced from Medicare patient records only and, therefore, is based solely on an elderly population that does not represent the total activity of a hospital or doctor. Proponents of the use of such volume data agree that it is not perfect, but suggest it can be one useful criterion in selecting the best places to receive care for these specific problems. While recognizing the limitations of such data, the healthcare consumer may, nonetheless, find it of interest and use.

The one type of experience you should specifically want to know about is that dealing with any special procedure, particularly a surgical one, that has recently been developed and introduced into practice. For example, in the 1980's many doctors using laparoscopic cholecystectomy, a then new, minimally invasive surgical technique for removing gallbladders, experienced a high percentage of problems because they were not properly trained. This prompted the American Board of Surgery to promulgate new standards for the training of surgeons using this technique. Do not hesitate to ask about your doctor's training in a procedure and how frequently and with what degree of success he or she has performed it. Practice may not lead to perfection, but it does improve skills and enhance the probability of success.

In some cases, relatively young doctors have recently completed residency or fellowship training under recognized leaders who have developed new approaches or techniques for dealing with a particular problem. They may have learned the new techniques from their mentors and may be far ahead of the field (and ahead of more senior and distinguished colleagues) in using those

SECOND OPINIONS

Second opinions are a valuable medical tool, too infrequently used in many instances and overused in others. Clearly, you do not want to seek another doctor's opinion on every ailment or problem that you face, but a second opinion should be pursued in the following situations:

- *before major surgery*

- *if a rare disease is diagnosed*

- *if a diagnosis is uncertain*

- *if the number of tests or procedures recommended might seem excessive*

- *if a test result has serious implications (e.g., a positive Pap smear)*

- *if the treatment suggested is risky or expensive*

- *if you are uncomfortable with the diagnosis and/or treatment*

- *if a course of treatment is not successful*

- *if you question your doctor's competence*

- *if your insurance company requires it*

approaches. So age and experience must be considered and weighed along with other factors when choosing a physician.

Most doctors will be supportive if you request a second opinion and many will recommend it. In many cases, insurance companies will pay for second opinions, but check ahead of time to make sure your insurance plan does cover them. In an HMO you may have to be more assertive because one way HMOs control costs is by limiting second opinions. Often, the opinion of a second doctor will confirm the opinion of the first, but the reassurance may be worth the time and extra cost. On the other hand, if the second opinion differs from the first, you have two alternatives: seek the opinion of a third doctor, or educate yourself as much as possible by talking to both doctors, reading up on the problem, and trusting your instincts about which diagnosis is correct. Sometimes obtaining a second opinion can be a major challenge. Occasionally, a physician may be offended. Nonetheless, you should not be dissuaded.

The simple logistics of getting a second opinion can be an obstacle. Tara Parker-Pope related in her column (Health Journal) in the *Wall Street Journal* the difficulty gathering her mother's records from five doctors, two radiology offices and the pathology lab. She also cited, in the same piece, a Northwestern University review of 340 breast cancer patients who sought second opinions. They reported that 20% of second opinions had no change in pathology or prognosis, but in the remaining 80% of patients some change did occur.

OFFICE AND PRACTICE ARRANGEMENTS

Some specialists will only see new patients who are referred to them by another doctor. Therefore, you may need to have your treating physician contact the specialist's office to arrange for your initial visit. Your health plan may also require that your primary care doctor provide a referral.

If English is not your first language, it may be advisable to determine whether someone in the specialist's office speaks your primary language or if a translator can be present during appointments or, perhaps take a bilingual person with you. This will ease communication and assure that all questions, responses and instructions are understood.

QUESTIONS CONCERNING PAYMENT

Other arrangements that may need to be made in advance of your first visit or discussed with the specialist's office staff concern payment. You may wish to ask the following:

- *Is the specialist within your plan's network and will you need to make a co-payment? Or, is the specialist out-of-network and will you have to pay for your care out-of-pocket, meet a deductible or submit a form for reimbursement?*

- *Are credit cards an acceptable mode of payment?*

- *Does the specialist accept Medicare or Medicaid?*

Accessibility of a physician's office may be a concern if you are wheelchair-bound, are elderly or cannot climb stairs or negotiate narrow corridors. Convenient parking may also be important to you.

When you are choosing a top specialist, these issues may be of lesser or greater importance, depending on the problem and type of care warranted. If you are traveling a great distance to have a specific procedure performed by a top specialist at a major medical center, continuing long-term monitoring or follow-up care by that physician may not be required or may not be feasible and such things as office practice arrangements are of less importance. On the other hand, if your disease needs to be monitored with follow-up care provided by the same top specialist, then such issues as accessibility of the doctor's office, appointment hours, waiting times and courtesy and professionalism of the staff become more significant.

INTRODUCTION

PERSONAL CHEMISTRY

One element of the doctor-patient relationship that we stress in our Guides is chemistry between doctor and patient, a part of which is often referred to as a doctor's "bedside manner." While this factor is of major importance in a long-term relationship such as you would have with your primary care physician, it is of less importance when you see a specialist only once or twice.

It is vital that there is a sense of mutual trust and respect between patient and doctor; this is a judgment that individuals must make for themselves. Among the many talented doctors listed in this Guide, there are very likely some to whom you would relate well and others with whom you may not feel as comfortable.

> *It is vital that there is a sense of mutual trust and respect between patient and doctor; this is a judgment that individuals must make for themselves.*

Patients prefer doctors who listen, demonstrate concern, are responsive to patient needs and spend sufficient time with them. The qualities of physicians in this regard, even the excellent ones in this Guide, vary widely.

You, the patient, are the only one who can assess these qualities because individuals react differently to various personalities. It is important for you to carefully judge your feelings towards a physician, especially if you are embarking on a long-term relationship. You should feel you can be open, trusting and responsive to your physician and that your relationship will be a positive one. Otherwise, find another doctor, since not doing so could adversely affect your care.

Once you have used this guide to identify the top specialist(s) best suited to treat your condition, there is much you can do to maximize the value of your first visit.

32

· 5 ·

MAXIMIZING YOUR FIRST APPOINTMENT WITH A TOP DOCTOR

After your research is done and you've secured an appointment for an initial consultation with a top doctor, known for his or her expertise in the diagnosis or treatment of your particular medical condition, what should you do?

A specialist becoming newly involved in your care needs to learn as much as possible about the state of your health in a very limited time. Since top doctors are extremely busy people with many demands on their time, you should make certain that all relevant records and case summaries are obtained and sent to the specialist well in advance of your appointment.

Lastly, it may be advisable to take a relative or close friend with you for support.

OBTAINING YOUR RECORDS

All healthcare providers, including hospitals, doctors and their staffs, are under legal obligation to maintain the privacy of your medical records. In order to obtain release of those records, you must make a request in writing. If you need to obtain records from a number of providers, you should write one clear and concise letter authorizing release of your records and including your name, address, telephone number, date of birth, and hospital patient I.D. number. You then can make photocopies of this letter, but be sure to sign and date each copy as if it were an original. You also may want to specifically name those test results (e.g., pathology slides) or X-ray films (not just written reports or summaries) that must be included in addition to making a general request for your records. It's also a good idea to indicate the date of your appointment so the office staff can respond in a timely manner.

Although state laws require the timely release of medical records, hospital medical records departments and doctors' offices often take several weeks to pull and review patient charts and get them in the mail either to you or to another doctor. In addition to written authorization, you may be asked to pay the costs involved in copying your records, test results and X-ray films because many doctors' offices will not release the originals. Consider placing a call in advance to determine the procedure for releasing your records, how long you can expect it to take, and the costs involved so that you can save time by including payment with your release authorization letter. Be sure to allow sufficient time in advance of your consultation appointment for your request to be processed. Since you often must wait several weeks for an appointment with a specialist, allow at least that amount of time to obtain your records.

You should make certain that all relevant records and case summaries are obtained and sent to the specialist well in advance of your appointment.

Even after making your written requests, you should follow up each letter with a telephone call to be sure that your records actually are sent. You should not assume that your request for records will be promptly fulfilled by an often overburdened, although well-intentioned, office staff.

Remember, the more information the specialist has about your condition, the fewer repeat or additional tests or procedures you will need to undergo. This will lower the costs of your consultation and enable the specialist to more easily assess your condition.

THE FACTS AND ONLY THE FACTS

Be thorough and organized in documenting your personal and familial medical histories, the medications you take and in relaying information about your condition. Even seemingly minor bits of information may provide subtle clues to the nature of your medical problem and the optimal way in which to treat it. It's also advisable to bring a list with you of names, addresses and telephone numbers of all physicians who have cared for you, especially those you have seen regarding your current medical problem.

Even though thoroughness is essential to presenting a clear picture of your medical condition, bear in mind that the specialist needs to get to your core health concerns as quickly as possible. Therefore, if you have a complex medical history, you may want to ask your current doctors to provide treatment summaries in addition to copies of your medical records. Hospital records should include your admission history and physical exam, dictated consultation and operation notes and discharge summaries for all hospitalizations. You may also be able to get a cumulative lab and X-ray summary for your hospital stays.

Remember, the more information the specialist has about your condition, the fewer repeat or additional tests or procedures you will need to undergo.

Unlike X-rays, which can be copied at reasonable cost, original pathology slides must be transported by mail or hand-carried. Your specialist may wish to have the pathologist with whom he or she works speak directly with the pathologist who initially interpreted your slides as part of the process of evaluating your case.

BEING PREPARED

To avoid leaving out important details of your condition or past treatment, prepare a concise, chronological summary before your consultation takes place. You may wish to type it and provide a copy to the specialist for

GATHERING THE FACTS

Have you done everything you can to prepare yourself and the specialist for the consultation? The following checklist will help you maximize the value of your visit to the specialist and will go a long way toward focusing you on the task at hand—getting the best advice or treatment for your health problem from one of the top doctors in the medical specialty related to your condition.

- *Does the specialist have all the information needed to make a diagnosis of or treatment plan for your condition?*

- *Have your medical records, test results and X-rays been sent ahead of time to allow for their review by the specialist in advance of your first appointment?*

- *Have you written out your medical history, including that of your siblings, parents and grandparents, emphasizing the particular problem for which you are visiting this specialist?*

- *Are you prepared with a written list of questions?*

- *When you ask your questions, have you understood the answers?*

inclusion in your chart. Highlight major medical results or significant events in the course of an illness or treatment if these will enlighten the doctor about your condition. Your personal perspective on the state of your health is vital to a full understanding of your medical problem.

It is possible that the specialist will use terminology that you do not understand or may speak quickly assuming certain knowledge on your part about your condition or its treatment. Don't hesitate to ask for clarification as often or repeatedly as you may need to in order to fully comprehend what you are being told. If you are concerned that you may forget what the doctor tells you, ask the doctor's permission to take notes or ask if you might bring along a tape recorder so you can later replay what was said, especially any instructions you are given. You may prefer to bring along a relative or close friend to serve as a "second set of ears," but, again, seek the doctor's permission to do so in advance of your appointment.

Your personal perspective on the state of your health is vital to a full understanding of your medical problem.

Following this process will assure that you and the specialist you are consulting get the most from your appointment. After all, you both have the same goal: restoring you to optimal health and well being.

WHAT TO DO IF YOU CAN'T GET AN APPOINTMENT

At times it may be difficult, perhaps even impossible, to secure an appointment with the specific specialist you have identified. There are a number of reasons why this may occur. For example, the specialist may not be taking any new patients or may have such a busy schedule that it takes several weeks or months to get an appointment. He or she may only see patients during very limited hours because of teaching, research or other responsibilities or currently may have other limitations related to the acceptance of new patients.

However, bear in mind that the doctors in this guide are the leaders in their fields and therefore they work with and train the very best and brightest

If you are unable to consult with a particular doctor, consider making an appointment with one of his or her outstanding colleagues

in their specialties. So, if you are unable to consult with a particular doctor, consider making an appointment with one of his or her outstanding colleagues. You can do this by asking a member of the doctor's office staff to refer you to an associate who is a member of the practice group or to another excellent physician who is specially trained to address your particular medical issue.

You can be comfortable knowing that you will receive high quality care from another specialist who practices in the same top setting.

• 6 •

CLINICAL TRIALS

The following information on special resources has been included to meet the needs of cancer patients and their families. These patients and their physicians may need to search for very new, cutting-edge, perhaps even experimental and not yet approved therapies. In such cases the search may lead to clinical trials, tests of new drugs and new medical devices, or innovative therapeutic approaches. Fortunately, these situations are rare, but when they do occur they are critical.

In addition to the outstanding private and public hospitals recognized in this guide, the U.S. government maintains its own unique, expert source of patient care and clinical research at the National Institutes of Health (NIH). In fact, the NIH operates its own hospital at which the care provided is usually related to clinical studies its researchers are undertaking.

In addition to those at the NIH, clinical trials also are conducted at leading medical centers and other organizations throughout the country. These facilities may be testing a new drug therapy, a new use for an existing medication or a medical device to deal with a problem that is not being resolved through the use of more traditional approaches.

This section will guide you in utilizing these special resources. These is also a listing of selected cancer resources in Appendix E.

THE CLINICAL TRIAL AS A TREATMENT OPTION

For some patients the best medical treatment may only be available through clinical trials (also called treatment studies), which are designed to develop improved ways to use current medical treatments or to find new medical treatments by studying their effects on humans. Treatments are studied to determine if they are safe, effective and better treatments than conventional or standard therapies. Only if they meet all three of these criteria are they made available to the general public.

Many people are frightened by the term "clinical trial" because it conveys the notion of being a "guinea pig" in an experiment. Contrary to popular belief, however, new treatments are extensively studied by scientists in the laboratory before they are ever tested by physicians in clinical settings. Among the factors that keep patients from participating in clinical trials are: lack of awareness about clinical trials as a treatment option; fear of side effects or adverse reactions to treatment; refusal of insurance companies to pay for experimental treatments; failure of a physician to inform the patient about clinical trials; difficulty finding suitable clinical trials; unavailability of clinical trials for certain medical problems; distance of the patient from major medical centers conducting clinical trials; disruption of personal and family life; and the decision to stop medical treatment altogether.

The National Cancer Institute sponsors clinical trials at more than 1,000 sites in the United States

Despite these and other obstacles, many people do seek out clinical trials. New medical treatments can offer participants hope for a cure, an extended lifespan, or an improvement in how they feel. Some participants also take comfort in knowing that others may benefit from their contribution to medical knowledge.

Deciding if a clinical trial is the right treatment option for you is no simple matter. Certainly, you will want to talk about it with your doctor(s) and other professionals involved in your care, as well as with family members and friends. But in order to fully benefit from what others have to say — based on either their professional knowledge or personal experience — you need to understand exactly what a clinical trial is and what your role as a volunteer will be.

UNDERSTANDING CLINICAL TRIALS

Clinical trials are conducted for just about every medical condition, including life-threatening diseases such as AIDS or cancer; chronic illnesses such as diabetes and asthma; psychiatric disorders such as depression or anxiety; behavioral problems such as smoking and substance abuse; and even common ailments such as hair loss and acne. Chances are there is at least one trial (and probably more) that may be appropriate for you.

With more than 100 different types of cancer, it is understandable that a large number of clinical trials are cancer-related. Extensive information about clinical trials for cancer can be found on www.cancer.gov, the Web site of the National Cancer Institute (NCI). NCI is part of the NIH. CenterWatch, an online clinical trials listing service, identifies over 14,000 clinical trials that are actively recruiting patients. Veritas Medicine, another useful online organization, allows individuals to perform personalized searches of its clinical trials database. See "Selected Cancer Resources" in Appendix E for more information on clinical trials.

One of the most pressing reasons to participate in clinical trials is the opportunity to obtain treatment that might not be available otherwise

Most clinical trials study new medical treatments, combinations of treatments, or improvements in conventional treatments using drugs, surgery and other medical procedures, medical devices, radiation or other therapies. Newer types of clinical trials, called screening or prevention trials, study how to prevent the incidence or recurrence of disease through the use of medicines, vitamins, minerals or other supplements; and how to screen for disease, especially in its early stages. Another type of trial studies how to improve the quality of life for patients, including both their physical and emotional well-being.

Clinical trials are sponsored both by the federal government (through the National Institutes of Health, the National Cancer Institute and many others) and by private industry through pharmaceutical and biotechnology

QUESTIONS TO ASK YOUR DOCTOR AND THE TRIAL'S RESEARCH TEAM IF YOU ARE CONSIDERING PARTICIPATING IN A CLINICAL TRIAL:

- *Who is sponsoring the trial?*

- *How many patients will be involved?*

- *Will the trial be testing a single treatment or a combination of treatments?*

- *Will there be one treatment group or more than one treatment group?*

- *If more than one treatment group, how are patients assigned to each group?*

- *Has this treatment been studied in previous clinical trials? What were the findings?*

- *What are the requirements for patient eligibility?*

companies, and through healthcare institutions (hospitals or health maintenance organizations) and community-based physician-investigators. The National Cancer Institute sponsors clinical trials at more than 1,000 sites in the United States. Trials are carried out in major medical research centers such as teaching hospitals as well as in community hospitals, specialized medical clinics and in doctors' offices.

Though clinical trials often involve hospitalized patients, a fair number of trials are conducted on an outpatient basis. Many trials are part of a cooperative network which may include as few as one or two sites or hundreds of locations, although one center generally assumes responsibility for overall coordination of the research. More than 45 research-oriented institutions, recognized for their scientific excellence, have been designated by the NCI as comprehensive or clinical cancer centers. See "Selected Cancer Resources" in Appendix E to find out how to locate these centers.

Clinical research is based on a protocol (established rules or procedures) describing who will be studied, how and when medications, procedures and/or treatments will be administered and how long the study will last. Trials that are conducted simultaneously at different sites use the same protocol to ensure that all patients are treated identically and all data are collected uniformly so that study findings can be compared.

Some participants also take comfort in knowing that others may benefit from their contribution to medical knowledge

Clinical trials generally are conducted in three phases, as outlined in the study protocol. The first phase begins testing of the treatment on a small group of human subjects after rigorous and successful animal testing has been concluded. The interim phase varies, but usually involves a broader test group and is designed to further evaluate the treatment's safety and more accurately determine appropriate dosage, application methods and side effects. In some trials there may be a fourth phase, conducted after the treatment is in widespread use, to monitor the results of long-term use and the occurrence of any serious side effects.

Some clinical trials test one treatment on one group of subjects, while others compare two or more groups of subjects. In such comparison studies participants are divided into two groups: the control group that receives the standard treatment and the experimental or treatment group which receives the new treatment. For example, the control group may undergo a surgical procedure while the experimental or treatment group undergoes a surgical procedure *plus* radiation to determine which treatment modality is more effective.

To ensure that patient characteristics do not unduly influence the study findings, patients may be randomly assigned to either the control or the experimental group, meaning that each patient's assignment is based purely on chance. In cases in which a standard treatment does not exist for a particular disease, the experimental group of patients receives the new treatment and the control group receives no treatment at all, or receives a placebo, an inactive medicine or procedure that has no treatment value. It is important to keep in mind that patients are never put into a control group without any treatment if

QUESTIONS TO ASK THE RESEARCH TEAM ABOUT THE BENEFITS AND RISKS OF A CLINICAL TRIAL:

- *What other treatment option(s) do I have at this time?*

- *What are the short and long-term benefits and risks as compared with standard treatment?*

- *Will I experience any known side effects or adverse reactions? Will these be temporary, long-term or permanent? Relatively minor or perhaps life-threatening?*

- *If I am harmed in any way by the new treatment, what other treatments will I be entitled to? Who will pay for subsequent treatment?*

there is a known treatment that could help them. Also, whether a patient is receiving an investigational drug or a placebo, he/she receives the same level and quality of medical care as those receiving the investigational treatment.

PROTECTING THE RIGHTS OF PARTICIPANTS

The safety of those who participate in clinical trials is a serious matter and is the number one priority of medical investigators. All clinical research, regardless of type of sponsorship results of long-term use and the occurrence of any serious side effect is guided by the same ethical and legal codes that govern the medical profession and the practice of medicine. Most clinical research is federally funded or federally regulated (at least in part) with built-in safeguards for patients. According to federal government regulations (and some state laws), every clinical trial in the United States must be approved and monitored by an Institutional Review Board (IRB), which is an independent committee of physicians, statisticians, community advocates and others (representing at least five distinct disciplines) to ensure that the protocol is being followed.

It is important to keep in mind that patients are never put into a control group without any treatment if there is a known treatment that could help them

Government regulations require researchers to fully inform participants about all aspects of a clinical trial before they agree to participate through a process called informed consent. To be sure that you understand your role in a clinical trial, you should jot down any questions beforehand so as not to forget them. You should also consider bringing along a friend or family member for support and additional input, and perhaps even tape recording the conversation (after asking permission to do so) to make sure you do not forget or misunderstand anything. Each participant in a clinical trial must be given a written consent form, which should be available in English and other languages. The consent form explains the issues listed in the box on page 47.

QUESTIONS TO ASK THE SPONSORS ABOUT YOUR RIGHTS AS A PARTICIPANT IN A CLINICAL TRIAL:

- *Who is responsible for approving and monitoring this research? Is there an IRB?*

- *Who informs me about the trial process? Do I sign a consent form? Will I receive a copy?*

- *May I leave the trial at any time? Have previous patients dropped out?*

- *Whom do I contact if I am experiencing any difficulty with this trial?*

Patients also are informed that they may leave the trial, or exclude themselves from any part of it, at any time. Informed consent means exactly what the term implies: you agree to join a clinical trial only after you completely understand exactly what your participation will involve for the duration of the study. By law, each patient must be provided with a copy of the signed consent form, which also must include the name and telephone number of a contact person for questions or additional information. Informed consent is a continuous process, so do not hesitate to ask questions before, during or after the trial.

The investigators must protect the privacy of each participant in a clinical trial by ensuring that all medical records are kept confidential except for inspection by the sponsoring agency, the Food and Drug Administration and other agencies involved in regulating the drug or treatment, and all data are collected anonymously by assigning a numeric code or initials to each individual.

During the course of the trial, participants are regularly seen by members of the research team to monitor their health and well-being. Participants also should be responsible for their own health by following the treatment plan (such as taking the proper dosage of medications on time), keeping all scheduled visits and informing members of the healthcare team about any symptoms that occur. If, during the course of the trial, the treatment proves to be ineffective or harmful, the patient is free to leave the study and still obtain conventional care. Conversely, as soon as there is evidence that one treatment modality is better than another, all patients in the trial are given the benefit of the new information.

THE CONSENT FORM SHOULD EXPLAIN THE FOLLOWING:

- *Why the research is being done.*

- *What the researchers hope to accomplish.*

- *What types of treatment interventions (and other test or procedures) will be performed?*

- *How long the study will continue.*

- *What the expected benefits and the possible risks are.*

- *What other treatments are available.*

- *What costs will be covered by the study, by the patient or by third-party payers such as Medicare, Medicaid or private insurance.*

INTRODUCTION

ENROLLING IN CLINICAL TRIALS

Each clinical trial has its own guidelines, called eligibility criteria, for determining who can participate. Treatment studies recruit participants who have a disease or other medical condition, while screening and prevention studies generally recruit healthy volunteers. Inclusion criteria (those that allow you to participate in a study) and exclusion criteria (those that keep you from participating in a study) ensure that the study will answer the research questions posed in the research protocol while maintaining the safety of participants. The disease being studied is a primary factor in selecting suitable patients, but other factors such as the patient's gender, age, treatment history and other diagnosed medical conditions may also be important. Unfortunately, eligibility also may depend upon ability to pay. Many health plans do not cover all of the costs associated with clinical trials because they define these trials as experimental procedures. However, trials sometimes pay volunteers for their time and/or reimburse them for travel, childcare, meals and lodging.

> *The investigators must protect the privacy of each participant in a clinical trial by ensuring that all medical records are kept confidential*

To prevent people who qualify from being excluded from clinical trials for financial reasons, agencies such as the National Cancer Institute are working with health plans to find solutions and a growing number of states require insurance companies to pay for all routine patient care costs in cancer trials. To encourage more senior citizens to participate in cancer trials, Medicare plans to revise its payment policy to cover those trials.

When choosing a clinical trial you should determine the factors that are most important to you. For instance, patients generally prefer to participate in trials near their homes so that they can maintain their usual day-to-day activities, be surrounded by family and friends and avoid travel and lodging costs. If travel or temporary relocation becomes necessary, try to find a trial site that is near to some family member or friend or one that is in a locale similar to your own city or town. Many

48

QUESTIONS TO ASK THE TRIAL'S SPONSOR ABOUT ELIGIBILITY CRITERIA:

- *What are the inclusion and exclusion criteria for the clinical trial(s) I am considering?*

- *How can I improve my chances of being accepted? Can I change my health plan to one that will cover the trial's costs? Can I relocate to another city or state?*

- *If I am not eligible for one trial, what other trials being conducted for my condition?*

- *Will I be paid for my time or reimbursed for my out-of-pocket expenses?*

organizations, such as the National Cancer Institute, will work with patients and their families to identify support networks for them wherever they participate.

PARTICIPATING IN A CLINICAL TRIAL

Clinical trials are conducted by a research team led by a principal investigator (usually a physician) and are comprised of physicians, nurses and other health professionals such as social workers, psychologists and nutritionists. As a participant you may be required to commit a fair amount of time to a clinical trial, often within more than one geographic region and states.

Participants in clinical trials should remain under the care of their regular physician(s) since clinical trials tend to provide short-term treatment for a specific medical condition and do not generally provide comprehensive primary care. In fact, some trials require that a patient's regular physician sign

INTRODUCTION

a consent form before the patient is enrolled. In addition, your regular physician can collaborate with the research team to make sure there are no adverse reactions between your other medications or treatments and the investigational treatment.

WEIGHING THE BENEFITS AND RISKS OF A CLINICAL TRIAL

To encourage more senior citizens to participate in cancer trials, Medicare plans to revise its payment policy to cover those trials

If you are considering participation in a clinical trial, you need to consider the medical, emotional and financial ramifications of participation. Of course, the obvious benefit of a clinical trial is the chance that a new treatment may improve your health and prognosis. You will have access to drugs and other medical interventions before they are widely available to the public and you will obtain expert and specialized medical care at leading healthcare facilities. Many patients receive an added psychological benefit by taking an active role in their treatment.

It is important to bear in mind that some medical interventions used in clinical trials may carry potential risks depending upon the type of treatment and the patient's condition. While many side effects or adverse reactions are temporary (such as hair loss and nausea caused by some anti-cancer drugs), other more serious reactions can be permanent and even life-threatening (for example, heart, liver or kidney damage).

Deciding whether or not to participate in a clinical trial is often a matter of determining if the trial's potential benefits outweigh its possible risks. This is a highly personal decision that may be difficult to make in situations involving experimental treatment in which limited medical information may be available.

QUESTIONS TO ASK THE RESEARCH TEAM OR YOUR PHYSICIAN ABOUT YOUR ROLE IN A CLINICAL TRIAL:

- *Who are the members of the health team? Who will be in charge of my care?*

- *How long will the trial last?*

- *How does treatment in the trial compare with or differ from the standard treatment?*

- *Will I be hospitalized? How often? For how long a period of time?*

- *What will occur during each visit? What treatments or procedures will I be given?*

- *Will I still be able to see my regular physician(s)?*

- *Will my doctor and the research team collaborate?*

- *Can I be put in touch with other patients who have participated in this trial?*

GETTING INFORMATION ON CLINICAL TRIALS

The more information you have about a clinical trial, the easier it will be to make a decision about whether or not it is right for you, and the more confident you will be that you made an appropriate decision. In addition to the "Selected Cancer Resources," Appendix E in this guide, the staff at your local public library, community hospital, or major medical center can assist you in locating the information you need from books, consumer organizations and on the Internet.

LEARNING ABOUT THE NATIONAL INSTITUTES OF HEALTH (NIH)

The National Institutes of Health (NIH) comprise one the world's leading medical research centers and the Federal government's principal agency for biomedical research. An agency of the United States Department of Health, United States Public Health Service, NIH encompasses 25 separate institutions and centers with its main campus located in Bethesda, Maryland. Research is also conducted at several field units across the country and abroad.

PATIENT CARE AT THE NIH

The Warren Grant Magnuson Clinical Center, NIH's principal medical research center and hospital located in Bethesda, Maryland, provides medical care only to patients participating in clinical research programs. Two categories of patients participate in the Clinical Center studies: children and adults who wish to improve their own health, such as those with newly diagnosed medical problems, ongoing medical problems or family history of disease; and healthy volunteers wishing to advance knowledge about the causes, progress and treatment of disease. The patient's case must fit into an ongoing NIH research project for which the patient has the precise kind or stage of illness under investigation. General diagnostic and treatment services common to community hospitals are not available.

It is important to bear in mind that some medical interventions used in clinical trials may carry potential risks depending upon the type of treatment and the patient's condition.

The Magnuson Clinical Center is the world's largest biomedical research hospital and ambulatory care facility, housing 1,600 laboratories conducting basic and clinical research. There are 1,200 tenured physicians, dentists and researchers on staff along with 660 nurses and 570 allied healthcare professionals (dieticians, imaging technologists, medical technologists, medical records and clerical staff, pharmacists and therapists).

The Center's hospital is specially designed for medical research and accommodates 540 carefully selected patients who are participating in clinical research programs. Its 350-bed facility has 24 inpatient care units to which 7,000 patients are admitted annually. The Center also has an Ambulatory Care Research Facility (ACRF) that serves 68,000 outpatient visits each year. A new facility, called the Mark O. Hatfield Clinical Research Center, which began accepting patients in early 2005, has 242 beds for inpatient care and 90 day-hospital stations for outpatient care. The Mark O. Hatfield Center carries out the latest biomedical research that results in new forms of disease diagnosis, prevention and treatment, which is then incorporated into improved methods of patient care.

Deciding whether or not to participate in a clinical trial is often a matter of determinng if the potential benefits outweigh its possible risks

This is a fine example of Translational Medicine where excellent research discoveries are translated into new and improved methods of clinical treatment. In other words, the laboratory discoveries are brought to the bedside.

The Clinical Center also maintains a Children's Inn for pediatric outpatients and their families. This family-centered residence operates 24 hours a day, 7 days a week, 365 days a year.

In an effort to bring clinical research to the community, NIH supports approximately 80 General Clinical Research Centers (GCRCs) around the country, located within hospitals of major academic medical centers.

It is important to note that, as part of the federal government, the Warren Grant Magnuson Clinical Center provides treatment in clinical trials at no cost to its patients. In some cases, patients receive a stipend to help cover the

IF YOUR PHYSICIAN CONCURS THAT A CLINICAL STUDY MIGHT BE APPROPRIATE FOR YOU, THE NIH RECOMMENDS THAT THE FOLLOWING STEPS BE TAKEN:

- *Contact NCI's Clinical Studies Support Center (CSSC), which is staffed by trained oncology (cancer) nurses who can identify appropriate clinical studies for you. Summaries of these trials and other pertinent information about the type of treatment being offered and the type of patients eligible for inclusion can be mailed or faxed to you and/or your physician.*

- *Review the clinical trials summaries and other information with your physician to decide which study or studies you should consider. Your physician also can contact the CSSC to communicate directly with the investigator in charge of the study.*

- *In cases in which you meet the initial eligibility requirements, it may be necessary for you to schedule a screening visit at the Clinical Center to learn more about the trial and possibly undergo some medical tests.*

- *If accepted for a clinical trial, make sure that you understand the details about the treatment and any possible risks and benefits.*

costs of traveling to Bethesda for treatment and follow-up care. Travel costs for the initial screening visit, however, are not covered.

AREAS OF CLINICAL STUDY AT THE NIH

At the Magnuson Clinical Center alone, NIH physician-scientists conduct nearly 1,000 studies each year. Among the areas of study are cancer and related diseases.

Not all of these clinical areas are under investigation at any given time, however. The Patient Recruitment and Public Liaison Office (PRPL) at the NIH Clinical Center assists patients, their families and their physicians in obtaining information about participation in NIH clinical trials. Trained nurses are available to answer questions about the research programs and admission procedures.

CANCER CARE AT THE WARREN GRANT MAGNUSON CLINICAL CENTER

The National Cancer Institute (NCI) is the largest of the biomedical research institutes and centers at NIH. There, clinical studies are designed to evaluate new and promising ways to prevent, detect, diagnose and treat cancer. The Warren Grant Magnuson Clinical Center provides a separate outpatient division for cancer patients and also has several designated inpatient units.

The Magnuson Clinical Center is the world's largest biomedical research hospital and ambulatory care facility

If you are interested in entering a cancer study at the Magnuson Clinical Center (or at the General Clinical Research Centers), you should first discuss treatment options with a physician. As a general rule, patients interested in participating in clinical studies must be referred by a physician. However, in some instances, self-referral may be permitted.

INTRODUCTION

Patients with medical problems other than cancer or healthy volunteers who wish to participate in a clinical study should contact the particular NIH institute responsible for the clinical area involved.

CANCER CARE AT THE NCI CLINICAL CENTERS AND COMPREHENSIVE CANCER CENTERS

You may also obtain clinical oncology services (education, screening, diagnosis or treatment) or participate in clinical trials at one of the 21 Cancer Centers or 39 Comprehensive Cancer Centers designated by the NCI for their scientific excellence and extensive resources devoted to cancer and cancer-related problems. Centers are located in 32 states, with the majority of sites in California, New York and Pennsylvania. You can find out about clinical trials at the NCI-designated centers by contacting NCI's Clinical Studies Support Center (CSSC) or by calling each center directly (See Appendix E for contact information). Information about other cancer-related services at these centers also may be obtained from the center itself. For more information, you can visit the National Cancer Institute's website at www.cancer.gov.

SECTION II

USING THIS GUIDE TO FIND A DOCTOR

• 7 •

HOW TO USE THIS BOOK

We assume most people who purchase this book have either received a diagnosis of cancer, or know someone who has. Although it would have been possible to arrange the listings by type of cancer, e.g. lung, breast, prostate, etc., that would not have been practical. For any particular type of cancer, a patient may be seeking one or more of a variety of different specialists. For example, any of the cancers mentioned could require, among other specialists, the involvement of pathologists, medical oncologists, surgeons, urologists, radiation oncologists and, possibly, psychiatrists.

Therefore, this guide and its list of physicians is organized first by specialty. Then, because many patients may prefer care as close to home as possible, we organized the lists by region. (See map on page 63)

The Special Expertise index included in the book may also be of great help in locating the best specialists to meet a patients' needs. We asked physicians making nominations to recommend individuals who were nationally recognized as leaders in the prevention, diagnosis and treatment of particular types of cancer, as well as leaders in various treatment modalities. When physicians selected for inclusion in *America's Top Doctors for Cancer* completed and submitted their professional biographies, we also asked them to list their areas of special expertise. As a result, the Special Expertise Index lists hundreds of these areas.

HOW TO USE THIS BOOK

The physicians are listed alphabetically within their specialties and then within their regions. A sample biography is presented and explained below.

SAMPLE PHYSICIAN LISTING

Smith, John MD [Hem] - **Spec Exp:** Leukemia; **Hospital:** State Cancer Hosp (page 000);
Name [Specialty]   Special Expertise(s)   Admitting Hospital
      & Hospital Information Page

Address: 5 Ridge Road Boston, MA 12345; **Phone:** (617) 555-1234; **Board Cert:** IM 74;Hem 76
Office Address   Office Phone   Board Certification(s)

Med School: National Med Sch 70; **Resid:** IM, State Cancer Hosp 74;
Medical School   Residency(ies)

Fellow: Hem, State Cancer Hosp 76; **Fac Appt:** Assoc Prof Med, The Med Sch
Fellowship(s)   Faculty Appointment

LOCATING A SPECIALIST

This guide is organized to make finding the right specialists for you or your loved ones as simple as possible. Physicians' biographies are presented by specialty and are organized by geographic region within each specialty or subspecialty. Thus, you may search for a particular type of specialist or subspecialist in one or more regions or throughout the nation.

A second way to locate the right specialist is to use the SPECIAL EXPERTISE INDEX beginning on page 617. This index is organized according to diseases, conditions and procedures or techniques. For example, you can locate a top specialist for diabetes or for Mohs' surgery by looking for those terms in the SPECIAL EXPERTISE INDEX.

If you already know a specialist's name, you can find his/her listing by using the ALPHABETICAL LISTING OF DOCTORS beginning on page 657.

The information reported in each doctor's listing is, for the most part, provided by the doctor or his/her office staff. Castle Connolly attempts to verify the data through other sources but cannot guarantee that in all cases all data have been so verified or are accurate. All such information is subject to change from time to time due to changes in physician practices.

STEP-BY-STEP DIRECTIONS FOR FINDING THE SPECIALIST YOU NEED

1. **Look for a doctor first by specialty.** Turn to the Special Expertise Index on p. 617. Review the list which is organized alphabetically, and find the particular disease, organ, procedure or treatment of interest to you. Write down the page numbers of physicians with that expertise and turn to those pages.

2. **Look in the area of the country closest to you.** Each specialty lists doctors alphabetically within their geographical region. These regions start in New England (northeast) and go around the country in a consistent order to finish the West Coast and Pacific. Each state is grouped into one of these seven geographical regions. See map of the United States and the regions on page 63. If you don't find a doctor in that particular specialty in your first geographic preference, expand your search to other regions.

3. **Check further in the special expertise index.** If you don't find a doctor to meet your needs, the last chapter contains those specialties which include a small number of doctors. The Special Expertise index may include some diseases which are not related to cancer because a physician who treats cancer patients also may treat patients with these diseases.

GEOGRAPHIC REGIONS & STATES

To assist you in using *America's Top Doctors for Cancer* in the most efficient and effective manner, the Guide is divided into seven geographic regions. This will help you to locate a specialist in your local or neighboring region. For example, if you live in Mississippi in the Southeast region and you are willing and able to travel to Louisiana in the Southwest region to consult with a specialist in medical oncology, you can review just those two regions, under the section headed "Medical Oncology." However, if you prefer to review the information on medical oncologists throughout the country, you can search the entire medical oncology section. Or, you can consult the "SPECIAL EXPERTISE INDEX" in the back of this Guide and choose a medical oncologist who has specific expertise to meet your particular needs.

The geographic regions are as follows:

New England
Mid Atlantic
Southeast
Midwest
Great Plains and Mountains
Southwest
West Coast and Pacific

The states that are included in each region are listed on the following page and a map of the regions is also provided. Please note that not all regions are represented in all specialties. For example, in "Vascular and Interventional Radiology" there are no listings in the Great Plains and Mountains region.

GEOGRAPHIC REGIONS AND STATES

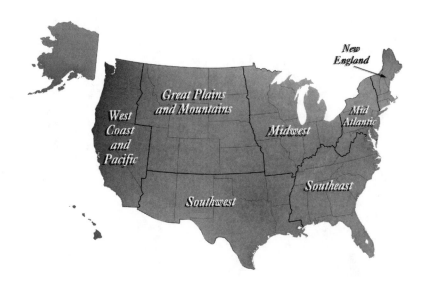

West Coast and Pacific:
Alaska
California
Hawaii
Nevada
Oregon
Washington

Great Plains and Mountains:
Colorado
Idaho
Kansas
Montana
Nebraska
North Dakota
South Dakota
Utah
Wyoming

Southwest:
Arizona
Arkansas
Louisiana
New Mexico
Oklahoma
Texas

Midwest:
Illinois
Indiana
Iowa
Michigan
Minnesota
Missouri
Ohio
Wisconsin

New England:
Connecticut
Maine
Massachusetts
New Hampshire
Rhode Island
Vermont

Mid Atlantic:
Delaware
Maryland
New Jersey
New York
Pennsylvania
Washington, DC
West Virginia

Southeast:
Alabama
Florida
Georgia
Kentucky
Mississippi
North Carolina
South Carolina
Tennessee
Virginia

• 8 •

MEDICAL SPECIALTIES

In the pages that follow, each list of doctors in a medical specialty or subspecialty is preceded by a brief description of that specialty (or subspecialty) and the training required for board certification.

Critical Care Medicine has been excluded because in emergency situations there is neither time nor opportunity for choice. A number of other specialities not relevant to most patients (e.g.Forensic Psychiatry) have not been included as well.

The following descriptions of medical specialties and subspecialties were provided by the American Board of Medical Specialties (ABMS), an organization comprised of the 24 medical specialty boards that provide certification in 25 medical specialties. A complete listing of all specialists certified by the ABMS can be found in The Official ABMS Directory of Board Certified Medical Specialists, is published by *Marquis Who's Who*. It is available (either in a multi-volume directory or on CD-ROM) in most public libraries, hospital libraries, university libraries and medical libraries. The ABMS also operates a toll-free phone line at 1-866-275-2267 and a website at www.abms.org to verify the certification status of individual doctors.

The following important policy statement, approved by the ABMS Assembly on March 19, 1987, remains valid.

HOW TO USE THIS BOOK

THE PURPOSE OF CERTIFICATION:

The intent of the certification process, as defined by the member boards of the American Board of Medical Specialties, is to provide assurance to the public that a certified medical specialist has successfully completed an approved educational program and an evaluation, including an examination process designed to assess the knowledge, experience and skills requisite to the provision of high quality patient care in that specialty.

MEDICAL SPECIALTY AND SUBSPECIALTY ABBREVIATIONS

The following medical specialty and subspecialties are indicated in the doctors' listings by their abbreviations. Specialties are indicated in bold, subspecialties in italics, and the four primary care specialties in capital, bold italics. To review the official American Board of Medical Specialties (ABMS) organization of specialties, refer to Appendix A.

Adolescent Medicine   AM
Involves the primary care treatment of adolescents and young adults. Involves the primary care treatment of adolescents and young adults. Involves the primary care treatment of adolescents and young adults. Involves the primary care treatment of adolescents and young adults.

Allergy & Immunology   A&I
Diagnosis and treatment of allergies, asthma, and skin problems such as hives and contact dermatitis.

Anesthesiology   Anes
Provides pain relief in maintenance or restoration of a stable condition during and following an operation. Anesthesiologists also diagnose and treat acute and long standing pain problems.

Cardiac Electrophysiology (Clinical)   CE
Involves complicated technical procedures to evaluate heart rhythms and determine appropriate treatment for them.

Cardiovascular Disease   Cv
Involves the diagnosis and treatment of disorders of the heart, lungs, and blood vessels.

Child & Adolescent Psychiatry   ChAP
Deals with the diagnosis and treatment of mental diseases in children and adolescents.

Child Neurology   ChiN
Diagnosis and medical treatment of disorders of the brain, spinal cord, and nervous system in children.

Clinical Genetics   CG
Deals with identifying the genetic causes of inherited diseases and ailments and preventing, when possible, their occurrence.

Colon and Rectal Surgery   CRS
Surgical treatment of diseases of the intestinal tract, colon and rectum, anal canal, and peranal area.

Dermatology D

Diagnosis and treatment of benign and malignant disorders of the skin, mouth, external genitalia, hair and nails, as well as a number of sexually transmitted diseases.

Diagnostic Radiology DR

Involves the study of all modalities of radiant energy in medical diagnoses and therapeutic procedures utilizing radiologic guidance.

Endocrinology, Diabetes & Metabolism EDM

Involves the study and treatment of patients suffering from hormonal and chemical disorders.

FAMILY MEDICINE FP

Deals with and oversees the total healthcare of individual patients and their family members. Family practitioners are more common in rural areas and may perform procedures more commonly performed by specialists (e.g., minor surgery).

Gastroenterology Ge

The study, diagnosis and treatment of diseases of the digestive organs including the stomach, bowels, liver, and gallbladder.

Geriatric Medicine Ger

Deals with diseases of the elderly and the problems associated with aging.

Geriatric Psychiatry GerPsy

Involves the diagnosis, prevention, and treatment of mental illness in the elderly.

Gynecologic Oncology GO

Deals with cancers of the female genital tract and reproductive systems.

Hand Surgery HS

Involves the treatment of injury to the hand through surgical techniques.

Hematology Hem

Involves the diagnosis and treatment of diseases and disorders of the blood, bone marrow, spleen, and lymph glands.

Infectious Disease Inf

The study and treatment of diseases caused by a bacterium, virus, fungus, or animal parasite.

INTERNAL MEDICINE IM

Diagnosis and nonsurgical treatment of diseases, especially those of adults. Internists may act as primary care specialists, highly trained family doctors, or they may subspecialize in specialties such as cardiology or nephrology.

Maternal & Fetal Medicine MF

Involves the care of women with high-risk pregnancies and their unborn fetuses.

Medical Oncology — Onc
Refers to the study and treatment of tumors and other cancers.

Neonatal-Perinatal Medicine — NP
Involves the diagnosis and treatments of infants prior to, during, and one month beyond birth.

Nephrology — Nep
Concerned with disorders of the kidneys, high blood pressure, fluid and mineral balance, dialysis of body wastes when the kidneys do not function, and consultation with surgeons about kidney transplantation.

Neurological Surgery — NS
Involves surgery of the brain, spinal cord, and nervous system.

Neurology — N
Diagnosis and medical treatment of disorders of the brain, spinal cord, and nervous system.

Neurophysiology (Clinical) — C/NPh
The study of the makeup and functioning of the nervous system in patients as opposed to in a laboratory.

Neuroradiology — NRad
Involves the utilization of imaging procedures during diagnosis as they relate to the brain, spine and spinal cord, head, neck, and organs of special sense in adults and children.

Nuclear Medicine — NuM
Evaluation of the functions of all the organs in the body and treatment of thyroid disease, benign and malignant tumors, and radiation exposure through the use of radioactive substances.

OBSTETRICS & GYNECOLOGY — ObG
Deals with the medical aspects of and intervention in pregnancy and labor and the overall health of the female reproductive system.

Ophthalmology — Oph
Diagnosis and treatment of diseases of and injuries to the eye.

Orthopaedic Surgery — OrS
Involves operations to correct injuries which interfere with the form and function of the extremities, spine, and associated structures.

Otolaryngology — Oto
Explores and treats diseases in the interrelated areas of the ears, nose and throat.

Otology/Neurotology — ON
Concentrates on the management, prevention, cure and care of patients with diseases of the ear and temporal bone, including disorders of hearing and balance.

HOW TO USE THIS BOOK

Pain Medicine   **PM**

Involves providing a high level of care for patients experiencing problems with acute or chronic pain in both hospital and ambulatory settings.

Pediatric Allergy & Immunology   **PA&I**

Involves the diagnosis and treatment of allergies, asthma and skin problems in children.

Pediatric Cardiology   **PCd**

Involves the diagnosis and treatment of heart disease in children.

Pediatric Critical Care Medicine   **PCCM**

Involves the care of children who are victims of life threatening disorders such as severe accidents, shock, and diabetes acidosis.

Pediatric Endocrinology   **PEn**

Involves the study and treatment of children with hormonal and chemical disorders.

Pediatric Gastroenterology   **PGe**

The study, diagnosis, and treatment of diseases of the digestive tract in children.

Pediatric Hematology-Oncology   **PHO**

The study and treatment of cancers of the blood and blood-forming parts of the body in children.

Pediatric Infectious Disease   **PInf**

The study and treatment of diseases caused by a virus, bacterium, fungus, or animal parasite in children.

Pediatric Nephrology   **PNep**

Deals with the diagnosis and treatment of disorders of the kidneys in children.

Pediatric Otolaryngology   **POto**

Involves the diagnosis and treatment of disorders of the ear, nose, and throat which affect children.

Pediatric Pulmonology   **PPul**

Involves the diagnosis and treatment of diseases of the chest, lungs, and chest tissue in children.

Pediatric Radiology   **PR**

Involves diagnostic imaging as it pertains to the newborn, infant, child, and adolescent.

Pediatric Rheumatology   **PRhu**

Involves the treatment of diseases of the joints and connective tissues in children.

Pediatric Surgery   **PS**

Treatment of disease, injury, or deformity in children through surgical techniques.

PEDIATRICS   **Ped**

Diagnosis and treatment of diseases of childhood and monitoring of the growth, development, and well-being of preadolescents.

Physical Medicine & Rehabilitation   **PMR**

The use of physical therapy and physical agents such as water, heat, light electricity, and mechanical manipulations in the diagnosis, treatment, and prevention of disease and body disorders.

Plastic Surgery   **PlS**

Involves reconstructive and cosmetic surgery of the face and other body parts.

Preventive Medicine   **PrM**

A specialty focusing on the prevention of illness and on the health of groups rather than individuals.

Psychiatry   **Psyc**

Examination, treatment, and prevention of mental illness through the use of psychoanalysis and/or drugs.

Public Health & General Preventive Medicine   **PHGPM**

Involves the investigation of the causes of epidemic disease and the prevention of a wide variety of acute and chronic illness.

Pulmonary Disease   **Pul**

Involves the diagnosis and treatment of diseases of the chest, lungs, and airways.

Radiation Oncology   **RadRo**

Involves the use of radiant energy and isotopes in the study and treatment of disease, especially malignant cancer.

Radiology   **Rad**

The use of various types of radiation, including X-rays, in the diagnosis and treatment of disease. Some imaging techniques no longer use radiation equipment (e.g., MRI and ultrasound).

Reproductive Endocrinology   **RE**

Deals with the endocrine system (including the pituitary, thyroid, parathyroid, adrenal glands, placenta, ovaries, and testes) and how its failure relates to infertility.

Rheumatology   **Rhu**

Involves the treatment of diseases of the joints, muscles, bones and associated structures.

Spinal Cord Injury Medicine   **SpCdInj**

Involves the prevention, diagnosis, treatment and management of traumatic spinal cord injuries.

Surgery   **S**

Treatment of disease, injury, and deformity by surgical procedures.

Thoracic Surgery (includes open heart surgery) TS

Involves surgery on the heart, lungs, and chest area.

Urology U

Diagnosis and treatment of diseases of the genitals in men and disorders of the urinary tract and bladder in both men and women.

Vascular & Interventional Radiology VIR

Involves diagnosing and treating diseases by percutaneous methods guided by various radiologic imaging modalities.

Vascular Surgery VascS

Involves the operative treatment of disorders of the blood vessels excluding those to the heart, lungs, or brain.

THE TRAINING OF A SPECIALIST

Excerpted from "Which Medical Specialist For You?", American Board of Medical Specialties, Evanston, IL, Revised April 2002.

Everyone knows that a "medical doctor" is a physician who has had years of training to understand the diagnosis, treatment and prevention of disease. The basic training for a physician specialist includes four years of premedical education in a college or university, four years of medical school, and after receiving the M.D. degree, at least three years of specialty training under supervision (called a "residency"). Training in subspecialties can take an additional one to three years.

Some specialists are primary care doctors such as family physicians, general internists and general pediatricians. Other specialists concentrate on certain body systems, specific age groups, or complex scientific techniques developed to diagnose or treat certain types of disorders. Specialties in medicine developed because of the rapidly expanding body of knowledge about health and illness and the constantly evolving new treatment techniques for disease.

A subspecialist is a physician who has completed training in a general medical specialty and then takes additional training in a more specific area of that specialty called a subspecialty. This training increases the depth of knowledge and expertise of the specialist in that particular field. For example, cardiology is a subspecialty of internal medicine and pediatrics, pediatric surgery is a subspecialty of surgery and child and adolescent psychiatry is a subspecialty of psychiatry. The training of a subspecialist within a specialty requires an additional one or more years of full-time education.

The training, or residency, of a specialist begins after the doctor has received the M.D. degree from a medical school. Resident physicians dedicate themselves for three to seven years to full-time experience in hospital and/or ambulatory care settings, caring for patients under the supervision of experienced specialists. Educational conferences and research experience are often part of that training. In years past, the first year of post-medical school training was called an internship, but is now called residency.

HOW TO USE THIS BOOK

LICENSURE

The legal privilege to practice medicine is governed by state law and is not designed to recognize the knowledge and skills of a trained specialist. A physician is licensed to practice general medicine and surgery by a state board of medical examiners after passing a state or national licensure examination. Each state or territory has its own procedures to license physicians and sets the general standards for all physicians in that state or territory.

WHO CREDENTIALS A SPECIALIST AND/OR SUBSPECIALIST?

Specialty boards certify physicians as having met certain published standards. There are 24 specialty boards that are recognized by the American Board of Medical Specialties (ABMS) and the American Medical Association (AMA). All of the specialties and subspecialties recognized by the ABMS and the AMA are listed in the brief descriptions that follow. Remember, a subspecialist first must be trained and certified as a specialist.

In order to be certified as a medical specialist by one of these recognized boards a physician must complete certain requirements. See box on page 76.

All of the ABMS Member Boards now, or will soon, issue only time-limited certificates which are valid for six to ten years. In order to retain certification, diplomates must become "recertified," and must periodically go through an additional process involving continuing education in the specialty, review of credentials and further examination. Boards that may not yet require recertification have provided voluntary recertification with similar requirements.

HOW TO DETERMINE IF A PHYSICIAN IS A CERTIFIED SPECIALIST

Certified specialists are listed in The Official ABMS Directory of Board Certified Medical Specialists published by *Marquis Who's Who*. The ABMS Directory can be found in most public libraries, hospital libraries, university libraries and medical libraries, and is also available on CD-ROM. Alternatively, you could ask for that information from your county medical society, the American Board of Medical Specialties, or one of the specialty boards.

The ABMS operates a toll free number (1-866-275-2267) to verify the certification status of individual physicians. Additionally, information about the ABMS organization and links to an electronic directory of certified specialists can be accessed through the ABMS Web site at www.abms.org.

Almost all board certified specialists also are members of their medical specialty societies. These societies are dedicated to furthering standards, practice and professional and public education within individual medical specialties. Some, such as the American College of Surgeons and the American College of Obstetricians and Gynecologists, require board certification for full membership. A physician who has attained full membership is called a "Fellow" of the society and is entitled to use this designation in all formal communications such as certificates, publications, business cards, stationery and signage. Thus, "John Doe, M.D., F.A.C.S. (Fellow of the American College of Surgeons) is a board certified surgeon. Similarly, F.A.A.D. (Fellow of the American Academy of Dermatology) following the M.D. or D.O. in a physician's title would likely indicate board certification in that specialty

TO BE CERTIFIED AS A MEDICAL SPECIALIST BY A RECOGNIZED BOARD, A PHYSICIAN MUST COMPLETE CERTAIN REQUIREMENTS, THESE INCLUDE:

1 Completion of a course of study leading to the M.D. or D.O. (Doctor of Osteopathy) degree from a recognized school of medicine.

2 Completion of three to seven years of full-time training in an accredited residency program designed to train specialists in the field.

3 Many specialty boards require assessments and documentation of individual performance from the residency training director, or from the chief of service in the hospital where the specialist has practiced.

4 All of the ABMS Member Boards require that a person seeking certification have an unrestricted license to practice medicine in order to take the certification examination.

5 Finally, each candidate for certification must pass a written examination given by the specialty board. Fifteen of the 24 specialty boards also require an oral examination conducted by senior specialists in that field. Candidates who have passed the exams and other requirements are then given the status of "Diplomate" and are certified as specialists.

• 9 •

THE PARTNERSHIP FOR EXCELLENCE PROGRAM

Among the more than 6,000 acute care and specialty hospitals in the United States, many have extraordinary capabilities for superior patient care. These hospitals, renowned for their use of state-of-the-art equipment and up-to-the-minute technology, also attract outstanding physicians and other healthcare professionals. Many of their physicians are among those in the listings in this Guide.

To assist you in your search for top specialists and to supplement the information contained in the physician listings that follow, we invited a select group of these fine institutions to profile their services, special programs and centers of excellence in the *Partnership for Excellence* program. This special section contains pages sponsored by the included hospitals. This paid sponsorship program is totally separate from the physician selection process, which is based upon a completely independent review.

The *Partnership for Excellence* program provides an overview of the programs and services offered by the included hospitals with information related to their accreditation and sponsorship. Most also provide their physician referral numbers, should you wish to ask the hospitals for recommendations of doctors not listed in *America's Top Doctors for Cancer.*

In addition to the *Partnership for Excellence* program, profiled hospitals were also invited to highlight their special programs or services that focus on a particular disease or medical condition. These can be found in the "Centers of Excellence" sections that are interspersed throughout this book following the medical specialties and/or subspecialties to which they relate. Sponsored pages in the centers of excellence sections reflect the depth of commitment of these hospitals, which provide the staff, resources and financial support necessary to develop these special programs.

We believe you will find this information helpful in your search for the best healthcare—from both physicians and hospitals—throughout the United States!

PARTICIPATING HOSPITALS

HOW TO USE THIS BOOK

HOW TO USE THIS BOOK

By visiting our website **www.AmericasTopDoctorsforCancer.com**, you may also link to the websites of these outstanding hospitals for even more detailed information on their cancer programs.

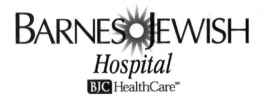

216 S. Kingshighway
St. Louis, MO 63110
314-TOP-DOCS
(314-867-3627)
or toll free 1-866-867-3627
www.BarnesJewish.org

Advancing Medicine. Touching Lives.

A 1,374-bed hospital,
fully accredited by the Joint Commission on Accreditation of Healthcare Organizations.

A LEADING HOSPITAL IN THE UNITED STATES

Barnes-Jewish Hospital ranks consistently among the top 10 hospitals nationally in *U.S. News & World Report* ratings. Recognized internationally as a premier teaching and research facility, Barnes-Jewish Hospital:

- is the primary, adult teaching hospital of Washington University School of Medicine, one of the top three schools of medicine in the country
- offers more than 10,000 dedicated physicians and staff members who are committed to providing exceptional patient care
- is revered for its hospital-based research programs, which are among the top recipients of funding from the National Institutes of Health.
- is the first adult hospital in Missouri to be certified as a "Magnet Hospital" by the American Nurses Credentialing Center (ANCC).

OFFERING UNPARALLELED CLINICAL EXCELLENCE

Barnes-Jewish Hospital has a superior reputation for compassionate patient care as well as its exceptional clinical programs including cancer, cardiology, cardiothoracic surgery, dermatology, endocrinology, gastroenterology, general medicine, general surgery, geriatrics, infectious disease, nephrology, neurology, neurosurgery, obstetrics/gynecology, ophthalmology, orthopaedic surgery, otolaryngology, pain management, plastic & reconstructive surgery, psychiatry, pulmonary disease, radiology, rehabilitation, rheumatology, transplantation, trauma, urology and vascular surgery. Today, Barnes-Jewish Hospital:

- is the largest hospital in Missouri with 557,044 inpatient admissions, outpatient visits and emergency department visits from patients around the world
- is home to many clinical firsts, including the world's first successful double lung transplant and the world's first laparoscopic nephrectomy, using a minimally invasive technique developed at the hospital
- is home of the Center for Advanced Medicine, a multidisciplinary outpatient center, and Siteman Cancer Center, the only NCI-designated cancer center in a 240-mile radius of St. Louis.

"The commitment, compassion and talent of our staff and physicians continue to earn this hospital a world-class reputation."

— Ronald G. Evens, MD, President, Barnes-Jewish Hospital

If you need a physician, go straight to the top.
Call **314-TOP-DOCS** (314-867-3627) or toll free 1-866-867-3627.
www.BarnesJewish.org

BAYLOR UNIVERSITY
MEDICAL CENTER AT DALLAS

3500 Gaston Avenue, Dallas, Texas 75246
Tel: 1-800-4BAYLOR (422-9567) • www.BaylorHealth.edu

BAYLOR
University Medical Center
at Dallas

Beds: 1,029
Sponsorship/Affiliation: Baylor University Medical Center at Dallas is a not-for-profit, medical center and serves as the flagship hospital for Baylor Health Care System.

A TRADITION OF EXCELLENCE

In 1903, the hospital opened with 25 beds; today it is a major patient care, teaching and research center for the southwest. It is home to more than 20 specialty centers and encompasses more than 30 city blocks. Specialty centers include Baylor Charles A. Sammons Cancer Center, Baylor Heart and Vascular Institute/Baylor Jack and Jane Hamilton Heart and Vascular Hospital, Baylor Regional Transplant Institute, Baylor Radiosurgery Center, Baylor George Truett James Orthopaedic Institute.

MEDICAL EDUCATION

Baylor University Medical Center (Baylor Dallas) offers 14 fellowship and 9 residency program opportunities for physicians with about 185 interns, residents, and fellows annually enroll in Baylor's training programs to acquire medical knowledge and experience. Through these educational programs, residents and fellows gain clinical and academic training to prepare them for a lifetime of serving the communities in which they will practice. Additional educational programs include a radiology allied health school, pharmacy residency, dietetic internship and administrative fellowship. The medical staff of Baylor Dallas consists of 1,265 physicians and 2,029 nurses. About 85 percent of the active physicians at the medical center are board certified.

RESEARCH AND INNOVATIVE TREATMENTS

Baylor Research Institute (BRI) promotes and supports research bringing innovative treatments from the laboratory workbench to the patient bedside. To achieve this bench-to-bedside concept, the institute focuses on basic science, clinical trials, health care effectiveness and quality of care research. Investigators at Baylor are conducting more than 500 active research protocols spanning more than 20 medical specialties.

NATIONALLY RECOGNIZED

Baylor Dallas cares for more than 300,000 people each year. Through our many specialty care centers, comprehensive medical services are provided including nationally recognized programs in cancer care, heart and vascular care, transplantation sciences, orthopaedic surgery and limb salvage, gastroenterology, radiosurgery using Gamma Knife® and CyberKnife® technologies, and rehabilitation services.

COMPREHENSIVE SERVICES

As an integral part of the city of Dallas, Texas, Baylor University Medical Center at Dallas is privileged to treat patients from around the world. The staff is multilingual and can link physicians and patients with translators who represent more than 40 languages. The downtown campus offers lodging services through the Baylor Plaza Hotel, and also the Baylor Twice Blessed apartments for transplant patients undergoing care at our medical center. Baylor Dallas is also one of only two level one trauma centers serving the North Texas region.

LOCALLY RENOWNED, NATIONALLY RECOGIZED

Baylor Dallas nurses earned the Magnet Award for "Excellence in Nursing Services" from the American Nurses Credentialing Center in January 2004. The 2004 *U.S. News & World Report* "America's Best Hospitals" guide marked the 12th consecutive year Baylor University Medical Center at Dallas is ranked. Baylor Dallas also received the 2004 Consumer Choice Award for Overall Quality and Image from the National Research Corporation (NRC). Baylor Dallas was chosen in the NRC survey as having the best doctors, nurses, and overall quality.

PHYSICIAN REFERRAL
Call 1-800-4BAYLOR (422-9567) for a physician referral or for more information.

DANA-FARBER/BRIGHAM AND WOMEN'S
CANCER CENTER

75 FRANCIS STREET • 44 BINNEY STREET
BOSTON, MA 02115
1-877-DFCI-BWH • WWW.DFBWCANCER.ORG

Trusted Expertise

Dana-Farber/Brigham and Women's Cancer Center brings widely recognized experts in every form of adult oncology to each patient's fight against cancer. The Center combines the clinical expertise, focus, and innovation of Dana-Farber Cancer Institute, rated by *U.S. News & World Report* as one of the top cancer centers in the nation, and Brigham and Women's Hospital, a leading teaching hospital consistently included on the *U.S. News & World Report* Honor Roll of "America's Best Hospitals." Dana-Farber/Brigham and Women's Cancer Center offers 12 specialized treatment centers—each devoted to the treatment of a major type of cancer. Dana-Farber Cancer Institute and Brigham and Women's Hospital are teaching affiliates of Harvard Medical School.

World-Class Treatment Centers

Each multidisciplinary treatment center brings together the clinical expertise at both Dana-Farber Cancer Institute and Brigham and Women's Hospital to diagnose and treat the full spectrum of cancers in the disease category. Experts at Dana-Farber/Brigham and Women's Cancer Center provide advanced care for patients with breast and gynecologic cancer, cutaneous cancer, endocrine cancer, gastrointestinal cancer, genitourinary cancer, head and neck cancer, hematologic oncology, hematology, neuro-oncology, sarcoma, and thoracic cancer.

Comprehensive and Coordinated Care

Our medical staff works as a team to provide expert evaluation and the most advanced care possible. This coordinated approach makes it possible for many patients to see all of their specialists in a single visit. Dedicated, multidisciplinary teams of disease-specific specialists include surgeons, radiologists, pathologists, medical oncologists, radiation oncologists, nurses, psycho-oncologists, dietitians, nurses, and social workers.

Innovative Clinical Trials

Researchers and clinicians at Dana-Farber/Brigham and Women's Cancer Center work together to offer patients the most advanced care, including hundreds of innovative clinical trials designed to improve patient outcomes and quality-of-life. Clinical trials are offered through Dana-Farber/Harvard Cancer Center, a National Cancer Institute-designated Comprehensive Cancer Center.

Comprehensive Support Services

At Dana-Farber/Brigham and Women's Cancer Center, we recognize that patients and families benefit from comprehensive support services in addition to clinical care while fighting their disease. Our patient and family-focused approach to care includes a wide range of complementary therapies and support services, such as social work, support groups, pain and palliative care, pastoral care, international patient assistance, disability services, financial information services, nutrition services, and recreational resources.

CALL **1-877-DFCI-BWH** FOR MORE INFORMATION, OR TO MAKE AN APPOINTMENT WITH A SPECIALIST AT DANA-FARBER/BRIGHAM AND WOMEN'S CANCER CENTER.

DANA-FARBER / PARTNERS CANCERCARE

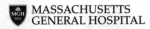 MASSACHUSETTS GENERAL HOSPITAL

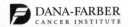 DANA-FARBER CANCER INSTITUTE

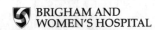 BRIGHAM AND WOMEN'S HOSPITAL

C|S CEDARS-SINAI MEDICAL CENTER®

8700 Beverly Blvd., Los Angeles, CA 90048
Tel: 1-800-CEDARS-1 (1-800-233-2771) • Fax: (310) 423-0499
www.cedars-sinai.edu

Beds: 877
Sponsorships/Network Affiliation: A nonprofit, independent healthcare organization

INNOVATION AND LEADERSHIP

For more than a century, Cedars-Sinai has been at the forefront of medical and scientific advancement. As one of the largest nonprofit hospitals in the western United States, we have built our nationally renowned reputation on distinguished programs and services of excellence.

COMPREHENSIVE MEDICAL CARE

With a medical staff that represents the full spectrum of specialty services, Cedars-Sinai offers comprehensive, state-of-the-art care ranging from obstetrics to trauma services and multiple organ transplantation. Many of the Medical Center's specialty services, including our highly-regarded cancer care program, are centralized to provide multidisciplinary diagnosis and treatment in one location.

COMPREHENSIVE CANCER CARE

Under the umbrella of the Samuel Oschin Comprehensive Cancer Institute are many specialized cancer programs and a team of experts that performs more oncological surgeries than any other medical center in Los Angeles County.

Dozens of nationally recognized programs and services are all available at the institute under one interconnected medical "roof." And, our unique 24-hour Cedars-Sinai Outpatient Cancer Center provides treatment day and night, a considerable convenience for our patients. Cedars-Sinai is the only center in Southern California to offer such flexibility.

ONE OF AMERICA'S BEST

Cedars-Sinai is highly regarded both nationally and locally. In addition to the hard-earned accreditations and licenses required of all hospitals, the Medical Center has been awarded numerous prestigious honors, including:

- Two consecutive four-year designations as a Magnet hospital, nursing's highest award of excellence
- Number two ranking among leading metropolitan hospitals nationwide as designated by the American Association of Retired Persons (AARP)
- Los Angeles-area consumers' choice as "Most Preferred Hospital for All Health Needs" for 17 consecutive years, according to National Research Corporation's annual Healthcare Market Guide®

A LEADING RESEARCH CENTER

Through its Burns and Allen Research Institute, Cedars-Sinai has been responsible for advancing diagnostic and treatment technologies and making a difference in the future of medicine. The institute is ranked among the top tier of non-university hospitals nationwide receiving competitive research funding from the National Institutes of Health.

TRAINING FUTURE LEADERS

Cedars-Sinai is training healthcare leaders today to ensure continued quality care tomorrow. In addition to a comprehensive nurse training program, the Medical Center supports residency and fellowship programs in eleven major specialty areas.

PHYSICIAN REFERRAL

Call 1-800-CEDARS-1 (1-800-233-2771) for a no-cost referral to a Cedars-Sinai physician, or visit us online at www.cedars-sinai.edu/find.

CITY OF HOPE CANCER CENTER

City of
Hope®

Where the Power of Knowledge Saves Li

1500 East Duarte Road
Duarte, California 91010
Tel. 800-826-HOPE (4673)
www.cityofhope.org

A LEADER IN CANCER CARE

City of Hope National Medical Center and Beckman Research Institute holds **the highest status awarded by the National Cancer Institute: the designation of Comprehensive Cancer Center**, recognizing excellence in cancer research and treatment. As **a founding member of the National Comprehensive Cancer Network**, City of Hope helps set standards of care for cancer treatment nationwide.

A FULL SPECTRUM OF CANCER CARE SERVICES

City of Hope offers a full spectrum of services provided by clinical experts in:

- Hematology
- Medical Oncology
- Surgery
- Supportive Care and Education

- Diagnostic Radiology
- Pediatrics
- Radiation Oncology

Supporting this expertise are premier services such as pathology and genetic risk assessment.

RESEARCH EXPERTISE

City of Hope is committed to developing new and better approaches to diagnosing, preventing, and treating disease, as well as improving quality of life. City of Hope research has contributed directly to the development of numerous new therapeutic agents to enhance length and quality of life.

Approximately **40 percent of City of Hope patients participate in clinical trials**—the national average is 3 to 4 percent.

STATE-OF-THE-ART CANCER CARE

Helford Clinical Research Hospital, a state-of-the-art, $200 million facility scheduled to open in 2005, enables City of Hope to provide **the safest and most effective patient care** while continuing our tradition of breakthrough research.

NATIONALLY RECOGNIZED

City of Hope is well recognized as a leader among health care organizations in the United States. Recognition includes:

- Ranking by *U.S. News & World Report* as one of America's 50 best cancer hospitals in 2003 and 2004;
- Ranking in the top 1 percent of hospitals by the Joint Commission on Accreditation of Healthcare Organizations (JCAHO); and
- The highest score possible in all applicable categories in the California Hospital Experience Survey (formerly known as PEP-C).

For more information, call 800-826-4673.

CLARIAN HEALTH PARTNERS

Methodist Hospital • Indiana University Hospital • Riley Hospital for Children Indianapolis, Indiana

Physician-to-Physician 800-622-4989 • Consumers 800-265-3220

www.clarian.org

Clarian Health Partners and its statewide affiliates make up the leading hospital system in the state and one of the busiest and most highly regarded in the nation. There are nearly 12,000 staff members at Clarian Health, including over 1,300 board-certified specialists and over 450 board-certified primary care physicians. Clarian is home to multiple centers of excellence, in areas ranging from cardiovascular care, organ transplantation, total joint replacement, cancer to pediatric medicine.

COMPREHENSIVE CLINICAL CARE

Clarian Health was created in 1997 by bringing together the comprehensive resources of three of central Indiana's strongest medical facilities: Methodist Hospital of Indiana, Indiana University Hospital and Riley Hospital for Children. Clarian's mission is to improve the health of our patients and community through innovation and excellence in care, education, research, and service. Our range of services covers virtually every patient need, from complex cardiac procedures and bone marrow transplants to patient self-care education. Clarian physicians are supported by our commitment to evidence-driven medicine, a key concept for the future of health care that provides improved outcomes through rigorous adherence to clinically proven treatment.

RESEARCH IMPROVES TREATMENT

Clarian's superb research capabilities allow us to move new treatment possibilities from laboratory bench to the patient's bedside at a remarkable rate. Indiana University School of Medicine educates the second largest medical student body in the country, and its research efforts– which includes focused activities in 19 research centers and institutes — is supported by more than $205 million in annual grants. The Methodist Research Institute conducts research that enhances Clarian's clinical mission, and research at Riley Hospital for Children is focused on improving pediatric medicine.

MULTIPLE CENTERS OF EXCELLENCE

Clarian's numerous centers of excellence combine the highest levels of physician expertise with advanced medical technologies. Among these centers are the Clarian Cardiovascular Center and the Level I Trauma Center on the Methodist Hospital campus. Riley Hospital offers Indiana's only Level I Regional Pediatric Trauma Center, its only pediatric burn unit, the Riley Burn Center, and one of the nation's largest autism treatment centers.

Clarian is also a recognized national center for transplantation procedures ranging from heart, liver, lung, and kidney to bone-marrow transplantations. The Indiana University Cancer Center has been designated a Cancer Center by the National Cancer Institute. The latest technological advances can often be found first in the state or nation at Clarian hospitals, including the *daVinci* Surgical System, Philips Brilliance CT 64-slice scanner, Novalis Shaped Beam Surgery, Mobetron and IMRT radiation therapy advances and Gamma Knife technology.

NATIONAL RECOGNITION, PATIENT SATISFACTION

For six consecutive years, Clarian flagship hospitals have been named among the "Best Hospitals in America" by *U.S. News & World Report* magazine, which consistently ranks a number of Clarian's clinical specialties among the top 50 nationwide. In last year's Top Doctors ranking, 43 of 54 physicians recognized in Indiana were from Clarian Health. Also, 2004 patient satisfaction survey data indicates that 97% of our patients say that they would choose Clarian again for their care and would recommend us to family members and friends. In 2004, Clarian Health Partners became the first Magnet hospital system in Indiana.

CANCER PROGRAM

INDIANA UNIVERSITY HOSPITAL

A CLARIAN HEALTH PARTNER

550 University Boulevard • Indianapolis, Indiana 46202
317-274-5000 • www.clarian.org

A CLARIAN HEALTH PARTNER

As a member of Clarian Health Partners, Indiana University Hospital is part of the leading hospital system in Indiana and one of the busiest and most highly regarded in the nation.

PUTTING RESEARCH INTO PRACTICE

The physicians at Indiana University Hospital are faculty members of the Indiana University School of Medicine and participate in extensive teaching and research programs that are internationally recognized. Their expertise is based on the transfer of research discoveries to clinical trials and into accepted practice. Research is conducted in most basic science and clinical areas, as well as in highly specialized areas including cancer, arthritis, medical genetics, pharmacology, and behavioral oncology.

CANCER PROGRAM

Indiana University Hospital's multidisciplinary cancer programs maintain perennial standing within the top 40 cancer programs in the United States, according to *U.S. News & World Report*. Further, the National Cancer Institute has designated the Indiana University Cancer Center as a Cancer Center, the only such center providing cancer care in Indiana. Special services and features include:

- Bone Marrow Transplant Program
- Multidisciplinary research and treatment programs, surgery, and radiation therapy
- Coleman Center for Women, offering research and patient care for women with gynecological cancers
- Clinical research and trials for breast, prostate, testicular, lung, gastrointestinal and hematologic cancers
- Together with the Indiana University Department of Radiation Oncology, co-sponsor of the Indiana Lions Gamma Knife Center. Use of Gamma Knife technology allows physicians to non-invasively treat abnormal areas in the brain such as tumors or vascular disorders
- Bone Marrow Transplant Program
- Founders and scientific base for the Hoosier Oncology Group, one of the most successful, independent cancer groups in the country

PIONEERING CANCER TREATMENT

Indiana University Hospital has pioneered numerous medical firsts. Significant achievements from Indiana University Hospital include:

- Development of the cure for testicular cancer by Lawrence Einhorn, MD
- First to use "nerve sparing" surgical techniques to successfully treat testis cancer while preserving fertility
- First multidisciplinary breast cancer care program in the region
- First hospital in Indiana to use Gamma Knife to treat hard to reach brain lesions
- First human clinical trials of Bevacizumab (trade name Avastin) now used to extend the lives of patients with advanced colon cancer
- First human clinical trials of Oprelvekin (trade name Neumega) now used to prevent low platelet counts caused by certain types of chemotherapy
- Pioneering studies of new anti-emetics that improved patient tolerance of chemotherapy
- Pivotal registration trials for at least four commercially available cancer drugs (cisplatin, ifosfamide, etoposide, gemcitabine)
- Development of groundbreaking chemotherapy regimens for several diseases still in use today (testis cancer, ovarian cancer, thymoma, ovarian germ cell tumors, lung cancer)

ACCREDITATION AND NATIONAL RECOGNITION

Indiana University Hospital is accredited by the Joint Commission on Accreditation of Healthcare Organizations. Its clinical programs continue to be listed among the best in *U.S. News & World Report*'s "America's Best Hospitals Guide." The Indiana University School of Medicine is nationally evaluated and accredited by the Liaison Committee on Medical Education.

THE CLEVELAND CLINIC

9500 Euclid Avenue • Cleveland, OH 44195
Tel. 216/444-CARE (2273) Outside of Cleveland, 800/223-2273
www.clevelandclinic.org

THE CLEVELAND CLINIC

One of the largest and busiest health centers in America. Number one in heart care. National leaders in urology and digestive diseases. Treating all illnesses and disorders of the body. Second opinions a specialty.

GENERAL OVERVIEW

Founded in 1921, The Cleveland Clinic is a 934-staffed-bed hospital that integrates clinical and hospital care with research and education in a private, non-profit group practice. This group practice model provides an environment that allows our physicians to stay at the cutting edge of medical technology. Additionally, there is no financial incentive for any of our physicians to overtreat patients.

VITAL STATISTICS

In 2003, more than 1,100 full-time salaried physicians representing more than 120 medical specialties and subspecialties provided for 2.5 million outpatient visits, 51,000 hospital admissions and 65,000 surgeries for patients from throughout the United States and more than 80 countries.

ONE OF AMERICA'S BEST

In 2003, The Cleveland Clinic was named one of the five best hospitals in America in the *U.S. News & World Report* annual "Best Hospitals" survey. In cardiology and cardiac surgery, we lead the nation. Our Heart Center has been ranked number one in America for nine years in a row by *U.S. News & World Report*. The Cleveland Clinic Glickman Urological Institute is rated second in the United States, and our Digestive Disease Center is ranked second. Additional specialities rated among America's best include Cancer, Endocrinology, Geriatrics, Gynecology, Nephrology, Neurology and Neurological Surgery, Ophthalmology, Orthopaedics, Otolaryngology, Pediatrics, Psychiatry, Pulmonary, Rehabilitation, and Rheumatology.

OUTSTANDING CARE FOR CHILDREN

The Children's Hospital at The Cleveland Clinic offers highly specialized pediatric care in a family-centered atmosphere. It has been ranked the best children's hospital in Ohio by *Child magazine*.

EXPANDING MEDICAL CARE

Over the past several years, The Cleveland Clinic has opened additional state-of-the-art facilities, including the Lerner Research Institute, the Cole Eye Institute, and the Taussig Cancer Center. A web-based program, e-Cleveland Clinic, provides specialist consultations and second opinions using the Internet for patients with life-threatening and life-altering diagnoses.

INTERNATIONAL SERVICES

The Cleveland Clinic's reputation draws patients from all over the world. The International Center is a full-service department dedicated to meeting the needs and requirements of international patients who receive their care at The Cleveland Clinic. The center is staffed by dedicated professionals who offer a variety of services designed to make patients feel welcome and ensure that their visit goes as smoothly as possible.

"Better care of the sick, investigation of their problems, and further education of those who serve."

CONTINUUM HEALTH PARTNERS

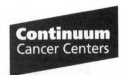

Beth Israel Medical Center
Roosevelt Hospital
St. Luke's Hospital
Long Island College Hospital
New York Eye and Ear Infirmary

Continuum Cancer Centers of New York

Phone 800-420-4004
www.chpnyc.org

Sponsorship: Voluntary Not-for-Profit

Beds: 2,761 certified beds

Accreditation: Joint Commission of Accreditation of Healthcare Organizations (JCAHO). Accreditation Council for Graduate Medical Education. Medical Society of New York, in conjunction with the Accreditation Council for Continuing Medical Education.

A STRONG PARTNERSHIP WITH A PROUD HERITAGE

Continuum Health Partners, Inc. is a partnership of five venerable health care providers, Beth Israel Medical Center, St. Luke's Hospital, Roosevelt Hospital, Long Island College Hospital, and the New York Eye and Ear Infirmary. Each of the five partner institutions was established more than a century ago by individuals committed to improving health and health care in their communities. Today, the system represents more the 4,000 physicians and dentists and is superbly equipped to respond to the health care needs of the populations we serve. Continuum providers also see patients in group and private practice settings and in ambulatory centers in New York City and Westchester County.

LOCATIONS

Continuum Health Partners has campuses throughout Manhattan and Brooklyn. Beth Israel Medical Center has two divisions: the Milton and Caroll Petrie Division on the East Side and the Kings Highway Division in Brooklyn. The Phillips Ambulatory Care Center, a state-of-the art outpatient center, is located at Union square. St Luke's Hospital is in Morningside Heights and Roosevelt Hospital is in the Columbus Circle and Lincoln Center neighborhoods on the West Side. Long Island College Hospital is located in the Brooklyn Heights/Cobble Hill section of Brooklyn. The New York Eye and Ear Infirmary is located on Second Avenue and 14th Street.

ACADEMIC AFFILIATIONS

Beth Israel Medical Center is University Hospital and Manhattan Campus for the Albert Einstein College of Medicine. St. Luke's-Roosevelt Hospital Center is University Hospital for Columbia University College of Physicians and Surgeons. Long Island College Hospital is the primary teaching affiliate of the SUNY-Health Science Center a Brooklyn. The New York Eye and Ear Infirmary is the primary teaching center of the New York Medical College and Affiliated teaching hospitals in the areas of ophthalmology and otolaryngology.

Physician Referral

For a referral to a doctor in your neighborhood, call (800) 420-4004 Continuum's Referral Service can help you to find a primary care physician or specialist affiliated with Beth Israel, St. Luke's, Roosevelt, Long Island College Hospital, or the New York Eye and Ear Infirmary. Visit our website at www.chpnyc.org.

DUKE UNIVERSITY HEALTH SYSTEM

Durham, North Carolina 27710
1-888-ASK-DUKE • dukehealth.org

Beds	Duke University Hospital: 989; Durham Regional Hospital: 369; Duke Health Raleigh Hospital: 205
Accreditation	Accredited by the Joint Commission on Healthcare Accreditation in 2004 for three years

OVERVIEW

Duke University Health System is a world-class health care network dedicated to providing outstanding patient care, educating tomorrow's health care leaders, and discovering better ways to treat disease through biomedical research. Duke offers every level of health service—from wellness and prevention programs to the most advanced specialty services to hospice care—in an atmosphere of caring and compassion.

DUKE UNIVERSITY MEDICAL CENTER

Duke University Medical Center, the hub of the Health System, is consistently rated among the top 10 hospitals in the country by *U.S.News & World Report*. It is the leading medical center in the Southeast, with a medical school ranked among the top three in the nation. For the past five years, Duke has received the National Research Corporation Consumer Choice Award after being ranked by area residents as the region's top health care facility.

A national leader in biomedical research, Duke quickly translates advances in technology and medical knowledge into improved patient care. Duke is playing a significant role in advancing understanding of the genetic aspects of human disease through its Center for Human Genetics and the creation of the Institute for Genome Sciences & Policy.

CLINICAL PROGRAMS

Duke provides a range of respected clinical programs to meet every patient's needs. Among them are the *Duke Comprehensive Cancer Center*, known for its multidisciplinary approach to treating large tumors and its innovative therapies using bone marrow transplantation and hyperthermia; the *Duke Heart Center*, which has conducted many leading-edge studies to advance our understanding of heart disease and improve cardiac care; a highly experienced organ transplant team; Duke Women's Services, offering comprehensive care for women at every stage of life; *Duke Neuroscience Services* delivering skilled, compassionate care for those with brain, spine, and nervous system disorders; and the *Duke Musculoskeletal Center*, providing expert bone, joint, and muscle care in such areas as major joint reconstruction, sports medicine, and reconstructive microsurgery. *The Duke Eye Center* treats challenging problems, such as glaucoma, retinal disease, diseases of the cornea, cataracts, eye muscle disorders, cancer of the eye and various forms of macular and retinal degeneration.

The Health System provides high-quality clinical services in convenient locations throughout the region. Care settings include three hospitals, ambulatory surgery centers, primary and specialty care clinics, home care, hospice, skilled nursing care, wellness centers, partnerships with several community hospitals and practices, and mobile cardiac catheterization services.

To make an appointment with a Duke physician, call 1-888-ASK-DUKE.

FOX CHASE CANCER CENTER

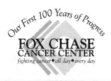

Our First 100 Years of Progress

FOX CHASE
CANCER CENTER
fighting cancer • all day • every day

333 Cottman Avenue
Philadelphia, Pennsylvania 19111-2497
Phone: 1-888-FOX CHASE
Fax: 215-728-2702
www.fccc.edu

Sponsorship	Independent Nonprofit
Beds	100 licensed beds
Accreditation	Joint Commission on Accreditation of Healthcare Organizations; American Hospital Association; American College of Surgeons, Commission on Cancer; College of American Pathology; American College of Radiology

U.S. News & World Report has named Fox Chase Cancer Center the leading cancer center serving Pennsylvania, New Jersey and Delaware and 11th in the entire nation. Fox Chase is also the first hospital in Pennsylvania and the nation's first cancer hospital to earn the Magnet Award for Nursing Excellence from the American Nurses Credentialing Center.

OVERVIEW

Fox Chase Cancer Center was founded in 1904 in Philadelphia as the nation's first cancer hospital. In 1974, Fox Chase became one of the first institutions designated as a National Cancer Institute Comprehensive Cancer Center. The mission of Fox Chase is to reduce the burden of human cancer through the highest-quality programs in basic, clinical, population and translational research; programs of prevention, detection and treatment of cancer; and community outreach.

- Fox Chase's 100-bed hospital is one of the few in the country devoted entirely to adult cancer care.
- Annual hospital admissions average about 4,000 and outpatient visits to physicians exceed 67,000 a year.
- Fox Chase's board-certified specialists are recognized nationally and internationally in medical, radiation and surgical oncology, diagnostic imaging, diagnostic pathology, pain management, oncology nursing and oncology social work.
- The multidisciplinary staff provides a coordinated approach to meet the treatment needs of each patient. Special multidisciplinary centers provide consultations and treatment recommendations for specific types of cancer.
- The nursing staff of specially trained oncology nurses provides one of the best nurse-to-patient ratios in the area.
- Fox Chase investigators have received numerous awards and honors, including Nobel Prizes in medicine and chemistry; a Kyoto Prize, a Lasker Clinical Research Award, memberships in the National Academy of Sciences and General Motors Cancer Research Foundation Prizes.
- Fox Chase is a founding member of the National Comprehensive Cancer Network, an alliance of the nation's leading academic cancer centers, and the hub of the 30-member Fox Chase Network of community cancer centers.

For more about Fox Chase physicians and services, visit our web site, www.fccc.edu,
or call 1-888-FOX CHASE

HACKENSACK UNIVERSITY MEDICAL CENTER

30 Prospect Avenue
Hackensack, NJ 07601
phone (201) 996-3760
fax (201) 996-3452

www.humc.com

Sponsorship	A not-for-profit, teaching and research hospital affiliated with the University of Medicine and Dentistry of New Jersey – New Jersey Medical School.
Beds	A 683-bed, Level II Trauma Center, providing tertiary and regional services for the New York/New Jersey metropolitan area.
Accreditation	Joint Commission on the Accreditation of Healthcare Organizations.

BACKGROUND

Founded in 1888 as Bergen County's first hospital, Hackensack University Medical Center has demonstrated more than a century of growth and progress in response to the needs of the communities it serves. The medical center continues to be the largest provider of inpatient and outpatient services in New Jersey and has been ranked as the seventh largest healthcare facility in the nation by number of inpatient admissions. Hackensack University Medical Center is Bergen County's largest employer with a work force of more than 7,200 employees and an annual budget of more than $1 billion.

MEDICAL AND DENTAL STAFF

There are nearly 1,400 members on the medical and dental staff. These physicians and dentists represent a full spectrum of medical and dental specialties and subspecialties.

HealthGrades® – The national healthcare quality firm honored HUMC with the 2003, 2004, and 2005 HealthGrades Distinguished Hospital Award for Clinical Excellence™. The award places HUMC among a group of less than 200 hospitals or five percent nationally who are at the pinnacle of quality performance across numerous clinical service lines. HealthGrades is the only consumer-oriented, national rating system strictly focused on clinical quality outcomes that rates every hospital in the country.

J.D. Power and Associates Distinguished Hospital Program℠ – HUMC was also recognized for service excellence under the new J.D. Power and Associates Distinguished Hospital Program.℠ This distinction acknowledges a strong commitment from HUMC to provide an outstanding patient experience. The service excellence distinction was determined by surveying a random sample of recently discharged patients from HUMC on their perceptions of their hospital stay and comparing the results to the national benchmark established by the J.D. Power and Associates Hospital Service Performance Study.℠

Nursing Excellence – Honored since 1995 as the first hospital in New Jersey to receive the Magnet Award for Nursing Excellence from the American Nurses Credentialing Center. The medical center became the second hospital in the country to receive redesignation of this prestigious award and continues to have this highly honored recognition. HUMC was redesignated again in 2003.

ACCOMPLISHMENTS

Hackensack University Medical Center is Ranked Number Three in the Nation for Hospital Safety and Quality in the Consumers Digest/Leapfrog Group List of "50 Exceptional Hospitals" – Hackensack University Medical Center has been ranked number three in the U.S. for hospital safety and quality in the April 2005 issue of *Consumers Digest*. The article, entitled "Hospital Safety: Where To Get the Best Care," includes a list of America's 50 exceptional hospitals, derived from a nationwide survey conducted by The Leapfrog Group. The New Jersey-based medical center came in third, following Massachusetts General Hospital (No. 1) and Brigham and Women's Hospital (No. 2).

Hackensack University Medical Center Receives "Hospital of Choice" Award –For a second consecutive year, The American Alliance of Healthcare Providers (AAHCP) selected Hackensack University Medical Center (HUMC) as a "Hospital of Choice." The AAHCP was founded in 1992 with the goal of establishing practical, effective, and efficient methods of improving patient care. AAHCP bestows this honor on organizations that meet their standards of being a physician-friendly institution, as well as one with a high level of customer satisfaction.

JOHNS HOPKINS
M E D I C I N E

600 North Wolfe Street • Baltimore, MD 21287
www.hopkinsmedicine.org

JOHNS HOPKINS MEDICINE

At its founding in 1889, The Johns Hopkins Hospital revolutionized medical practice in the United States. With the opening of the School of Medicine four years later, Hopkins became America's first true teaching hospital. Together, they are called Johns Hopkins Medicine.

Ranked as America's top hospital and medical school year after year, Johns Hopkins sets the standard for medical care, education, and discovery around the world.

Johns Hopkins practices a unique brand of medicine – pursuing three interwoven goals in a way that makes us extraordinarily effective as an incubator for innovation:

We heal. Johns Hopkins is a beacon of hope for people with the most complex and puzzling conditions. The care we provide is exceptional. In the clinic, in the classroom, and in the laboratory, we focus always on our patients.

We discover. Hopkins physicians and staff are active researchers, receiving more research grants from the National Institutes of Health than faculty at any other institutions. When discoveries are made, we move rapidly to apply our knowledge to the care of people who are suffering.

We teach. Medical professionals from around the world seek us out for consultation and training on everything from new techniques in transplantation to patient safety.

Our history and our heritage are the foundation of a culture that persists to this day and enables us to make discoveries and advances that are nothing short of remarkable.

Among our Centers of Excellence:

- Asthma & Allergy Center
- Brady Urologic Institute
- Children's Center
- Comprehensive Transplant Center
- Heart Center
- Meyer Neurosciences Center
- Meyerhoff Digestive Disease Center
- McKusick-Nathans Institute for Genetic Medicine
- Phipps Psychiatric Institute
- Sidney Kimmel Comprehensive Cancer Center
- Wilmer Eye Institute

The Marburg Pavilion, a special group of patient rooms offering five star hotel-like accommodations and amenities, is available to many patients at The Johns Hopkins Hospital. An executive physical program also is available.

To find a specialist at Johns Hopkins, call:
410-955-5464 for calls in Baltimore • 410-847-3582 for calls from outside the Baltimore area
+01-410-847-3580 for calls from outside the United States

LOYOLA UNIVERSITY HEALTH SYSTEM

Cardinal Bernardin Cancer Center
2160 S. First Avenue
Maywood, Ill. 60153
Tel. (888) LUHS-888
www.luhs.org/cancer

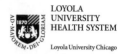

LOYOLA
UNIVERSITY
HEALTH SYSTEM
Loyola University Chicago

We also treat the human spirit.®

Sponsorship: Not-for-profit hospital system affiliated with Loyola University Chicago Stritch School of Medicine

Accreditation: Recipient of National Cancer Institute (NCI) Cancer Center Planning Grant and full member of the Southwest Oncology Group.

A PLACE OF HEALING

Celebrating its 10th anniversary, the Cardinal Bernardin Cancer Center of Loyola University Health System is one of the country's only freestanding facilities dedicated to cancer research and treatment. Ranked among the nation's best by U.S. News & World Report, this multidisciplinary environment fosters constant collaboration between doctors and researchers, with the common goal of providing the best possible patient care. Both doctor visits and high-end care, such as outpatient stem-cell transplants and chemotherapy, are available at the same state-of-the-art facility. The Cancer Center even provides programs, such as support groups, complementary medicine, acupuncture and art therapy, to augment Loyola's holistic approach to health care.

PIONEERING RESEARCH MEETS QUALITY PATIENT CARE

Last year, approximately 50,000 patients were treated at the Cardinal Bernardin Cancer Center, and all were given access to one of the country's leading cancer research facilities, located right inside the Center. Our patients also are offered participation in some of the world's most groundbreaking clinical trials. With all disciplines of cancer treatment under one roof, the Center facilitates an open exchange of ideas and collaborative efforts to transform what is learned in the laboratory into more effective methods of fighting cancer – bringing innovative bench research to practical bedside use. A new outreach center in Hickory Hills, Ill., now brings this cancer care to the south suburbs of Chicago.

GOING BEYOND THE ILLNESS

At Loyola, we pride ourselves on going beyond the illness to treat the whole person. Cancer patients have very specific needs, and our goal is to educate them so they can make the best possible choices. This spring, the Coleman Center for Image Renewal will open, providing complementary massage and acupuncture, personal services such as manicures and pedicures, beauty treatments, wigs and skin products designed specifically for cancer patients, nutritional counseling and meditation. Loyola recognizes the importance that a patient's attitude plays in recovery, and our goal is to give patients every advantage possible. Our comprehensive approach also targets helping patients' families.

The Cardinal Bernardin Cancer Center is recognized as one of the best cancer programs in the country. It remains the only all-inclusive cancer facility in Illinois, bringing researchers and clinicians under one roof.

For Cancer Information: A special cancer information line is available to handle questions and provide direction to the appropriate specialist. Please call (708) CAN-HELP to speak with a Cancer Center coordinator, M-F, 8:30 a.m. – 5 p.m. After-hours, a message center will take your information for a return call the next business day.

MAIMONIDES MEDICAL CENTER

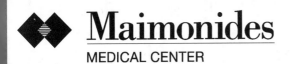

4802 Tenth Avenue
Brooklyn, New York 11219
phone: (718) 283-6000

Physician Referral: 1-888 MMC DOCS
http://www.maimonidesmed.org

Sponsorship:	Voluntary, Not-for-Profit
Beds:	705 acute, 70 psychiatric
Accreditation:	Joint Commission on Accreditation of Healthcare Organizations (JCAHO)
	American College of Surgeons
	American Council of Graduate Medical Education (ACGME)

GENERAL DESCRIPTION

Maimonides Medical Center is the nation's third largest independent teaching hospital. A conductor of numerous national trials for new treatments and technology, Maimonides is known for its investment in the welfare of patients and advanced medical technology and systems. It is among the five percent of hospitals in the nation whose physicians and nurses use computers to record patient information, thereby reducing the risk of errors, increasing efficiency, and speeding the healing process.

Its excellence in cardiac care spans decades. The first successful human heart transplant in the nation was performed at Maimonides in 1967, and *Modern Healthcare* magazine recently reported its selection as one of the nation's Top 100 Cardiovascular Hospitals in 2002, by Solucient, a health research company. Known as one of the nation's *Most Wired* hospitals, it also recently won the prestigious Nicholas E. Davies Award from the Healthcare Information and Management Systems Society. It is one of the few hospitals in the region to meet the criteria for excellence in healthcare established by the Leapfrog Group, a coalition of some of the nation's leading employers.

Cardiac Institute	Is world-renowned for its cardiac surgeons, who perform more than 1,000 operations annually including robotic surgeries, and its interventional cardiologists, who do more than 5,000 procedures a year.
Orthopaedic Institute	Undertakes complex procedures such as limb-lengthening, correction of congenital deformities, endoscopic spinal surgery, kyphoplasty, and repair of traumatic sports injuries.
Vascular Institute	Operates the largest and busiest vascular diagnostic lab in the state; sets the standard for stroke prevention and vascular surgery, and operates a Wound Center for those with chronic non-healing wounds.
Infants & Children's Hospital	Encompasses Pediatric ICU, Inpatient and Ambulatory Surgery units, Neonatal ICU, Outpatient Pavilion, Pediatric Emergency Center. A full range of pediatric subspecialties is provided.
Genesis Fertility & Reproductive Medicine	Known for diagnostic testing and intervention, including hormone and genetic screening, ovulation induction, in-vitro fertilization, use of donor eggs and other assisted reproductive techniques.
Stella & Joseph Payson Birthing Center	Offers a home-like setting combined with new technology; is staffed by 40 physicians and 27 midwives, and features perinatal testing with 3-D ultrasound. More than 6,800 babies were born here in 2003.
Weinberg Emergency Center	Handles more than 85,000 visits annually. It is a designated Heart Center, has a separate Chest Pain Observation Unit and Fast Track Care Center; is equipped for events involving hazardous materials (Hazmat).
Community Mental Health Center	Features specialized programs to meet community needs, including weekly "recovery" meetings; a Latino Day Program; services for the developmentally disabled; and FACES, an innovative teen theater network.

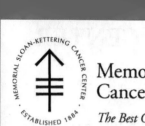

Memorial Sloan-Kettering Cancer Center

The Best Cancer Care. Anywhere.

1275 York Avenue
New York, NY 10017
Phone: 1-212-639-2000
Physician Referral: 1-800-525-2225
www.mskcc.org

Beds: 432
Sponsorship/Network Affiliation: Private, Non-Profit

THE MSKCC ADVANTAGE: CANCER IS OUR ONLY FOCUS

At Memorial Sloan-Kettering Cancer Center, our sole focus is cancer, and it has been for more than a century. Our doctors have unparalleled expertise in diagnosing and treating all types of cancer, using the latest technology and the most innovative, advanced therapies to increase the chances of a cure. Our designation as a National Cancer Institute (NCI) Comprehensive Cancer Center conveys our position as one of the nation's premier cancer centers.

A MULTIDISCIPLINARY, TEAM APPROACH TO CANCER CARE

Our Disease Management Program features multidisciplinary teams, defined by cancer type, whose members work together to guide each patient through diagnosis, treatment and recovery. These teams have a depth and breadth of experience that is unsurpassed. Using this approach, treatment plans reflect the combined expertise of many doctors—surgeons, medical oncologists, radiologists, radiation oncologists and pathologists. This approach also ensures that patients who need several different therapies to treat their cancer will receive the best combination for them.

GREATER PRECISION IN DIAGNOSIS

At Memorial Sloan-Kettering, highly sophisticated imaging techniques are used to accurately diagnose and stage cancers. In addition to MRI and CT, we offer the most advanced imaging technologies, such as combination PET/CT imaging, which can more accurately detect cancer and pinpoint its exact location in the body. Our highly specialized pathologists analyze tumor samples to determine a precise diagnosis. They are increasingly able to identify the molecular differences among tumors, providing even greater precision in diagnosis, which means physicians are able to determine the optimal therapy that is available to treat each individual's cancer.

UNPARALLELED SURGICAL EXPERTISE

Recent studies have shown that, for many cancers, patients who have their operations at a hospital that performs large numbers of the procedures are more likely to survive and have fewer complications. Because of their sole focus on cancer, our surgeons are among the most experienced cancer surgeons in the world. Over the years, they have pioneered scores of surgical innovations, including the use of minimally invasive techniques for many cancers. Using several small incisions instead of one large one, this approach results in less post-surgical pain and faster recovery. Our surgeons are also at the forefront of developing surgical procedures to spare organs and preserve function.

LEADERS IN RADIATION THERAPY

Memorial Sloan-Kettering's radiation oncologists pioneered intensity-modulated radiation therapy, a system for delivering radiation that permits unparalleled precision in the shaping and targeting of radiotherapy beams. This allows higher, more effective doses of radiation to be delivered to tumors while minimizing the exposure of surrounding healthy tissues and organs. Our doctors have also developed the use of radiation therapy combined with chemotherapy, which makes tumor cells more sensitive to the effects of radiation, thereby enhancing the success of the treatment.

THE MOUNT SINAI MEDICAL CENTER

One Gustave L. Levy Place (Fifth Avenue and 98th Street)
New York, NY 10029-6574
Phone: (212) 241-6500
Physician Referral: 1-800-MD-SINAI (637-4624)
www.mountsinai.org

Sponsorship	Voluntary Not-for-Profit
Beds	1,171
Accreditation	Joint Commission on Accreditation of Healthcare Organization (JCAHO)
	Commission for Accreditation of Rehabilitation Facilities (CARF)

Founded in 1852, The Mount Sinai Medical Center is one of the country's oldest and largest voluntary teaching hospitals. Mount Sinai is internationally acclaimed for excellence in clinical care, education, and scientific research in nearly every aspect of medicine.

Recognized for excellence in numerous specialties, The Mount Sinai Medical Center and its medical staff have been consistently ranked among the best in New York City and the country by such respected magazines as *U.S. News & World Report*, and *New York* magazine. Among the departments and services most frequently singled out for excellence are:

- **The Zena and Michael A. Wiener Cardiovascular Institute and the Marie-Josée and Henry R. Kravis Center for Cardiovascular Health**, under the direction of Dr. Valentin Fuster, provide tertiary and quaternary care for those at risk for heart disease and those who suffer from acute cardiac illnesses. A team of physicians and surgeons works with a full complement of rehabilitation experts and special services designed to help patients live life to the fullest.

- Mount Sinai's **Cardiothoracic Surgery Center** brings together one of the nation's most renowned teams of cardiothoracic surgeons, headed by Dr. David Adams. They work in collaboration with their colleagues in cardiovascular care to deliver the best in cardiothoracic surgery, including mitral valve repair, beating heart coronary bypass surgery, minimally invasive valve surgery and pediatric cardiac surgery. Another team member, Dr. Scott Swanson, brings world-class expertise in thoracic surgery to Mount Sinai, including thoracic oncology, swallowing disorders and gastroesophageal reflux disease.

- The **Recanati/Miller Transplantation Institute** is recognized across the country in organ transplantation, and one of the few to successfully provide combined organ transplantation. Renowned for its long-term experience in the field, The Mount Sinai Hospital was the site of the first liver transplant surgery in New York State.

- The **Minimally-Invasive Surgery** program offers an ever-expanding expertise in laparoscopic procedures: aortic valve replacement, mitral valve repair and replacement, abdominal aortic aneurysm repair, radical prostatectomy, nephrectomy, cystectomy, gastric bypass, treatments for endometriosis, uterine fibroids, ovarian cysts, as well as for cervical, ovarian, and uterine cancers.

Physician Referral (800) MD-SINAI / (800) 637-4624
The Mount Sinai Medical Center provides a free physician referral and health resource service from 8:30 a.m. to 6 p.m. weekdays, staffed exclusively by registered nurses. Consumers can also select a Mount Sinai physician by visiting the Find A Doctor section of our website, www.mountsinai.org

THE NEW YORK EYE & EAR INFIRMARY

310 East 14th Street • New York, New York 10003
Tel.: 212.979.4000 • Fax.: 212.228.0664
Web: www.nyee.edu

NY Eye & Ear Infirmary

Affiliated Teaching
Hospital of New York
Medical College

Continuum Health Partners, Inc.

Sponsorship: Voluntary Not-for-Profit
Accreditation: Joint Commission on Accreditation of Healthcare Organizations, College of
American Pathologists

ABOUT THE NEW YORK EYE AND EAR INFIRMARY

The New York Eye and Ear Infirmary is one of the world's leading facilities for the diagnosis and treatment of diseases of the eyes, ears, nose, throat and related conditions. A voluntary, not-for-profit institution, the Infirmary is an affiliated teaching hospital of New York Medical College and a member of Continuum Health Partners, Inc.

THE MEDICAL STAFF

The Medical Staff includes more than 500 attending physicians and surgeons throughout the metropolitan area. Many are renowned for their breakthrough research introducing widely practiced techniques.

RESEARCH AND EDUCATION

The New York Eye and Ear Infirmary is a national and international leader in research in its specialties, achieving many "firsts" in successful procedures and medical treatments. Laboratories include Cell Culture, Ocular Imaging, and Microsurgical Education.

SPECIALTIES

Ophthalmology: Within this area are subspecialties of cataract, glaucoma, retina, cornea and refractive surgery, ocular plastic surgery, pediatric ophthalmology and strabismus, neuro-ophthalmology and ocular tumor. Laser, photography, fluorescein angiography and electro-physiological testing are among the most advanced services available anywhere.

Otolaryngology: The department is in the forefront of treatment modalities using highly sophisticated endoscopic and laser equipment, Subspecialties include allergy, voice, rhinology, head & neck surgery, otology, neurotology, pediatric otolaryngology, audiology, speech therapy and hearing aid dispensing.

Plastic & Reconstructive Surgery: Microsurgical capabilities and premium patient accommodations provide an optimum environment for facial plasty, liposuction and repair of defects from disease or trauma.

RELATED SERVICES

New York Eye Trauma Center: An advanced program for emergency treatment of eye injuries, it also is the Eye Injury Registry of New York State and leading collector of data which will help develop preventative strategies.

Vision Correction Center: State-of-the-art facility dedicated to all forms of laser refractive surgery performed in an academic medical center in the forefront of teaching and research in vision correction.

Ambulatory Surgery: A comprehensive Ambulatory Surgery Center is designed to expedite admission testing, pre-op preparation and post-op recovery in an efficient and comfortable setting.

Pediatric Specialty Care: The city's only such center coordinating the services of eye and ear, nose and throat specialists with other staff especially sensitive to the youngest patients.

Physician Referral: Call 1-800-449-HOPE (4673)

⌐ NewYork Presbyterian
⌐ The University Hospital of Columbia and Cornell

Affiliated with Columbia University College of Physicians and Surgeons and Weill Medical College of Cornell University

NewYork-Presbyterian Hospital
Weill Cornell Medical Center
525 East 68th Street
New York, NY 10021

NewYork-Presbyterian Hospital
Columbia University Medical Center
622 West 168th Street
New York, NY 10032

Sponsorship: Voluntary Not-for-Profit
Beds: 2,369
Accreditation: Joint Commission on Accreditation of Healthcare Organizations (JCAHO), Commission on Accreditation of Rehabilitation Facilities (CARF) and College of American Pathologists (CAP)

The *U.S. News & World Report* has ranked NewYork-Presbyterian Hospital higher in more specialties than any other hospital in the New York area. NewYork-Presbyterian Hospital was named to the *Honor Roll of America's Best Hospitals.*

OVERVIEW:

NewYork-Presbyterian Hospital is the largest hospital in New York and one of the most comprehensive health-care institutions in the world with 5,500 physicians, approximately 96,000 discharges and nearly 1 million out-patient visits annually, and with its affiliated medical schools, more than $330 million in research support.

AMONG ITS RENOWNED CENTERS OF EXCELLENCE ARE:

Morgan Stanley Children's Hospital and the Komansky Center for Children's Health – One of the largest, most comprehensive provider of children's healthcare in the world providing highly sophisticated pediatric medical, surgical and intensive care, including a pediatric cardiovascular center, in a compassionate environment.

NewYork-Presbyterian Cancer Centers – Coordinated, multidisciplinary care and the latest therapeutic options and clinical trials available for all types of cancer.

NewYork-Presbyterian Heart – Expert diagnostic capabilities and medical and surgical innovations for simple to complex heart conditions.

NewYork-Presbyterian Neuroscience Centers – Latest research, diagnosis and treatment capabilities in Alzheimer's disease, Multiple Sclerosis, Parkinson's disease, aneurysms, epilepsy, brain tumors, stokes and other neurological disorders.

NewYork-Presbyterian Psychiatry – World-renowned center of excellence in psychiatric treatment, research and education.

NewYork-Presbyterian Transplant Institute – Adult and pediatric heart, liver, and kidney and adult pancreas and lung transplantation and cutting-edge research.

NewYork-Presbyterian Vascular Care Center – Comprehensive and integrated preventive, diagnostic and treatment program for diverse problems related to arteries and veins throughout the body.

NewYork-Presbyterian Digestive Disease Services – Expert capabilities in the broad range of conditions that affect the organs as well as other components of the digestive system.

William Randolph Hearst Burn Center – Largest and busiest burn center in the nation which also conducts research to improve survival and enhance quality of life for burn victims.

In addition, the Hospital offers extraordinary expertise, comprehensive programs and specialized resources in the fields of AIDS, Complementary Medicine, Gene Therapy, Reproductive Medicine and Infertility, Trauma Center and Women's Health Care.

ACADEMIC AFFILIATIONS:

NewYork-Presbyterian is the only hospital in the world affiliated with two Ivy League medical schools; The Joan and Sanford I Weill Medical College of Cornell University and the Columbia University College of Physicians & Surgeons.

Physician Referral: To find a NewYork-Presbyterian Hospital affiliated physician to meet your needs, call toll free 1-877-NYP-WELL (1-877-697-9355) or visit our website at www.nyp.org

NYU MEDICAL CENTER

550 First Avenue (at 31st Street)
New York, NY 10016
Physician Referral:
1-888-7-NYU-MED
www.nyumc.org

Sponsorship:	Private, Not-for-Profit
Beds:	878 beds
Accreditation:	Joint Commission on Accreditation of Healthcare Organizations (JCAHO), Commission for Accreditation of Rehabilitation Facilities (CARF)

A LEADER IN PATIENT CARE

NYU Medical Center is one of the nation's leading biomedical resources, combining excellence in patient care, research and medical education. A not-for-profit institution, NYU Medical Center includes **Tisch Hospital**, a voluntary 704-bed tertiary care facility serving more than 28,000 inpatients annually, and the **Rusk Institute of Rehabilitation Medicine**, which has 174 beds and serves 2,816 inpatients and more than 53,900 outpatients annually. **The NYU Cancer Institute** specializes in Medical Oncology, GYN Oncology, Surgical Oncology, Radiation Oncology, Diagnostic Imaging, Pathology, and Hematology. The Medical Center also includes the **Hospital for Joint Diseases Orthopaedic Institute,** which has 220 beds and is one of the nation's premier hospitals for treating orthopaedic and rheumatological disorders.

SPECIAL PROGRAMS AT NYU

Cancer The NYU Cancer Institute's Clinical Cancer Center meets the outpatient needs of people with cancer and provides the latest cancer prevention, screening, diagnostic, treatment, genetic counseling, and support services in one convenient and comfortable facility.

Cardiac Surgery A leader in minimally invasive techniques and robotic procedures

Cardiology A full range of diagnostic, prognostic and treatment services for patients of all ages

Epilepsy   One of the largest facilities of its kind on the East Coast

Obstetrics & Gynecology   NYU Medical Center offers unparalleled diagnostic techniques and surgical innovations to treat women of all ages, with world-class expertise in infertility treatment and management of high-risk pregnancies.

Plastic Surgery The largest facility of its kind in the world

The Rusk Institute of Rehabilitation Medicine is the world's first and one of the largest university centers for the treatment of adults and children with disabilities.

Transplant Some of the nation's best patient and graft survival outcomes

Urology Leaders in treating prostate disorders and other urological problems

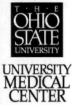

The Ohio State University Medical Center

Fred Sanfilippo, MD, PhD
Chief Executive Officer

370 West 9th Avenue
Columbus, Ohio 43210
Phone: 1-800-293-5123
www.medicalcenter.osu.edu

Part of the most comprehensive health sciences campus in the United States, The Ohio State University Medical Center includes a college of medicine and public health, five hospitals, two free-standing research institutes and a network of more than 30 community-based primary and specialty care facilities throughout central Ohio. Our three-part mission of patient care, teaching and research sets us apart as the only academic medical center in the area.

PATIENT CARE

The Ohio State University Hospitals is a 923-bed hospital consistently named one of "America's Best" by *U.S. News &World Report*. We specialize in cardiac care, organ transplantation, rehabilitation, neurosciences, and women's health and house a Level I Trauma Center and Level III neonatal intensive care unit.

University Hospital East extends the medical center's mission with a unique blend of academic and community-based medicine in Columbus' east side. University Hospital East is a full-service hospital with areas of emphasis in Orthopaedics, Family Medicine, Emergency Services, Addiction Services and Wound Care.

The Arthur G. James Cancer Hospital and Richard J. Solove Research Institute is a 160-bed cancer hospital and research institute consistently ranked among "America's Best" by *U.S. News & World Report*. The James is one of only 39 organizations in the U.S. designated as a Comprehensive Cancer Center by the National Cancer Institute.

The Richard M. Ross Heart Hospital, opening in late 2004, will be central Ohio's first hospital dedicated exclusively to heart disease. Complementing the 100-bed hospital's private patient rooms and state-of-the-art imaging technologies will be an advanced conference center for consulting with and training heart-care professionals worldwide.

OSU Harding is central Ohio's most comprehensive inpatient and outpatient service for persons with depression, post-trauma, family conflict, personality disorders, anxiety, sexual abuse and related conditions. Children and adults are treated in a caring and supportive environment by the region's leading psychiatrists, psychologists, nurses, therapists, and counselors.

The OSU Primary Care Network is a group of nearly 100 physicians located in dozens of offices throughout greater Columbus who offer individuals and families a broad range of preventive and routine healthcare services. Together, these offices see more than 375,000 patient visits each year.

TEACHING

The Ohio State University College of Medicine and Public Health, consistently ranked among the nation's best, is well known for its curricular innovation, world-renowned faculty, pioneering research and clinical training opportunities. In addition to the MD degree, the College offers combined degrees, dozens of CME opportunities annually, and more than 60 residency programs. The College includes Schools of Public Health, Allied Medical Professions, and Biomedical Sciences.

RESEARCH

OSU Medical Center has seen tremendous growth in research funding over the past two years, surpassing $100 million annually for the first time in 2002. Our goal is to be among the top quartile of academic medical centers in research funding by 2008.

The OSU Comprehensive Cancer Center is a network of seven interdisciplinary cancer research programs that collectively comprise 223 scientists from 12 Ohio State University colleges.

The Dorothy M. Davis Heart and Lung Research Institute houses more than 100 clinicians and researchers and the laboratories for 50 investigators conducting the gamut of heart and vessel research, from basic science studies to clinical trials.

For additional information, please call 1-800-293-5123 or visit our Web site at www.medicalcenter.osu.edu

ROBERT WOOD JOHNSON UNIVERSITY HOSPITAL

One Robert Wood Johnson Place,
New Brunswick, NJ 08903-2601
General Information (732) 828-3000. Physician Referral 888-44-RWJUH
www.rwjuh.edu

Accreditation	Joint Commission of Healthcare Organizations (JCAHO); American Nurses Credential Center-Magnet Recognition Award
Affiliations:	Principal hospital for the University of Medicine and Dentistry of New Jersey—Robert Wood Johnson Medical School; The Cancer Institute of New Jersey; New Jersey Council of Teaching Hospitals; flagship hospital of the Robert Wood Johnson Health System and Network.

GENERAL OVERVIEW

Robert Wood Johnson University Hospital is one of the nation's leading academic health centers, offering a full range of health care services from preventative to specialty and subspecialty diagnosis and treatment.

A 572-bed tertiary and quaternary care facility, the hospital treats the most severely ill patients referred from community hospitals around the state and around the country. More than 1,100 physicians and surgeons in every specialty are affiliated with the hospital. We are a site for medical residency and medical student training.

CENTERS OF EXCELLENCE

The Heart Center of New Jersey offers complete diagnostic capabilities and treatment options for heart disease, including the latest in minimally invasive techniques. Home to one of the busiest cardiac catheterization programs in the nation, the Heart Center performs more than 1,200 cardiac surgeries and 11,000 cardiac interventional procedures annually. The Advanced Heart Failure and Transplant Program offers specialized care for patients with heart failure, including medical management, surgically implanted assist devices, and a Medicare-certified heart transplantation program.

The Center for Kidney and Pancreas Transplantation is one of a select few programs in the state to offer kidney and pancreas transplantation. A team of physicians, surgeons, nurses and health professionals offer adult and pediatric patients the full spectrum of care.

The Cancer Hospital of New Jersey is the flagship hospital of The Cancer Institute of New Jersey, the state's only National Cancer Institute-designated Comprehensive Cancer Center. This 123-bed hospital has an outpatient chemotherapy treatment area, a bone marrow transplant unit, medical oncology unit, surgical oncology unit, as well as an urgent-care center. The hospital offers oncology-focused services including diagnostic, laboratory, pain management and psychosocial services.

The Bristol-Myers Squibb Children's Hospital is a state-designated acute care children's hospital providing the region's first state-designated Pediatric Intensive Care Unit, pediatric Level I trauma and a full range of pediatric specialties and subspecialties, including cardiac surgery, hematology-oncology, orthopaedics and neurosurgery. It staffs a dedicated pediatric critical care transport vehicle.

Regional Perinatal Services: Designated a Regional Perinatal Center, the hospital offers the latest technology to treat high-risk pregnancies, as well as the most critically ill newborns. The Center's renowned maternal-fetal medicine and neonatology specialists provide a full array of services and surgical support for babies and families. The Center has a new neonatal intensive care unit, special care nursery, labor and delivery suite, private post-partum unit and a well baby nursery.

Level I Trauma Center provides a skilled shock/trauma team composed of general surgeons, orthopaedic surgeons, neurosurgeons and anesthesiologists. The Center provides care for adults and children.

ROSWELL PARK
CANCER INSTITUTE (RPCI)

A National Cancer Institute Designated-Comprehensive Cancer Center
Elm & Carlton Streets • Buffalo, NY 14263
Tel. 716.845.2300 Toll Free 1-800-ROSWELL (1-800-767-9355)
www.roswellpark.org

PATIENT-CENTERED CARE INSPIRES INNOVATIVE TREATMENTS

Roswell Park Cancer Institute's efforts emanate from the needs of the cancer patients who are at the center of its work. RPCI provides a complete range of services: a customized treatment plan for all types of cancers, supportive services to help patients with spiritual and emotional issues, pain management, physical and occupational therapy and continued evaluation after discharge. Because cancer affects the patient's family as well as the patient, RPCI provides support services for both, extending the circle to help as it broadens its power to heal.

Over 95% of Roswell Park patients consistently rate the care at Roswell Park as "excellent" or "very good" and say they would recommend Roswell Park Cancer Institute to other cancer patients.

MULTIDISCIPLINARY CENTERS

Breast Center
Chemotherapy and Infusion Center
Dermatology, Sarcoma and Melanoma Center
Gastrointestinal Center
Gynecology Center
Head and Neck/Dental Center
Hematology Center
Neuro-Oncology Center
Pain Management Center
Pediatric Center
Thoracic Center
Urology Center

SPECIALIZED TREATMENTS

Clinical Trials • Blood & Marrow Transplantation • Clinical Genetics Testing and Counseling • High-dose Chemotherapy • Photodynamic Therapy • Gamma Knife • Follow-up Clinic for Long-Term Survivors of Childhood Cancer • Minimally Invasive Surgical Procedures • Regional Center for Maxillofacial Prosthetics • Buffalo-Niagara Prostate Cancer Consortium • Center for HIV-related Malignancies

NURTURING HOPE AT THE CENTER AND BEYOND

Call today for your free educational kit, which includes a video on "Caring the Roswell Park Way" -   1-877-ASK-RPCI.

(1-877-275-7724)

GENERATING IDEAS THAT CARRY US CLOSER TO A CURE

Roswell Park Cancer Institute was the first facility in the nation dedicated to the understanding and treatment of cancer. It remains one of the world's foremost cancer research centers, developing new therapies, technologies, diagnostics, and pharmaceuticals that are changing the lives of cancer patients globally. Founded in 1898, RPCI is the only National Cancer Institute-designated Comprehensive Cancer Center in Upstate New York. Its 25-acre campus, located between the shores of Lake Erie and Lake Ontario, consists of 15 buildings with a new 119-bed hospital building, a comprehensive diagnostic and treatment center and a newly built medical research complex.

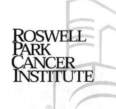

ROSWELL
PARK
CANCER
INSTITUTE

SAINT VINCENT CATHOLIC MEDICAL CENTERS

Saint Vincent Catholic Medical Centers serves nearly 600,000 people each year with treatments ranging from prenatal to hospice care. We deliver the care our patients' need, along with the attention they deserve, throughout every stage of life.

Saint Vincent's Hospitals serve as the academic medical center for New York Medical College in New York City.

Hospitals – Call 1-800-CARE-421 for information or physician referral

St. Vincent's Manhattan, St. Vincent's Staten Island and St. Vincent's Westchester, along with Mary Immaculate and St. John's Hospital in Queens and St. Mary's Hospital Brooklyn

Nursing Homes – Call 1-866-NURSE-28 for more information

Monsignor Fitzpatrick Pavilion in Queens, Bishop Mugavero and Holy Family Home in Brooklyn and St. Elizabeth Ann's Health Care and Rehabilitation Center on Staten Island

Home Care – Serving the New York metropolitan area-- Call 1-866-NURSE-28

Specialized Services Throughout the Greater New York Area

Behavioral Health – We treat people with mental illness or chemical dependency. Services include one of the few inpatient programs for children in New York City, geriatric programs that deliver medical and psychiatric services, chemical dependency detoxification and rehabilitation programs and bilingual, bicultural Latino Treatment Services.

Cancer Services – Our cancer centers, St. Vincent's Comprehensive Cancer Center in Manhattan, the I. Joseph Aprile Cancer Institute at Mary Immaculate Hospital in Queens and the Cancer Center on Staten Island help people meet the challenges of living with cancer while delivering the highest quality care. These centers work together to offer the most advanced treatment options along with access to the latest clinical trials.

Cardiovascular Services – We offer comprehensive services to prevent and treat heart disease. Our Cardiovascular Services for Women is a program that recognizes women's unique needs and teaches them how the symptoms of heart disease may manifest differently in them than in men.

Orthopaedic Services – We offer the most advanced treatments for musculoskeletal problems, including arthritis, fractures and dislocations, hip and knee replacement, spine and sports injuries, and many more.

For more information, or to find a primary or specialty care physician, please call 1-800-CARE-421 or log onto www.svcmc.org.

SHANDS HEALTHCARE

www.shands.org

Sponsorship: Non-profit hospital system with two academic medical centers affiliated with the University of Florida
Accreditation: Joint Commission on Accreditation of HealthCare Organizations

A COMPREHENSIVE HEALTHCARE RESOURCE FOR THE SOUTHEAST

Shands HealthCare, affiliated with the University of Florida, is one of the premier health systems in the Southeast. Shands includes nine not-for-profit hospitals and more than 80 affiliated UF Physicians clinical practices. Shands delivers advanced diagnostic and medical treatments and provides highly specialized, complex health services that draw patients from every county in Florida, throughout the United States and beyond.

ACADEMIC MEDICAL CENTERS

Shands HealthCare is a unique health system with two academic medical centers. At the system's core is Shands at the University of Florida (Shands at UF) located in Gainesville. It is a 618-bed medical center that includes a children's hospital, a regional burn center, a level 1 Trauma Center and a transplant center. Shands at UF is consistently ranked in *U.S. News & World Report's* "Guide to America's Best Hospitals." Shands Jacksonville, located in Jacksonville, has 760 beds and is home to a Level 1 Trauma Center, a Neuroscience Institute and Cardiovascular Institute. Shands HealthCare campuses are linked with the University of Florida Shands Cancer Center and draw on the expertise of UF research centers such as the McKnight Brain Institute and Genetics Institute.

SPECIALIZED PATIENT CARE

More than 700 University of Florida faculty physicians representing 110 medical specialties work with teams of highly skilled nurses and healthcare professionals to provide quality patient care.

Shands Healthcare is a regional resource for patients who have complex health problems or are challenged with a chronic disease. Such high acuity needs require advanced technical equipment and state-of-the-art facilities.

PIONEERING RESEARCH

As one of the Southeast's most comprehensive centers for basic and clinical research, Shands HealthCare is involved in more than 1,500 investigations into promising technologies and therapies aimed at improving outcomes for disease prevention, diagnosis and treatment. By rapidly transferring knowledge from the "bench to bedside," UF physicians help to bring a higher level of care to patients.

Physician Referral

The Shands Consultation Center is your link to University of Florida physicians and the numerous programs and services offered by Shands HealthCare. For more information or to schedule an appointment, please call **800.749.7424** or visit our Web site at **shands.org**.

THOMAS JEFFERSON UNIVERSITY HOSPITALS

111 S. 11th Street
Philadelphia, PA 19107-5098
Tel. 215-955-6000
www.JeffersonHospital.org

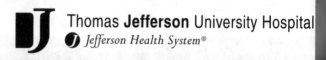

SERVING OUR COMMUNITY CONVENIENTLY

Begun in 1825, the Thomas Jefferson University Hospitals with 925 licensed acute care beds offers major programs for a wide range of clinical specialties. Services are delivered at several locations - Center City, Jefferson Hospital for Neuroscience, Methodist Hospital, which is located in South Philadelphia, Ford Road, Jefferson HealthCARE—Voorhees, in New Jersey, and several ambulatory care satellites and radiation therapy centers.

JEFFERSON HOSPITAL'S OUTSTANDING ACADEMIC AND RESEARCH PROGRAMS

Jefferson Hospitals' 588 residents participate in 20 residency programs with 137 fellows in 36 fellowships in partnership with Thomas Jefferson University. Also benefiting from the hospitals' academic programs are 563 undergraduate students, 408 master's level students, 933 medical students, and 125 doctoral candidates. Research is conducted in all clinical departments and divisions.

A STAFF OF MEDICAL EXPERTS

Jefferson Hospitals' medical staff consists of 866 active full-time physicians, many of whom are world renowned, and 1,272 full-time Registered Nurses. In addition to their clinical responsibilities, these medical leaders enjoy academic appointments at Thomas Jefferson University's three colleges.

ADVANCED MEDICINE, SUPERIOR CARE

The Jefferson Heart Institute's Advanced Heart Failure and Cardiac Transplant Program offers leading-edge cardiology services, from drug therapy to heart transplantation. • A National Cancer Institute-designated clinical cancer center, the Kimmel Cancer Center at Jefferson offers innovative therapies and clinical trial participation opportunities for breast, brain, lung, prostate, colon and rectal, and head and neck cancer.• Rothman Institute at Jefferson orthopaedic surgeons form one of the 10 busiest departments in the U.S. performing more than 8,000 annual procedures including hip, knee, shoulder and elbow and spine surgeries. • The Jefferson Hospital for Neuroscience (JHN) neurosurgical team treats more cerebral aneurysms than any other in the U.S. or Canada and more brain tumors than any team in the Delaware Valley. To precisely treat brain tumors while sparing healthy tissue, JHN recently introduced Shaped Beam™ Stereotactic Radiosurgery. The Surgical Epilepsy Center at JHN performs nearly 100 epilepsy surgeries each year. Neuroscientist/ researchers at our Farber Institute for Neurosciences focus on basic and clinical research in Alzheimer's disease, amyotrophic lateral sclerosis (ALS) and other neurodegenerative disorders.

RECENT ACCOLADES

Thomas Jefferson University Hospital has been rated as one of "America's Best Hospitals" for many specialties by *U.S. News & World Report* for 15 years in a row. The Hospital received the Consumer Choice Award for Healthcare recognizing innovation and leadership in healthcare services in Philadelphia for six years in a row. In recent years, Jefferson University Hospital ranked among the nation's 100 Top Hospitals™ for patient care, teaching, management, stroke care and ICUs by Solucient. Our doctors are consistently listed in "Best Doctors in America," and *Philadelphia Magazine*.

RECOGNIZED QUALITY CARE

Jefferson University Hospital is one of only a few hospitals in the United States that is both a Regional Trauma Center and a federally designated regional Spinal Cord Injury Center. The Hospital is fully accredited by the Joint Commission on Accreditation of Healthcare Organizations (JCAHO) and licensed by the Department of Health of the Commonwealth of Pennsylvania.

UCLA MEDICAL CENTER

10883 Le Conte Avenue • Los Angeles, CA 90024
1-800-UCLA-MD1 (1-800-825-2631)
www.healthcare.ucla.edu

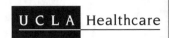

Beds: 668
Sponsorship/Network Affiliation: **UCLA Medical Center is a non-profit hospital and part of UCLA Healthcare.**

UCLA HEALTHCARE

For nearly half a century, UCLA has been recognized as a leader in patient care, medical research and teaching. The legacy that began in 1955 when UCLA Medical Center opened its doors in Westwood has grown to include four hospitals and a network of community offices, known together as UCLA Healthcare.

UCLA HEALTHCARE HOSPITALS

- UCLA Medical Center, located in Westwood, offers patients of all ages comprehensive care, from routine to highly specialized medical and surgical treatment.
- Santa Monica-UCLA Medical Center, which became a part of UCLA Healthcare in 1995, continues to provide primary and specialty care to the local community and beyond.
- Mattel Children's Hospital at UCLA, located within UCLA Medical Center, offers a wide range of services from well-child care to treating the most difficult and life-threatening illnesses.
- UCLA Neuropsychiatric Hospital offers programs in geriatric, adult, adolescent and child psychiatry.

HONORS AND RECOGNITION

- For the 15th consecutive year, UCLA Medical Center ranks number one in the West in *U.S. News & World Report*'s America's Best Hospitals survey.
- *U.S. News* ranks UCLA Jonsson Cancer Center best in the western United States.
- 275 UCLA physicians are cited in Best Doctors, which is based on an extensive poll of medical specialists worldwide.

SPECIALTIES AND RESEARCH

- Cancer care through UCLA's Jonsson Comprehensive Cancer Center
- Integrative healthcare through UCLA's East-West Medicine Center
- Advanced care for all neurological disorders, including Alzheimer's disease and neuromuscular diseases and disorders
- Full range of comprehensive cardiology services from prevention to rehab
- Ophthalmology services through Jules Stein Eye Institute and the Doris Stein Eye Research Center
- World-renowned adult and pediatric organ transplant programs
- Treatment of disorders of the spine and brain through UCLA's neurosurgery services
- The UCLA AIDS Institute for state-of-the-art treatment
- Comprehensive women's health services
- Innovative surgical approaches, including minimally invasive and robotic procedures

PHYSICIAN REFERRAL:
To find the UCLA doctor who best meets your needs, call the UCLA Physician Referral Service at 1-800-UCLA-MD1 (1-800-825-2631)

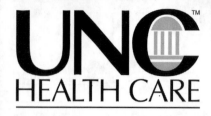

The University of North Carolina Health Care System
101 Manning Drive Chapel Hill, NC 27514
www.unchealthcare.org

Beds: 688   Accreditation: Accredited by JCAHO

GENERAL OVERVIEW

UNC Hospitals – a medical center consisting of four separate hospitals and a burn center – is the cornerstone of UNC Health Care. More than 30,000 people each year are patients at UNC Hospitals, coming from across North Carolina, the rest of the United States and other countries. More than 2,900 infants are born each year at UNC Hospitals. In 2002, UNC Health Care opened two new state-of-the-art hospitals: North Carolina Children's Hospital and North Carolina Women's Hospital. Design planning is currently under way to build a fifth hospital on the UNC campus, the North Carolina Cancer Hospital.

ACADEMIC AND CLINICAL APPLICATIONS

The University of North Carolina at Chapel Hill School of Medicine relies on UNC Hospitals as its teaching hospital. This partnership has enabled the School of Medicine to become one of only four medical schools in the United States that is ranked in the top 20 percent by the Association of American Medical Colleges both in production of primary care physicians and in receiving research grants from the National Institutes of Health.

MEDICAL STAFF

UNC Hospitals has more than 900 attending physicians, 49 of whom were listed in the fourth edition of *America's Top Doctors*, and more than 500 residents. Many of the attending physicians also teach and conduct research in the UNC School of Medicine.

UNC Health Care extends beyond Chapel Hill and into the greater Triangle region of North Carolina through its network of primary care and specialty physician practices located in Orange, Wake, Durham, Chatham Lee, Vance and Alamance counties. These offices, in addition to the UNC Family Practice Center and Ambulatory Care Center, provide the basic health care outpatient services most families need, in convenient neighborhood locations. Nearly a half-million people are cared for at UNC practices and clinics each year.

PIONEERING, COMPREHENSIVE MEDICAL CARE

Specialized patient care services include the Breast Center, Cardiovascular Program, Diabetes Care Center, Lung Center, Rehabilitation Center, Spine Center, Wound Management Program and Comprehensive Transplant Center. The medical center's extensive expertise in arthritis, digestive diseases, endocrinology, ENT, gynecology, hemophilia, infertility, rheumatology, and orthopaedics has achieved both regional and national recognition. And UNC is home to the Lineberger Comprehensive Cancer Center, one of a small number of National Cancer Institute-designated centers in the United States.

ACCREDITATION, COMMENDATIONS AND NATIONAL RECOGNITION

UNC Hospitals is accredited by the Joint Commission on Accreditation of Healthcare Organizations. *AARP Modern Maturity* magazine identified UNC Hospitals as one of the top 20 in the United states. For the last 11 years in a row, multiple clinical programs at UNC Hospitals were ranked among the top 50 programs of their kind nationwide in *U.S. News & World Report's* annual "America's Best Hospitals" issue.

OVERVIEW

For more than two centuries, Penn physicians and scientists have been committed to the highest standards of patient care, education and research. Our commitment has been recognized by our peers and by others throughout the Philadelphia region and across the nation.

U.S. News & World Report has named the Hospital of the University of Pennsylvania to its Honor Roll of the best hospitals in the nation for the seventh straight year. Our hospital is one of just 17 hospitals nationwide -- and the only hospital in Pennsylvania, New Jersey and Delaware - named to the list. *U.S. News* also consistently ranks our School of Medicine and School of Nursing among the nation's best.

The University of Pennsylvania Medical Center ranks second nationally in special grant funding from the National Institutes of Health. Four departments - Dermatology, Pathology and Laboratory Medicine, Radiology and Radiation Oncology - are ranked first nationally. Overall, Penn has more individual departments ranked in the top five than any other academic medical center.

THE FUTURE OF MEDICINE

Our physicians and scientists are united in the institution's mission to expand the frontiers of medicine through new discoveries in the detection, treatment and prevention of human disease. Because we develop and test new treatments through clinical trials, our patients gain access to the very latest advances, and future generations benefit from the work we do today.

Penn continues to lead the way in discovering new treatment methods for diseases once considered incurable. Groundbreaking research in cancer, neurosciences, genetics and imaging are just a few areas in which Penn has brought the future of medicine closer.

Over the past 30 years, Penn physicians and scientists have participated in many important discoveries, including:
- The first general vaccine against pneumonia.
- The introduction of total intravenous feeding.
- The development of magnetic resonance imaging and other imaging technologies.
- The discovery of the Philadelphia chromosome, which revolutionized cancer research by making the connection between genetic abnormalities and cancer.

LOCATIONS

Patients can be seen at Hospital of the University of Pennsylvania, Presbyterian - University of Pennsylvnia Medical Center, Pennsylvania Hospital, Phoenixville Hospital or our outpatient setting at Penn Medicine at Radnor, Cherry Hill or Limerick. Through our primary care physicians, patients can be seen at a location close to home either in Bucks, Montgomery and Philadelphia counties in Pennsylvania or in Southern New Jersey. We also provide hospice and homecare services through PENN Home Care and Hospice Services.

ON THE WEB

Visit pennhealth.com for the latest patient education with explanation of surgical procedures and follow-up care, screening tools, drug interactions and descriptions as well as an encyclopedia of information for you and your patients.

For direct connection to one of our Penn physicians, call PennLine 1-800-635-7780.

NATIONAL EXCELLENCE IN A FULL RANGE OF HEALTH CARE SERVICES

University of Pittsburgh Medical Center (UPMC), affiliated with the University of Pittsburgh, is the premier health care system in western Pennsylvania and one of the largest nonprofit health care systems in the country. UPMC is dedicated to providing exemplary patient care, educating the next generation of health care professionals, and advancing biomedical research.

Consistently ranking among the nation's top hospitals according to *U.S. News & World Report*, UPMC's 19 tertiary care, specialty, and community hospitals provide some of the finest care in the country. UPMC also comprises a wide network of doctors' offices, cancer centers, outpatient satellites, specialized imaging and surgery facilities, in-home care, rehabilitation sites, behavioral health care, and nursing homes—encompassing more than 350 health care sites.

DEVELOPING TOMORROW'S TREATMENTS

UPMC programs treat patients with virtually every human illness, no matter how complex, often taking on cases that are considered too complicated or even untreatable elsewhere. With UPMC's support, the University of Pittsburgh conducts robust research programs designed to develop tomorrow's treatments. In fact, the University and affiliated research programs attract more than $375 million each year in National Institutes of Health funding, ranking among the top 10 in the country.

UPMC's prominence is not restricted to the United States; patients have come to UPMC for care from dozens of countries. An international transplantation center in Palermo, Italy, has imported UPMC clinical excellence to patients throughout the Mediterranean region, and has generated funds for continuing UPMC research and clinical care.

PHYSICIAN REFERRAL
For more information, call 800-533-UPMC (8762).

THE UNIVERSITY OF TEXAS
MD ANDERSON
CANCER CENTER
Making Cancer History™

1515 Holcombe Blvd.

Houston, Texas 77030-4095

Tel. 713-792-6161

Toll Free 800-392-1611

www.mdanderson.org

Beds: 475

Deciding where to seek cancer treatment is difficult. We know you have many options. Here are some of the reasons why M. D. Anderson is your best hope for cancer care.

EXPERTISE

- We're one of the largest cancer centers in the world. We've been working to eliminate cancer for more than six decades. Our depth of experience informs every aspect of your care.

- We focus exclusively on cancer and have seen cases of every kind. Our doctors treat more rare cancers in a single day than most physicians see in a lifetime. That means you receive expert care no matter what your diagnosis.

- We are the top-ranked cancer hospital in the United States according to the 2004 *U.S. News and World Report* annual survey of hospitals.

- Our physicians are frequently recognized as among the best in the nation by services including Best Doctors in America.

- We have more nurses per patient than many hospitals in the country, so you receive the utmost attention and quality care.

- We're world-renowned for using and developing front-line diagnostic technology. That lets physicians pinpoint each patient's unique cancer and tailor treatment for the best possible outcome.

CUTTING-EDGE RESEARCH

- One of our greatest strengths is our ability to translate today's most promising laboratory findings into tomorrow's new, more effective and less traumatic treatments. We've pioneered countless medical advances over the years. Our patients benefit from that quest by receiving not only the best treatments to minimize or eliminate their cancer, but those treatments that will also give them the best chance at a high quality of life afterwards.

- New and innovative therapies generally are available at M. D. Anderson several years before they become standard in the community. Our clinical trials incorporate state-of-the-art patient care, while evaluating the most recent developments in cancer medicine. They also offer treatment opportunities for difficult or aggressive tumors.

- M. D. Anderson ranks first in the number and amount of research grants awarded by the National Cancer Institute. By studying how cancer begins and responds to various treatments, we can help patients overcome disease and prevent recurrence.

SUPPORT AND EDUCATION

At M. D. Anderson, we understand that cancer is not just a physical disease. To help you cope with every aspect of cancer, we provide a number of programs including:

- The Place...*of wellness* - more than 75 complementary programs, free of charge, to help with the non-medical dimensions of living with cancer.

- The Anderson Network - a unique cancer support group of more than 1,300 current and former patients and can offer the right patient-to-patient advice and encouragement when you need it most.

- Life After Cancer Care - a comprehensive medical program that can anticipate, recognize and manage potential health problems that may arise from cancer or its treatments.

- The M. D. Anderson Learning Center - provides books and other learning materials for reference and checkout by patients and their families.

- M. D. Anderson's Cancer Prevention Center - offers programs, counseling services and information to help people make healthy lifestyle choices to prevent cancer or its recurrence.

- The Jesse Jones Rotary House International – a hotel that provides a home-like environment with personnel who understand our patients' health care needs.

Every day, we at M. D. Anderson renew our commitment to our core values of caring, integrity and discovery. As we continue Making Cancer History, you can rest assured we'll be both at the forefront and by your side.

♥ Vanderbilt Medical Center

1313 21st Avenue South, Suite 405, Nashville, Tennessee 37232-4335
Tel. 615.936.0301 Fax. 615.936.0320 www.mc.vanderbilt.edu

Beds: 661
Vanderbilt University Medical Center (VUMC) is a major not-for-profit academic medical center affiliated with Vanderbilt University located in Nashville, Tennessee. VUMC is a member of the Association of Academic Medical Centers and the University Hospital Consortium.

A HISTORY OF EXCELLENCE

Throughout its history, Vanderbilt University Medical Center (VUMC) has been dedicated to excellence in patient care, medical and nursing education and biomedical research. Founded in 1875, VUMC has grown to become a comprehensive, multi-faceted institution that touches thousands of lives throughout the nation every day.

COMPREHENSIVE MEDICAL CARE

With a medical staff of 793 board certified physicians, and more than 95 specialty services, VUMC offers the most comprehensive range of patient care services of any hospital in the area. VUMC's reputation for excellence has made Vanderbilt a major patient referral center for the Mid-South.

UNIQUE SERVICES

VUMC offers many services that are unique to the region. VUMC has the region's only **Level I trauma center, burn center, voice center, poison control center and liver transplant program**. VUMC's cancer center, the **Vanderbilt-Ingram Cancer Center** is the only National Cancer Institute (NCI)-designated **Comprehensive Cancer Center** in Tennessee and one of only 38 nationwide. Opened in February of 2004, **Vanderbilt Children's Hospital** is the only comprehensive provider of Children's specialty services in Middle Tennessee. VCH offers the region's only level IV neonatal intensive care unit, pediatric cardiology and the only emergency department totally devoted to children.

ACCREDITATION, COMMENDATIONS AND NATIONAL RECOGNITION

Vanderbilt Medical Center has been recognized as one of the *U.S. News & World Report* 17 Honor Roll hospitals, and for nine consecutive years is ranked among the nation's *top 50* American hospitals in more than 9 specialties including: **Cancer; Ear Nose and Throat, Hormonal Disorders, Gynecology, Kidney Disease, Neurology and Neurosurgery, Orthopaedics; Respiratory Care** and **Urology**. Solucient has again named Vanderbilt among the nation's *100 Top Hospitals* list. For the fourth year in a row, VUMC is the top hospital in the **National Research Corporation's** annual survey and earned the **NRC's Consumer Choice Award**. Vanderbilt is fully accredited by the JCAHO.

Wake Forest University Baptist
MEDICAL CENTER ®

Medical Center Boulevard • Winston-Salem, NC 27157
Health On-Call® (Patient access) 1-800-446-2255
PAL® (Physician-to-physician calls) 1-800-277-7654
www.wfubmc.edu • www.brennerchildrens.org • www.besthealth.com

OVERVIEW

Wake Forest University Baptist Medical Center encompasses **North Carolina Baptist Hospital**, a tertiary care facility ranked among the nation's best, and **Wake Forest University School of Medicine**, whose reputation for excellence attracts some of the nation's top doctors to its faculty practice. A major research center, Wake Forest Baptist is renowned for state-of-the-art medical treatment and technology, innovation and teaching excellence.

WORLD-CLASS CARE

U.S.News & World Report ranks N.C. Baptist Hospital of Wake Forest University Baptist Medical Center among the nation's top 50 hospitals in six specialties (July '04). Services include: Brenner Children's Hospital, offering highly specialized neonatal and pediatric care in a new, child-friendly facility; the Heart Center, renowned for innovative diagnostic technologies and treatments, and transplant services; the NCI-designated Comprehensive Cancer Center of WFU, offering N.C.'s only Gamma Knife and other state-of-the-art treatments in a new outpatient setting; and Neurology and Neurosurgery Services, including Stroke, ALS and Epilepsy Centers and leading edge treatments such as deep brain stimulator implants for Parkinson's disease. The Medical Center is home to North Carolina's only Level I Adult and Pediatric Trauma Center accredited by the American College of Surgeons and handles more trauma cases than any other N.C. hospital.

RESEARCH

With outside research funding exceeding $186 million and nearly 1,000 research studies and clinical trials underway, Wake Forest Baptist is expanding frontiers of medical knowledge. Outstanding centers include: the Comprehensive Cancer Center, with more than 220 clinical trials; a highly active, NIH-funded General Clinical Research Center; Center for Human Genomics; Centers for Neurobehavioral Study of Alcohol and Neurobiological Investigation of Drug Abuse; Claude D. Pepper Older Americans Center and the Hypertension and Vascular Disease Center, to name a few.

INNOVATION

Providing patients with the latest technology and treatment - such as North Carolina's only Gamma Knife - is a Wake Forest University Baptist Medical Center tradition. Experts here were first in the world to successfully use magnetic resonance imaging to diagnose heart blockages and to treat a brain tumor patient with a new GliaSite radiation therapy, as well as first in the U.S. to detect prostate cancer with ultrasound.

CONSUMER CHOICE

In an independent National Research Corporation survey, Piedmont Triad residents named Wake Forest University Baptist Medical Center as their preferred hospital since 1999, citing the best doctors, nurses and overall care. Patient satisfaction scores are in the top 1% in the nation, according to Press Ganey reports (2003). Outstanding nursing earned Wake Forest Baptist one of the nation's first 15 Magnet Awards for nursing excellence, awarded by the American Nurses Credentialing Center.

a world of difference in the world of medicine™

To make an appointment or find a specialist at Wake Forest University Baptist Medical Center, call
Health On-Call® at 1-800-446-2255.

SECTION III

PHYSICIAN LISTINGS BY MEDICAL SPECIALTY

COLON & RECTAL SURGERY

A colon and rectal surgeon is trained to diagnose and treat various diseases of the intestinal tract, colon, rectum, anal canal and perianal area by medical and surgical means. This specialist also deals with other organs and tissues (such as the liver, urinary and female reproductive system) involved with primary intestinal disease.

Colon and rectal surgeons have the expertise to diagnose and often manage anorectal conditions such as hemorrhoids, fissures (painful tears in the anal lining), abscesses and fistulae (infections located around the anus and rectum) in the office setting. They also treat problems of the intestine and colon and perform endoscopic procedures to evaluate and treat problems such as cancer, polyps (pre-cancerous growths) and inflammatory conditions.

Training Required: *Six Years (including general surgery)*

PHYSICIAN LISTINGS

NYU Medical Center
550 1st Avenue (at 31st St
New York, NY 10016
Physician Referral:
1-888-7-NYU-MED
www.nyumc.org

SCHOOL OF
MEDICINE

NEW YORK UNIVERSITY

NYU Cancer Institute
at the **NYU Clinical Cancer Center**
160 East 34th Street
New York, NY 1001
1-212-731-6000
www.nyuci.org

COLON AND RECTAL SURGERY

The gastrointestinal surgery program is a division of the Department of Surgery, whose surgeons perform over 5,000 outpatient and inpatient procedures each year using laser, laparoscopic, endoscopic, and other minimally invasive techniques. It maintains a nationally-regarded residency training program in Surgery through the NYU School of Medicine. Candidates for gastrointestinal surgery receive same-day care that includes imaging, radiation, and nutritional support.

The program provides an integrated team approach based on communication between surgeons and caregivers. The result is cancer care in a full service environment that offers a complete, patient-centered approach.

VIRTUAL COLONOSCOPIES – a noninvasive method of cancer screening that uses the same techniques as a CT scan

LAPAROSCOPIC TECHNIQUES – surgeons use tiny incisions to remove a segment of the colon; this dramatically speeds recovery and reduces the need for pain medication

LIVER LESIONS – these are effectively treated using painless radiofrequency ablation

Specialists at the NCI-designated NYU Cancer Institute seek to enhance and coordinate the extensive resources of NYU Medical Center to optimize research, treatment, and the ultimate control of cancer.

Our new NYU Clinical Cancer Center is located at 160 East 34th Street. This state-of-the-art 13-level, 85,000-square-foot building serves as "home base" for patients, by providing the latest cancer prevention, screening, diagnostic treatment, genetic counseling, and support services in one central location. The NYU Clinical Cancer Center stands to dramatically improve the lives of people with cancer. As part of NYU Medical Center, patients can access a variety of other non-cancer services throughout the institution.

PHYSICIAN REFERRAL
1-888-7-NYU-MED
(1-888-769-8633)
www.nyumc.org
www.nyuci.org

COLON & RECTAL SURGERY

New England

Bleday, Ronald MD [CRS] - **Spec Exp:** Colon Cancer; **Hospital:** Brigham & Women's Hosp (page 87); **Address:** Brigham & Women's Hosp, Dept Genl Surg, 75 Francis St, ASB II, Boston, MA 02115; **Phone:** 617-732-8460; **Board Cert:** Surgery 99; Colon & Rectal Surgery 03; **Med School:** McGill Univ 82; **Resid:** Surgery, Brown Univ-RI Hosp 89; Surgical Oncology, Brigham & Women's Hosp 86; **Fellow:** Endoscopy, Mass Genl Hosp; Colon & Rectal Surgery, Univ Minn 91; **Fac Appt:** Asst Prof S, Harvard Med Sch

Coller, John MD [CRS] - **Spec Exp:** Colon Cancer; Laparoscopic Surgery; Incontinence-Fecal; **Hospital:** Lahey Clin; **Address:** Colon & Rectal Surg, 41 Mall Rd, Burlington, MA 01805; **Phone:** 781-744-8581; **Board Cert:** Surgery 73; Colon & Rectal Surgery 73; **Med School:** Univ Pennsylvania 65; **Resid:** Surgery, Hosp Univ Penn 72; **Fellow:** Colon & Rectal Surgery, Lahey Clinic Fdn 73; **Fac Appt:** Asst Clin Prof S, Tufts Univ

Longo, Walter E MD [CRS] - **Spec Exp:** Colon & Rectal Cancer; Gastrointestinal Surgery; Inflammatory Bowel Disease; **Hospital:** Yale - New Haven Hosp; **Address:** Yale Univ Sch Med, Dept Surg, Box 208062, New Haven, CT 06520-8062; **Phone:** 203-785-2616; **Board Cert:** Surgery 01; Colon & Rectal Surgery 04; **Med School:** NY Med Coll 84; **Resid:** Surgery, Yale-New Haven Hosp 87; **Fellow:** Gastrointestinal Surgery, Yale-New Haven Hosp 90; Colon & Rectal Surgery, Cleveland Clinic 91; **Fac Appt:** Prof S, Yale Univ

Opelka, Frank MD [CRS] - **Spec Exp:** Colon & Rectal Cancer; Crohn's Disease & Ulcerative Colitis; Diverticulitis; **Hospital:** Beth Israel Deaconess Med Ctr - Boston; **Address:** BIDMC, Div Colon & Rectal Surg, 330 Brookline Ave, Stoneman 932, Boston, MA 02215; **Phone:** 617-667-4159; **Board Cert:** Colon & Rectal Surgery 02; **Med School:** Univ Hlth Sci/Chicago Med Sch 81; **Resid:** Surgery, Eisenhower AMC 86; Colon & Rectal Surgery, Ochsner Clinic 90

Roberts, Patricia L MD [CRS] - **Spec Exp:** Diverticulitis; Colon & Rectal Cancer; Inflammatory Bowel Disease; **Hospital:** Lahey Clin; **Address:** 41 Mall Rd, Burlington, MA 01805; **Phone:** 781-744-8243; **Board Cert:** Surgery 96; Colon & Rectal Surgery 03; **Med School:** Boston Univ 81; **Resid:** Surgery, Boston Univ-Boston City Hosp 86; **Fellow:** Colon & Rectal Surgery, Lahey Clinic 88; **Fac Appt:** Assoc Prof S, Tufts Univ

Schoetz, David MD [CRS] - **Spec Exp:** Inflammatory Bowel Disease/Crohn's; Colon & Rectal Cancer; Incontinence-Fecal; **Hospital:** Lahey Clin; **Address:** Lahey Clinic Med Ctr, Dept Colon & Rectal Surg, 41 Mall Rd, Burlington, MA 01805-0001; **Phone:** 781-744-8889; **Board Cert:** Surgery 01; Colon & Rectal Surgery 83; **Med School:** Med Coll Wisc 74; **Resid:** Surgery, Boston Univ Med Ctr. 81; **Fellow:** Colon & Rectal Surgery, Lahey Clin Med Ctr 82; **Fac Appt:** Prof S, Tufts Univ

Shellito, Paul C MD [CRS] - **Spec Exp:** Colon & Rectal Cancer; Ulcerative Colitis; Anorectal Disorders; **Hospital:** Mass Genl Hosp; **Address:** 15 Parkman St, Ste 336, Boston, MA 02114-3117; **Phone:** 617-724-0365; **Board Cert:** Surgery 92; Colon & Rectal Surgery 94; **Med School:** Harvard Med Sch 77; **Resid:** Surgery, Mass Genl Hosp 83; Surgery, Auckland Univ Med Sch; **Fellow:** Colon & Rectal Surgery, Univ Minn 85; **Fac Appt:** Asst Prof S, Harvard Med Sch

Mid Atlantic

Eisenstat, Theodore E MD [CRS] - **Spec Exp:** Colon Cancer; Inflammatory Bowel Disease; **Hospital:** Robert Wood Johnson Univ Hosp - New Brunswick (page 106); **Address:** 3900 Park Ave, Ste 101, Edison, NJ 08820-3032; **Phone:** 732-494-6640; **Board Cert:** Surgery 74; Colon & Rectal Surgery 94; **Med School:** NY Med Coll 68; **Resid:** Surgery, Thomas Jefferson Univ Hosp 71; Surgery, Pennsylvania Hosp 73; **Fellow:** Colon & Rectal Surgery, Muhlenberg Med Ctr 78; **Fac Appt:** Clin Prof S, UMDNJ-RW Johnson Med Sch

Fry, Robert Dean MD [CRS] - **Spec Exp:** Rectal Cancer; Inflammatory Bowel Disease/Crohn's; Colon Cancer; **Hospital:** Hosp Univ Penn - UPHS (page 113); **Address:** Hosp Univ Pennsylvania, Div Colon & Rectal Surgery, 3400 Spruce St, 4 Silverstein, Philadelphia, PA 19104; **Phone:** 215-662-2664; **Board Cert:** Surgery 96; Colon & Rectal Surgery 98; **Med School:** Washington Univ, St Louis 72; **Resid:** Surgery, Jewish Hosp 77; **Fellow:** Colon & Rectal Surgery, Cleveland Clin Fdn 78; **Fac Appt:** Prof S, Univ Pennsylvania

Gorfine, Stephen MD [CRS] - **Spec Exp:** Anal Fissure; Hemorrhoids; Rectal Cancer; **Hospital:** Mount Sinai Med Ctr (page 101); **Address:** 25 E 69th St, New York, NY 10021-4925; **Phone:** 212-517-8600; **Board Cert:** Internal Medicine 81; Surgery 96; Colon & Rectal Surgery 88; **Med School:** Univ Mass Sch Med 78; **Resid:** Internal Medicine, Mount Sinai Hosp 81; Surgery, Mount Sinai Hosp 85; **Fellow:** Colon & Rectal Surgery, Ferguson Hosp 87; **Fac Appt:** Clin Prof S, Mount Sinai Sch Med

Guillem, Jose MD [CRS] - **Spec Exp:** Colon & Rectal Cancer; Anal Sphincter/Bladder Preservation; Colon & Rectal Cancer-Familial; **Hospital:** Meml Sloan Kettering Cancer Ctr (page 100); **Address:** Meml Sloan Kettering Cancer Ctr, 1275 York Ave, rm C1077, New York, NY 10021; **Phone:** 212-639-8278; **Board Cert:** Colon & Rectal Surgery 04; Surgery 04; **Med School:** Yale Univ 83; **Resid:** Surgery, Columbia-Presby Med Ctr 90; **Fellow:** Colon & Rectal Surgery, Lahey Clinic 91; **Fac Appt:** Assoc Prof CRS, Cornell Univ-Weill Med Coll

Medich, David MD [CRS] - **Spec Exp:** Colon & Rectal Cancer; Ulcerative Colitis; Inflammatory Bowel Disease/Crohn's; **Hospital:** Allegheny General Hosp; **Address:** 320 E North Ave, Fl 5 South Tower, Pittsburgh, PA 15212; **Phone:** 412-359-3901; **Board Cert:** Surgery 94; Colon & Rectal Surgery 95; **Med School:** Ohio State Univ 87; **Resid:** Surgery, Univ Pittsburgh Med Ctr 90; **Fellow:** Research, Univ Pittsburgh 93; Colon & Rectal Surgery, Cleveland Clin Fdn 94; **Fac Appt:** Assoc Prof CRS, Drexel Univ Coll Med

Milsom, Jeffrey W MD [CRS] - **Spec Exp:** Inflammatory Bowel Disease; Laparoscopic Colon & Rectal Surgery; Colon & Rectal Cancer; **Hospital:** NY-Presby Hosp - NY Weill Cornell Med Ctr (page 103); **Address:** Weill Med Coll, Div Colon & Rectal Surgery, 525 E 68th St, Payson 717A, Box 172, New York, NY 10021; **Phone:** 212-746-6030; **Board Cert:** Surgery 92; Colon & Rectal Surgery 86; **Med School:** Univ Pittsburgh 79; **Resid:** Surgery, Roosevelt Hosp 81; Surgery, Univ Virginia Med Ctr 84; **Fellow:** Colon & Rectal Surgery, Ferguson Hosp 85; **Fac Appt:** Prof S, Columbia P&S

Rombeau, John L MD [CRS] - **Spec Exp:** Colon & Rectal Cancer; Crohn's Disease; Ulcerative Colitis; **Hospital:** Hosp Univ Penn - UPHS (page 113); **Address:** Hosp Univ Penn, Dept Surg, 3400 Spruce St, 4 Silverstein, Philadelphia, PA 19104; **Phone:** 215-662-2050; **Board Cert:** Surgery 92; Colon & Rectal Surgery 77; **Med School:** Loma Linda Univ 67; **Resid:** Surgery, Good Samaritan Hosp 71; Surgery, LAC-USC Med Ctr 75; **Fellow:** Colon & Rectal Surgery, Cleveland Clinic 76; **Fac Appt:** Prof S, Univ Pennsylvania

Smith, Lee MD [CRS] - **Spec Exp:** Colon & Rectal Cancer; Inflammatory Bowel Disease/Crohn's; Anorectal Disorders; **Hospital:** Washington Hosp Ctr; **Address:** 106 Irving St NW, Ste 2100, Washington, DC 20010-2975; **Phone:** 202-877-8484; **Board Cert:** Surgery 71; Colon & Rectal Surgery 73; **Med School:** UCSF 62; **Resid:** Surgery, Naval Hosp 70; Colon & Rectal Surgery, Univ Minn 73; **Fac Appt:** Prof S, Georgetown Univ

Steinhagen, Randolph MD [CRS] - **Spec Exp:** Colostomy Avoidance; Colon & Rectal Cancer; Inflammatory Bowel Disease/Crohn's; **Hospital:** Mount Sinai Med Ctr (page 101); **Address:** Surgical Associates, 5 E 98th St Fl 11, Box 1263, New York, NY 10029-6501; **Phone:** 212-241-3547; **Board Cert:** Surgery 02; Colon & Rectal Surgery 85; **Med School:** Wayne State Univ 77; **Resid:** Surgery, Mount Sinai Hosp 82; **Fellow:** Colon & Rectal Surgery, Cleveland Clinic 83; **Fac Appt:** Assoc Prof S, Mount Sinai Sch Med

Whelan, Richard L MD [CRS] - **Spec Exp:** Laparoscopic Surgery; Colon Cancer; **Hospital:** NY-Presby Hosp - Columbia Presby Med Ctr (page 103); **Address:** 161 Ft Washington Ave, rm 820, New York, NY 10032; **Phone:** 212-342-1155; **Board Cert:** Surgery 97; Colon & Rectal Surgery 89; **Med School:** Columbia P&S 82; **Resid:** Surgery, Columbia Presby Hosp 87; **Fellow:** Colon & Rectal Surgery, Univ Minn Med Ctr 88; **Fac Appt:** Assoc Clin Prof S, Columbia P&S

Wong, Westley Douglas MD [CRS] - **Spec Exp:** Endorectal Ultrasound; Anal Disorders; Rectal Cancer/Sphincter Preservation; **Hospital:** Meml Sloan Kettering Cancer Ctr (page 100); **Address:** Meml Sloan Kettering Cancer Ctr, 1275 York Ave, rm C-1067, New York, NY 10021-6094; **Phone:** 212-639-5117; **Board Cert:** Surgery 97; Colon & Rectal Surgery 04; **Med School:** Canada 72; **Resid:** Surgery, Univ Manitoba Hosp 77; **Fellow:** Colon & Rectal Surgery, Univ Minn Med Ctr 84; **Fac Appt:** Assoc Prof S, Cornell Univ-Weill Med Coll

Southeast

Cohen, Alfred M MD [CRS] - **Spec Exp:** Colon & Rectal Cancer; Liver Cancer; **Hospital:** Univ Kentucky Med Ctr; **Address:** Markey Cancer Center, 800 Rose St, Ste 140, Lexington, KY 40536; **Phone:** 859-323-6556; **Board Cert:** Surgery 76; **Med School:** Johns Hopkins Univ 67; **Resid:** Surgery, Mass General Hosp 73; Surgical Oncology, Natl Cancer Inst 75; **Fac Appt:** Prof S, Univ KY Coll Med

Foley, Eugene F MD [CRS] - **Spec Exp:** Colon & Rectal Surgery; Colon & Rectal Cancer; Ulcerative Colitis; **Hospital:** Univ Virginia Med Ctr; **Address:** Univ Va Hlth Sys, Dept Surg, PO Box 800709, Charlottesville, VA 22908; **Phone:** 434-924-9304; **Board Cert:** Surgery 93; Colon & Rectal Surgery 94; **Med School:** Harvard Med Sch 85; **Resid:** Surgery, New England Deaconess Hosp 91; **Fellow:** Colon & Rectal Surgery, Lahey Clinic 93; **Fac Appt:** Assoc Prof S, Univ VA Sch Med

Galandiuk, Susan MD [CRS] - **Spec Exp:** Colon & Rectal Cancer; Inflammatory Bowel Disease/Crohn's; **Hospital:** Univ of Louisville Hosp; **Address:** Univ Surg Assoc PSC, 6001 S Floyd St, Louisville, KY 40202; **Phone:** 502-583-8303; **Board Cert:** Surgery 98; Colon & Rectal Surgery 99; **Med School:** Germany 82; **Resid:** Surgery, Cleveland Clinic Fdtn 88; **Fellow:** Research, Univ Louisville Hosp 89; Colon & Rectal Surgery, Mayo Clinic 90; **Fac Appt:** Prof CRS, Univ Louisville Sch Med

Golub, Richard MD [CRS] - **Spec Exp:** Colon & Rectal Cancer; Laparoscopic Surgery; Hemorrhoids; **Hospital:** Sarasota Meml Hosp; **Address:** 3333 Cattlemen Rd, Ste 206, Sarasota, FL 34232; **Phone:** 941-341-0042; **Board Cert:** Surgery 00; Colon & Rectal Surgery 03; **Med School:** Albert Einstein Coll Med 84; **Resid:** Surgery, Univ Hosp Stony Brook 90; **Fellow:** Colon & Rectal Surgery, Grant Medical Center 91

Larach, Sergio MD [CRS] - **Spec Exp:** Colon Cancer; Inflammatory Bowel Disease/Crohn's; **Hospital:** Orlando Regl Med Ctr; **Address:** 2501 N Orange Ave, Ste 309, Orlando, FL 32804; **Phone:** 407-228-4141; **Board Cert:** Colon & Rectal Surgery 79; **Med School:** Chile 68; **Resid:** Surgery, Hosp de Salvador 73; Surgery, Orlando Reg Med Ctr 76; **Fellow:** Colon & Rectal Surgery, Univ Texas 77; **Fac Appt:** Assoc Prof S, Univ Fla Coll Med

Nogueras, Juan J MD [CRS] - **Spec Exp:** Colon & Rectal Cancer; Inflammatory Bowel Disease/Crohn's; Incontinence-Fecal; **Hospital:** Cleveland Clin - Weston (page 92); **Address:** Cleveland Clinic, Dept Colorectal Surgery, 2950 Cleveland Clinic Blvd, Weston, FL 33331; **Phone:** 954-659-5251; **Board Cert:** Surgery 97; Colon & Rectal Surgery 93; **Med School:** Jefferson Med Coll 82; **Resid:** Surgery, Columbia Presby Med Ctr 87; **Fellow:** Colon & Rectal Surgery, Univ Minn 91

Vernava III, Anthony M MD [CRS] - **Spec Exp:** Colon & Rectal Cancer; Incontinence-Fecal; Inflammatory Bowel Disease; **Hospital:** Cleveland Clin - Naples (page 92); **Address:** Cleveland Clinic, Dept Surgery, 6101 Pine Ridge Rd, Naples, FL 34119; **Phone:** 239-348-4000; **Board Cert:** Surgery 97; Colon & Rectal Surgery 89; **Med School:** St Louis Univ 82; **Resid:** Surgery, St Louis Univ Med Ctr 88; Colon & Rectal Surgery, Univ Minnesota Med Ctr 89; **Fellow:** Colon & Rectal Surgery, St Marks Hosp 90; **Fac Appt:** Prof S, Univ Fla Coll Med

Wexner, Steven MD [CRS] - **Spec Exp:** Rectal Cancer; Inflammatory Bowel Disease/Crohn's; Laparoscopic Surgery; **Hospital:** Cleveland Clin - Weston (page 92); **Address:** 2950 Cleveland Clinic Blvd, Weston, FL 33331-3609; **Phone:** 954-659-5251; **Board Cert:** Surgery 96; Colon & Rectal Surgery 89; **Med School:** Cornell Univ-Weill Med Coll 82; **Resid:** Surgery, Roosevelt Hosp 87; **Fellow:** Colon & Rectal Surgery, Univ Minn 88; **Fac Appt:** Prof S, Univ S Fla Coll Med

Midwest

Abcarian, Herand MD [CRS] - **Spec Exp:** Rectal Cancer/Sphincter Preservation; Inflammatory Bowel Disease; Anorectal Disorders & Incontinence; **Hospital:** Univ of IL Med Ctr at Chicago; **Address:** 675 W NW Ave, rm 406, Melrose Park, IL 60160; **Phone:** 708-450-5075; **Board Cert:** Surgery 72; Colon & Rectal Surgery 72; **Med School:** Iran 65; **Resid:** Surgery, Cook County Hosp 71; Colon & Rectal Surgery, Cook County Hosp 72; **Fac Appt:** Prof S, Univ IL Coll Med

Fleshman, James MD [CRS] - **Spec Exp:** Colon & Rectal Cancer; Laparoscopic Surgery; Inflammatory Bowel Disease; **Hospital:** Barnes-Jewish Hosp (page 85); **Address:** Washington Univ Sch Med, 660 S Euclid Ave, Box 8109, St Louis, MO 63110; **Phone:** 314-454-7177; **Board Cert:** Colon & Rectal Surgery 88; Surgery 96; **Med School:** Washington Univ, St Louis 80; **Resid:** Surgery, Jewish Hospital 86; **Fellow:** Colon & Rectal Surgery, Univ Toronto 87; **Fac Appt:** Prof S, Washington Univ, St Louis

Kodner, Ira J MD [CRS] - **Spec Exp:** Colon & Rectal Cancer; Inflammatory Bowel Disease/Crohn's; Laparoscopic Surgery; **Hospital:** Barnes-Jewish Hosp (page 85); **Address:** Wash Univ Sch Med, Div Colon & Rectal Surgery, 660 S Euclid Ave, Queeny Twr, Box 8109, St. Louis, MO 63110; **Phone:** 314-454-7177; **Board Cert:** Surgery 75; Colon & Rectal Surgery 75; **Med School:** Washington Univ, St Louis 67; **Resid:** Surgery, Barnes-Jewish Hosp 74; **Fellow:** Colon & Rectal Surgery, Cleveland Clinic 75; **Fac Appt:** Prof S, Washington Univ, St Louis

Lavery, Ian C MD [CRS] - **Spec Exp:** Colon & Rectal Cancer; Inflammatory Bowel Disease; Pediatric Gastrointestinal Surgery; **Hospital:** Cleveland Clin Fdn (page 92); **Address:** Cleveland Clinic, Desk A30, 9500 Euclid Ave, Cleveland, OH 44195; **Phone:** 216-444-6930; **Board Cert:** Colon & Rectal Surgery 98; **Med School:** Australia 67; **Resid:** Surgery, Princess Alexandra Hosp 74; Colon & Rectal Surgery, Cleveland Clinic 77

MacKeigan, John MD [CRS] - **Spec Exp:** Rectal Cancer; Anal Surgery; Ulcerative Colitis; **Hospital:** Spectrum Hlth Blodgett Campus; **Address:** The Ferguson Clinic, 4100   Lake Dr SE, Ste 205, Grand Rapids, MI 49546-8292; **Phone:** 616-356-4100; **Board Cert:** Colon & Rectal Surgery 74; **Med School:** Dalhousie Univ 69; **Resid:** Surgery, Dalhousie Univ 73; Colon & Rectal Surgery, Ferguson Hosp 74; **Fac Appt:** Assoc Prof S, Mich State Univ

Madoff, Robert D MD [CRS] - **Spec Exp:** Colon & Rectal Cancer; Inflammatory Bowel Disease; Incontinence/Pelvic Floor Disorders; **Hospital:** Fairview-Univ Med Ctr - Univ Campus; **Address:** 420 Delaware St SE, MMC 450, Minneapolis, MN 55455; **Phone:** 651-626-6666; **Board Cert:** Surgery 95; Colon & Rectal Surgery 02; **Med School:** Columbia P&S 79; **Resid:** Surgery, Univ Minn Hosps 87; **Fellow:** Colon & Rectal Surgery, Univ Minn Hosps 88; **Fac Appt:** Prof S, Univ Minn

Nelson, Heidi MD [CRS] - **Spec Exp:** Colon & Rectal Cancer; Gastrointestinal Cancer; **Hospital:** Mayo Med Ctr & Clin - Rochester; **Address:** Mayo Clinic, Div Colon & Rectal Surg, 200 First St SW, Rochester, MN 55905; **Phone:** 507-284-3329; **Board Cert:** Surgery 95; Colon & Rectal Surgery 89; **Med School:** Univ Wash 81; **Resid:** Surgery, Oregon Hlth Sci Univ Hosp 87; Colon & Rectal Surgery, Oregon Hlth Sci Univ Hosp 85; **Fellow:** Colon & Rectal Surgery, Mayo Clinic 88; **Fac Appt:** Prof S, Mayo Med Sch

Nivatvongs, Santhat MD [CRS] - **Spec Exp:** Colon & Rectal Cancer; Anorectal Disorders; Inflammatory Bowel Disease; **Hospital:** Mayo Med Ctr & Clin - Rochester; **Address:** Mayo Clinic, Div Colon & Rectal Surg, 200 First St SW, Rochester, MN 55905-0002; **Phone:** 507-284-4985; **Board Cert:** Surgery 71; Colon & Rectal Surgery 71; **Med School:** Thailand 64; **Resid:** Surgery, Harper Hosp 67; Surgery, United Hosp 70; **Fellow:** Colon & Rectal Surgery, Univ Minn 71; **Fac Appt:** Prof S, Mayo Med Sch

Pemberton, John MD [CRS] - **Spec Exp:** Rectal Surgery; Inflammatory Bowel Disease/Crohn's; Colon & Rectal Cancer; **Hospital:** St Mary's Hosp - Rochester; **Address:** Mayo Clinic, Div Colon & Rectal Surg, 200 First St SW, Gonda 9-S, Rochester, MN 55905; **Phone:** 507-284-2359; **Board Cert:** Surgery 01; Colon & Rectal Surgery 85; **Med School:** Tulane Univ 76; **Resid:** Surgery, Mayo Clinic 83; **Fellow:** Colon & Rectal Surgery, Mayo Clinic 84; **Fac Appt:** Prof S, Mayo Med Sch

Rothenberger, David A MD [CRS] - **Spec Exp:** Colon & Rectal Cancer; **Hospital:** Fairview-Univ Med Ctr - Univ Campus; **Address:** Fairview-UMC, Dept Colon & Rectal Surg, 420 Delaware St SE, MMC 450, Minneapolis, MN 55455; **Phone:** 612-625-3288; **Board Cert:** Colon & Rectal Surgery 95; **Med School:** Tufts Univ 73; **Resid:** Surgery, St Paul-Ramsey Med Ctr 78; **Fellow:** Colon & Rectal Surgery, Univ Minnesota Hosps 79; **Fac Appt:** Clin Prof S, Univ Minn

Saclarides, Theodore John MD [CRS] - **Spec Exp:** Rectal Cancer/Sphincter Preservation; Incontinence-Fecal; Inflammatory Bowel Disease; **Hospital:** Rush Univ Med Ctr; **Address:** Univ Surgeons, 1725 W Harrison St, Ste 810, Chicago, IL 60612-3832; **Phone:** 312-942-6543; **Board Cert:** Surgery 96; Colon & Rectal Surgery 89; **Med School:** Univ Miami Sch Med 82; **Resid:** Surgery, Rush Presby-St Luke's Hosp 87; **Fellow:** Colon & Rectal Surgery, Mayo Clinic 88; **Fac Appt:** Prof S, Rush Med Coll

Senagore, Anthony MD [CRS] - **Spec Exp:** Laparoscopic Surgery; Colon & Rectal Cancer; Anorectal Disorders; **Hospital:** Cleveland Clin Fdn (page 92); **Address:** Cleveland Clinic Fdn, 9500 Euclid Ave, Crile Bldg, rm A30, Cleveland, OH 44195-0002; **Phone:** 216-445-7882; **Board Cert:** Surgery 95; Colon & Rectal Surgery 01; **Med School:** Mich State Univ 81; **Resid:** Surgery, Butterworth Hospital 87; Colon & Rectal Surgery, Ferguson Hospital 89

Stryker, Steven J MD [CRS] - **Spec Exp:** Colon & Rectal Cancer; Inflammatory Bowel Disease; Laparoscopic Surgery; **Hospital:** Northwestern Meml Hosp; **Address:** 676 N St Clair St, Ste 1525A, Chicago, IL 60611-2862; **Phone:** 312-943-5427; **Board Cert:** Surgery 92; Colon & Rectal Surgery 86; **Med School:** Northwestern Univ 78; **Resid:** Surgery, Northwestern Meml Hosp 83; **Fellow:** Colon & Rectal Surgery, Mayo Clinic 85; **Fac Appt:** Assoc Clin Prof S, Northwestern Univ

Wolff, Bruce MD [CRS] - **Spec Exp:** Inflammatory Bowel Disease; Crohn's Disease; Colon & Rectal Cancer; **Hospital:** Mayo Med Ctr & Clin - Rochester; **Address:** Mayo Clinic, Div Colon & Rectal Surg, 200 First St SW, Rochester, MN 55905; **Phone:** 507-284-2472; **Board Cert:** Surgery 00; Colon & Rectal Surgery 83; **Med School:** Duke Univ 73; **Resid:** Surgery, Cornell Med Ctr 81; **Fellow:** Colon & Rectal Surgery, Mayo Med Sch 82; **Fac Appt:** Prof S, Mayo Med Sch

Great Plains and Mountains

Thorson, Alan MD [CRS] - **Spec Exp:** Colon & Rectal Cancer; Laparoscopic Surgery; Incontinence-Fecal; **Hospital:** Nebraska Meth Hosp; **Address:** 9850 Nicholas St, Ste 100, Omaha, NE 68114-2191; **Phone:** 402-343-1122; **Board Cert:** Surgery 94; Colon & Rectal Surgery 99; **Med School:** Univ Nebr Coll Med 79; **Resid:** Surgery, Univ Nebraska 84; Colon & Rectal Surgery, Univ Minn 85; **Fac Appt:** Assoc Clin Prof S, Creighton Univ

Southwest

Bailey, Harold Randolph MD [CRS] - **Spec Exp:** Rectal Cancer/Sphincter Preservation; Inflammatory Bowel Disease; Incontinence-Fecal; **Hospital:** Methodist Hosp - Houston; **Address:** Colon & Rectal Clinic, Smith Twr, 6550 Fannin St, Ste 2307, Houston, TX 77030-2717; **Phone:** 713-790-9250; **Board Cert:** Surgery 74; Colon & Rectal Surgery 94; **Med School:** Univ Tex SW, Dallas 68; **Resid:** Surgery, Hermann Hosp-Univ Tex Med Sch 73; **Fellow:** Colon & Rectal Surgery, Ferguson-Droste- Hosp 74; **Fac Appt:** Clin Prof S, Univ Tex, Houston

Beck, David E MD [CRS] - **Spec Exp:** Colon & Rectal Cancer; Minimally Invasive Surgery; Inflammatory Bowel Disease; **Hospital:** Ochsner Fdn Hosp; **Address:** Ochsner Clinic Fdn, Colorectal Surgery, 04East, 1514 Jefferson Hwy, 4th Fl, New Orleans, LA 70121; **Phone:** 504-842-4060; **Board Cert:** Colon & Rectal Surgery 87; **Med School:** Univ Miami Sch Med 79; **Resid:** Surgery, Wilford Hall USAF Med Ctr 84; **Fellow:** Colon & Rectal Surgery, Cleveland Clinic Fdn 86; **Fac Appt:** Assoc Prof S, Louisiana State Univ

Huber Jr, Philip J MD [CRS] - **Spec Exp:** Colon & Rectal Cancer; Inflammatory Bowel Disease; **Hospital:** St Paul Univ Hosp; **Address:** 5920 Forest Park Rd, Ste 500, Dallas, TX 75235; **Phone:** 214-956-6802; **Board Cert:** Surgery 97; Colon & Rectal Surgery 93; **Med School:** Columbia P&S 72; **Resid:** Surgery, Parkland Hosp 77; Colon & Rectal Surgery, Presby Hosp

West Coast and Pacific

Beart Jr, Robert W MD [CRS] - **Spec Exp:** Colon & Rectal Cancer; Inflammatory Bowel Disease/Crohn's; **Hospital:** USC Norris Canc Comp Ctr; **Address:** 1441 Eastlake Ave, Ste 7418, Los Angeles, CA 90033; **Phone:** 323-865-3690; **Board Cert:** Surgery 93; Colon & Rectal Surgery 95; **Med School:** Harvard Med Sch 71; **Resid:** Surgery, Univ Colo Med Ctr 76; Colon & Rectal Surgery, Mayo Clinic 78; **Fellow:** Transplant Surgery, Univ Colo Med Ctr 75; **Fac Appt:** Prof S, USC Sch Med

Stamos, Michael J MD **(CRS)** - **Spec Exp:** Rectal Cancer/Sphincter Preservation; Colon Cancer; Laparoscopic Surgery; **Hospital:** UC Irvine Med Ctr; **Address:** UC Irivne Med Ctr - Div Colon & Rectal Surg, 101 The City Drive, Bldg 55 - Ste 110, Rt 81, Orange, CA 92868; **Phone:** 714-456-8511; **Board Cert:** Surgery 00; Colon & Rectal Surgery 03; **Med School:** Case West Res Univ 85; **Resid:** Surgery, Jackson Meml Hosp 90; Colon & Rectal Surgery, Ochsner Clinic 91; **Fac Appt:** Prof S, UC Irvine

Volpe, Peter A MD **(CRS)** - **Spec Exp:** Colon Cancer; **Hospital:** CA Pacific Med Ctr - Pacific Campus; **Address:** 3838 California St, Ste 616, San Francisco, CA 94118; **Phone:** 415-668-0411; **Board Cert:** Surgery 70; Colon & Rectal Surgery 71; **Med School:** Ohio State Univ 61; **Resid:** Surgery, UCSF Hosps 69; Colon & Rectal Surgery, ABCRS Preceptorship 71; **Fac Appt:** Clin Prof S, UCSF

Welton, Mark L MD **(CRS)** - **Spec Exp:** Ulcerative Colitis; Crohn's Disease; Colon & Rectal Cancer & Surgery; **Hospital:** Stanford Univ Med Ctr; **Address:** Stanford Univ - Colon & Rectal Surgery, 300 Pasteur Drive, rm H 3680, Stanford, CA 94305-5655; **Phone:** 650-723-5461; **Board Cert:** Surgery 00; Colon & Rectal Surgery 05; **Med School:** UCLA 84; **Resid:** Surgery, UCLA Med Ctr 92; **Fellow:** Colon & Rectal Surgery, Barnes Jewish Hosp 93; **Fac Appt:** Assoc Prof S, Stanford Univ

DERMATOLOGY

A *dermatologist is trained to diagnose and treat pediatric and adult patients with benign and malignant disorders of the skin, mouth, external genitalia, hair and nails, as well as a number of sexually transmitted diseases. The dermatologist has had additional training and experience in the diagnosis and treatment of skin cancers, melanomas, moles and other tumors of the skin, the management of contact dermatitis and other allergic and non allergic skin disorders, and in the recognition of the skin manifestations of systemic (including internal malignancy) and infectious diseases.*

Dermatologists may have special training in dermatopathology and in the surgical techniques used in dermatology. They also have expertise in the management of cosmetic disorders of the skin such as hair loss and scars, and the skin changes associated with aging.

Training Required: *Four years*

PHYSICIAN LISTINGS

133

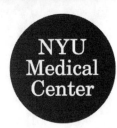

NYU Medical Center

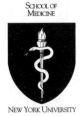

SCHOOL OF MEDICINE

NEW YORK UNIVERSITY

DERMATOLOGY:
Taking Care of Skin Problems

The Ronald O. Perelman Department of Dermatology at NYU Medical Center is recognized nationally and internationally as a leader in dermatology. Through the Charles C. Harris Skin and Cancer Pavilion, the Medical Center's general and specialty clinics, the Faculty Group Practice, and affiliated hospital facilities, the staff members of the Department provide primary and consultative dermatologic care for over 100,000 ambulatory and hospitalized patients yearly. In addition, faculty members of the Department train many students, residents and fellows each year, and conduct major research projects aimed at the most significant dermatologic problems of our day.

The expertise of NYU Medical Center's dermatologists encompasses all facets of medical, surgical, pediatric and cosmetic dermatology, including diseases of the hair, nails, and mucuous membranes. Laser surgery is performed for a wide variety of pigmented and nonpigmented skin lesions, and Mohs micrographic surgery is available for cutaneous tumors.

Dermatologists at NYU Medical Center work closely with researchers trying to better understand and help alleviate dermatologic conditions, so their care of even common dermatological problems, such as acne, eczema, psoriasis, and warts, takes advantage of the most up-to-date breakthroughs in clinical medicine and science.

AREAS OF BASIC AND CLINICAL RESEARCH

Allergic Diseases:
Hives and vasculitis

Bullous Diseases:
Epidermolysis bullosas pemphigus, and related diseases

Dermatopharmacology

Dermatopathology:
Clinical drug evaluations

Dermatologic Manifestations of Systemic Diseases

Epithelial Biology:
Psoriasis, eczema and ichthyosis

Dermatologic Surgery:
Cosmetic and cancer surgery

Hair: Alopecia and hirsutism

Immunodermatology:
Contact dermatitis

Infectious Diseases:
Bacterial, fungal, viral diseases of the skin, hair and nails including sexually transmitted diseases.

Laser: Birthmarks, skin tumors, pigmentary disorders

Oncology: Melanoma, basal cell carcinoma, squamous cell carcinoma, cutaneous lymphoma

Pediatric Dermatology:
Inherited pigmentary disorders and birthmarks

Photomedicine: Psoriasis, vitiligo, eczema and lymphoma of the skin

DERMATOLOGY
New England

Braverman, Irwin MD **[D]** - **Spec Exp:** Psoriasis; Lupus/SLE; Cutaneous Lymphoma; **Hospital:** Yale - New Haven Hosp; **Address:** Yale Dermatology, 2 Church St S Fl 3, New Haven, CT 06510; **Phone:** 203-789-1249; **Board Cert:** Dermatology 63; Dermatopathology 82; **Med School:** Yale Univ 55; **Resid:** Internal Medicine, Yale-New Haven Hosp 56; Internal Medicine, Yale-New Haven Hosp 59; **Fellow:** Dermatology, Yale-New Haven Hosp 62; **Fac Appt:** Prof D, Yale Univ

Edelson, Richard MD **[D]** - **Spec Exp:** Cutaneous T Cell Lymphoma; Skin Diseases-Immunologic; Cutaneous Lymphoma; **Hospital:** Yale - New Haven Hosp; **Address:** 800 Howard Ave, New Haven, CT 06519-1369; **Phone:** 203-785-4632; **Board Cert:** Dermatology 77; **Med School:** Yale Univ 70; **Resid:** Dermatology, Mass Genl Hosp 72; Dermatology, Natl Inst Hlth 75; **Fac Appt:** Prof D, Yale Univ

Gilchrest, Barbara MD **[D]** - **Spec Exp:** Photoaging; Melanoma; Skin Cancer; **Hospital:** Boston Med Ctr; **Address:** 609 Albany St Bldg J - Ste 507, Boston, MA 02118-2394; **Phone:** 617-638-5538; **Board Cert:** Internal Medicine 75; Dermatology 78; **Med School:** Harvard Med Sch 71; **Resid:** Internal Medicine, Boston City Hosp 73; Dermatology, Harvard Med Sch 76; **Fellow:** Photo Biology, Harvard Med Sch 75; **Fac Appt:** Prof D, Boston Univ

Leffell, David J MD **[D]** - **Spec Exp:** Mohs' Surgery; Melanoma & Skin Cancer; Skin Laser Surgery; **Hospital:** Yale - New Haven Hosp; **Address:** 40 Temple St, Ste 5A, New Haven, CT 06510; **Phone:** 203-785-3466; **Board Cert:** Internal Medicine 84; Dermatology 87; **Med School:** McGill Univ 81; **Resid:** Internal Medicine, New York Hosp 84; Dermatology, Yale-New Haven Hosp 86; **Fellow:** Dermatology, Yale-New Haven Hosp 87; Dermatologic Surgery, Univ Michigan Med Ctr 88; **Fac Appt:** Prof D, Yale Univ

Maloney, Mary MD **[D]** - **Spec Exp:** Mohs' Surgery; Skin Laser Surgery; **Hospital:** UMass Memorial Med Ctr; **Address:** Univ Mass Med Ctr, Div Derm, 281 Lincoln St Fl 4, Worcester, MA 01605; **Phone:** 508-334-5962; **Board Cert:** Dermatology 82; **Med School:** Univ VT Coll Med 77; **Resid:** Internal Medicine, Hartford Hospital 79; Dermatology, Dartmouth-Hitchcock Med Ctr 82; **Fellow:** Dermatologic Surgery, UCSF Med Ctr; **Fac Appt:** Prof D, Univ Mass Sch Med

McDonald, Charles J MD **[D]** - **Spec Exp:** Lymphoma; Autoimmune Diseases; Psoriasis; **Hospital:** Rhode Island Hosp; **Address:** RI Hospital, APC Bldg, Dept Derm, 593 Eddy St, APC-10, Providence, RI 02903-4923; **Phone:** 401-444-7959; **Board Cert:** Dermatology 66; **Med School:** Howard Univ 60; **Resid:** Internal Medicine, Hosp St Raphael 63; Dermatology, Yale New Haven Hosp 65; **Fellow:** Clinical Oncology, Yale New Haven Hosp 66; **Fac Appt:** Prof D, Brown Univ

Mihm Jr., Martin C MD **[D]** - **Spec Exp:** Melanoma & Lymphoma; Vascular Birthmarks; Dermatopathology; **Hospital:** Mass Genl Hosp; **Address:** Mass General Hosp, 55 Fruit St, Warren Bldg 827, Boston, MA 02114-2926; **Phone:** 617-724-1350; **Board Cert:** Dermatology 69; Dermatopathology 74; Anatomic Pathology 74; **Med School:** Univ Pittsburgh 61; **Resid:** Internal Medicine, Mt Sinai Hosp 64; Dermatology, Mass Genl Hosp 67; **Fellow:** Anatomic Pathology, Mass Genl Hosp 72; **Fac Appt:** Clin Prof Path, Harvard Med Sch

Sober, Arthur MD **[D]** - **Spec Exp:** Melanoma; Skin Cancer; **Hospital:** Mass Genl Hosp; **Address:** Mass General Hospital, ACC4, Rm 477, 55 Fruit St, Boston, MA 02114; **Phone:** 617-726-2914; **Board Cert:** Dermatology 75; Internal Medicine 74; **Med School:** Geo Wash Univ 68; **Resid:** Internal Medicine, Beth Israel Hosp 70; Dermatology, Mass General Hosp 74; **Fellow:** Immunology, Peter Bent Brigham Hosp 76; **Fac Appt:** Prof D, Harvard Med Sch

Mid Atlantic

Ackerman, A Bernard MD [D] - **Spec Exp:** Dermatopathology; Melanoma Consultation; Inflammatory Diseases of Skin; **Hospital:** St Luke's - Roosevelt Hosp Ctr - Roosevelt Div (page 93); **Address:** 145 E 32nd St Fl 10, New York, NY 10016; **Phone:** 212-889-6225; **Board Cert:** Dermatology 70; Dermatopathology 74; **Med School:** Columbia P&S 62; **Resid:** Dermatology, Hosp Univ Penn 67; Dermatology, Mass Genl Hosp 68; **Fellow:** Dermatopathology, Mass Genl Hosp 69

Braun III, Martin MD [D] - **Spec Exp:** Mohs' Surgery; Skin Cancer; **Hospital:** G Washington Univ Hosp; **Address:** 2112 F St NW, Ste 701, Washington, DC 20037; **Phone:** 202-293-7618; **Board Cert:** Dermatology 77; Dermatopathology 82; **Med School:** Univ MD Sch Med 70; **Resid:** Dermatology, Univ MichMed Ctr 76; **Fellow:** Mohs Surgery, Precept w/ Dr Frederic Mohs; **Fac Appt:** Clin Prof D, Geo Wash Univ

Brodland, David MD [D] - **Spec Exp:** Mohs' Surgery; Skin Cancer; Reconstructive Surgery-Skin; **Hospital:** UPMC Shadyside (page 114); **Address:** South Hills Med Bldg, 575 Coal Valley Rd, Ste 360, Clairton, PA 15025; **Phone:** 412-466-9400; **Board Cert:** Dermatology 89; **Med School:** Southern IL Univ 85; **Resid:** Dermatology, Mayo Grad Sch Med 89; **Fellow:** Mohs Surgery, John A Zitelli MD 90; **Fac Appt:** Asst Clin Prof D, Univ Pittsburgh

Bystryn, Jean-Claude MD [D] - **Spec Exp:** Melanoma; Blistering Diseases; **Hospital:** NYU Med Ctr (page 104); **Address:** 530 1st Ave, Ste 7F, New York, NY 10016; **Phone:** 212-889-3846; **Board Cert:** Dermatology 70; Clinical & Laboratory Dematologic Immunology 85; **Med School:** NYU Sch Med 62; **Resid:** Internal Medicine, Montefiore Hosp 64; Dermatology, NYU Med Ctr 69; **Fellow:** Immunology, New York Univ 72; **Fac Appt:** Prof D, NYU Sch Med

Dzubow, Leonard MD [D] - **Spec Exp:** Mohs' Surgery; Skin Laser Surgery; Reconstructive Surgery-Skin; **Hospital:** Bryn Mawr Hosp; **Address:** 101 Chesley Drive, Media, PA 19063; **Phone:** 484-621-0082; **Board Cert:** Internal Medicine 78; Dermatology 80; **Med School:** Univ Pennsylvania 75; **Resid:** Internal Medicine, Hosp Univ Penn 78; Dermatology, NYU-Skin Cancer Unit 80; **Fellow:** Mohs Surgery, NYU-Skin Cancer Unit 8; **Fac Appt:** Clin Prof D, Univ Pennsylvania

Fisher, Michael MD [D] - **Hospital:** Montefiore Med Ctr - Weiler-Einstein Div; **Address:** 1575 Blondell Ave, Ste 200, Bronx, NY 10461; **Phone:** 718-405-8300 x7441; **Board Cert:** Dermatology 70; **Med School:** SUNY Downstate 63; **Resid:** Dermatology, Mass Genl Hosp 69; **Fac Appt:** Prof D, Albert Einstein Coll Med

Geronemus, Roy MD [D] - **Spec Exp:** Skin Laser Surgery; Cosmetic Dermatology; Mohs' Surgery; **Hospital:** NYU Med Ctr (page 104); **Address:** 317 E 34 St, Ste 11N, New York, NY 10016-4974; **Phone:** 212-686-7306; **Board Cert:** Dermatology 83; **Med School:** Univ Miami Sch Med 79; **Resid:** Dermatology, NYU-Skin Cancer Unit 83; **Fellow:** Mohs Surgery, NYU-Skin Cancer Unit 84; **Fac Appt:** Clin Prof D, NYU Sch Med

Gordon, Marsha MD [D] - **Spec Exp:** Cosmetic Dermatology-Botox & Collagen; Acne; Skin Cancer; **Hospital:** Mount Sinai Med Ctr (page 101); **Address:** 5 E 98th St Fl 5, New York, NY 10029-6501; **Phone:** 212-241-9728; **Board Cert:** Dermatology 88; **Med School:** Univ Pennsylvania 84; **Resid:** Dermatology, Mount Sinai Hosp 88; **Fac Appt:** Assoc Clin Prof D, Mount Sinai Sch Med

Granstein, Richard MD [D] - **Spec Exp:** Autoimmune Disorders of Skin; Skin Cancer; Acne; **Hospital:** NY-Presby Hosp - NY Weill Cornell Med Ctr (page 103); **Address:** 520 E 70th St Fl 3 - Ste 326, New York, NY 10021; **Phone:** 212-746-2007; **Board Cert:** Dermatology 83; Clinical & Laboratory Dermatologic Immunology 85; **Med School:** UCLA 78; **Resid:** Dermatology, Mass Genl Hosp 81; **Fellow:** Research, Natnl Cancer Inst-Frederick Cancer Resch Facilitys 82; Dermatology, Mass Genl Hosp 83; **Fac Appt:** Prof D, Cornell Univ-Weill Med Coll

Halpern, Allan C MD [D] - **Spec Exp:** Skin Cancer; Melanoma; Melanoma Early Detection/Prevention; **Hospital:** Meml Sloan Kettering Cancer Ctr (page 100); **Address:** 160 E 53rd St, New York, NY 10022; **Phone:** 212-610-0766; **Board Cert:** Dermatology 88; Internal Medicine 84; **Med School:** Albert Einstein Coll Med 81; **Resid:** Dermatology, Hosp U Penn 88; **Fellow:** Epidemiology, Hosp U Penn 89; **Fac Appt:** Assoc Prof Med, Cornell Univ-Weill Med Coll

Lebwohl, Mark MD [D] - **Spec Exp:** Skin Cancer; Psoriasis; **Hospital:** Mount Sinai Med Ctr (page 101); **Address:** 5 E 98th St Fl 5, New York, NY 10029-6501; **Phone:** 212-241-9728; **Board Cert:** Internal Medicine 81; Dermatology 83; **Med School:** Harvard Med Sch 78; **Resid:** Internal Medicine, Mount Sinai Hosp 81; **Fellow:** Dermatology, Mount Sinai Hosp 83; **Fac Appt:** Prof D, Mount Sinai Sch Med

Lessin, Stuart R MD [D] - **Spec Exp:** Melanoma; Skin Cancer; Cutaneous Lymphoma; **Hospital:** Fox Chase Cancer Ctr (page 95); **Address:** Fox Chase Cancer Ctr, Dept Dermatology, 333 Cottman Ave, Philadelphia, PA 19111; **Phone:** 215-728-2191; **Board Cert:** Dermatology 86; **Med School:** Temple Univ 82; **Resid:** Dermatology, Univ Penn Med Ctr 86; **Fac Appt:** Prof D, Temple Univ

Miller, Stanley MD [D] - **Spec Exp:** Dermatologic Surgery; Skin Cancer; **Hospital:** Johns Hopkins Hosp - Baltimore (page 97); **Address:** Charles Towson Bldg, Ste 201, 1104 Kenilworth Drive, Baltimore, MD 21204; **Phone:** 443-279-0340; **Board Cert:** Dermatology 89; **Med School:** Univ VT Coll Med 84; **Resid:** Dermatology, UCSD Med Ctr 89; **Fellow:** Dermatologic Surgery, Hosp Univ Penn 91; **Fac Appt:** Prof D, Johns Hopkins Univ

Nigra, Thomas P MD [D] - **Spec Exp:** Hair Problems; Psoriasis; Skin Cancer; **Hospital:** Washington Hosp Ctr; **Address:** Washington Hosp Ctr, Derm Assocs, 110 Irving St NW, 2B44, Washington, DC 20010-2976; **Phone:** 202-877-6227; **Board Cert:** Dermatology 73; **Med School:** Univ Pennsylvania 67; **Resid:** Dermatology, Mass Genl Hosp 73; **Fac Appt:** Clin Prof D, Geo Wash Univ

Ramsay, David L MD [D] - **Spec Exp:** Cutaneous Lymphoma; **Hospital:** NYU Med Ctr (page 104); **Address:** 530 1st Ave, Ste 7G, New York, NY 10016; **Phone:** 212-683-6283; **Board Cert:** Dermatology 74; **Med School:** Indiana Univ 69; **Resid:** Dermatology, New York Univ Med Ctr 73; **Fellow:** Nat Inst Health 73; **Fac Appt:** Clin Prof D, NYU Sch Med

Rigel, Darrell S MD [D] - **Spec Exp:** Melanoma; Skin Cancer; Cosmetic Dermatology; **Hospital:** NYU Med Ctr (page 104); **Address:** 35 E 35th Street, Ste 208, New York, NY 10016-3823; **Phone:** 212-684-5964; **Board Cert:** Dermatology 83; **Med School:** Geo Wash Univ 78; **Resid:** Dermatology, NYU Med Ctr 82; **Fellow:** Dermatologic Surgery, NYU Med Ctr 83; **Fac Appt:** Clin Prof D, NYU Sch Med

Robins, Perry MD [D] - **Spec Exp:** Mohs' Surgery; Skin Cancer; Melanoma; **Hospital:** NYU Med Ctr (page 104); **Address:** 530 First Ave, Ste 7H, New York, NY 10016; **Phone:** 212-263-7222; **Med School:** Germany 61; **Resid:** Dermatology, VA Med Ctr 64; **Fellow:** Dermatology, NYU Med Ctr 67; **Fac Appt:** Prof D, NYU Sch Med

Rook, Alain H MD [D] - **Spec Exp:** Cutaneous Lymphoma; Immune Disorders of Skin; Mycosis Fungoides; **Hospital:** Hosp Univ Penn - UPHS (page 113); **Address:** Hosp Univ Penn, Dept Dermatology, 3600 Spruce St, Philadelphia, PA 19104-4204; **Phone:** 215-662-6751; **Board Cert:** Internal Medicine 79; Nephrology 80; Dermatology 91; **Med School:** Univ Mich Med Sch 75; **Resid:** Internal Medicine, McGill Univ Med Ctr 77; Dermatology, Hosp Univ Penn 89; **Fellow:** Nephrology, McGill Univ Med Ctr 79; Immunology, NIH 86; **Fac Appt:** Prof D, Univ Pennsylvania

Safai, Bijan MD [D] - **Spec Exp:** Dermatologic Surgery; Skin Cancer; Laser & Cosmetic Dermatology; **Hospital:** Metropolitan Hosp Ctr - NY; **Address:** 625 Park Ave, New York, NY 10021; **Phone:** 212-988-8918; **Board Cert:** Dermatology 74; **Med School:** Iran 65; **Resid:** Internal Medicine, VA Med Ctr 70; Dermatology, NYU Med Ctr 73; **Fellow:** Immunology, Mem Sloan-Kettering Cancer Ctr 74; **Fac Appt:** Prof D, NY Med Coll

Zitelli, John MD [D] - **Spec Exp:** Mohs' Surgery; Skin Cancer; Melanoma; **Hospital:** UPMC Shadyside (page 114); **Address:** Shadyside Med Ctr, 5200 Centre Ave, Ste 303, Pittsburgh, PA 15232-1312; **Phone:** 412-681-9400; **Board Cert:** Dermatology 80; **Med School:** Univ Pittsburgh 76; **Resid:** Dermatology, Univ Hlth Ctr Hosp 79; **Fellow:** Mohs Surgery, Univ Wisconsin

Southeast

Amonette, Rex A MD [D] - **Spec Exp:** Skin Cancer; Mohs' Surgery; **Hospital:** Meth Healthcare Central - Univ Hosp; **Address:** Memphis Dermatology Clinic, 1455 Union Ave, Memphis, TN 38104-6727; **Phone:** 901-726-6655; **Board Cert:** Dermatology 74; **Med School:** Univ Ark 66; **Resid:** Dermatology, Univ Tenn Med Ctr 71; **Fellow:** Mohs Surgery, NYU Med Ctr 72; **Fac Appt:** Clin Prof D, Univ Tenn Coll Med, Memphis

Eichler, Craig MD [D] - **Spec Exp:** Skin Cancer; Dermatologic Surgery; **Hospital:** Cleveland Clin - Naples (page 92); **Address:** 6101 Pine Ridge Rd, Naples, FL 34119; **Phone:** 239-348-4000; **Board Cert:** Dermatology 93; **Med School:** Univ Fla Coll Med 89; **Resid:** Dermatology, Univ Texas Med Branch 93

Elmets, Craig A MD [D] - **Spec Exp:** Phototherapy in Skin Disease; Psoriasis; Skin Cancer; **Hospital:** Univ of Ala Hosp at Birmingham; **Address:** Univ of Alabama-Birmingham-Derm Dept, 1530 Third Ave S, Birmingham, AL 35294; **Phone:** 205-934-5189; **Board Cert:** Dermatology 80; Internal Medicine 78; Diagnostic Lab Immunology 89; **Med School:** Univ Iowa Coll Med 75; **Resid:** Internal Medicine, Kansas Med Ctr 78; Dermatology, Univ Iowa Hosps 80; **Fellow:** Immunological Dermatology, Univ Texas Hlth Sci Ctr 82; **Fac Appt:** Prof D, Univ Ala

Fenske, Neil A MD [D] - **Spec Exp:** Skin Cancer; Melanoma; Psoriasis; **Hospital:** H Lee Moffitt Cancer Ctr & Research Inst; **Address:** 12901 Bruce B Downs Blvd, MDC-79, Tampa, FL 33612-4742; **Phone:** 813-974-2920; **Board Cert:** Dermatology 77; Dermatopathology 84; **Med School:** St Louis Univ 73; **Resid:** Dermatology, Wisconsin Hlth Sci Ctr 77; **Fac Appt:** Prof Med, Univ S Fla Coll Med

Flowers, Franklin P MD [D] - **Spec Exp:** Mohs' Surgery; Dermatopathology; **Hospital:** Shands Hlthcre at Univ of FL (page 109); **Address:** 2000 SW Archer Rd, Ste 3151, Gainesville, FL 32610; **Phone:** 352-265-8001; **Board Cert:** Dermatology 76; Dermatopathology 81; **Med School:** Univ Fla Coll Med 71; **Resid:** Dermatology, Ohio State Univ 75; **Fellow:** Mohs Surgery, Univ Alabama 93; **Fac Appt:** Prof Med, Univ Fla Coll Med

Green, Howard MD [D] - **Spec Exp:** Mohs' Surgery; Skin Cancer; **Hospital:** St Mary's Med Ctr - W Palm Bch; **Address:** 120 Butler St, Ste A, West Palm Beach, FL 33407-6106; **Phone:** 561-659-1510; **Board Cert:** Internal Medicine 88; Dermatology 04; **Med School:** Boston Univ 85; **Resid:** Internal Medicine, Jefferson Univ Hosp 88; Dermatology, Harvard Med Sch 92; **Fellow:** Mohs Surgery, Boston Univ Med Ctr 93

Johr, Robert MD [D] - **Spec Exp:** Pigmented Lesions; Melanoma; Pediatric Dermatology; **Hospital:** Univ of Miami Hosp & Clins/Sylvester Comp Canc Ctr; **Address:** 1050 NW 15th St, Ste 201A, Boca Raton, FL 33486-1341; **Phone:** 561-368-4545; **Board Cert:** Dermatology 81; **Med School:** Mexico 75; **Resid:** Dermatology, Roswell Park Cancer Ctr 77; Dermatology, Metro Med Ctr/Case Western Reserve 79; **Fac Appt:** Clin Prof D, Univ Miami Sch Med

Leshin, Barry MD [D] - **Spec Exp:** Skin Cancer; Mohs' Surgery; Dermatologic Surgery; **Address:** 125 Sunnynoll Ct, Ste 100, Winston-Salem, NC 27106; **Phone:** 336-724-2434; **Board Cert:** Dermatology 85; **Med School:** Univ Tex, Houston 81; **Resid:** Dermatology, Univ IA Hosp 85; **Fellow:** Dermatologic Surgery, Univ IA Hosp 86

Olsen, Elise A MD [D] - **Spec Exp:** Hair loss; Cutaneous Lymphoma; **Hospital:** Duke Univ Med Ctr (page 94); **Address:** Duke University Medical Ctr, Box 3294, Durham, NC 27710; **Phone:** 919-668-5613; **Board Cert:** Dermatology 83; **Med School:** Baylor Coll Med 78; **Resid:** Internal Medicine, U NC Meml Hosp 80; Dermatology, Duke U Med Ctr 83; **Fac Appt:** Prof D, Duke Univ

Sobel, Stuart MD [D] - **Spec Exp:** Skin Cancer; Blistering Diseases; **Hospital:** Meml Regl Hosp - Hollywood; **Address:** 4340 Sheridan St, Ste 101, Hollywood, FL 33021-3511; **Phone:** 954-983-5533; **Board Cert:** Dermatology 77; **Med School:** Tufts Univ 72; **Resid:** Dermatology, Mt Sinai Hosp 76

Midwest

Bailin, Philip L MD [D] - **Spec Exp:** Mohs' Surgery; Skin Laser Surgery; **Hospital:** Cleveland Clin Fdn (page 92); **Address:** 9500 Euclid Ave, Desk A61, Cleveland, OH 44195-5032; **Phone:** 216-444-2115; **Board Cert:** Dermatology 75; **Med School:** Northwestern Univ 68; **Resid:** Dermatology, Cleveland Clin Fdn 74; **Fellow:** Dermatopathology, Armed Forces Inst Pathology 75; Mohs Surgery, Univ Wisc Hosp & Clin

Cornelius, Lynne A MD [D] - **Spec Exp:** Melanoma; **Hospital:** Barnes-Jewish Hosp (page 85); **Address:** 660 S Euclid, Box 8123, St Louis, MO 63110; **Phone:** 314-362-8187; **Board Cert:** Dermatology 89; **Med School:** Univ MO-Columbia Sch Med 84; **Resid:** Dermatology, Barnes Jewish Hosp-Wash Univ 89; **Fellow:** Immunological Dermatology, Emory Univ Med Ctr 92; **Fac Appt:** Assoc Prof D, Washington Univ, St Louis

Hanke, C William MD [D] - **Spec Exp:** Mohs' Surgery; Skin Laser Surgery; Cosmetic Surgery; **Hospital:** St Vincent Carmel Hosp; **Address:** Laser & Skin Surgery Ctr of Indiana, 13450 N Meridian St, Ste 355, Carmel, IN 46032-1486; **Phone:** 317-582-8484; **Board Cert:** Dermatology 78; Dermatopathology 82; **Med School:** Univ Iowa Coll Med 71; **Resid:** Dermatology, Cleveland Clinic 78; Dermatopathology, Indiana Univ 82; **Fellow:** Cutaneous Oncology, Cleveland Clinic 79; **Fac Appt:** Clin Prof D, Indiana Univ

Hruza, George J MD [D] - **Spec Exp:** Skin Laser Surgery; Mohs' Surgery; Cosmetic Surgery; **Hospital:** St Luke's Hosp - Chesterfield, MO; **Address:** Laser & Derm Surg Ctr, 14377 Woodlake Drive, Ste 111, St. Louis, MO 63017-5735; **Phone:** 314-878-3839; **Board Cert:** Dermatology 86; **Med School:** NYU Sch Med 82; **Resid:** Dermatology, NYU Med Ctr-Skin Cancer Unit 86; **Fellow:** Laser Surgery, Mass Genl Hosp-Harvard 87; Surgery, Univ Wisc 88; **Fac Appt:** Assoc Clin Prof D, St Louis Univ

Johnson, Timothy M MD [D] - **Spec Exp:** Melanoma; Mohs' Surgery; **Hospital:** Univ Michigan Hlth Sys; **Address:** Univ of Michigan Hlth System, Dept Dermatology, 1910 Taubman Ctr, Ann Arbor, MI 48109-0314; **Phone:** 734-936-4190; **Board Cert:** Dermatology 88; **Med School:** Univ Tex, Houston 84; **Resid:** Dermatology, Univ Texas Med Ctr 88; **Fellow:** Mohs Surgery, Univ Mich Med Ctr 89; Mohs Surgery, Univ Oregon Hlth Sci Ctr 90; **Fac Appt:** Prof D, Univ Mich Med Sch

Lim, Henry W MD [D] - **Spec Exp:** Phototherapy in Skin Disease; Vitiligo; Cutaneous Lymphoma; **Hospital:** Henry Ford Hosp; **Address:** Henry Ford Hosp, Dept Derm, 2799 W Grand Blvd, Detroit, MI 48202-2689; **Phone:** 313-916-4060; **Board Cert:** Dermatology 79; Clinical & Laboratory Dematologic Immunology 85; **Med School:** SUNY Downstate 75; **Resid:** Dermatology, NYU Med Ctr 79; **Fellow:** Immunological Dermatology, NYU Med Ctr 80

Lowe, Lori MD [D] - **Spec Exp:** Dermatopathology; Skin Cancer; **Hospital:** Univ Michigan Hlth Sys; **Address:** Univ Mich, Med Sci I, 1301 Catherine, rm M5226, Ann Arbor, MI 48109-0602; **Phone:** 734-764-4460; **Board Cert:** Dermatology 90; Dermatopathology 91; **Med School:** Univ Tex, Houston 85; **Resid:** Dermatology, Univ Tex Hlth Sci Ctr 90; **Fellow:** Dermatopathology, Univ Colo Hlth Sci Ctr 91; **Fac Appt:** Assoc Clin Prof D, Univ Mich Med Sch

Neuburg, Marcy MD [D] - **Spec Exp:** Mohs' Surgery; Skin Cancer; Pigmented Lesions; **Hospital:** Froedtert Meml Lutheran Hosp; **Address:** Dept Dermatology, 9200 W Wisconsin Ave, Milwaukee, WI 53226; **Phone:** 414-805-3666; **Board Cert:** Internal Medicine 85; Dermatology 88; **Med School:** Oregon Hlth Sci Univ 82; **Resid:** Internal Medicine, Georgetown Univ Hosp 85; Dermatology, Boston Univ Sch Med Ctr 88; **Fellow:** Mohs Surgery, Tufts New England Med Ctr 90; **Fac Appt:** Assoc Prof D, Med Coll Wisc

Otley, Clark C MD [D] - **Spec Exp:** Mohs' Surgery; Skin Cancer; Skin Cancer in Transplant Patients; **Hospital:** Mayo Med Ctr & Clin - Rochester; **Address:** Mayo Clinic, 200 1st St SW, Rochester, MN 55905; **Phone:** 507-284-3579; **Board Cert:** Dermatology 95; **Med School:** Duke Univ 91; **Resid:** Dermatology, Mass Genl Hosp 95; **Fellow:** Dermatologic Surgery, Mayo Clinic 96; **Fac Appt:** Assoc Prof D, Mayo Med Sch

Wood, Gary S MD [D] - **Spec Exp:** Cutaneous Lymphoma; Melanoma; Skin Cancer; **Hospital:** Univ WI Hosp & Clins; **Address:** University of Wisconsin Health, Dept Dermatology, 1 S Park St Fl 7, Madison, WI 53715-1375; **Phone:** 608-287-2620; **Board Cert:** Anatomic Pathology 83; Dermatology 86; Dermatopathology 87; **Med School:** Univ IL Coll Med 79; **Resid:** Anatomic Pathology, Stanford Univ Med Ctr 83; Dermatology, Stanford Univ Med Ctr 85; **Fellow:** Immunopathology, Stanford Univ Med Ctr 81; **Fac Appt:** Prof D, Univ Wisc

Great Plains and Mountains

Bowen, Glen M MD [D] - **Spec Exp:** Melanoma; Cutaneous Lymphoma; Clinical Trials; **Hospital:** Univ Utah Hosps and Clins; **Address:** Huntsman Cancer Inst, 2000 Circle of Hope, Ste 2400, Salt Lake City, UT 84112; **Phone:** 801-585-0197; **Board Cert:** Dermatology 95; **Med School:** Univ Utah 90; **Resid:** Dermatology, Univ Michigan Med Ctr 93; **Fellow:** Immunological Dermatology, Univ Michigan Med Ctr 95; Mohs Surgery, Univ Utah 01; **Fac Appt:** Asst Prof D, Univ Utah

Southwest

Butler, David F MD [D] - **Spec Exp:** Skin Cancer; **Hospital:** Scott & White Mem Hosp; **Address:** Scott & White Memorial Hospital, Dept Dermatology, 2401 S 31st St, Temple, TX 76508-0001; **Phone:** 254-742-3725; **Board Cert:** Dermatology 85; **Med School:** Univ Tex Med Br, Galveston 80; **Resid:** Dermatology, Walter Reed Army Med Ctr 85; **Fac Appt:** Assoc Prof D, Texas Tech Univ

Duvic, Madeleine MD [D] - **Spec Exp:** Cutaneous Lymphoma; Skin Cancer; **Hospital:** UT MD Anderson Cancer Ctr, The (page 115); **Address:** MD Anderson Cancer Ctr, Dept Derm, 1515 Holcombe Blvd, Unit 434, Houston, TX 77030; **Phone:** 713-745-1113; **Board Cert:** Dermatology 81; Internal Medicine 82; **Med School:** Duke Univ 77; **Resid:** Dermatology, Duke Univ Med Ctr 80; Internal Medicine, Duke Univ Med Ctr 82; **Fellow:** Geriatric Medicine, Duke Univ Med Ctr 84; **Fac Appt:** Prof D, Univ Tex, Houston

Horn, Thomas D MD [D] - **Spec Exp:** Graft vs Host Disease; Skin Cancer; **Hospital:** UAMS Med Ctr; **Address:** UAMS, Dept Derm, 4301 W Markham Drive, Slot 576, Little Rock, AR 72205; **Phone:** 501-686-5110; **Board Cert:** Dermatology 01; Dermatopathology 88; **Med School:** Univ VA Sch Med 82; **Resid:** Dermatology, Univ Maryland Med Ctr 87; **Fellow:** Dermatopathology, Johns Hopkins Hosp 89; **Fac Appt:** Prof D, Univ Ark

Orengo, Ida F MD [D] - **Spec Exp:** Melanoma; Mohs' Surgery; **Hospital:** St Luke's Episcopal Hosp - Houston; **Address:** Baylor College of Medicine, 6560 Fannin St, Ste 802, Houston, TX 77030; **Phone:** 713-798-6925; **Board Cert:** Dermatology 01; **Med School:** Harvard Med Sch 88; **Resid:** Dermatology, Baylor Coll Med 91; **Fac Appt:** Assoc Prof D, Baylor Coll Med

Taylor, R Stan MD [D] - **Spec Exp:** Mohs' Surgery; Melanoma; Skin Cancer; **Hospital:** Zale Lipshy Univ Hosp - Dallas; **Address:** Univ Tex SW Med Sch, Dept Derm, 5323 Harry Hines Blvd, DF3 608, Dallas, TX 75390-9192; **Phone:** 214-648-0620; **Board Cert:** Dermatology 89; **Med School:** Univ Tex Med Br, Galveston 85; **Resid:** Dermatology, Univ Mich 89; **Fellow:** Immunological Dermatology, Univ Mich 90; Mohs Surgery, Oregon Hlth Sci Univ 91; **Fac Appt:** Assoc Prof D, Univ Tex SW, Dallas

Wheeland, Ronald MD [D] - **Spec Exp:** Skin Laser Surgery; Mohs' Surgery; Cosmetic Dermatology; **Hospital:** Univ Med Ctr - Tucson; **Address:** Univ Arizona, Sect Dermatology, 535 N Wilmot, Ste 101, Tucson, AZ 85711; **Phone:** 505-694-0690; **Board Cert:** Dermatology 77; Dermatopathology 78; **Med School:** Univ Ariz Coll Med 73; **Resid:** Dermatology, Univ Ok Hlth Sci Ctr 77; **Fellow:** Dermatopathology, Univ Ok Hlth Sci Ctr 78; Dermatologic Surgery, Cleveland Clin Fnd 84; **Fac Appt:** Prof D, Univ Ariz Coll Med

West Coast and Pacific

Bastian, Boris C MD [D] - **Spec Exp:** Melanoma; Skin Cancer; **Hospital:** UCSF Med Ctr; **Address:** UCSF, Box 0808, San Francisco, CA 94143; **Phone:** 415-476-5132; **Med School:** Germany 88; **Resid:** Dermatology, University of Wurzburg 94; **Fellow:** Hematology, Ludwig-Maximilian-University 89; **Fac Appt:** Asst Prof D, UCSF

Bennett, Richard G MD [D] - **Spec Exp:** Mohs' Surgery; Skin Cancer; **Hospital:** UCLA Med Ctr (page 111); **Address:** 1301 20th St, Ste 570, Santa Monica, CA 90404-2053; **Phone:** 310-315-0171; **Board Cert:** Dermatology 75; **Med School:** Case West Res Univ 70; **Resid:** Dermatology, Univ Penn Hosp 74; **Fellow:** Chemosurgery, NYU Med Ctr 77; **Fac Appt:** Clin Prof D, UCLA

Berg, Daniel MD [D] - **Spec Exp:** Skin Laser Surgery; Skin Cancer; **Hospital:** Univ Wash Med Ctr; **Address:** 4225 Roosevelt Way NE, Seattle, WA 98105; **Phone:** 206-598-6647; **Board Cert:** Dermatology 99; **Med School:** Univ Toronto 85; **Resid:** Internal Medicine, Sunnybrook Med Ctr 88; Dermatology, Duke Univ Med Ctr 91; **Fellow:** Dermatologic Surgery, Univ Toronto 93; Dermatologic Surgery, Univ British Columbia 94; **Fac Appt:** Prof D, Univ Wash

Conant, Marcus A MD [D] - **Spec Exp:** AIDS/HIV-Kaposi's Sarcoma; **Hospital:** UCSF Med Ctr; **Address:** 74 Hartford St, San Francisco, CA 94114; **Phone:** 415-661-2613; **Board Cert:** Dermatology 69; **Med School:** Duke Univ 61; **Resid:** Dermatology, UCSF Med Ctr 67; **Fac Appt:** Clin Prof D, UCSF

Glogau, Richard G MD **[D]** - **Spec Exp:** Mohs' Surgery; Cosmetic Dermatology; Skin Laser Surgery; **Hospital:** UCSF Med Ctr; **Address:** 350 Parnassus Ave, Ste 400, San Francisco, CA 94117; **Phone:** 415-564-1261; **Board Cert:** Dermatology 78; Dermatopathology 82; **Med School:** Harvard Med Sch 73; **Resid:** Dermatology, UCSF Med Ctr 77; **Fellow:** Chemosurgery, UCSF Med Ctr 78; **Fac Appt:** Clin Prof D, UCSF

Greenway, Hubert T MD **[D]** - **Spec Exp:** Skin Cancer; Mohs' Surgery; **Hospital:** Scripps Green Hosp; **Address:** Scripps Clinic, Dept Mohs' Surgery, 10666 N Torrey Pines Rd, MS 112A, La Jolla, CA 92037; **Phone:** 858-554-8646; **Board Cert:** Dermatology 82; **Med School:** Med Coll GA 74; **Resid:** Dermatology, Naval Hosp 82; **Fellow:** Chemosurgery, Univ Wisconsin Med Ctr 83

Kim, Youn-Hee MD **[D]** - **Spec Exp:** Cutaneous Lymphoma; Skin Cancer; **Hospital:** Stanford Univ Med Ctr; **Address:** 900 Blake Wilbur Drive, rm W0010, MC 5334, Stanford University Medical Ctr, Dept Dermatology, Stanford, CA 94305-5334; **Phone:** 650-723-4000; **Board Cert:** Dermatology 89; **Med School:** Stanford Univ 85; **Resid:** Dermatology, Metropolitan Hospital 89

Lowe, Nicholas J MD **[D]** - **Spec Exp:** Psoriasis; Cosmetic Dermatology; Skin Cancer; **Hospital:** UCLA Med Ctr (page 111); **Address:** S Calif Derm/Psoriasis Ctr, 2001 Santa Monica Blvd, Ste 490W, Santa Monica, CA 90404-2102; **Phone:** 310-828-8969; **Board Cert:** Dermatology 78; **Med School:** England 68; **Resid:** Dermatology, Univ Southhampton 74; Dermatology, Univ Liverpool 77; **Fellow:** Dermatology, Scripps Clin 76; **Fac Appt:** Clin Prof D, UCLA

Swanson, Neil MD **[D]** - **Spec Exp:** Skin Cancer; Cosmetic Dermatology; **Hospital:** OR Hlth & Sci Univ; **Address:** Oregon Hlth & Sci Univ, Dept Derm, 3181 SW Sam Jackson Park Rd, OP06, Portland, OR 97239; **Phone:** 503-418-3376; **Board Cert:** Dermatology 80; **Med School:** Univ Rochester 76; **Resid:** Dermatology, Univ Michigan Med Ctr 79; **Fellow:** Dermatology, UCSF Med Ctr 80; **Fac Appt:** Prof D, Oregon Hlth Sci Univ

Tabak, Brian MD **[D]** - **Spec Exp:** Skin Cancer; **Hospital:** Long Beach Meml Med Ctr; **Address:** 2699 Atlantic Ave, Long Beach, CA 90806; **Phone:** 562-426-3333; **Board Cert:** Dermatology 81; **Med School:** McGill Univ 77; **Resid:** Dermatology, USC Med Ctr 81; **Fac Appt:** Asst Clin Prof Med, USC Sch Med

ENDOCRINOLOGY

---

a subspecialty of INTERNAL MEDICINE

---

*A*n internist who concentrates on disorders of the internal (endocrine) glands such as the thyroid and adrenal glands. This specialist also deals with disorders such as diabetes, metabolic and nutritional disorders, pituitary diseases, menstrual and sexual problems.

Training required: *Three years in internal medicine plus additional training and examination for certification in endocrinology, diabetes, and metabolism.*

INTERNAL MEDICINE: *An internist is a personal physician who provides long-term, comprehensive care in the office and the hospital, managing both common and complex illness of adolescents, adults and the elderly. Internists are trained in the diagnosis and treatment of cancer, infections and diseases affecting the heart, blood, kidneys, joints and digestive, respiratory and vascular systems. They are also trained in the essentials of primary care internal medicine, which incorporates an understanding of disease prevention, wellness, substance abuse, mental health and effective treatment of common problems of the eyes, ears, skin, nervous system and reproductive organs.*

PHYSICIAN LISTINGS

145

ENDOCRINOLOGY

Mid Atlantic

Hurley, James R MD [EDM] - **Spec Exp:** Thyroid Disorders; Graves' Disease; Thyroid Cancer; **Hospital:** NY-Presby Hosp - NY Weill Cornell Med Ctr (page 103); **Address:** 525 E 68th St, Box 136, New York, NY 10021-4870; **Phone:** 212-746-6290; **Board Cert:** Internal Medicine 68; Nuclear Medicine 72; **Med School:** Cornell Univ-Weill Med Coll 61; **Resid:** Internal Medicine, New York Hosp 64; **Fellow:** Endocrinology, New York Hosp 65; **Fac Appt:** Assoc Prof Med, Cornell Univ-Weill Med Coll

Ladenson, Paul W MD [EDM] - **Spec Exp:** Thyroid Disorders; Thyroid Cancer; **Hospital:** Johns Hopkins Hosp - Baltimore (page 97); **Address:** Div Endocrinology & Metabolism, 1830 E Monument St, Ste 333, Baltimore, MD 21287-0003; **Phone:** 410-955-3663; **Board Cert:** Internal Medicine 78; Endocrinology, Diabetes & Metabolism 81; **Med School:** Harvard Med Sch 75; **Resid:** Internal Medicine, Mass Genl Hosp 78; **Fellow:** Endocrinology, Diabetes & Metabolism, Mass Genl Hosp 80; **Fac Appt:** Prof Med, Johns Hopkins Univ

Robbins, Richard MD [EDM] - **Spec Exp:** Thyroid Cancer; Pituitary Cancer & Disorders; **Hospital:** Meml Sloan Kettering Cancer Ctr (page 100); **Address:** Memorial Sloan Kettering Cancer Ctr, 1275 York Ave, Box 296, New York, NY 10021; **Phone:** 212-639-2888; **Board Cert:** Internal Medicine 78; Endocrinology, Diabetes & Metabolism 83; **Med School:** Creighton Univ 75; **Resid:** Internal Medicine, NY Hosp-Cornell Med Ctr 78; **Fellow:** Endocrinology, New England Med Ctr 81; **Fac Appt:** Prof Med, Cornell Univ-Weill Med Coll

Snyder, Peter Joseph MD [EDM] - **Spec Exp:** Pituitary Tumors; Reproductive Endocrinology-Male; **Hospital:** Hosp Univ Penn - UPHS (page 113); **Address:** Univ Pennsylvania Med Group, 3400 Spruce St, Philadelphia, PA 19104; **Phone:** 215-898-0208; **Board Cert:** Internal Medicine 72; Endocrinology, Diabetes & Metabolism 72; **Med School:** Harvard Med Sch 65; **Resid:** Internal Medicine, Beth Israel Hosp 67; Internal Medicine, Beth Israel Hosp 70; **Fellow:** Endocrinology, Diabetes & Metabolism, Hosp Univ Penn 71; **Fac Appt:** Prof Med, Univ Pennsylvania

Wartofsky, Leonard MD [EDM] - **Spec Exp:** Thyroid Cancer; Thyroid Disorders; **Hospital:** Washington Hosp Ctr; **Address:** 110 Irving St NW, Ste 2A62, Washington, DC 20010-2975; **Phone:** 202-877-3109; **Board Cert:** Internal Medicine 71; Endocrinology, Diabetes & Metabolism 72; **Med School:** Geo Wash Univ 64; **Resid:** Internal Medicine, Barnes Hosp 66; Internal Medicine, Bronx Muni Hosp Ctr 67; **Fellow:** Endocrinology, Diabetes & Metabolism, Boston City Hosp 69; **Fac Appt:** Prof Med, Uniformed Srvs Univ, Bethesda

Southeast

Earp III, H Shelton MD [EDM] - **Spec Exp:** Cancer-Hormonal Influences; **Hospital:** Univ NC Hosps (page 112); **Address:** UNC Lineberger Comprehensive Cancer Center, CB 7295, Chapel Hill, NC 27599-7295; **Phone:** 919-966-3036; **Board Cert:** Internal Medicine 76; Endocrinology, Diabetes & Metabolism 77; **Med School:** Univ NC Sch Med 70; **Resid:** Internal Medicine, NC Memorial Hosp 75; **Fellow:** Endocrinology, Diabetes & Metabolism, Univ North Carolina Hosp 77; **Fac Appt:** Prof Med, Univ NC Sch Med

Midwest

Clutter, William E MD **(EDM)** - **Spec Exp:** Endocrine Disorders & Cancer; Calcium Disorders; Metabolic Bone Disease; **Hospital:** Barnes-Jewish Hosp (page 85); **Address:** Barnes Jewish Hospital, Dept Internal Medicine, 660 S Euclid, Box 8121, St Louis, MO 63110; **Phone:** 314-362-8094; **Board Cert:** Internal Medicine 78; Endocrinology, Diabetes & Metabolism 81; **Med School:** Ohio State Univ 75; **Resid:** Internal Medicine, Barnes Jewish Hosp 78; **Fellow:** Endocrinology, Diabetes & Metabolism, Barnes Jewish Hosp 80; **Fac Appt:** Prof Med, Washington Univ, St Louis

Great Plains and Mountains

Ridgway, E Chester MD **(EDM)** - **Spec Exp:** Thyroid Cancer; Thyroid Disorders; Pituitary Disorders; **Hospital:** Univ Colorado Hosp; **Address:** UCHSC at Fitzsimons, Endocrinology, MS 8106, PO Box 6511, Aurora, CO 80045; **Phone:** 303-724-3921; **Board Cert:** Internal Medicine 72; Endocrinology 73; **Med School:** Univ Colorado 68; **Resid:** Internal Medicine, Mass Genl Hosp 70; **Fellow:** Endocrinology, Mass Genl Hosp 72; **Fac Appt:** Prof Med, Univ Colorado

Southwest

Gagel, Robert F MD **(EDM)** - **Spec Exp:** Thyroid Cancer; **Hospital:** UT MD Anderson Cancer Ctr, The (page 115); **Address:** MD Anderson Cancer Ctr, 1515 Holcombe Blvd, Unit 433, Houston, TX 77030; **Phone:** 713-792-6517; **Board Cert:** Internal Medicine 75; Endocrinology 77; **Med School:** Ohio State Univ 71; **Resid:** Internal Medicine, New England Med Ctr 73; **Fellow:** Endocrinology, New England Med Ctr 75; Research, Harvard Med Sch 81; **Fac Appt:** Prof Med, Univ Tex, Houston

Rubenfeld, Sheldon MD **(EDM)** - **Spec Exp:** Thyroid Cancer; Thyroid Disorders; Diabetes; **Hospital:** St Luke's Episcopal Hosp - Houston; **Address:** 7515 S Main St, Ste 690, Houston, TX 77030; **Phone:** 713-795-5750; **Board Cert:** Infectious Disease 76; Endocrinology, Diabetes & Metabolism 79; **Med School:** Georgetown Univ 71; **Resid:** Internal Medicine, Baylor Affil Hosps 76; **Fellow:** Endocrinology, Baylor Affil Hosps 78; **Fac Appt:** Assoc Clin Prof Med, Baylor Coll Med

Sherman, Steven I MD **(EDM)** - **Spec Exp:** Thyroid Cancer; **Hospital:** UT MD Anderson Cancer Ctr, The (page 115); **Address:** MD Anderson Cancer Ctr, 1515 Holcombe Blvd, Unit 435, Houston, TX 77030; **Phone:** 713-792-2840; **Board Cert:** Internal Medicine 88; Endocrinology 91; **Med School:** Johns Hopkins Univ 85; **Resid:** Internal Medicine, Johns Hopkins Hosp 88; **Fellow:** Endocrinology, Diabetes & Metabolism, Johns Hopkins Hosp 91; **Fac Appt:** Assoc Prof Med, Univ Tex, Houston

West Coast and Pacific

Chait, Alan MD **(EDM)** - **Spec Exp:** Cholesterol/Lipid Disorders; Diabetes; Nutrition & Cancer/Disease Prevention; **Hospital:** Univ Wash Med Ctr; **Address:** Univ Washington Med Ctr, 1959 NE Pacific St, Box 356166, Seattle, WA 98195; **Phone:** 206-598-4615; **Med School:** South Africa 67; **Resid:** Internal Medicine, Hammersmith Hosp 71; **Fellow:** Endocrinology, Diabetes & Metabolism, Hammersmith Hosp 73; Endocrinology, Diabetes & Metabolism, Univ Washington 77; **Fac Appt:** Prof Med, Univ Wash

Darwin, Christine H MD **(EDM)** - **Spec Exp:** Pituitary Tumors; Diabetes; **Hospital:** UCLA Med Ctr (page 111); **Address:** 200 Medical Plaza, Ste 365 C1, Los Angeles, CA 90095-1622; **Phone:** 310-794-5584; **Board Cert:** Geriatric Medicine 94; Endocrinology, Diabetes & Metabolism 97; **Med School:** India 80; **Resid:** Internal Medicine, UC Irvine Med Ctr 87; **Fellow:** Endocrinology, VA Hosp 88; Endocrinology, USC Med Ctr 93; **Fac Appt:** Assoc Prof Med, UCLA

Fitzgerald, Paul Anthony MD [EDM] - **Spec Exp:** Diabetes; Thyroid Disorders & Cancer; Pituitary/Adrenal Disorders & Cancer; **Hospital:** UCSF Med Ctr; **Address:** 350 Parnassus Ave, Ste 710, San Francisco, CA 94117; **Phone:** 415-665-1136; **Board Cert:** Internal Medicine 75; Endocrinology, Diabetes & Metabolism 81; **Med School:** Jefferson Med Coll 72; **Resid:** Internal Medicine, Presby Med Ctr-Univ Colo 75; **Fellow:** Endocrinology, Diabetes & Metabolism, UC San Francisco Med Ctr 78; **Fac Appt:** Clin Prof EDM, UCSF

Heber, David MD [EDM] - **Spec Exp:** Nutrition & Disease Prevention/Control; Nutrition & Cancer Prevention; **Hospital:** UCLA Med Ctr (page 111); **Address:** 900 Veteran Ave, Rm 12-217, UCLA Center for Human Nutrition, Los Angeles, CA 90095-1742; **Phone:** 310-206-1987; **Board Cert:** Internal Medicine 76; Endocrinology, Diabetes & Metabolism 77; **Med School:** Harvard Med Sch 73; **Resid:** Internal Medicine, LA Co Harbor Genl Hosp 75; **Fellow:** Endocrinology, Diabetes & Metabolism, LA Co Harbor Genl Hosp 78; **Fac Appt:** Prof Med, UCLA

Hoffman, Andrew R MD [EDM] - **Spec Exp:** Pituitary Disorders; Pituitary Tumors; Neuro-Endocrinology; **Hospital:** Stanford Univ Med Ctr; **Address:** 900 Blake Wilbur Drive, rm W2030, Palo Alto, CA 94304; **Phone:** 650-723-6961; **Board Cert:** Internal Medicine 79; Endocrinology 81; **Med School:** Stanford Univ 76; **Resid:** Internal Medicine, Mass Genl Hosp 78; **Fellow:** Pharmacology, Mass Genl Hosp 80; Endocrinology, Diabetes & Metabolism, Mass Genl Hosp 82; **Fac Appt:** Prof Med, Stanford Univ

Melmed, Shlomo MD [EDM] - **Spec Exp:** Pituitary Tumors; Acromegaly; **Hospital:** Cedars-Sinai Med Ctr (page 88); **Address:** Cedars Sinai Med Ctr, 8700 Beverly Blvd, rm 2015, Los Angeles, CA 90048; **Phone:** 310-423-4691; **Board Cert:** Internal Medicine 79; Endocrinology, Diabetes & Metabolism 83; **Med School:** South Africa 70; **Resid:** Internal Medicine, Sheba Med Ctr 76; **Fellow:** Endocrinology, Diabetes & Metabolism, Wadsworth VA Hosp 80; **Fac Appt:** Prof Med, UCLA

GASTROENTEROLOGY

a subspecialty of INTERNAL MEDICINE

A n internist who specializes in diagnosis and treatment of diseases of the digestive organs including the stomach, bowels, liver, and gallbladder. This specialist treats conditions such as abdominal pain, ulcers, diarrhea, cancer and jaundice and performs complex diagnostic and therapeutic procedures using endoscopes to see internal organs.

Training required: *Three years in internal medicine plus additional training and examination for certification in gastroenterology.*

INTERNAL MEDICINE: *An internist is a personal physician who provides long-term, comprehensive care in the office and the hospital, managing both common and complex illness of adolescents, adults and the elderly. Internists are trained in the diagnosis and treatment of cancer, infections and diseases affecting the heart, blood, kidneys, joints and digestive, respiratory and vascular systems. They are also trained in the essentials of primary care internal medicine, which incorporates an understanding of disease prevention, wellness, substance abuse, mental health and effective treatment of common problems of the eyes, ears, skin, nervous system and reproductive organs.*

PHYSICIAN LISTINGS

GASTROINTESTINAL CANCER PROGRAM
CITY OF HOPE CANCER CENTER

City of
Hope®

Where the Power of Knowledge Saves Lives®

1500 East Duarte Road
Duarte, California 91010
Tel. 800-826-HOPE (4673)
www.cityofhope.org

With over 250,000 new gastrointestinal cancer cases reported in the United States every year, the Gastrointestinal Cancer Program at City of Hope employs multidisciplinary strategies for dealing with malignancies of the digestive system, including the esophagus, stomach, liver, biliary tract, pancreas, colon, rectum and anus.

A COLLABORATIVE TEAM OF EXPERTS

City of Hope focuses on the prevention, early detection, diagnosis and treatment for those individuals who are at risk for developing gastrointestinal cancer or for those individuals who have already been diagnosed and are looking for treatment opportunities. Individuals are treated by a world-class team of physicians including

- Gastroenterologists
- Medical Oncologists
- Radiation Oncologists
- Surgeons

Physicians combine their skills and knowledge to provide patients with the highest quality of multidisciplinary care. The result is a personal, comprehensive treatment plan for those suffering from all forms of gastrointestinal cancer.

MINIMALLY INVASIVE AND ROBOTIC SURGICAL TECHNIQUES AVAILABLE

Surgery is an important treatment for localized tumors. Our specialists utilize minimally invasive surgery with advanced technologies such as laparoscopy for anal and rectal cancers, and the new *daVinci Surgical System®* with robotic capabilities for greater precision. These same experts continue to refine the art of minimally invasive surgery by developing new, innovative surgery techniques.

CLINICAL TRIALS MAY OFFER PROMISING NEW TREATMENTS

Physicians participate in a broad range of both intra- and extramural studies.

- Targeted Therapeutics: In the Yttrium labeled anti-CEA antibody trials, radiolabeled antibodies are given in combination with radiosensitizing doses of chemotherapy. These trials, requiring close cooperation among radiation therapy, medical oncology, and surgery, demonstrate the multidisciplinary nature of treatment.

- Multi-drug Therapy: Another trial involves the use of agent GTI-2040 combined with the chemotherapeutic drugs capectibine and oxaliplatin. GTI-2040 is an antisense molecule designed to disrupt the mRNA of ribonucleotide reductase, a key enzyme in DNA and cancer metabolism. This study is being conducted in cooperation with the National Cancer Institute and CTEP, and represents a potential treatment for colorectal and other gastrointestinal cancers.

EARLY DETECTION HELPS CONQUER COLORECTAL CANCER

Early detection, diagnosis and treatment of colorectal cancer (CRC), the second deadliest cancer in the U.S., is at the forefront of the program's mission. Our specialists offer an individualized approach to CRC screenings by offering an array of diagnostics, including colonoscopies. Each procedure is tailored to the individual patient's needs.

City of Hope is a National Cancer Institute (NCI)-designated Comprehensive Cancer Center–the highest accolade given by the NCI.

Other distinctions include:

- Founding member of the National Comprehensive Cancer Network, setting national standards of care for cancer;

- Scoring in the top 1 percent of hospitals surveyed by the Joint Commission on Accreditation of Healthcare Organizations (JCAHO); and

- Receiving the highest score possible in all applicable categories in the California Hospital Experience Survey (formerly known as PEP-C).

Helford Clinical Research Hospital, opened in 2005, continues City of Hope's tradition of progress and further substantiates City of Hope's ranking by *U.S. News & World Report* as one of America's 50 best cancer hospitals.

For more information, call 800-826-4673.

Patients choosing care through the Gastrointestinal Cancer Program at Indiana University Hospital can count on a comprehensive, multidisciplinary approach to cancer treatment. The program offers the most advanced diagnostic and treatment options for gastrointestinal malignancies, including esophageal, gastric, pancreatic, liver, gallbladder, appendix, biliary tract, small and large bowel and rectal cancers. Our physicians also treat individuals with familial cancer syndromes.

RELIABLE DIAGNOSIS AND EVALUATION

An accurate diagnosis is the first step in battling any type of cancer. The highly trained physicians affiliated with IU Hospital's Gastrointestinal Cancer Program employ the most reliable diagnostic tools available today, including:

- Radiographic studies
- Spiral CT and PET scanning
- Endoscopy
- Colonoscopy
- Endoscopic ultrasound
- Fine needle aspiration
- ERCP (endoscopic retrograde cholangiopancreatography)
- Genetic screening and counseling
- Endoscopic Mucosal Resection
- Management of Barrett's Esophagus

PROVEN TREATMENT OPTIONS

Our physicians tailor a treatment program to each patient's individual diagnosis and needs. Some of the therapeutic options offered to gastrointestinal patients are: surgery, chemotherapy, radiotherapy, photodynamic therapy (PDT) and palliative procedures, such as celiac axis block, ERCP and stent placement. These treatments may be used alone or in combination, depending upon the most current treatment recommendations and the needs of the patient.

Eligible patients also have access to innovative clinical trials and information about ongoing clinical studies taking place across the United States.

COMPREHENSIVE CARE IN ONE LOCATION

IU Hospital and the Indiana University Cancer Center offer interdisciplinary clinical programs that allow patients to see—in one simple visit—a variety of specialists who work as a team to provide complete cancer care. The IU Cancer Center was the first cancer center in Indiana to truly operate as a multidisciplinary center. IU Hospital and IU Cancer Center have full representation of all medical and surgical specialties, giving patients access to the range of services they may need throughout their course of treatment.

WORLD-CLASS CANCER CARE

The IU Gastrointestinal Cancer Program is a leader in cancer diagnosis and treatment, making it one of the most widely recognized cancer programs in the U.S. and the world. The program brings together the talents, strengths and resources of a diverse group of individuals and organizations with a single focus: to reduce cancer incidence, suffering and mortality in Indiana and beyond.

AMONG AN ELITE GROUP

Based on its record of groundbreaking research and superior clinical patient care, the IU Cancer Center has been designated a Cancer Center by the National Cancer Institute. The IU Cancer Center is the only such designated cancer center providing patient care in Indiana, placing it among an elite group of centers focusing on excellent clinical care and the rapid implementation of new discoveries into the treatment of cancer.

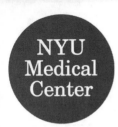

NYU Medical Center

550 First Avenue (at 31st Street)
New York, NY 10016
Physician Referral:
1-888-7-NYU-MED
www.nyumc.org

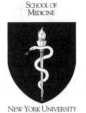

SCHOOL OF MEDICINE

NEW YORK UNIVERSITY

GASTROENTEROLOGY

The mission of the Division of Gastroenterology at NYU Medical Center is excellence in the delivery of patient care, research, and education in diseases of the gastrointestinal tract. Its physicians bring with them a rich body of knowledge in the diagnosis and management of inflammatory bowel disease, peptic ulcer disease, esophageal disorders, gastrointestinal cancer, and liver, biliary, and pancreatic diseases. Their multidisciplinary approach insures the greatest possible patient care at NYU's three acclaimed, academically-integrated teaching hospitals: Tisch Hospital (New York University Hospital), Bellevue Hospitals Center, and the New York Harbor Health Care System (Manhattan Veterans Hospital).

Members of the Division of Gastroenterology are nationally recognized leaders who are involved in numerous studies in the field of gastroenterology and hepatology, including clinical research in liver diseases (especially hepatitis C), endoscopy, colon cancer screening, acute and chronic GI bleeding, and Helicobacter pylori.

Always at the forefront of new technologies, NYU's gastroenterologists work side-by-side with radiologists to perform virtual colonoscopies, a new minimally invasive technique for finding early-stage cancers in the colon.

Virtual colonoscopy is a new screening test in which a radiologist uses a CAT (Computer Assisted Tomography) scanner and sophisticated image processing computers to actually recreate and evaluate the inner surface of the colon. The CAT scanner provides the x-ray images; the image-processing computers create the 3-D display for the final interpretation by the referring gastroenterologist. The study gives a complete evaluation of the entire surface of the colon and can be performed quickly, with little discomfort and extremely accurate readings.

The colon and the rectum are the final sections of the large intestine. In the United States, approximately 150,000 people are diagnosed with colorectal cancer every year and of these, approximately 55,000 will die of the disease. Cancer of the colon is the second leading cause of cancer death in the United States. Most experts agree that it is preventable, and NYU is on the cutting edge of 21st century research into quicker, safer, and more accurate diagnosis and treatment, with its advanced video colonoscopy and non-invasive radiologic techniques.

PHYSICIAN REFERRAL
1-888-7-NYU-MED
(1-888-769-8633)
www.nyumc.org

THE UNIVERSITY OF TEXAS
MD ANDERSON
CANCER CENTER

Making Cancer History™

1515 Holcombe Blvd.
Houston, Texas 77030-4095
Tel. 713-792-6161
Toll Free 800-392-1611
www.mdanderson.org

GASTROINTESTINAL ONCOLOGY

M. D. Anderson's Gastrointestinal Center diagnoses, treats and manages cancers of the digestive system and allied diseases. This multidisciplinary facility has specialized teams of oncologists to handle malignancies of the liver, pancreas, bowels, stomach and esophagus. Endocrine tumors in the pancreas, adrenal glands, thyroid and parathyroid are also treated here. Specialized services include medical, surgical, and radiation oncology; hepatology; enterostomal therapy; intra-arterial therapy; nutritional support; and diagnostic and therapeutic gastrointestinal endoscopic procedures.

Standard treatment available from our Gastrointestinal Oncologists include:

- Sphincter-sparing surgery for patients with rectal cancer
- Resection and adjuvant regional chemotherapy for patients with primary and metastatic liver malignances
- Radio-frequency ablation of liver tumors for patients with unresectable liver tumors, with very low complication and recurrence rates
- Preoperative chemoradiation therapy for patients with pancreatic, rectal and gastric cancers
- Videoendoscopy facility offering the latest in endoscopic diagnosis and treatment, including esophageal, biliary, small bowel, and rectal stent placement; photodynamic therapy for esophageal cancer and Barrett's esophagus; endoscopic ultrasonography with high-frequency probes and fine-needle aspiration; endoscopic argon plasma coagulation with an Erbe electrosurgical generator
- Laparoscopic adrenalectomy for selected patients with adrenal tumors
- Rapid intraoperative parathyroid hormone assay and intraoperative gamma-probe identification of sestamibi-labeled parathyroid glands to facilitate minimally invasive parathyroidectomy in selected patients
- Genetic testing and a comprehensive approach to evaluaton, counseling and disease management for multiple endocrine neoplasia

CLINICAL TRIALS

The Gastrointestinal Oncology Center offers an extensive array of clinical trials. A clinical trial is one of the most advanced stages of a long careful research process. Clinical trials are designed to test the effectiveness of new treatment, including novel drugs, surgical procedures, or combinations of therapy.

New and Innovative therapies generally are available at M.D. Anderson several years before they become standard in the community. Our clinical trials incorporate state-of-the-art patient care, while evaluating the most recent developments in cancer medicine. They also offer treatment opportunities for difficult or aggressive tumors.

M. D. Anderson is one of the largest cancer centers in the world. We've been working to eliminate cancer for more than six decades. Our depth of experience informs every aspect of your care.

We focus exclusively on cancer and have seen cases of every kind. Our doctors treat more rare cancers in a single day than most physicians see in a lifetime. That means you receive expert care no matter what your diagnosis.

We are the top-ranked cancer hospital in the United States according to the 2004 *U.S.News & World Report* annual survey of hospitals.

M. D. Anderson ranks first in the number and amount of research grants awarded by the National Cancer Institute. By studying how cancer begins and responds to various treatments, we can help patients overcome disease and prevent recurrence.

At M. D. Anderson, we understand that cancer is not just a physical disease. To help you cope with every aspect of cancer, we provide a number of support programs.

GASTROENTEROLOGY
New England

Mason, Joel B MD [Ge] - **Spec Exp:** Nutrition in Acute Illness; Nutrition in Bowel Disorders; Nutrition & Cancer Prevention; **Hospital:** Tufts-New England Med Ctr; **Address:** Tufts-New England Medical Ctr, Dept Gastroenterology, 750 Washington St, Boston, MA 02111; **Phone:** 617-636-1621; **Board Cert:** Internal Medicine 84; Gastroenterology 87; **Med School:** Univ Chicago-Pritzker Sch Med 81; **Resid:** Internal Medicine, Univ Iowa Hosps 84; **Fellow:** Gastroenterology, U Chicago Hosps 86; **Fac Appt:** Assoc Prof Med, Tufts Univ

Mid Atlantic

Goggins, Michael MD [Ge] - **Spec Exp:** Pancreatic Cancer-Early Detection; **Hospital:** Johns Hopkins Hosp - Baltimore (page 97); **Address:** Johns Hopkins Univ Sch Med, Dept Med-GE, 720 Rutland Ave Bldg Ross - rm 632, Baltimore, MD 21205; **Phone:** 410-955-3511; **Med School:** Ireland 88; **Resid:** Internal Medicine, St Jame's Hosp 90; **Fellow:** Gastroenterology, St Jame's Hosp 92; **Fac Appt:** Assoc Prof Med, Johns Hopkins Univ

Haluszka, Oleh MD [Ge] - **Spec Exp:** Pancreatic/Biliary Endoscopy (ERCP); Gastrointestinal Cancer Diagnosis; Endoscopic Ultrasound; **Hospital:** Fox Chase Cancer Ctr (page 95); **Address:** Fox Chase Cancer Ctr, 333 Cottman Ave, Ste C307, Philadelphia, PA 19111; **Phone:** 215-214-1424; **Board Cert:** Internal Medicine 87; Gastroenterology 01; **Med School:** Uniformed Srvs Univ, Bethesda 82; **Resid:** Internal Medicine, US Naval Hosp 87; **Fellow:** Gastroenterology, US Naval Hosp 90; Endoscopy, Med Coll Wisconsin 93; **Fac Appt:** Assoc Clin Prof Med, Temple Univ

Holt, Peter R MD [Ge] - **Spec Exp:** Diarrheal Diseases; Ulcerative Colitis/Crohn's; Nutrition & Cancer Prevention; **Hospital:** St Luke's - Roosevelt Hosp Ctr - Roosevelt Div (page 93); **Address:** 1111 Amsterdam Ave, Ste 1216, New York, NY 10025-1716; **Phone:** 212-523-3679; **Board Cert:** Internal Medicine 66; **Med School:** England 54; **Resid:** Internal Medicine, London Hosp 55; Internal Medicine, St Luke's Hosp 59; **Fellow:** Gastroenterology, Mass Genl Hosp 61; **Fac Appt:** Prof Emeritus Med, Columbia P&S

Lightdale, Charles MD [Ge] - **Spec Exp:** Barrett's Esophagus; Gastrointestinal Cancer; Endoscopic Ultrasound; **Hospital:** NY-Presby Hosp - Columbia Presby Med Ctr (page 103); **Address:** Columbia-Presbyterian Medical Ctr, 161 Fort Washington Ave, Irving Pavilion, rm 812, New York, NY 10032-3713; **Phone:** 212-305-3423; **Board Cert:** Internal Medicine 72; Gastroenterology 73; **Med School:** Columbia P&S 66; **Resid:** Internal Medicine, Yale-New Haven Hosp 68; Internal Medicine, New York Hosp 69; **Fellow:** Gastroenterology, New York Hosp-Cornell 73; **Fac Appt:** Prof Med, Columbia P&S

Lipshutz, William H. MD [Ge] - **Spec Exp:** Inflammatory Bowel Disease/Crohn's; Colon Cancer; Esophageal Disorders; **Hospital:** Pennsylvania Hosp (page 113); **Address:** 230 W Washington Sq, Farm Journal Bldg, Fl 4, Philadelphia, PA 19106; **Phone:** 215-829-3561; **Board Cert:** Internal Medicine 72; Gastroenterology 73; **Med School:** Univ Pennsylvania 67; **Resid:** Internal Medicine, Pennsylvania Hosp 72; **Fellow:** Gastroenterology, Hosp Univ Penn 71; **Fac Appt:** Clin Prof Med, Univ Pennsylvania

Pochapin, Mark B MD [Ge] - **Spec Exp:** Pancreatic Disease; Endoscopic Ultrasound (EUS); **Hospital:** NY-Presby Hosp - NY Weill Cornell Med Ctr (page 103); **Address:** NY Presbyterian-Cornell Medical Ctr, 520 E 70th St, Ste J314, New York, NY 10021; **Phone:** 212-746-4014; **Board Cert:** Internal Medicine 91; Gastroenterology 93; **Med School:** Cornell Univ-Weill Med Coll 86; **Resid:** Internal Medicine, NY Hosp-Cornell Med Ctr 91; **Fellow:** Gastroenterology, Montefiore Med Ctr/Albert Einstein 93; **Fac Appt:** Assoc Clin Prof Med, Cornell Univ-Weill Med Coll

Shike, Moshe MD [Ge] - **Spec Exp:** Gastrointestinal Cancer; Nutrition; Endoscopy; **Hospital:** Meml Sloan Kettering Cancer Ctr (page 100); **Address:** 1275 York Ave, rm S-536, New York, NY 10021; **Phone:** 212-639-7230; **Board Cert:** Internal Medicine 77; Gastroenterology 81; **Med School:** Israel 75; **Resid:** Internal Medicine, Mt Auburn Hosp 77; **Fellow:** Gastroenterology, Toronto Genl Hosp 81; **Fac Appt:** Prof Med, Cornell Univ-Weill Med Coll

Waye, Jerome MD [Ge] - **Spec Exp:** Endoscopy; Colon Cancer; Colonoscopy; **Hospital:** Mount Sinai Med Ctr (page 101); **Address:** 650 Park Ave, New York, NY 10021-6115; **Phone:** 212-439-7779; **Board Cert:** Internal Medicine 65; Gastroenterology 70; **Med School:** Boston Univ 58; **Resid:** Internal Medicine, Mount Sinai Hosp 61; **Fellow:** Gastroenterology, Mount Sinai Hosp 62; **Fac Appt:** Clin Prof Med, Mount Sinai Sch Med

Winawer, Sidney J MD [Ge] - **Spec Exp:** Colonoscopy; Colon Cancer; Cancer Prevention; **Hospital:** Meml Sloan Kettering Cancer Ctr (page 100); **Address:** 1275 York Ave, Box 90, New York, NY 10021-6094; **Phone:** 212-639-7678; **Board Cert:** Internal Medicine 65; Gastroenterology 73; **Med School:** SUNY Downstate 56; **Resid:** Internal Medicine, VA Hosp 61; Internal Medicine, Maimonides Hosp 62; **Fellow:** Gastroenterology, Boston City Hosp 64; **Fac Appt:** Prof Med, Cornell Univ-Weill Med Coll

Southeast

Barkin, Jamie S MD [Ge] - **Spec Exp:** Pancreatic & Biliary Disease; Gastrointestinal Cancer; Endoscopy; **Hospital:** Mount Sinai Med Ctr - Miami; **Address:** Mount Sinai Medical Center, Gumenick Bldg, 4300 Alton Rd, Ste 2522, Miami Beach, FL 33140-2800; **Phone:** 305-674-2240; **Board Cert:** Internal Medicine 73; Gastroenterology 75; **Med School:** Univ Miami Sch Med 70; **Resid:** Internal Medicine, Univ Miami Hosp 73; **Fellow:** Gastroenterology, Univ Miami Hosp 75; **Fac Appt:** Prof Med, Univ Miami Sch Med

Boyce Jr, H Worth MD [Ge] - **Spec Exp:** Swallowing Disorders; Barrett's Esophagus; Esophageal Cancer; **Hospital:** H Lee Moffitt Cancer Ctr & Research Inst; **Address:** Ctr for Swallowing Disorders, 12901 Bruce B Downs Blvd, MC-72, Tampa, FL 33612; **Phone:** 813-974-3374; **Board Cert:** Internal Medicine 77; Gastroenterology 65; **Med School:** Wake Forest Univ 55; **Resid:** Internal Medicine, Brooke Army Hosp 59; Gastroenterology, Brooke Army Hosp 60; **Fac Appt:** Prof Med, Univ S Fla Coll Med

Liddle, Rodger Alan MD [Ge] - **Spec Exp:** Gastrointestinal Cancer; Pancreatic Disease; Hormone Secreting Tumors; **Hospital:** Duke Univ Med Ctr (page 94); **Address:** Duke University Medical Ctr, Div Gastroenterology, Box 3913, Durham, NC 27710; **Phone:** 919-681-6380; **Board Cert:** Internal Medicine 81; Gastroenterology 83; **Med School:** Vanderbilt Univ 78; **Resid:** Internal Medicine, UCSF Med Ctr 81; **Fellow:** Gastroenterology, UCSF Med Ctr 84; **Fac Appt:** Prof Med, Duke Univ

Raiford, David S MD [Ge] - **Spec Exp:** Liver Disease; Drug Toxicity in Liver; Liver Tumors; **Hospital:** Vanderbilt Univ Med Ctr (page 116); **Address:** Vanderbilt Hepatology, 1501 The Vanderbilt Clinic, Nashville, TN 37232-5280; **Phone:** 615-322-0128; **Board Cert:** Internal Medicine 89; Gastroenterology 91; **Med School:** Johns Hopkins Univ 85; **Resid:** Internal Medicine, Johns Hopkins Hosp 88; **Fac Appt:** Prof Med, Vanderbilt Univ

Midwest

Brown, Kimberly A MD [Ge] - **Spec Exp:** Liver Cancer & Disease; Transplant Medicine-Liver; Hepatitis C; **Hospital:** Henry Ford Hosp; **Address:** Henry Ford Hosp, Dept Gastroenterology, 2799 W Grand Blvd Bldg K Fl 7, Detroit, MI 48202-2608; **Phone:** 313-916-8865; **Board Cert:** Internal Medicine 88; Gastroenterology 02; **Med School:** Wayne State Univ 85; **Resid:** Internal Medicine, Univ Michigan Med Ctr 89; **Fellow:** Gastroenterology, Univ Michigan Med Ctr 92

Crippin, Jeffrey S MD [Ge] - **Spec Exp:** Transplant Medicine-Liver; Liver Disease; Gastrointestinal Cancer; **Hospital:** Barnes-Jewish Hosp (page 85); **Address:** Barnes Jewish Hosp, Div Gastroenterology, One Barnes Jewish Hospital Plaza, St Louis, MO 63110; **Phone:** 314-454-8160; **Board Cert:** Internal Medicine 87; Gastroenterology 01; **Med School:** Univ Kans 84; **Resid:** Internal Medicine, Kansas Univ Med Ctr 88; **Fellow:** Gastroenterology, Mayo Clinic 91; **Fac Appt:** Assoc Prof Med, Washington Univ, St Louis

Di Bisceglie, Adrian Michael MD [Ge] - **Spec Exp:** Hepatitis C; Hepatitis; Liver Cancer; **Hospital:** St Louis Univ Hosp; **Address:** St Louis Univ Hosp, Dept. Gastroenterology, 3635 Vista Ave, PO Box 15250, St. Louis, MO 63110-0250; **Phone:** 314-577-8764; **Board Cert:** Internal Medicine 02; Gastroenterology 02; **Med School:** South Africa 77; **Resid:** Internal Medicine, Baragwanath Hosp 84; **Fellow:** Hepatology, Natl Inst Hlth 88; **Fac Appt:** Prof Med, St Louis Univ

Goldberg, Michael MD [Ge] - **Spec Exp:** Colon Cancer; Inflammatory Bowel Disease; Pancreatic & Billiary Disease; **Hospital:** Evanston Hosp; **Address:** 2600 Ridge Ave, Ste G-208, Evanston, IL 60201; **Phone:** 847-657-1900; **Board Cert:** Internal Medicine 78; Gastroenterology 81; **Med School:** Univ IL Coll Med 75; **Resid:** Internal Medicine, Univ Illinois Hosp 78; **Fellow:** Gastroenterology, Tufts-New England Med Ctr 80; **Fac Appt:** Assoc Clin Prof Med, Northwestern Univ

Waxman, Irving MD [Ge] - **Spec Exp:** Gastrointestinal Cancer; Pancreatic Cancer; Endoscopy; **Hospital:** Univ of Chicago Hosps; **Address:** University of Chicago Hospitals, 5758 S Maryland Ave, MC 9028, Chicago, IL 60637; **Phone:** 773-702-1459; **Board Cert:** Internal Medicine 88; Gastroenterology 03; **Med School:** Mexico 86; **Resid:** Internal Medicine, New England Deaconess Hosp 88; **Fellow:** Gastroenterology, Georgetown Univ Med Ctr 91; Endoscopy, Academic Med Ctr-Univ Amsterdam; **Fac Appt:** Prof Med, Univ Chicago-Pritzker Sch Med

Great Plains and Mountains

Burt, Randall W MD [Ge] - **Spec Exp:** Colon Cancer; Familial Adenomatous Polyposis (FAP); **Hospital:** Univ Utah Hosps and Clins; **Address:** Huntsman Cancer Inst At Univ Utah, 2000 Circle of Hope, Salt Lake City, UT 84112; **Phone:** 801-585-3281; **Board Cert:** Internal Medicine 77; Gastroenterology 79; **Med School:** Univ Utah 74; **Resid:** Internal Medicine, Barnes Hosp 77; **Fellow:** Gastroenterology, Univ Utah Med Ctr 79; **Fac Appt:** Prof Med, Univ Utah

Southwest

Boland, C. Richard MD [Ge] - **Spec Exp:** Colon Cancer Detection/Risk Asseessment; Colon & Rectal Cancer-Hereditary; Cancer Genetics; **Hospital:** Baylor Univ Medical Ctr (page 86); **Address:** Gastroenterology Dept, 3500 Gaston Ave, Dallas, TX 75246; **Phone:** 214-820-2692; **Board Cert:** Internal Medicine 78; Gastroenterology 81; **Med School:** Yale Univ 73; **Resid:** Internal Medicine, USPHS Hosp 78; **Fellow:** Gastroenterology, UCSF 81

Bresalier, Robert MD **[Ge]** - **Spec Exp:** Gastrointestinal Cancer; Peptic Acid Disorders; **Hospital:** UT MD Anderson Cancer Ctr, The (page 115); **Address:** UT MD Anderson Canc Ctr, Dept GI Med & Nutrition, 1515 Holcombe Blvd - Unit 436, Houston, TX 77030-4009; **Phone:** 713-745-4340; **Board Cert:** Internal Medicine 81; Gastroenterology 83; **Med School:** Univ Chicago-Pritzker Sch Med 78; **Resid:** Internal Medicine, Barnes Hosp-Washington Univ 81; **Fellow:** Gastroenterology, UCSF Med Ctr 83; **Fac Appt:** Prof Med, Univ Tex, Houston

Cunningham, John MD **[Ge]** - **Spec Exp:** Biliary Disease; Pancreatitis; Pancreatic Tumors; **Hospital:** Univ Med Ctr - Tucson; **Address:** Univ Arizona, Div Gastroenterology, 1501 N Campbell Ave, PO Box 245028, Tuscon, AZ 85724-5028; **Phone:** 520-626-6119; **Board Cert:** Internal Medicine 75; Gastroenterology 77; **Med School:** Med Coll VA 70; **Resid:** Internal Medicine, Med Univ South Carolina 75; **Fellow:** Gastroenterology, Med Univ South Carolina 77; **Fac Appt:** Prof Med, Univ Ariz Coll Med

Fleischer, David MD **[Ge]** - **Spec Exp:** Barrett's Esophagus; Esophageal Cancer; **Hospital:** Mayo Clin Hosp - Scottsdale; **Address:** Mayo Clinic - Scottsdale, 13400 E Shea Blvd, Div Gastroenterology 2A, Scottsdale, AZ 85259; **Phone:** 480-301-8484; **Board Cert:** Internal Medicine 75; Gastroenterology 77; **Med School:** Vanderbilt Univ 70; **Resid:** Internal Medicine, Metro General Hosp 75; **Fellow:** Gastroenterology, LA Co Harbor-UCLA Med Ctr 77; **Fac Appt:** Prof Med, Mayo Med Sch

Levin, Bernard MD **[Ge]** - **Spec Exp:** Gastrointestinal Cancer; Colon & Rectal Cancer; Cancer Prevention; **Hospital:** UT MD Anderson Cancer Ctr, The (page 115); **Address:** Univ Tex MD Anderson Cancer Ctr, 1515 Holcombe Blvd Unit #1370, Houston, TX 77030-4095; **Phone:** 713-792-3900; **Board Cert:** Internal Medicine 72; Gastroenterology 72; **Med School:** South Africa 64; **Resid:** Internal Medicine, Rush Presby-St Lukes Hosp 68; **Fellow:** Pathology, Univ Chicago 70; Gastroenterology, Univ Chicago 72

HEMATOLOGY &
MEDICAL ONCOLOGY

a subspecialty of
INTERNAL
MEDICINE

Hematology: An internist with additional training who specializes in diseases of the blood, spleen and lymph glands. This specialist treats conditions such as anemia, clotting disorders, sickle cell disease, hemophilia, leukemia and lymphoma.

Medical Oncology: An internist who specializes in the diagnosis and treatment of all types of cancer and other benign and malignant tumors. This specialist decides on and administers chemotherapy for malignancy, as well as consulting with surgeons and radiotherapists on other treatments for cancer.

Training Required: Three years in internal medicine plus additional training and examination for certification in hematology or medical oncology.

PHYSICIAN LISTINGS

Hematology:

Medical Oncology:

INTERNAL MEDICINE: *An internist is a personal physician who provides long-term, comprehensive care in the office and the hospital, managing both common and complex illness of adolescents, adults and the elderly. Internists are trained in the diagnosis and treatment of cancer, infections and diseases affecting the heart, blood, kidneys, joints and digestive, respiratory and vascular systems. They are also trained in the essentials of primary care internal medicine, which incorporates an understanding of disease prevention, wellness, substance abuse, mental health and effective treatment of common problems of the eyes, ears, skin, nervous system and reproductive organs.*

BLOOD AND MARROW TRANSPLANTATION
BAYLOR UNIVERSITY MEDICAL CENTER AT DALLAS

3500 Gaston Avenue, Dallas, Texas 75246
Tel: 1-800-4BAYLOR (422-9567) • www.BaylorHealth.edu

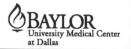

A HISTORY OF SUCCESS

Since its beginning in 1983, the blood and marrow transplant program at Baylor University Medical Center (Baylor Dallas) has performed more than 2,800 transplants, ranking it among the largest in the country. The program has vast expertise in autologous, allogeneic-related and allogeneic-unrelated donor transplantation. Treatment is available for the following principal diseases: acute and chronic leukemia, Hodgkin's lymphoma, non-Hodgkin's lymphoma, myeloma and related diseases, and selected solid tumors. Patients of the Baylor blood and marrow program are cared for in our 25-bed inpatient marrow transplant/intensive care unit and 32-bed oncology unit. Both units were designed to meet patient, family and nursing needs. All rooms are high-efficiency particulate air (HEPA)-filtered to provide optimal isolation from infection.

RESEARCH: A KEY COMPONENT

Research in the blood and marrow transplant program at Baylor Dallas focuses on the unique treatments such as non-myeloablative transplants, cancer vaccines and the use of radiopharmaceuticals in cancer treatment. Researchers also have studies on graft-versus-host disease, induction of immune tolerance, studies of supportive care for transplant recipients, and studies in the prevention and treatment of infectious complications of blood or marrow transplantation. The program currently has eleven IRB approved research protocols enrolling patients.

NATIONAL MARROW DONOR PROGRAM

As a member of the National Marrow Donor Program (NMDP), Baylor Dallas is able to search national and international registries to seek suitable matches for our patients. Our program is one of only 6 programs nationwide that maintains a transplant center, donor center, and collection center. In 2003, 125 donor recruitment events were held, bringing the total number of potential donors on Baylor's registry to 32,710, including 571 minority donors. Baylor's unrelated transplant center has facilitated more than 400 stem cell transplants since inception, and continues to perform 40-50 unrelated donor transplants each year.

ACCREDITATION

In 1998, Baylor University Medical Center at Dallas became one of the first centers in the United States to receive initial accreditation by the Foundation for the Accreditation of Cellular Therapy (FACT), and in 2001, received accreditation renewal with high marks for overall performance and level of quality.

BAYLOR CHARLES A. SAMMONS CANCER CENTER AT DALLAS

Baylor Charles A. Sammons Cancer Center provides a full array of oncology services, including surgical and gynecologic consultation, radiation oncology, medical oncology-hematology, blood/marrow transplantation. The center also offers therapy and prevention trials, screening and genetic risk evaluation programs, a patient education and support centers and a boutique designed to meet the cosmetic needs of cancer patients.

Physicians at the Baylor Sammons Cancer Center treat all forms of cancer with particular emphasis on breast, prostate, lung, colon, and gynecologic cancers as well as hematologic malignancies (leukemia, lymphoma and myeloma).

Multidisciplinary interaction among doctors from different specialties is the focus of cancer center activities. These specialists and researchers work together to provide patients with personalized, high quality care and to conduct educational and research programs that continue the quest for a cure.

DANA-FARBER/BRIGHAM AND WOMEN'S
CANCER CENTER
STEM CELL/BONE MARROW TRANSPLANT PROGRAM

75 FRANCIS STREET • 44 BINNEY STREET • BOSTON, MA 02115

1-877-DFCI-BWH • WWW.DFBWCANCER.ORG

TRUSTED EXPERTISE

The Stem Cell/Bone Marrow Transplant Program is part of the Center for Hematologic Oncology, a specialized treatment center at Dana-Farber/Brigham and Women's Cancer Center. The Center combines the clinical expertise, focus, and innovation of Dana-Farber Cancer Institute, one of the nation's leading cancer centers, with the world-class care and services of Brigham and Women's Hospital, one of the nation's leading teaching hospitals. Dana-Farber Cancer Institute and Brigham and Women's Hospital are teaching affiliates of Harvard Medical School. One of the oldest and largest transplant centers in the world, more than 4,000 stem cell/bone marrow transplants have been performed since our program began in 1972.

DISEASES TREATED

Our physicians perform approximately 300 transplants each year for the treatment of adult cancers and disorders, including acute lymphoblastic leukemia (ALL), acute myeloid leukemia (AML), chronic lymphocytic leukemia (CLL), chronic myelogenous leukemia (CML), Hodgkin's Lymphoma, Non-Hodgkin's Lymphoma, multiple myeloma, myelodysplastic syndrome, Waldenstrom's Macroglobulinemia, hematological disorders, myeloproliferative disorders, and testicular cancer.

COMPREHENSIVE AND COORDINATED CARE

The collaboration and integration of services at Dana-Farber Cancer Institute and Brigham and Women's Hospital enables us to provide superior patient care in the field of stem cell transplantation. Drawing on many years of experience, our scientists, physicians, and the entire patient care team are able to solve diagnostic dilemmas, evaluate new transplant techniques and supportive therapies, identify targeted treatment options, and serve as leaders and educators.

ADVANCED TREATMENT

The Stem Cell/Bone Marrow Transplant Program at Dana-Farber/Brigham and Women's Cancer Center offers a comprehensive range of stem cell/bone marrow transplant services, including allogeneic transplants (with matched family member, unrelated donor, or umbilical cord blood), autologous transplants, and identical twin transplantation. The Center provides identification of matched related or unrelated donors and coordination of stem cell collection for transplantation, as well as identification of umbilical cord blood stem cell products and coordination of stem cell collection for transplantation. With a state-of-the-art cell manipulation core facility, services include outpatient care, consultations and services, such as chemotherapy, inpatient care, including stem cell transplantation, laboratory services, imaging, radiation oncology, support services, and post-transplant care, including collaboration with patients' local physicians.

INNOVATIVE CLINICAL TRIALS

The Center for Hematologic Oncology offers patients access to a growing number of innovative clinical trials for hematologic malignancies and transplant through Dana-Farber/Harvard Cancer Center, at National Cancer Institute-designated Comprehensive Cancer Center.

CALL **1-877-DFCI-BWH** FOR MORE INFORMATION, OR TO MAKE AN APPOINTMENT WITH A SPECIALIST AT DANA-FARBER/BRIGHAM AND WOMEN'S CANCER CENTER.

DANA-FARBER / PARTNERS CANCERCARE

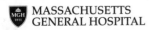
MASSACHUSETTS GENERAL HOSPITAL

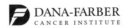
DANA-FARBER CANCER INSTITUTE

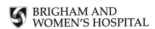
BRIGHAM AND WOMEN'S HOSPITAL

CEDARS-SINAI MEDICAL CENTER.
Samuel Oschin Comprehensive Cancer Institute

8700 Beverly Blvd.
Los Angeles, CA 90048
Tel: 1-800-CEDARS-1
(1-800-233-2771)
Fax: (310) 423-0499
www.cedars-sinai.edu/cancer

INNOVATION AND LEADERSHIP

Innovation underlies the medical care provided at the Samuel Oschin Comprehensive Cancer Institute at Cedars-Sinai Medical Center. That's one of many reasons more oncological surgeries are performed at our institute than at any other facility in Los Angeles County.

In addition, our clinical trials and research studies offer renewed hope to thousands every year. Thanks to ongoing research and leadership by some of the most knowledgeable and creative minds in medical research today, new treatments are introduced as quickly as they are determined to be safe and effective.

PATIENT-FOCUSED, MULTIDISCIPLINARY CARE

At the institute, dozens of nationally recognized programs and services are all available under one, interconnected medical "roof"—an important benefit to cancer patients. Every resource of this remarkable organization is at the disposal of top physicians and scientists from various specialties, who blend their knowledge and skills to provide leading-edge healthcare services customized to meet the unique needs of each patient.

OUTPATIENT CARE WHEN YOU NEED IT

We understand that not all healthcare needs fall during business hours, so we make our treatment services fit patients' daily lives. That's why our Cedars-Sinai Outpatient Cancer Center offers a uniquely responsive, round-the-clock schedule, the only center in Southern California to do so.

ONE OF AMERICA'S BEST

The institute is part of Cedars-Sinai Medical Center, a nationally renowned 877-bed facility, one of the largest medical centers in the western United States. Deemed the most preferred hospital in Los Angles County every year since 1987, Cedars-Sinai has been awarded numerous prestigious national honors as well. These include Magnet hospital status, nursing's highest award of excellence, and AARP's ranking as the number two metropolitan hospital nationwide

SPECIALIZED SERVICES

Because cancer takes many forms, each calling for different prevention, diagnostic and treatment techniques, the Samuel Oschin Comprehensive Cancer Institute serves as a hub for a wide array of cancer specialty centers and treatment programs, including:

- Maxine Dunitz Neurosurgical Institute
- Minimally Invasive Urology Institute
- Cedars-Sinai Outpatient Cancer Center
- Cedars-Sinai Center for Chest Diseases
- Louis Warschaw Prostate Cancer Center
- Saul and Joyce Brandman Breast Center, a Project of Women's Guild
- Carcinoid and Neuroendocrine Tumor Center
- Head and Neck Cancer Center
- Blood and Marrow Transplant Program
- Gilda Radner Cancer Detection Program
- Gynecologic Oncology Program
- Colorectal Cancer Program
- Multiple Myeloma and Bone Metastases Programs
- Sarcoma Program
- General and Pediatric Hematology/Oncology

HEMATOLOGY & HEMATOPOIETIC CELL TRANSPLANTATION AND MEDICAL ONCOLOGY
CITY OF HOPE CANCER CENTER

Where the Power of Knowledge Saves Lives®

1500 East Duarte Road
Duarte, California 91010
Tel. 800-826-HOPE (4673)
www.cityofhope.org

TREATING CANCERS OF THE BLOOD AND MARROW

The Hematologic Neoplasia Program at City of Hope Cancer Center has a long history of success in developing novel therapies for patients with:

- acute leukemia
- chronic leukemia
- malignant lymphoma
- Hodgkin's disease
- myelodysplasia
- myeloproliferative disorders

In 1976, City of Hope was one of the first medical centers in the nation to successfully perform bone marrow transplantation for leukemia. It now has one of the largest, most successful programs in the world. As respected leaders in hematologic cancer research and treatment, City of Hope physicians and investigators are working to expand the application of transplant for treatment of other diseases.

MEDICAL ONCOLOGY AND EXPERIMENTAL THERAPEUTICS

City of Hope is a leader in the translation of laboratory research into innovative clinical care. Patients have the widest possible range of therapeutic options and receive new treatments with a unique focus on the their entire well-being, not just the disease. City of Hope evaluates anticancer agents in their earliest stage of development. Among these are antiangiogenic molecules, chemotherapeutic drugs, and targeted therapies for all types of cancer, including breast, lung, prostate, gastrointestinal, brain and spinal cord.

ADVANCING PATIENT-FOCUSED MEDICINE

City of Hope is committed to developing better approaches to diagnosing, preventing, and treating disease, as well as improving quality of life. Approximately **40 percent of patients at City of Hope participate in clinical trials**, far surpassing the national average of 3 to 4 percent.

CITY OF HOPE is a National Cancer Institute (NCI)-designated Comprehensive Cancer Center–the highest accolade given by the NCI.

Other distinctions include:

- Founding member of the National Comprehensive Cancer Network, setting national standards of care for cancer;

- Scoring in the top 1 percent of hospitals surveyed by the Joint Commission on Accreditation of Healthcare Organizations (JCAHO); and

- Receiving the highest score possible in all applicable categories in the California Hospital Experience Survey (formerly known as PEP-C).

Helford Clinical Research Hospital, opened in 2005, continues City of Hope's tradition of progress and further substantiates City of Hope's ranking by U.S. News & World Report as one of America's 50 best cancer hospitals.

For more information, call 800-826-4673.

BONE MARROW AND STEM CELL TRANSPLANT
INDIANA UNIVERSITY HOSPITAL
A Clarian Health Partner

550 University Boulevard
Indianapolis, Indiana 46202
317-274-5000
www.clarian.org

A nationally recognized group of health care professionals, the Bone Marrow and Stem Cell Transplant Team at Indiana University Hospital provides exceptional care for adults and children with life-threatening diseases. Bone marrow and stem cell transplantation – procedures that restore immature, blood-producing stem cells – can be done as a first line of treatment for disease such as cancer, or to replenish stem cells destroyed by high doses of chemical and/or radiation therapy.

Through collaboration in national and local clinical trials, our team combines multidisciplinary research, education and patient care to offer hope and cure to bone marrow and stem cell transplant patients and their families.

ADVANCING TREATMENT THROUGH RESEARCH
The specific research goals of our program include:

- Stem cell biology – the scientific study of cells from which other blood cell types can develop
- Wide variety of stem cell sources, including cord blood
- Germ cell tumors – at tumor that begins in cells that produce sperm or eggs (testical/ovarian)
- Gene therapy – the treatment of cancer by altering a gene

A GROWING, PROGRESSIVE PROGRAM
IU Hospital performed its first allogeneic (taken from a human donor) bone marrow transplant in January 1985 and its first autologous (taken from a patient's own tissues) in July 1986. Since then, the number of bone marrow transplants accomplished at IU Hospital has steadily increased.

COMPREHENSIVE CARE IN ONE LOCATION
IU Hospital and the Indiana University Cancer Center offer interdisciplinary clinical programs that allow patients to see – in one simple visit – a variety of specialists who work as a team to provide complete cancer care. The Indiana University Cancer Center was the first cancer center in Indiana to truly operate as a multidisciplinary center. IU Hospital and IU Cancer Center have full representation of all medical and surgical specialties, giving patients access to the range of services they may need throughout their course of treatment.

WORLD-CLASS CANCER CARE
The IU Bone Marrow and Stem Cell Transplant Program is a leader in cancer diagnosis and treatment, making it one of the most widely recognized cancer programs in the U.S. and the world. The program brings together the talents, strengths and resources of a diverse group of individuals and organizations with a single focus: to reduce cancer incidence, suffering and mortality in Indiana and beyond.

AMONG AN ELITE GROUP
Based on its record of groundbreaking research and superior clinical patient care, the Indiana University Cancer Center has been designated a Cancer Center by the National Cancer Institute. The IU Cancer Center is the only such designated cancer providing patient care in Indiana, placing it among an elite group of centers focusing on excellent clinical care and the rapid implementation of new discoveries into the treatment of cancer.

TAUSSIG CANCER CENTER
THE CLEVELAND CLINIC

9500 Euclid Avenue • Cleveland, OH 44195
www.clevelandclinic.org/cancer
For appointments or second opinions,
call toll-free 866/CCF-8100

THE CLEVELAND CLINIC
Taussig Cancer Center

THE CLEVELAND CLINIC TAUSSIG CANCER CENTER: PUSHING THE LIMITS OF MEDICINE

At the Cleveland Clinic Taussig Cancer Center, we're fighting the battle against cancer and winning. Every day, our team of cancer experts pushes the limits of medicine – within the region, across the country and around the world.

Under the direction of Derek Raghavan, M.D., Ph.D., the Taussig Cancer Center annually serves more than 24,000 cancer patients, making it the largest cancer treatment center in the region. A team of 250 cancer specialists cares for patients with breast, colorectal, lung, urologic, endocrine, gastrointestinal, gynecologic, head and neck, musculoskeletal and ophthalmic cancers; cancers of the brain and spinal cord; skin cancer and melanoma; and hematologic malignancies. "Our treatment strategies are based on an emerging definition of molecular targets and of the genes and proteins that control cancer growth. We can now tailor treatments that are more effective and have fewer side effects," says Dr. Raghavan.

The center offers the latest advances in cancer diagnosis and treatments, including clinical trials of new therapies. For pediatric cancer patients, clinical-trials research has led to a high rate of cure, as well as the development of safer treatments for all persons with cancer.

The center also is one of just a few hospitals in the region to offer different technologies for administering stereotactic radiosurgery. Novalis and the Peacock/Corvus system are used for extracranial lesions, and Gamma Knife is used to treat primary and metastatic brain tumors.

"To stay at the forefront of cancer research, we continue to recruit world-renowned investigators," says Dr. Raghavan. "This focus on discovery and innovation is leading us toward a vision of cure for cancer in the 21st century."

To schedule an appointment or second opinion, call the Cancer Answer Line toll-free at 866/CCF-8100.

HOW DO YOU MEASURE QUALITY?

Visit our Web site at www.clevelandclinic.org /quality for information on the criteria most often used to measure quality in health care; data on how The Cleveland Clinic compares to other health care centers; patient satisfaction data; and quality measures for numerous specific diseases and conditions, including cancer.

SPECIAL SERVICE FOR OUT-OF-STATE PATIENTS

The Cleveland Clinic offers a complimentary concierge service exclusively for out-of-state patients and their families. Among other things, Cleveland Clinic Medical Concierge staff assist with coordinating multiple appointments; schedule or confirm air and ground transportation; and assist with hotel and housing reservations. Call 800/ 223-2273, ext. 55580, or send an e-mail to medicalconcierge@ccf.org.

CONTINUUM CANCER CENTERS OF NEW YORK

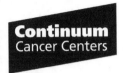

Beth Israel Medical Center
Roosevelt Hospital
St. Luke's Hospital
Long Island College Hospital
New York Eye and Ear Infirmary

Phone: 212-844-6027

Continuum Cancer Centers of New York

The hospitals of Continuum – Beth Israel Medical Center, St. Luke's and Roosevelt Hospitals, Long Island College Hospital and the New York Eye and Ear Infirmary – are leading providers of cancer care through Continuum Cancer Centers of New York. Our integrated system allows us to build on the clinical strengths found at each of our partner hospitals.

The goal – and result – is delivery of care in ways that are more efficient, more attractive and more convenient for patients. Specifically, it means that cancer patients at any Continuum hospital can benefit from system-wide cancer expertise, facilities and resources. Continuum Cancer Centers feature world-renowned cancer specialists, including top-rated surgeons, medical oncologists, radiation oncologists, radiologists, pathologists, and oncology nurses.

Comprehensive diagnostic and treatment services are available for breast cancer, prostate cancer, head and neck cancers, skin cancer, lung cancer, colorectal and other gastrointestinal cancers, Lymphoma/Hodgkin's Disease, gynecological cancers, and cancers of the brain and central nervous system. Delivered efficiently in a friendly and supportive environment, services include prevention programs - such as community education, screenings and early detection – expert diagnosis, outpatient treatment, inpatient services and home care. In addition, the Research Program offers patients access to investigational protocols through a wide number of clinical trials. Our physicians are leaders in both non-invasive and minimally invasive cancer treatments that focus on maximizing both the cure rate and the quality of life.

Support services play an important role at Continuum Cancer Centers. Nurses, social workers, psychiatrists, chaplin's, pharmacists, rehabilitation therapists and nutritionists -each with specialized knowledge and expertise in the field of oncology -work together to ensure that patients' medical, emotional and family needs are addressed appropriately and in a timely manner.

Duke Comprehensive Cancer Center
DUKE UNIVERSITY HEALTH SYSTEM

Durham, North Carolina • *1-888-ASK-DUKE* • *dukehealth.org*

The Duke Comprehensive Cancer Center (DCCC) was established in 1972 and has benefited from continuous recognition and funding from the National Cancer Institute (NCI) as one of the original eight centers. Today, Duke is one of only 38 NCI recognized Comprehensive Cancer Centers nationwide. The Duke Comprehensive Cancer Center treats close to 5,000 new patients with cancer in over 120,000 clinic visits annually and cares for 11% of all cancer patients in North Carolina. Thirty percent of Duke's cancer patients come from outside of North Carolina.

DCCC was ranked seventh among the nation's best cancer treatment hospitals in 2003 by *U.S.News & World Report*.

PROGRAM HIGHLIGHTS

The Brain Tumor Center at Duke has received one of only two brain tumor grants from the National Institute of Neurological Disorders and Stroke and is internationally recognized as a leader in the research and treatment of brain tumors.

The Duke Pediatric Bone Marrow Transplant Unit pioneered the use of umbilical cord blood to replace bone marrow destroyed by chemotherapy.

The Duke Oncology Network is a collaborative effort by the Duke University Health System and the Duke Comprehensive Cancer Center to affiliate with hospitals and private practices throughout North Carolina and the Southeast in order to provide patients in these communities with the highest quality cancer care.

The Duke Clinical Research Institute (DCRI) is the largest academic clinical trials group in the world focused on oncology. Today, the DCRI has nearly 900 employees and has enrolled more than 300,000 participants worldwide in its clinical trials.

Duke is home to the *American College of Surgeons Oncology Group*, a group of health professionals that was established to evaluate the surgical management of patients with malignant solid tumors.

Duke is a world leader in PET (positron emission tomography) scanning, which allows physicians to pinpoint hot spots of cancer throughout the body and more easily distinguish benign from malignant tumors.

DUKE
COMPREHENSIVE
CANCER CENTER

RESEARCH LEADERSHIP

The DCCC is a leader in translational research. The large volume of patients treated at Duke, combined with the extensive laboratory research programs, enable the Cancer Center to bring more new therapeutic treatments to patients faster.

A national clinical trial led by researchers at the DCCC was the first to show that the anti-angiogenesis drug, Avastin™, shrinks tumors by choking off their blood supply.

DCCC researchers were involved in the discovery of the BRCA 2 gene, which is associated with hereditary breast cancer. The discovery is considered a major breakthrough in breast cancer research.

In one of the clearest models of cancer metastasis, Duke scientists first demonstrated that spreading cancer cells receive growth-sustaining signals from nearby blood vessels telling them where to go for permanent nourishment and oxygen. These findings present a model of the earliest stages of cancer metastasis and bolster medicine's latest strategy of blocking blood vessel growth as a means of inhibiting cancer's spread.

MEDICAL ONCOLOGY
FOX CHASE CANCER CENTER

333 Cottman Avenue
Philadelphia, Pennsylvania 19111-2497
Phone: 1-888-FOX CHASE • Fax: 215-728-2702 • www.fccc.edu

Medical oncologists at Fox Chase Cancer Center specialize in all major adult solid tumors as well as cancers of the blood and bone marrow and rare tumors such as sarcomas. Major clinical interests include breast, gastrointestinal, genitourinary, lung, neuroendocrine and ovarian cancers; adult leukemias and lymphomas; mesothelioma; gastroenterology; pain management; and palliative care. Bone-marrow and blood stem-cell transplants are available through the Fox Chase-Temple Bone Marrow Transplant Program.

Fox Chase physicians and scientists are among the world's leaders in developing and testing new anticancer drugs and new methods of drug delivery and immunotherapy. Patients may receive state-of-the-art drugs alone or as part of a treatment plan using two or more therapies.

Medical oncology and pharmacology research focuses on creating more effective anticancer drugs and investigating the molecular mechanisms that allow some tumor cells to acquire drug resistance. New drug development includes not only drugs for treatment but also potential preventive agents and sensitizing agents that make cancer cells more responsive to drugs (chemosensitizers), to radiation therapy (radiosensitizers) or to light (photodynamic therapy agents).

Fox Chase medical oncologists are also leading the way in developing immunotherapy—treatments that activate the immune system to attack cancer cells. Several treatment approaches designed here combine such biologic agents as interferons and interleukins or team them with monoclonal antibodies or established anticancer drugs.

The development of new, "two-way" monoclonal antibodies has advanced the potential for immunotherapy to stimulate a patient's immune system and deliver activated immune cells directly to the cancer. Monoclonal antibody therapies have shown tremendous promise in clinical trials for people with chemotherapy-resistant lymphoma and for some women with breast cancer. Fox Chase medical oncologists continue to study combination therapies pairing this antibody treatment with other drugs or radioactive molecules that can be delivered directly to the tumor cells.

CLINICAL TRIALS HELP SCIENCE AND MEDICINE WORK TOGETHER

Fox Chase translates new research findings into medical applications that may become models for improved comprehensive cancer care. Along with trials designed and offered only at Fox Chase, the Center participates in many national studies.

More than 170 clinical trials of new cancer prevention, diagnostic and treatment techniques are under way at any one time, including phase I trials that are the first to test new treatment drugs in patients.

For healthy people who want to reduce their risk of cancer, Fox Chase conducts one-of-a-kind trials of agents that may prevent cancer in high-risk individuals. The Fox Chase advantage includes a leading role in national cancer prevention trials.

THE CANCER CENTER – HACKENSACK UNIVERSITY MEDICAL CENTER

20 Prospect Avenue, Hackensack, New Jersey 07601
Phone 201-996-5800; Fax 201-996-9246; www.humc.com

New Jersey's Largest Cancer Center – The Cancer Center at Hackensack University Medical Center is New Jersey's largest and most comprehensive cancer program and one of the top 10 in the nation in patient volume. Each week, more than 150 new patients come to The Cancer Center seeking services that are widely recognized for their innovation and attention to patients' needs and concerns. With one of the largest Blood and Marrow Transplantation Programs in the nation, The Cancer Center offers patients the most advanced treatments available.

Vision and Focus – The Cancer Center's mission is to provide the highest quality cancer care, preventive services, treatment, research, management, and screenings. Fourteen specialized cancer-care teams provide advanced care that combines state-of-the-art technology, skilled medical expertise, research breakthroughs, and compassionate care giving.

Bringing You Tomorrow's Breakthroughs Today™ – Most of today's cancer-care breakthroughs have come about from basic and clinical research into how cancer can be best detected, treated, or managed. Some of the most innovative cancer clinical trials are conducted at The Cancer Center, spearheaded by internationally renowned award-winning researchers. These trials give patients access to promising investigational medications, treatment protocols, and surgical techniques. This strong research component coupled with its patient care services elevates The Cancer Center to a world-class academic medical center.

Finding Answers – The first step in cancer care is to define the illness, determine its location, and find out whether it has spread. At The Cancer Center, pathologists, radiologists, and other physicians use precise, sophisticated technology to gain answers to these questions. Among the equipment and tests used are a dedicated PET scanner, ultrasonography, nuclear medicine, computerized tomography, magnetic resonance imaging, mammography, and angiography.

Today's Treatment Innovations – Physicians at The Cancer Center have pioneered some of the most promising treatments for cancer – including peripheral stem cell transplantation. Through its specialized divisions, The Cancer Center offers patients the most advanced treatment options, including intensity modulated radiation therapy, brachytherapy, stereotactic radiosurgery; the latest chemotherapy medications; innovative adjuvant therapy approaches; and state-of-the-art surgical techniques, including video-assisted thoracic surgery, radio-ablation therapy, and minimally invasive procedures that reduce pain, lessen side effects, decrease recovery time, and increase patients' mobility.

To receive information about all of The Cancer Center's services and 14 specialized divisions, please call 201-996-5800.

LIVING WITH CANCER

The Cancer Center provides an outstanding array of aftercare and support services to help patients manage their quality of life. These include:

• Support groups for adults, children, and family members to help them cope with the illness, treatment, and aftercare

• The Integrative Cancer Care Program at The Center for Health and Healing brings together a range of services to address the physical, emotional, and spiritual needs of patients with cancer, their family members, and friends

• The Ellen H. Lazar Shoppe on Fifth, provides high-quality products in a private setting for patients undergoing or who have completed treatment for cancer

• The Department of Social Services, provides crisis intervention, financial guidance, stress reduction sessions, psychosocial counseling, referrals to community resources, a floating library, and various educational workshops

• The Hospice Program offers pain- and symptom-relief services, spiritual support, skilled nursing care, social services, home healthcare, and bereavement

PHYSICIAN REFERRAL

Hackensack University Medical Center's Physician Referral Service representatives offer information on the nearly 1,400 medical and dental staff members representing more than 50 specialties. Call (201) 996-2020.

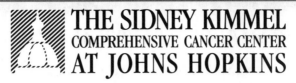

THE SIDNEY KIMMEL
COMPREHENSIVE CANCER CENTER
AT JOHNS HOPKINS

401 N. Broadway • Baltimore, MD 21231
www.hopkinskimmelcancercenter.org

THE SIDNEY KIMMEL COMPREHENSIVE CANCER CENTER at JOHNS HOPKINS

Best of the Best

The Sidney Kimmel Comprehensive Cancer Center at Johns Hopkins consistently ranks among the top three cancer centers nationwide by *US News & World Report*. We have internationally known experts in the treatment of cancers of the breast, lung, prostate, colon, pancreas, leukemia and lymphoma, plus cancer pain management, a state-of-the-art Gamma Knife Center for brain tumors, vaccine research, and treatment of childhood cancers.

30 Years of Discovery and Compassionate Care

The Kimmel Cancer Center is one of only 41 centers nationwide, and one of the first in the nation, designated by the National Cancer Institute as a Comprehensive Cancer Center. Among the prestigious awards the Center holds are seven spore (Specialized Programs of Research Excellence) grants to help speed the time between basic science discoveries in the laboratory and clinical trials in patients. In the fall of 2001, Johns Hopkins received an extraordinary gift – $150 million for patient care and cancer research – from Sidney Kimmel, founder and chairman of Jones Apparel Group. In recognition of Mr. Kimmel's gift, the largest in Hopkins' history, the center changed its name to become the Sidney Kimmel Comprehensive Cancer Center at Johns Hopkins.

Offering Patients Hope

Many clinical trials of novel drugs are currently under way at the Center, with approximately 150 studies available to patients. The Center conducts research studies funded by the National Cancer Institute and our physicians participate with other centers in large group trials across the country.

Call **410-955-8804** to speak with a cancer clinical trials specialist:

To find a specialist at Johns Hopkins call
410-955-5464 for calls in Baltimore
410-847-3582 for calls from outside the Baltimore area
+01-410-847-3580 for calls from outside the United States

SPECIALTY SERVICES

- Breast Center
- Bone Marrow Transplant
- Brain and Spinal Tumor Program (Neuro-Oncology)
- Colon Cancer Center
- Head and Neck Cancer
- HIV-Related Cancers
- Johns Hopkins Ovarian Cancer Center of Excellence
- Kelly Gynecologic Oncology Service
- Leukemia Service
- Liver Cancer Center
- Lymphoma Program and Clinic
- Melanoma and Cutaneous Oncology
- Myeloid Disorders Clinic
- Palliative Care Initiative
- Pancreatic Cancer
- Pediatric Oncology
- Prostate and Genitourinary Cancers
- Sarcoma and Soft Tissue
- Thyroid Tumor
- Thoracic Oncology and Lung Cancer

MAIMONIDES MEDICAL CENTER

COMPREHENSIVE CANCER CENTER

6300 Eighth Avenue, Brooklyn, New York
718 765-2500
www.maimonidesmed.org

Early 2004 saw the opening of the Women's Breast Center, the first element of Maimonides' new Comprehensive Cancer Center. When completed it will be the first such center in Brooklyn to offer a complete spectrum of services for the prevention, diagnosis, treatment and support of cancer patients and their families at one location. The Center will also serve as an educational resource for its patients and conduct community education and research.

Taking advantage of the latest imaging technologies and treatment modalities, the Center will offer state-of-the-art care through a full range of clinical and support services. A multidisciplinary team of outstanding oncologists, surgeons, radiologists, nurses, social workers and treatment specialists will provide care supported by a complementary range of services including: nutrition counseling, pain management, psychological and pastoral counseling, social work assistance and support groups. Consistent with the Maimonides philosophy of compassionate patient-centered care, the full needs of patients and their families will be addressed through ongoing communication.

The completed Cancer Center will provide the following services: medical oncology, infusion services, urologic oncology, women's breast services and radiation oncology. It will also be a resource center for patients and their families with computerized guided access to both local and national information and publications and a spectrum of support resources. The Center will also conduct clinical research and provide a referral service for information on clinical outcomes, research protocols, prevention and treatment.

All specialty centers are expected to be operational by 2005. For additional information about the Maimonides Comprehensive Cancer Center please call 718 765-2500.

COMPREHENSIVE CANCER CENTER

With the opening of the Women's Breast Center, the first phase of Maimonides new Comprehensive Cancer Center is complete. Over the next year, the Center will complete the introduction of medical oncology, infusion services, urologic oncology and radiation oncology, and will provide patient education and start clinical research.

By 2005, Maimonides will have attained its goal of providing at one location the first center offering comprehensive cancer care for the residents of Brooklyn.

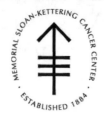

Memorial Sloan-Kettering Cancer Center

The Best Cancer Care. Anywhere.

1275 York Avenue • New York, NY 10017
Phone: 1-212-639-2000 • Physician referral: 1-800-525-2225
www.mskcc.org

Sponsorship:	Private, Non-Profit
Beds:	432
Accreditation:	Awarded Accreditation from the Joint Commission on Accreditation of Healthcare Organizations (JCAHO).

SUB-SPECIALIZED CLINICAL EXPERTISE

At Memorial Sloan-Kettering, the sole focus is cancer. Our physicians provide expert care in the hundreds of different subtypes of cancer. For patients, this specialization means a singular level of medical expertise, superb patient care, and an often dramatic effect on a patient's chances for a cure or control of his or her disease.

Our Disease Management Program features medical teams, defined by cancer type (breast, lung, etc.) whose members work together to guide each patient through every aspect of their care-diagnosis, treatment and recovery. These teams have a depth and breadth of experience that is unsurpassed. Using this approach, the treatment plans reflect the combined expertise of many medical professionals, including surgeons, medical oncologists, radiologists, radiation oncologists, pathologists, psychologists and social workers. This approach also ensures that patients who need several different therapies to treat their cancer will receive the best combination for them.

RESEARCH AND EDUCATION

One of Memorial Sloan-Kettering's great strengths is the close relationship between scientists and clinicians. The constant collaboration between our doctors and research scientists means that new drugs and therapies developed in the laboratory can be moved quickly to the bedside, offering patients improved treatment options. The Center's renowned training programs prepare today's physicians, scientists, nurses and other health professionals for tomorrow's leadership roles in science and medicine, especially as it relates to cancer.

SUPPORTING OUR PATIENTS

At Memorial Sloan-Kettering, we have long understood that cancer is not solely a physical disease. For more than 50 years, we have provided expert assistance in dealing with cancer-related distress, and have developed a range of comprehensive programs and services to help patients, families and caregivers manage the unique set of changes that often accompany illness. Many of our programs now serve as models for other cancer centers around the world.

A TRADITION OF EXCELLENCE

From its founding more than a century ago, Memorial Sloan-Kettering Cancer Center has been guided by a clear mission: to offer the best possible care for patients today, and to seek strategies to prevent, control and ultimately cure cancer in the future. We are proud of our designation as one of the few select National Cancer Institute Comprehensive Cancer Centers.

To see one of our specialized cancer experts, simply call us at (800)525-2225.

THE MOUNT SINAI MEDICAL CENTER
ONCOLOGY / CANCER CARE

One Gustave L. Levy Place (Fifth Avenue and 98th Street)
New York, NY 10029-6574   Phone: (212) 241-6500
Physician Referral: 1-800-MD-SINAI (637-4624)
www.mountsinai.org

A TRADITION OF COMMITMENT AND DEDICATION
Mount Sinai has dedicated itself to one of the most widespread life-threatening diseases.

SUPERB CARE
In an atmosphere of learning, clinical excellence, and superb patient care, Mount Sinai coordinates a full service diagnostic and treatment program for the cancer patient.

A WIDE RANGE OF PROGRAMS
Programs include medical chemotherapy, radiation, surgery, bone marrow and stem cell transplants, clinical trials for adults and children, and palliative care.

ADVANCED TECHNIQUES
Mount Sinai specialists use the most recent advances in the diagnosis and treatment of all cancers and especially, breast, colorectal, liver, lung, prostate, head and neck, gynecological and genitourinary cancers, and cancers of the blood and lymph systems.

TEAMWORK
Using a multi-disciplinary approach, The Hospital's cancer specialists work with their colleagues in Medical Oncology, Radiation Oncology, Radiology, Surgery, and Pathology to treat the wide spectrum of types and locations of cancer.

INNOVATION
In addition, the Medical Center takes innovative approaches to the treatment of cancer patients: minimal access, local therapy for endocrine tumors, high risk screening, genetics of breast cancer, multi-modality therapy for gastrointestinal cancer, melanoma screening, vaccine program, and minimal access surgery for cancer in the elderly. And with the knowledge gained through the Human Genome Project, Mount Sinai researchers are working on a gene therapy program for colon, prostate and breast cancer.

PROSTATE HEALTH CENTER
Under the auspices of the Barbara and Maurice A. Deane Prostate Health Center, patients can access the expertise of experienced urologists, medical oncologists, and radiation oncologists, so that a patient may ultimately choose his definitive therapy with full knowledge of the risks and benefits of each treatment option. The focus of the Integrated Prostate Cancer Program is the provision of care for patients for whom standard treatments for localized disease, locally advanced disease, or metastatic disease have failed.

THE DERALD H. RUTTERBERG CANCER CENTER

The mission of the **Derald H. Ruttenberg Cancer Center** at Mount Sinai School of Medicine is to reduce the burden of human cancer through its outstanding interdisciplinary programs in research and patient care, including cancer prevention, treatment, early detection, and education.

The **Ruttenberg Treatment Center** builds on this multidisciplinary model to provide state of the art ambulatory cancer care.

The members of the Cancer Center, scientists and medical professionals, are working together to develop cancer therapies and prevention strategies to improve cancer care. New translational cancer research initiatives, from "bench to bedside" are being developed in a number of research laboratories with funding from the National Cancer Institute.

For information on Thoracic Surgery, see the Thoracic Surgery page 501.

⌐ NewYork Presbyterian
⌐ The University Hospital of Columbia and Cornell
NewYork-Presbyterian Cancer Centers

Affiliated with Columbia University College of Physicians and Surgeons and Weill Medical College of Cornell University

Herbert Irving Comprehensive Cancer Center
At NewYork-Presbyterian Hospital
Columbia University Medical Center
161 Fort Washington Avenue
New York, NY 10032

Weill Cornell Cancer Center
At NewYork-Presbyterian Hospital
Weill Cornell Medical Center
525 East 68th Street
New York, NY 10021

OVERVIEW:

NewYork-Presbyterian Cancer Centers are dedicated to reducing cancer morbidity and mortality by providing

- a full continuum of multidisciplinary, state-of-the-art screening, diagnostic, treatment and support services for all phases of the disease process;
- cutting-edge basic, clinical, and public health research;
- full range of cancer-related educational programs and resources to clinicians, scientists, patients and survivors, families, and the cancer prevention community.

The Cancer Centers, which treat over 6,000 new patients annually, draw on the innovation and excellence of the NCI- designated Herbert Irving Comprehensive Cancer Center at NewYork-Presbyterian Hospital/Columbia University Medical Center and oncology services at NewYork-Presbyterian Hospital/Weill Cornell Medical Center. Programs include:

- AIDS-related Malignancies
- Bone Marrow Transplant
- Breast Cancer
- Dermatologic/Skin Cancer
- Gastrointestinal Cancers
- Genitourinary Cancers
- Gynecologic Cancers
- Head and Neck Cancers
- Hematologic Malignancies, such as lymphoma, myeloma and leukemias
- Lung Cancer
- Neurologic Cancer
- Ophthalmic Cancer
- Pediatric Hematology/Oncology
- Urologic Cancers, including bladder, kidney and prostate cancer
- Sarcomas and Mesotheiliomas

The Centers are frequent recipients of major grants and gifts to support research programs. Recent highlights include:

- Avon Products Foundation $10 million award to NewYork-Presbyterian Hospital/Columbia University Medical Center and Columbia University for establishment of the Avon Products Breast Center to support basic, clinical and public health research in breast cancer;
- The Leukemia and Lymphoma Society five-year $7.5 million grant to NewYork-Presbyterian Hospital/Weill Cornell Medical Center to study fundamental causes of multiple myeloma.

Physician Referral: For a physician referral call toll free **1-877-NYP-WELL** (1-877-697-9355) to learn more about our Cancer Centers visit our website at **www.nypcancer.org**

COMPREHENSIVE SERVICES INCLUDE:

- Access to over 400 clinical trials supported by the National Institutes of Health and many prominent pharmaceutical companies.

- Bone marrow and blood stem cell transplant, including New York State approval to perform transplants using unrelated donors for patients with hematologic malignancies

- CT screening for early lung cancer detection

- Sentinel node biopsy to assess spread of breast cancer

- Skin-sparing mastectomy and reconstruction

- Laparoscopic surgery for colon cancer

- Intraoperative brachytherapy for GI, prostate and other cancers

- Stereotactic biopsies for breast cancer and brain cancer

- Stereotactic gamma radiation for brain tumors

NYU MEDICAL CENTER
550 1st Avenue (at 31st Street)
New York, NY 10016
Physician Referral:
1-888-7-NYU-MED
www.nyumc.org

SCHOOL OF MEDICINE

NEW YORK UNIVERSITY

NYU CANCER INSTITUTE
at the NYU Clinical Cancer Center
160 East 34th Street
New York, NY 1001
1-212 731-6000
www.nyuci.org

HEMATOLOGY AND MEDICAL ONCOLOGY

- *RENOWNED EXPERTS. COMPASSIONATE CARE.*

Individualized treatment and a program of multidisciplinary care is provided for patients with a wide range of benign and malignant solid tumors as well as hematological disorders. In addition to the Bone Marrow Transplantation Program, our integrated programs focus on the breast, reproductive system, gastrointestinal tract, genitourinary system (such as prostate cancer), nervous system (including brain cancer), lung, and head and neck, as well as melanoma and hematologic cancer. Patients may seek treatment for a variety of conditions including anemia, white blood cell and platelet disorders, enlargement of the lymph nodes or spleen, bleeding and clotting disorders, leukemia, lymphoma, and lymphoproliferative and myeloproliferative disorders.

- *PROMPT SCREENING & DIAGNOSIS*

Advanced imaging procedures and other diagnostic tests are performed to detect cancer. Radiologists and pathologists located on site ensure accurate and prompt evaluation of imaging films and test results.

- *PATIENT-FOCUSED TREATMENT SETTINGS*

For patients receiving infusion, injection, and/or transfusion services, private treatment areas with television, telephone, and visitor space have been designed to maximize privacy, safety, and comfort.

- *ACCESS TO CLINICAL TRIALS*

A variety of investigator-initiated trials, as well as access to clinical trials via cooperative groups are available to evaluate new approaches for treating, diagnosing, or preventing specific diseases. To facilitate the application of promising laboratory findings, NYU Cancer Institute's Translational Research Task Force is designed to support the integration of basic sciences and clinical care.

- *SUPPORT FOR MIND AND SPIRIT*

Support services for patients and caregivers include referrals and on-site programs for patient education, nutrition, counseling, pain management, and social work services, as well as access to complementary therapies.

Specialists at the NCI-designated NYU Cancer Institute seek to enhance and coordinate the extensive resources of NYU Medical Center to optimize research, treatment, and the ultimate control of cancer.

Our new NYU Clinical Cancer Center is located at 160 East 34th Street. This state-of-the-art 13-level, 85,000-square-foot building serves as "home base" for patients, by providing the latest cancer prevention, screening, diagnostic treatment, genetic counseling, and support services in one central location. The NYU Clinical Cancer Center stands to dramatically improve the lives of people with cancer. As part of NYU Medical Center, patients can access a variety of other non-cancer services throughout the institution.

PHYSICIAN REFERRAL
1-888-7-NYU-MED
(1-888-769-8633)
www.nyumc.org
www.nyuci.org

Comprehensive Cancer Center (OSUCCC) – Arthur G. James Cancer Hospital and Richard J. Solove Research Institute (The James)

THE OHIO STATE UNIVERSITY

300 W. 10th Ave. • Columbus, Ohio 43210 • 1-800-293-5066
www.jamesline.com

RESEARCH

NCI Designation

As one of only 39 NCI-designated Comprehensive Cancer Centers in the nation, the OSUCCC's mission is to reduce cancer incidence, morbidity and mortality by conducting scientific studies that improve patient care.

Focus

OSUCCC researchers focus on cancer etiology, human cancer genetics, development of anticancer drugs, diagnostic methods, cancer prevention, and improving treatment methods through surgery, chemotherapy, genetics, molecular oncology, immunotherapy, radiotherapy and combinations of treatment modalities.

Clinical Trials

Utilizing the many resources of a large university, the OSUCCC is involved in dozens of clinical trials for the prevention, diagnosis and treatment of cancer. These trials offer patients some of the very latest cancer treatments.

PATIENT CARE

Facilities

The James is a 160-bed cancer hospital with 13 floors that accommodate such facilities as a 24-bed bone marrow transplantation unit, six specialized surgical suites, 21 chemotherapy suites with an accompanying pharmacy, and outpatient facilities featuring 40 physician examination and consultation rooms.

Radiotherapy

The James has a sophisticated radiotherapy unit that includes five linear accelerators, a gamma knife for stereotactic radiosurgery on brain tumors, and Intensity Modulated Radio Therapy, the most advanced method for treating malignant tumors with radiation.

NCCN

As a charter member of the National Comprehensive Cancer Network (NCCN) – an alliance of prestigious cancer centers established to more effectively fight cancer – The James provides input for NCCN printed practice guidelines for various forms of cancer.

OSUCCC/THE JAMES

Research contributing to global knowledge about cancer is conducted daily in the OSUCCC, a network of seven interdisciplinary cancer research programs that collectively comprise 223 scientists from 12 colleges at Ohio State.

OSU has been designated by the National Cancer Institute (NCI) as a Comprehensive Cancer Center since 1976. The James opened in 1990 as the patient-care component of the OSUCCC and has earned a reputation for outstanding patient care, research and education.

The hospital is consistently ranked by *U.S. News and World Report* as one of America's Best Hospitals for cancer care.

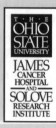

The Cancer Institute of New Jersey
195 Little Albany Street, New Brunswick, NJ 08903-2681
Tel. 732/235-CINJ (2465) www.cinj.org

Overview

As a Center of Excellence of the University of Medicine and Dentistry of New Jersey – Robert Wood Johnson Medical School, The Cancer Institute of New Jersey (CINJ) is the state's first and only National Cancer Institute-designated Comprehensive Cancer Center. It is dedicated to improving the prevention, detection, treatment, and care of patients with cancer, through the transformation of laboratory discoveries into clinical practice. CINJ is committed to the fight against cancer and being a leader in cancer care and treatment.

Treatment

Patients of CINJ can be treated in our New Brunswick, New Jersey facility or at a hospital close to home in one of our 17 partner and affiliate hospitals located throughout the state. During a visit, patients can meet with a dedicated team of nationally renowned specialists including medical oncologists, surgical oncologists, radiation oncologists, social workers, pharmacists and nurses. CINJ patients have unprecedented access to cancer clinical trials that may offer the best available treatment.

Each multidisciplinary team of healthcare providers at CINJ focuses on a particular disease and is led by an academic physician who is an expert in the etiology and treatment of that disease. CINJ faculty are involved in basic laboratory and clinical research in an effort to bring new understanding regarding the causes and mechanisms of cancer directly to the patient in the form of innovative treatment. Clinical Programs at CINJ include: Bone Marrow/Stem Cell Transplant Program; Breast Oncology Program/ New Jersey Comprehensive Breast Care Center; Cancer Risk Assessment and Genetic Counseling Program; Gastrointestinal/Hepatobiliary Oncology Program; General Oncology Services; Genitourinary Oncology Program; Gynecologic Oncology Program; Leukemia/Lymphoma Program; Melanoma and Soft Tissue Oncology Program; Neuro-Oncology Program; Pediatric Hematology-Oncology Program; Phase I/Developmental Therapeutics Program; Radiation Oncology; Symptom Management Supportive Care Program; and Thoracic Oncology Program.

Research

CINJ's physician-scientists engage in translational research, transforming their laboratory discoveries into clinical practice—quite literally bringing research to life. At CINJ, laboratory research is supported by more than $80 million annually in cancer-related research grants. CINJ researchers hold faculty positions at UMDNJ-Robert Wood Johnson Medical School, UMDNJ-School of Public Health, and Rutgers University. Basic scientist and clinical researchers meet regularly to exchange information and ensure that laboratory discoveries are refined and applied to clinical care as quickly as possible, and that clinical observations reach laboratory researchers on a continuing basis. Top-notch scientists are at the forefront of developing methods to treat and prevent cancer.

CINJ Network

CINJ's Network is composed of partner and affiliate hospitals and practicing oncologists throughout the state. It provides a mechanism to rapidly disseminate important, valid discoveries into the community. Through the Network, the member hospitals and physicians make clinical trials and new investigational treatments available in the communities they serve. Members of the Network include: Partner Hospitals - Robert Wood Johnson University Hospital; and Atlantic Health System (Morristown Memorial Hospital, Mountainside Hospital, and Overlook Hospital). Affiliate Hospitals - Bayshore Community Hospital; CentraState Healthcare System; Cooper University Hospital;* Jersey Shore University Medical Center; JFK Medical Center; Monmouth Medical Center; Raritan Bay Medical Center; Robert Wood Johnson University Hospital at Hamilton; Saint Peter's University Hospital; Southern Ocean County Hospital; The University Hospital/UMDNJ-New Jersey Medical School* and University Medical Center at Princeton

 * Academic Affiliate

ROSWELL PARK CANCER INSTITUTE

A National Cancer Institute Designated-Comprehensive Cancer Center

Elm & Carlton Streets
Buffalo, New York 14263
phone: (716) 845-2300

www.roswellpark.org

BRINGING HOPE TO PATIENTS WITH CANCER FOR MORE THAN A CENTURY

Roswell Park Cancer Institute began the 20th century as the nation's first cancer research, treatment and education center, and today is one of the nation's most preeminent Comprehensive Cancer Centers. It offers patients the best in cancer diagnosis, care and treatment. Roswell Park was one of three cancer facilities that served as the model for the 39 highly specialized National Cancer Institute-designated Comprehensive Cancer Centers that exist in the United States today. Its breakthroughs in techniques and treatments have played a commanding role in the war on cancer.

If you decide to have treatment at Roswell Park Cancer Institute, you will benefit from the caring and compassionate attitude exhibited by each and every member of the team. It takes a special person to work at a cancer center, and Roswell Park carefully chooses every staff member with its patients in mind.

You will be treated with dignity and confidentiality, by people who truly want to help make you comfortable and help you fight this disease. The staff is a source of hope, encouragement and information for all patients, and they encourage you to get to know them, so you will feel comfortable and can ask the questions that surely are on your mind.

At Roswell Park, a multidisciplinary team approach to care is taken, which means each and every staff member, as well as your family and friends are on your care team.

HERE ARE A FEW FREQUENTLY ASKED QUESTIONS.

What if I have or a family member has a general question about cancer or the types of services Roswell Park has to offer?

For information about cancer and the types of services Roswell Park offers, call the Information Center at 1-877-ASK RPCI (1-877-275-7724).

How do I become a Roswell Park patient?

Your physician may make the referral for you or you can make it yourself by calling 1-800 ROSWELL (1-800-767-9355). Our referral professionals will ask you to contact your physician for the appropriate authorization, which is required if you participate in a managed care plan.

Why should I choose Roswell Park for my cancer care?

When diagnosed with a life-threatening illness, you owe it to yourself to know all of your treatment options. If you receive one option through your community physician, you should ask for a second opinion at Roswell Park. There are several benefits for choosing care at a National Cancer Institute-designated Comprehensive Cancer Center. These include new therapies that may not otherwise be available elsewhere; a comprehensive and multidisciplinary approach to care from diagnosis to rehabilitation; and built-in resources to help you and your family with all your questions, whether simple or complex.

FOR MORE INFORMATION, VISIT
ROSWELL PARK CANCER INSTITUTE
AT WWW.ROSWELLPARK.ORG OR
CALL 1-877-ASK RPCI (1-877-275-7724).

ST. VINCENT'S
COMPREHENSIVE CANCER CENTER

325 West 15th Street
(Between 8th and 9th Avenue)
New York, NY 10011

With many of the top radiation oncologists, physicists, therapists and technicians in the country and the most advanced, state-of-the-art treatment technology, you can rest assured that patients are in good hands and are receiving the best care available.

Patients are the top priority at St. Vincent's Comprehensive Cancer Center (SVCCC). The Center was designed to provide medically superb, integrated care while enhancing the patient's comfort level and well-being. To ensure that patients are receiving the most comprehensive, well-rounded treatment possible, SVCCC clinicians continuously work with the patient's referring physician who is considered part of the patient's treatment team.

The Radiation Oncology Department at SVCCC has been designated a Varian Learning Center, where physicians from all over the world come to be trained on some of the most advanced treatment technology available. The Radiation Department provides a complete range of treatment options in one convenient location including IMRT, HDR (High Dose Rate) Brachytherapy, Respiratory Gating, and Cranial and Extra-Cranial Radiosurgery. PET/CT scans are also performed on site. Multidisciplinary teams of surgeons, medical oncologists, radiation oncologists, physicists and others specializing in breast, prostate and lung cancer treatment participate in designing a customized treatment plan for each individual patient. Patients also have access to a nutritionist, social worker and other support services to complement their medical treatment.

Refer your patient's to SVCCC—the Cancer Center with the most advanced technology, a top-notch staff and the compassionate care that will support your patients during this very difficult time

To refer a patient, to make an appointment, or for information call:

1-888-44-CANCER
(442-2623)

UNIVERSITY OF FLORIDA
SHANDS CANCER CENTER

2000 SW Archer Road, Gainesville, FL 32610
Patient referral: 800.749.7424
Physician-to-physician referral: 800.633.2122
www.shands.org

SPECIALIZED SERVICES

The UFSCC was among the first in the nation to perform many of the newest medical procedures, some of which were developed by UF physicians. The center combines personalized cancer treatment with access to advanced procedures and innovative research alternatives.

The UF faculty cancer specialists and their teams provide many services, including:

- Surgical procedures
- Chemotherapy
- Hematology/oncology
- Bone marrow transplantation
- Radiation oncology, including image guided treatment options; high-energy linear accelerators and advanced computer simulation
- Lymphography and sophisticated nuclear medicine studies
- Sentinel lymph node biopsy for breast cancer patients
- Gene therapy to attack tumors at a molecular level without destroying normal tissue
- Minimally invasive techniques to remove tumors

CLINICAL TRIALS AND RESEARCH

The UFSCC's research mission is to provide a multidisciplinary approach to the study of cancer that will result in improved outcomes for prevention, diagnosis and treatment. Enhancing translational research is the key to making progress toward improved outcomes, and linking basic and clinical scientists brings a new dimension to cancer research at UF. A variety of clinical trials, including numerous national clinical trials, are available to further advance understanding of cancer biology and create improved treatment options for patients.

PHYSICIAN REFERRAL

The Shands Consultation Center is your link to UF physicians at the UFSCC. For more information or to schedule an appointment, please call **800.749.7424** or visit our Web site at **shands.org**.

WORLD-CLASS CANCER CARE

The University of Florida Shands Cancer Center (UFSCC) is an interdisciplinary initiative at the UF Health Science Center's Gainesville and Jacksonville campuses, Shands at UF in Gainesville, and Shands Jacksonville. Clinicians and scientists affiliated with the UFSCC perform original scientific research and enhance clinical strategies for the diagnosis, treatment and prevention of cancer. Multidisciplinary teams work together to utilize the latest diagnostic and therapeutic innovations to optimize treatment outcomes. UFSCC cancer care services consistently are ranked among the nation's best by *U.S.News and World Report*.

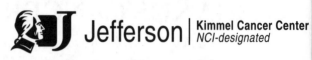

The UCLA Hematology/Oncology Program provides both investigative and standard-of-care therapy for adults and children with hematologic and oncology diseases.

Cancer researchers have long believed that the future of treatment rests in targeted therapies -"smart" drugs that, unlike the non-discriminating chemotherapy approach, take aim at the proteins, enzymes and pathways unique to cancer. Two drugs that utilize this strategy gained Federal Drug Administration approval after years of laboratory and clinical research at UCLA: the breast cancer drug Herceptin, which attacks a genetic mutation in breast cancer, and Gleevec, which is used to treat leukemia.

UCLA researchers are breaking new ground in cutting-edge gene therapy and with angiogenesis inhibitors, a class of drugs that attempt to fight cancer by cutting off the blood supply to tumors. And state-of-the-art molecular genetics provide the foundation for UCLA's Brain Tumor Program.

UCLA'S JONSSON CANCER CENTER

Designated by the National Cancer Institute as one of only 38 Comprehensive Cancer Centers in the United States, UCLA's Jonsson Cancer Center has earned an international reputation for developing new cancer therapies, providing the best in experimental and traditional treatments, and expertly guiding and training the next generation of medical researchers. The center's 250 physicians and scientists treat upwards of 20,000 patient visits per year and offer hundreds of clinical trials that provide the latest in experimental cancer treatments (www.cancer.mednet.ucla.edu). The center also offers patients and families psychological and support services.

UCLA's Jonsson Cancer Center has been ranked the best cancer center in the western United States by *U.S. News & World Report's* Annual Best Hospitals survey for the past five years. UCLA Medical Center, of which the Cancer Center is a part, has ranked best in the West for the past 15 years.

**Call 1-800-UCLA-MD1 (825-2631)
for a referral to a UCLA doctor.**

U C L A Healthcare

*THE UCLA
HEMATOLOGY/
ONCOLOGY
PROGRAM OFFERS
TREATMENTS FOR:*

Advanced malignancies

Breast cancer

Bone marrow/stem cell transplantation

Gastro-intestinal oncology

Genito-urinary oncology

Head and neck cancers

Leukemia

Lymphomas

Melanoma

Multiple myeloma

Neuro-Oncology

Thoracic oncology

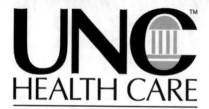

UNC Lineberger Comprehensive Cancer Center
CB# 7295 Chapel Hill, NC 27599-7295
http://cancer.med.unc.edu
1-866-828-0270

UNC LINEBERGER

The UNC Lineberger Comprehensive Cancer Center is one of 38 Comprehensive Cancer Centers designated by the National Cancer Institute. UNC Lineberger, the cancer center of the University of North Carolina Health System, is a national leader in research and care innovation. Design and planning is currently under way for the new North Carolina Cancer Hospital, to be built next to the existing UNC Hospitals complex.

PATIENT CARE

- Multidisciplinary approach means that a team of cancer specialists provides individualized treatment plans and care for each patient.
- Bone Marrow and Stem Cell Transplantation
- Breast Cancer
- Cancer Genetics
- Gastrointestinal Cancer
- Gynecologic Oncology
- Head and Neck Cancer
- Lung and Thoracic Cancer
- Lymphoma/Leukemia and Myelomas
- Melanoma
- Neuro-Oncology
- Pediatric Oncology
- Sarcomas
- Urologic Cancer

- Leading-edge technology – from early breast cancer detection, using digital mammography, to innovative clinical trials for late-stage cancers with molecular gene profiling of patients' tumors to analyze the best therapy
- Genetic counseling for patients and families at increased risk for cancer
- Patient programs including a Patient/Family Resource Center, support groups, patient and family counseling wig/scarves loan program, and free massages

RESEARCH

- Clinical trials for virtually all cancer types and stages, from UNC-developed studies to national trials offered through clinical cooperative groups
- UNC is ranked in the top 15 institutions nationally in cancer research funding
- Regional population studies to seek environmental causes of cancers
- Specialized Program of Research Excellence (SPORE) in breast cancer, one of nine in the country designated by the National Cancer Institute to provide leading-edge care using novel therapeutic strategies for cancer

PREVENTION

- Trials to prevent cancer in those at high risk
- Projects that work in communities with citizens and practitioners to reduce cancer risk by promoting early detection, screening, and healthy lifestyles

Patients coming to UNC receive individualized care from a multi-disciplinary team. A broad cancer genetics program extends from patient and family counseling and risk assessment to the use of leading-edge technol-ogies to plan therapy and evaluate the extent of the cancer. Innovative clinical trials are available for those with advanced cancer. For more information about UNC Lineberger's cancer programs or clinical trials, please visit: http://cancer.med.unc.edu. To make an appointment, please call toll-free 1-866-828-0270.

Established in 1975, the UNC Lineberger Comprehensive Cancer Center is part of the University of North Carolina at Chapel Hill and UNC Health Care. Center faculty treat patients, conduct research into the causes of cancer, direct programs in cancer prevention, and train future physicians and scientists.

PENN CANCER SERVICES
UNIVERSITY OF PENNSYLVANIA
HEALTH SYSTEM

Philadelphia, PA
1-800-635-7780, PENNLine
pennhealth.com

LEADERS IN CANCER

The Abramson Cancer Center of the University of Pennsylvania is one of a select group of cancer centers in the country awarded the prestigious designation of Comprehensive Cancer Center by the National Cancer Institute. This status reflects our outstanding research, clinical services, education and information services and community outreach. With more than 300 faculty actively involved in the diagnosis and treatment of cancer patients, the Cancer Center offers a team of experts who provide coordinated patient care.

As one of the nation's foremost cancer centers, the Abramson Cancer Center offers tremendous medical services and technological resources to meet any need throughout the course of treatment and follow-up care.

The Cancer Center has established a variety of interdisciplinary centers dedicated to specific cancers. Each center offers patients a complete oncologic evaluation and treatment options by a team of physicians with recognized expertise in their type of cancer. Each center is committed to excellence in clinical and patient and family support services.

The University of Pennsylvania Cancer Network, established in 1991, is a select group of community hospitals throughout Pennsylvania and New Jersey collaborating with the Abramson Cancer Center to provide excellence in patient care throughout the region. Penn's Cancer Network includes 25 hospitals that are recognized for excellence in patient care and commitment to improving the health and well being of the community. Penn physicians are highly supportive and maintain close communication with community-based physicians.

Pennsylvania Hospital, founded in 1751, offers a wide-ranging program that combines leading-edge technology and broad-based expertise with the intimacy of a personalized medical practice. At the Joan Karnell Cancer Center at Pennsylvania Hospital, patients have access to the latest cancer treatments, clinical trials and education programs through Penn's Cancer Network. A closely integrated team of medical, surgical, radiation and related cancer specialists use their knowledge and experience to bring patients a level of care that reflects the most current approaches to physical, emotional, family and social needs.

For direct connection to one of our Penn physicians, call PENNLine 1-800-635-7780.

OVERVIEW

The University of Pennsylvania Health System is one of the leading health care providers in the country, known for its innovative approaches to cancer diagnosis and treatment as well as the care and compassion of its staff. United in a commitment to clinical excellence and innovative research, the University of Pennsylvania

Health System has made enormous strides in under-standing cancer's underlying causes. Each new advance improves the chances for recovery and enhances the quality of life for patients.

LOCATIONS

- Hospital of the University of Pennsylvania
- Pennsylvania Hospital
- Presbyterian Medical Center
- Penn Medicine at Radnor
- Penn Medicine at Cherry Hill

THE UNIVERSITY OF TEXAS
MD ANDERSON
CANCER CENTER
Making Cancer History ™

1515 Holcombe Blvd.
Houston, Texas 77030-4095
Tel. 713-792-6161
Toll Free 800-392-1611
www.mdanderson.org

HEMATOLOGY AND MEDICAL ONCOLOGY

The Lymphoma and Myeloma Center at M. D. Anderson is one of the largest multidisciplinary programs in the nation. Using M. D. Anderson's renowned team approach to treatment, medical oncologists, radiation therapists, clinical pharmacists, radiologists, hemato-pathologists and translational researchers join the advanced nurse practitioners, research nurses, clinical nurses, and physician assistants to plan and implement optimal treatments for newly diagnosed and relapsed patients. The team is further supported by social workers, financial counselors, dieticians and patient advocates – all dedicated to helping patients and their families throughout their cancer care.

Diseases treated include both Hodgkin's and non-Hodgkin's lymphomas; B-cell and T-cell lymphomas, follicular cell lymphoma, small cleaved-cell lymphoma, Mantle Cell lymphoma, cutaneous T-cell lymphoma, Multiple Myeloma and Waldenstrom's macroglobulinemia. Cellular determination and extent of disease is critical in treatment planning so patients are often re-assessed and staged based on their M. D. Anderson workup reviewed by our multidisciplinary clinician teams.

The center also offers an ongoing array of clinical trials for new and improved therapies for this growing disease. New and innovative therapies generally are available at M. D. Anderson several years before they become standard in the community. Our clinical trials incorporate state-of-the-art patient care, while evaluating the most recent developments in cancer medicine. They also offer treatment opportunities for difficult or aggressive tumors.

The Leukemia and Bioimmunotherapy Center staff treats all leukemias (acute and chronic), myelodysplastic syndromes, aplastic and other anemias, specific lymphomas (lymphoblastic lymphoma, splenic lymphoma, Burkitt's lymphoma, large granular lymphocyte leukemia/lymphoma, and mantle cell lymphoma), myeloproliferative syndromes and other related hematologic malignancies. They also provide biological therapeutics and immunotherapeutic approaches to a wide variety of hematologic and solid tumor diseases.

Features include:
- The largest practice of leukemia subspecialists in the world
- Access to innovative new drugs and state-of-the art biological and immunotherapeutic therapies
- On-site full-service hematopathology laboratory and bone marrow aspiration clinic
- Fast-track clinic for patients that allows for timely evaluation and coordination of outpatient care
- Inpatient protective environment unit for high-risk patients undergoing induction chemotherapy.

M. D. Anderson is one of the largest cancer centers in the world. We've been working to eliminate cancer for more than six decades. Our depth of experience informs every aspect of your care.

We focus exclusively on cancer and have seen cases of every kind. Our doctors treat more rare cancers in a single day than most physicians see in a lifetime. That means you receive expert care no matter what your diagnosis.

We are the top-ranked cancer hospital in the United States according to the 2004 *U.S.News & World Report* annual survey of hospitals.

M. D. Anderson ranks first in the number and amount of research grants awarded by the National Cancer Institute. By studying how cancer begins and responds to various treatments, we can help patients overcome disease and prevent recurrence.

At M. D. Anderson, we understand that cancer is not just a physical disease. To help you cope with every aspect of cancer, we provide a number of support programs.

Vanderbilt-Ingram Cancer Center

Vanderbilt University Medical Center
691 Frances Williams Preston Building
Nashville, Tennessee 37232-6838
Tel. 615.936.5855 Fax. 615.936.5879 www.vicc.org

A Comprehensive Cancer Center

The Vanderbilt-Ingram Cancer Center is the only Comprehensive Cancer Center designated by the National Cancer Institute in Tennessee and one of only 38 nationwide. The designation, the highest distinction awarded to cancer centers, recognizes research excellence in cancer causes, development, treatment and prevention, as well as a demonstrated commitment to community education, information and outreach.

Clinical Trials and Research

Vanderbilt-Ingram conducts a full spectrum of research, from basic science to population-based studies that seek out cancer causes, to development of innovative treatment and prevention strategies. At any one time, the center offers more than 120 investigational therapies. Many of these studies are available to patients through Vanderbilt-Ingram's Affiliate Network, which includes more than a dozen hospitals throughout Tennessee, Kentucky and Georgia.

Care and Support for Patients and Families

In addition to providing the latest in cancer treatment and conducting world-class research, Vanderbilt-Ingram offers programs to care for patients and families facing emotional, symptomatic, psychological, and social issues related to cancer and cancer treatment. These include Patient and Family Care, which offers in-clinic refreshments, music and pet therapy, free wigs and other support; Pain and Symptom Management; Strength for Life, which assists patients who have recently completed treatment make the transition back to "normalcy," and the Family Cancer Risk Service, which consults with individuals and families concerned about inherited risks of cancer and genetic testing.

Vanderbilt-Ingram Team

Vanderbilt-Ingram includes more than 1,000 doctors, researchers, nurses, technicians and other staff, all dedicated to the vision of preventing most cancers and curing the rest with innovative therapies and few, if any, side effects. The center includes more than 100 laboratories throughout Vanderbilt University and Medical Center, as well as the Henry-Joyce Cancer Clinic and Clinical Research Center and inpatient units in the Vanderbilt Hospital and Children's Hospital.

The expertise of Vanderbilt Ingram's senior leadership has been recognized by medical and scientific peers across the country, who have elected three Vanderbilt-Ingram faculty to lead major cancer organizations in 2004-2005: Dr. Harold Moses, president of the American Association of Cancer Institutes; Dr. David Johnson, president of the American Society of Clinical Oncology, and Dr. Lynn Matrisian, president of the American Association for Cancer Research. This is the first time in history these organizations have been led simultaneously by faculty from the same center.

Wake Forest University Baptist
MEDICAL CENTER

– COMPREHENISVE CANCER CENTER –

Medical Center Boulevard • Winston-Salem, NC 27157
Health On-Call® (Patient Access) 1-800-446-2255
PAL® (Physician-to-physician calls) 1-800-277-7654
www.wfubmc.edu/cancer

TOP RANKINGS

U.S. News & World Report ranks the Comprehensive Cancer Center of Wake Forest University Baptist Medical Center among the nation's top hospitals for cancer care (7/04). It is among an elite group of only 1% of U.S. cancer centers designated by the National Cancer Institute as comprehensive, indicating excellence in research, patient care and education. With the 2004 opening of a new outpatient cancer center, patients benefit from a soothing, state-of-the-art setting as they receive the latest in treatment.

RESEARCH ADVANTAGES

Wake Forest Baptist offers more cancer-related clinical trials than any other hospital in western N.C. From gene therapy to vitamin and nutrition studies to new surgical and radiological treatments, patients benefit from the leading edge of cancer knowledge and care. Innovative basic science, public health and clinical research promote new discovery about prevention, detection and treatment of cancers. Wake Forest scientists were first in the world to discover cancer resistant cells in mice.

TECHNOLOGY AND TREATMENT STRENGTHS

Wake Forest University Baptist Medical Center is home to North Carolina's only Gamma Knife, a non-invasive, stereotactic radiosurgical tool used to treat malignant and benign brain tumors once considered inoperable. Operated by one of the nation's most experienced treatment teams, the Gamma Knife painlessly bombards tumors with perfectly focused beams of gamma energy—sparing normal tissue—and is performed on an outpatient basis. Extracranial body stereotactic radiosurgery offers new options for other types of cancers.

Wake Forest Baptist offers highly targeted Intensity Modulated Radiation Therapy (IMRT) for treatment of cancers of the prostate, brain, lung, and head and neck—the latest generation in 3-D conformal radiation treatment. Other treatment innovations include IPHC (intraperitoneal hyperthermic chemotherapy) for abdominal cavity cancers and radiofrequency ablation for liver malignancies.

MULTIDISCIPLINARY EXPERTISE

Expert, subspecialized oncology teams provide patients a consensus opinion on treatment. Multidisciplinary centers include the Thoracic Oncology Program, the Breast Care Center, and the Neuro-oncology Clinic.

**To make an appointment or find a specialist,
call Health On-Call® at 1-800-446-2255.**

HIGHLIGHTS OF EXCELLENCE

- Western North Carolina's only NCI-designated Comprehensive Cancer Center now offers the convenience and comfort of a new Outpatient Cancer Center. The nation's first Cancer Patient Support Group was developed here.

- The Cancer Center's Blood and Marrow Transplant Program operates the nation's second-largest collection site.

- The Breast Cancer Risk Assessment Clinic and the Hereditary Cancer Clinic help patients understand their risk profile.

- Treatments include high dose rate (HDR) and low dose rate (LDR) brachytherapy for cancers of the prostate, breast, cervix, uterus, vagina, head and neck, brain and eye.

HEMATOLOGY

New England

Benz Jr., Edward MD **[Hem]** - **Spec Exp:** Anemias & Red Cell Disorders; Bone Marrow Transplant; **Hospital:** Brigham & Women's Hosp (page 87); **Address:** 44 Binney St, rm D 1628, Boston, MA 02115; **Phone:** 617-632-2159; **Board Cert:** Hematology 82; Internal Medicine 79; **Med School:** Harvard Med Sch 73; **Resid:** Internal Medicine, Peter Bent Brigham Hosp 75; Hematology, Yale New Haven Hosp 80; **Fellow:** Hematology, Natl Inst of Hlth 78; **Fac Appt:** Prof Med, Harvard Med Sch

Dezube, Bruce J MD **[Hem]** - **Spec Exp:** AIDS Related Cancers; **Hospital:** Beth Israel Deaconess Med Ctr - Boston; **Address:** BIDMC-Division of Hematology/Oncology, 330 Brookline Ave, Shapiro 9, Boston, MA 02215; **Phone:** 617-667-7082; **Board Cert:** Internal Medicine 86; Medical Oncology 89; Hematology 88; **Med School:** Tufts Univ 83; **Resid:** Internal Medicine, New England Med Ctr 86; **Fellow:** Hematology and Oncology, Beth Israel Deaconess Hosp 89; **Fac Appt:** Assoc Prof Med, Harvard Med Sch

Groopman, Jerome E MD **[Hem]** - **Spec Exp:** AIDS/HIV; AIDS Related Cancers; **Hospital:** Beth Israel Deaconess Med Ctr - Boston; **Address:** Beth Israel Deaconess Medical Ctr, 330 Brookline Ave, Boston, MA 02215; **Phone:** 617-667-0070; **Board Cert:** Internal Medicine 79; Medical Oncology 81; Hematology 84; **Med School:** Columbia P&S 76; **Resid:** Internal Medicine, Mass Genl Hosp; **Fac Appt:** Prof Med, Harvard Med Sch

Meehan, Kenneth MD **[Hem]** - **Spec Exp:** Bone Marrow Transplant; **Hospital:** Dartmouth - Hitchcock Med Ctr; **Address:** Norris Cotton Cancer Center-Dartmouth-Hitchcock MC, 1 Medical Center Drive, Lebanon, NH 03756; **Phone:** 603-650-4628; **Board Cert:** Internal Medicine 89; Hematology 03; Medical Oncology 91; **Med School:** Georgetown Univ 86; **Resid:** Internal Medicine, Georgetown Univ 89; **Fellow:** Hematology and Oncology, Dartmouth-Hitchcock Med Ctr 92; **Fac Appt:** Assoc Prof Hem, Dartmouth Med Sch

Miller, Kenneth B. MD **[Hem]** - **Spec Exp:** Bone Marrow Transplant; Leukemia; **Hospital:** Beth Israel Deaconess Med Ctr - Boston; **Address:** 330 Brookline Ave, Kirstein Bldg, rm 121, Boston, MA 02215; **Phone:** 617-667-9920; **Board Cert:** Internal Medicine 76; Hematology 80; **Med School:** NY Med Coll 72; **Resid:** Internal Medicine, NYU Med Ctr/VA Hosp 76; Internal Medicine, NYU Med Ctr 76; **Fellow:** Hematology, New England Med Ctr 79; **Fac Appt:** Prof Med, Tufts Univ

Spitzer, Thomas R MD **[Hem]** - **Spec Exp:** Bone Marrow Transplant; Leukemia; **Hospital:** Mass Genl Hosp; **Address:** Mass Genl Hosp-Bone Marrow Tranplant Program, 100 Blossom St, Cox 640, Boston, MA 02114; **Phone:** 617-724-1124; **Board Cert:** Internal Medicine 77; Medical Oncology 83; Hematology 84; **Med School:** Univ Rochester 74; **Resid:** Internal Medicine, NY Hosp-Cornell Med Ctr 77; **Fellow:** Hematology and Oncology, Case West Res Univ 83; **Fac Appt:** Assoc Prof Med, Harvard Med Sch

Stone, Richard Maury MD **[Hem]** - **Spec Exp:** Leukemia-Adult; **Hospital:** Dana-Farber Cancer Inst (page 87); **Address:** Dana Farber Cancer Inst, Adult Leukemia Prog, 44 Binney St, rm D-840B, Boston, MA 02115-6084; **Phone:** 617-632-2214; **Board Cert:** Internal Medicine 84; Medical Oncology 87; Hematology 88; **Med School:** Harvard Med Sch 81; **Resid:** Internal Medicine, Brigham & Womens Hosp 84; **Fellow:** Medical Oncology, Dana Farber Cancer Inst 87; **Fac Appt:** Assoc Prof Med, Harvard Med Sch

Mid Atlantic

Cheson, Bruce D MD [Hem] - **Spec Exp:** Leukemia; Chronic Lymphocytic Leukemia (CLL); Hematologic Malignancies; **Hospital:** Georgetown Univ Hosp; **Address:** GUMC - Lombardi Cancer Ctr, 3800 Reservoir Rd NW, Podium A, Washington, DC 20007; **Phone:** 202-444-2223; **Board Cert:** Internal Medicine 74; Hematology 76; **Med School:** Tufts Univ 71; **Resid:** Internal Medicine, Univ Virginia Hosp 74; **Fellow:** Hematology, New England Med Ctr Hosp 76

Emerson, Stephen G MD/PhD [Hem] - **Spec Exp:** Leukemia; Lymphoma; **Hospital:** Hosp Univ Penn - UPHS (page 113); **Address:** Hospital U Penn, 510 Maloney Bldg, 3400 Spruce St, Philadelphia, PA 19104; **Phone:** 215-573-3002; **Board Cert:** Internal Medicine 83; Hematology 86; Medical Oncology 87; **Med School:** Yale Univ 80; **Resid:** Internal Medicine, Mass Genl Hosp 82; **Fellow:** Hematology and Oncology, Brigham & Women's Hosp 86; **Fac Appt:** Prof Med, Univ Pennsylvania

Fruchtman, Steven M MD [Hem] - **Spec Exp:** Myeloproliferative Disorders; Polycythemia Rubra Vera; Stem Cell Transplant; **Address:** 1111 Park Ave, New York, NY 10029; **Phone:** 212-427-7700; **Board Cert:** Internal Medicine 80; Hematology 84; **Med School:** NY Med Coll 77; **Resid:** Internal Medicine, Univ Hosp/SUNY 81; **Fellow:** Hematology, Mount Sinai Med Ctr 84; Hematology, Meml Sloan Kettering Cancer Ctr 85; **Fac Appt:** Assoc Prof Hem, NY Med Coll

Gewirtz, Alan M MD [Hem] - **Spec Exp:** Leukemia; Gene Therapy; **Hospital:** Hosp Univ Penn - UPHS (page 113); **Address:** Hosp Univ Penn - Div Hem/Onc, 3400 Spruce St, 15 Penn Tower, Philadelphia, PA 19104; **Phone:** 215-662-3914; **Board Cert:** Internal Medicine 79; Hematology 82; Medical Oncology 81; **Med School:** SUNY Buffalo 76; **Resid:** Internal Medicine, Mt Sinai Hosp 79; **Fellow:** Oncology, Yale New Haven Hosp 81; **Fac Appt:** Prof Med, Univ Pennsylvania

Kempin, Sanford Jay MD [Hem] - **Spec Exp:** Bleeding/Coagulation Disorders; Leukemia; Lymphoma; **Hospital:** St Vincent Cath Med Ctrs - Manhattan (page 108); **Address:** St Vincents Cancer Ctr, 325 W 15th St, Ground Fl, New York, NY 10011; **Phone:** 212-604-6010; **Board Cert:** Internal Medicine 76; Medical Oncology 77; Hematology 78; **Med School:** Belgium 71; **Resid:** Internal Medicine, Lemuel Shattuck Hosp 72; **Fellow:** Hematology, St Jude Chldns Hosp 75; Medical Oncology, Meml Sloan Kettering Cancer Ctr 76

Kessler, Craig M MD [Hem] - **Spec Exp:** Bleeding/Coagulation Disorders; Hemophilia; Hematologic Malignancies; **Hospital:** Georgetown Univ Hosp; **Address:** Georgetown Univ Med Ctr - Lombardi Cancer Ctr, 3800 Reservoir Rd, Washington, DC 20007; **Phone:** 202-444-7094; **Board Cert:** Internal Medicine 76; Hematology 80; **Med School:** Tulane Univ 73; **Resid:** Internal Medicine, Ochsner Fdn Hosp 76; **Fellow:** Hematology, Johns Hopkins Hosp 78; **Fac Appt:** Prof Med, Georgetown Univ

Kopel, Samuel MD [Hem] - **Spec Exp:** Hematologic Malignancies; **Hospital:** Maimonides Med Ctr (page 99); **Address:** MMC Hemoto/Oncol, 6323 7th Ave, Brooklyn, NY 11220; **Phone:** 718-283-6900; **Board Cert:** Internal Medicine 75; Hematology 78; Medical Oncology 79; **Med School:** Italy 72; **Resid:** Internal Medicine, Jewish Hosp 75; **Fellow:** Hematology and Oncology, Mt Sinai Med Ctr 78; **Fac Appt:** Asst Prof Med, SUNY Downstate

Mears, John Gregory MD [Hem] - **Spec Exp:** Breast Cancer; Lymphoma; Leukemia; **Hospital:** NY-Presby Hosp - Columbia Presby Med Ctr (page 103); **Address:** 161 Ft Washington Ave, New York, NY 10032-3713; **Phone:** 212-305-3506; **Board Cert:** Internal Medicine 76; Hematology 78; **Med School:** Columbia P&S 73; **Resid:** Internal Medicine, Boston Univ Med Ctr 75; **Fellow:** Hematology and Oncology, Columbia-Presby Med Ctr 78; **Fac Appt:** Clin Prof Med, Columbia P&S

Nimer, Stephen D MD [Hem] - **Spec Exp:** Bone Marrow & Stem Cell Transplant; Anemia-Aplastic; Leukemia, Multiple Myeloma; **Hospital:** Meml Sloan Kettering Cancer Ctr (page 100); **Address:** Memorial Sloan Kettering Cancer Ctr, 1275 York Ave, Box 575, New York, NY 10021; **Phone:** 212-639-7871; **Board Cert:** Internal Medicine 82; Hematology 86; Medical Oncology 85; **Med School:** Univ Chicago-Pritzker Sch Med 79; **Resid:** Internal Medicine, UCLA Med Ctr 82; **Fellow:** Hematology and Oncology, UCLA Med Ctr 86; **Fac Appt:** Assoc Prof Med, Cornell Univ-Weill Med Coll

Pecora, Andrew L MD [Hem] - **Spec Exp:** Stem Cell Transplant; Myelodysplastic Syndromes; Melanoma; **Hospital:** Hackensack Univ Med Ctr (page 96); **Address:** The Cancer Ctr at Hackensack Univ Med Ctr, 20 Prospect Ave, Ste 400, Hackensack, NJ 07601; **Phone:** 201-996-5900; **Board Cert:** Internal Medicine 86; Hematology 88; Medical Oncology 89; **Med School:** UMDNJ-NJ Med Sch, Newark 83; **Resid:** Internal Medicine, NY Hosp-Cornell Med Ctr 86; **Fellow:** Hematology and Oncology, Meml Sloan Kettering Cancer Ctr 88; **Fac Appt:** Prof Med, UMDNJ-NJ Med Sch, Newark

Porter, David L MD [Hem] - **Spec Exp:** Leukemia; Bone Marrow Transplant; **Hospital:** Hosp Univ Penn - UPHS (page 113); **Address:** Hosp Univ Penn, Div Hem/Onc, 3400 Spruce St, 16 Penn Twr, Philadelphia, PA 19104; **Phone:** 215-662-2862; **Board Cert:** Internal Medicine 90; Medical Oncology 93; Hematology 94; **Med School:** Brown Univ 87; **Resid:** Internal Medicine, Univ Hosp 90; **Fellow:** Hematology and Oncology, Brigham & Womens Hosp 92

Rai, Kanti MD [Hem] - **Spec Exp:** Leukemia; Lymphoma; **Hospital:** Long Island Jewish Med Ctr; **Address:** 270-05 76th Ave, New Hyde Park, NY 11040-1433; **Phone:** 718-470-7135; **Board Cert:** Pediatrics 61; **Med School:** India 55; **Resid:** Pediatrics, Lincoln Hosp 58; Pediatrics, North Shore Univ Hosp 59; **Fellow:** Hematology, LI Jewish Med Ctr 60; **Fac Appt:** Prof Med, Albert Einstein Coll Med

Raphael, Bruce MD [Hem] - **Spec Exp:** Lymphoma; Leukemia; Multiple Myeloma; **Hospital:** NYU Med Ctr (page 104); **Address:** 160 E 34th Street Ave Fl 7, New York, NY 10016-6402; **Phone:** 212-731-5185; **Board Cert:** Internal Medicine 78; Hematology 80; Medical Oncology 81; **Med School:** McGill Univ 75; **Resid:** Internal Medicine, Jewish Genl Hosp 77; **Fellow:** Medical Oncology, Meml Sloan Kettering Cancer Ctr 78; Hematology, NYU Med Ctr 80; **Fac Appt:** Assoc Prof Med, NYU Sch Med

Roodman, G David MD [Hem] - **Spec Exp:** Multiple Myeloma; **Hospital:** UPMC Shadyside (page 114); **Address:** Hillman Cancer Ctr, 5115 Center Ave Fl 2nd Outpatient Service, Pittsburgh, PA 15232; **Phone:** 412-692-4724; **Board Cert:** Internal Medicine 78; Hematology 80; **Med School:** Univ KY Coll Med 73; **Resid:** Internal Medicine, Univ Minn Hosp 78; **Fellow:** Hematology, Univ Minn Hosp 80

Savage, David G MD [Hem] - **Spec Exp:** Stem Cell Transplant; Multiple Myeloma; Lymphoma; **Hospital:** NY-Presby Hosp - Columbia Presby Med Ctr (page 103); **Address:** 177 Fort Washington Ave, rm 6-435, New York, NY 10032; **Phone:** 212-305-9783; **Board Cert:** Internal Medicine 77; Hematology 82; Medical Oncology 85; **Med School:** Columbia P&S 71; **Resid:** Internal Medicine, Harlem Hosp/Columbia Presby Med Ctr 75; **Fellow:** Hematology and Oncology, Harlem Hosp/Columbia Presby Med Ctr 77; **Fac Appt:** Assoc Prof Med, Columbia P&S

Schuster, Michael MD [Hem] - **Spec Exp:** Bone Marrow Transplant; **Hospital:** NY-Presby Hosp - NY Weill Cornell Med Ctr (page 103); **Address:** 525 E 68th St, Starr 341, New York, NY 10021; **Phone:** 212-746-2119; **Board Cert:** Internal Medicine 84; Hematology 86; **Med School:** Dartmouth Med Sch 80; **Resid:** Internal Medicine, New England Deaconess Hosp 83; **Fellow:** Hematology and Oncology, Beth Israel Hosp-Harvard 87; **Fac Appt:** Assoc Prof Med, Cornell Univ-Weill Med Coll

Spivak, Jerry L MD [Hem] - **Spec Exp:** Myeloproliferative Disorders; Polycythemia Rubra Vera; **Hospital:** Johns Hopkins Hosp - Baltimore (page 97); **Address:** 720 Rutland Ave Bldg Ross - Ste 1025, Baltimore, MD 21205; **Phone:** 410-614-0167; **Board Cert:** Internal Medicine 71; Hematology 74; **Med School:** Cornell Univ-Weill Med Coll 64; **Resid:** Internal Medicine, New York Hosp 69; Internal Medicine, Johns Hopkins Hosp 72; **Fellow:** Hematology, Johns Hopkins Hosp 71; **Fac Appt:** Prof Med, Johns Hopkins Univ

Wisch, Nathaniel MD [Hem] - **Spec Exp:** Lymphoma; Breast Cancer; Leukemia; **Hospital:** Lenox Hill Hosp; **Address:** 12 E 86th St, New York, NY 10028-0506; **Phone:** 212-861-6660; **Board Cert:** Internal Medicine 65; Hematology 72; Medical Oncology 77; **Med School:** Northwestern Univ 58; **Resid:** Internal Medicine, VA Hosp 60; Internal Medicine, Montefiore Hosp 61; **Fellow:** Hematology, Mount Sinai Hosp 62; **Fac Appt:** Assoc Prof Med, Mount Sinai Sch Med

Zalusky, Ralph MD [Hem] - **Spec Exp:** Anemia; Leukemia; Lymphoma; **Hospital:** Beth Israel Med Ctr - Petrie Division (page 93); **Address:** 1st Ave & 16th St, Fl 19, New York, NY 10003; **Phone:** 212-420-4185; **Board Cert:** Internal Medicine 64; Hematology 72; **Med School:** Boston Univ 57; **Resid:** Internal Medicine, Duke Univ Med Ctr 62; **Fellow:** Hematology, Boston Med Ctr/Harvard 61; **Fac Appt:** Prof Med, Albert Einstein Coll Med

Southeast

Abramson, Neil MD [Hem] - **Spec Exp:** Breast Cancer; Bleeding/Coagulation Disorders; Hematologic Malignancies; **Hospital:** Baptist Medical Center - Jacksonville; **Address:** 1235 San Marco Blvd, Jacksonville, FL 32207; **Phone:** 904-202-7051; **Board Cert:** Internal Medicine 70; Hematology 72; Medical Oncology 75; **Med School:** Albert Einstein Coll Med 63; **Resid:** Internal Medicine, Presbyterian Univ Hosp 65; **Fellow:** Hematology, Thorndike Meml Lab-Harvard 69; **Fac Appt:** Clin Prof Med, Univ Fla Coll Med

Djulbegovic, Benjamin MD [Hem] - **Spec Exp:** Multiple Myeloma; **Hospital:** H Lee Moffitt Cancer Ctr & Research Inst; **Address:** H Lee Moffitt Cancer Ctr, 12902 Magnolia Drive, MS SRB4, Tampa, FL 33612; **Phone:** 813-745-4605; **Board Cert:** Internal Medicine 02; Hematology 94; **Med School:** Bosnia 76; **Resid:** Internal Medicine, Univ Med Ctr 83; Internal Medicine, Univ Louisville Med Ctr 88; **Fellow:** Univ Manchester 85; Hematology and Oncology, Univ Louisville 90

Emanuel, Peter D MD [Hem] - **Spec Exp:** Lymphoma; Leukemia; **Hospital:** Univ of Ala Hosp at Birmingham; **Address:** 1824 6th Ave, Birmingham, AL 35294; **Phone:** 205-934-6195; **Board Cert:** Internal Medicine 88; Hematology 94; **Med School:** Univ Wisc 85; **Resid:** Internal Medicine, Univ Ala 88; **Fellow:** Hematology and Oncology, Univ Ala 91; **Fac Appt:** Prof Med, Univ Ala

Fields, Karen MD [Hem] - **Spec Exp:** Bone Marrow Transplant; Blood/Marrow Transplant Breast Cancer; **Hospital:** H Lee Moffitt Cancer Ctr & Research Inst; **Address:** 12902 Magnolia Dr, Tampa, FL 33612; **Phone:** 813-979-7202; **Board Cert:** Medical Oncology 89; Hematology 90; Internal Medicine 84; **Med School:** Ohio State Univ 81; **Resid:** Internal Medicine, The Jewish Hospital 84; Medical Oncology, University of Cincinnati 88; **Fellow:** Hematology and Oncology, University Hospital 89; **Fac Appt:** Prof Hem, Univ S Fla Coll Med

Greer, John P MD [Hem] - **Spec Exp:** Leukemia & Lymphoma; Myelodysplastic Syndromes; Stem Cell Transplant; **Hospital:** Vanderbilt Univ Med Ctr (page 116); **Address:** 2665 The Vanderbilt Clinic, 1301 22nd Ave S, Nashville, TN 37232-5505; **Phone:** 615-936-1803; **Board Cert:** Pediatrics 85; Internal Medicine 79; Hematology 84; Medical Oncology 85; **Med School:** Vanderbilt Univ 76; **Resid:** Internal Medicine, Tulane Univ Med Ctr 79; Pediatrics, Med Coll Virginia 81; **Fellow:** Hematology and Oncology, Vanderbilt Univ Med Ctr 84; **Fac Appt:** Prof Med, Vanderbilt Univ

Lilenbaum, Rogerio MD [Hem] - **Spec Exp:** Lung Cancer; **Hospital:** Mount Sinai Med Ctr - Miami; **Address:** Oncology Hematology Assocs, 4306 Alton Rd, Ste 3, Miami, FL 33140-2840; **Phone:** 305-535-3310; **Board Cert:** Internal Medicine 95; Hematology 98; Medical Oncology 97; **Med School:** Brazil 86; **Resid:** Internal Medicine, Univ Hosp-Rio de Janeiro 89; **Fellow:** Hematology and Oncology, Washington Univ Sch Med 92; Oncology, UCSD 94; **Fac Appt:** Assoc Clin Prof Med, Univ Miami Sch Med

List, Alan F MD [Hem] - **Spec Exp:** Myelodysplastic Syndromes; Leukemia; **Hospital:** H Lee Moffitt Cancer Ctr & Research Inst; **Address:** 12902 Magnolia Drive, SRB 4, Tampa, FL 33612-9497; **Phone:** 813-745-6086; **Board Cert:** Internal Medicine 83; Medical Oncology 85; Hematology 86; **Med School:** Univ Pennsylvania 80; **Resid:** Internal Medicine, Good Samaritan Hosp 83; Oncology, Vanderbilt Univ Med Ctr 85; **Fellow:** Hematology, Vanderbilt Univ Med Ctr 86

Solberg, Lawrence MD/PhD [Hem] - **Spec Exp:** Bone Marrow Transplant; Myeloproliferative Disorders; Porphyria; **Hospital:** St Luke's Hosp - Jacksonville; **Address:** Mayo Clinic, 4500 San Pablo Rd, Jacksonville, FL 32224; **Phone:** 904-953-7292; **Board Cert:** Internal Medicine 78; Hematology 80; **Med School:** St Louis Univ 75; **Resid:** Internal Medicine, Mayo Clinic 78; **Fellow:** Hematology, Mayo Clinic 80; **Fac Appt:** Prof Med, Mayo Med Sch

Zuckerman, Kenneth S MD [Hem] - **Spec Exp:** Myeloproliferative Disorders; Myelodysplasia, Leukemia, & Lymphoma; Thrombotic Disorders; **Hospital:** H Lee Moffitt Cancer Ctr & Research Inst; **Address:** H Lee Moffitt Cancer Ctr, 12902 Magnolia Drive, Ste 3157, Tampa, FL 33612-9416; **Phone:** 813-745-8090; **Board Cert:** Internal Medicine 75; Hematology 78; **Med School:** Ohio State Univ 72; **Resid:** Internal Medicine, Ohio State Univ Hosps 75; **Fellow:** Hematology, Peter Bent Brigham Hosp/Harvard Univ 78; **Fac Appt:** Prof Med, Univ S Fla Coll Med

Midwest

Baron, Joseph M MD [Hem] - **Spec Exp:** Bleeding/Coagulation Disorders; Lymphoma; Myeloproliferative Disorders; **Hospital:** Univ of Chicago Hosps; **Address:** 5841 S Maryland Ave, MC 2115, Chicago, IL 60637-1463; **Phone:** 773-702-6149; **Board Cert:** Internal Medicine 69; Hematology 72; Medical Oncology 75; **Med School:** Univ Chicago-Pritzker Sch Med 62; **Resid:** Internal Medicine, Univ Chicago Hosps 64; **Fellow:** Hematology, Univ Chicago Hosps 68; **Fac Appt:** Assoc Prof Med, Univ Chicago-Pritzker Sch Med

Bockenstedt, Paula MD [Hem] - **Spec Exp:** Bleeding/Coagulation Disorders; Leukemia; Von Willebrand's Disease; **Hospital:** Univ Michigan Hlth Sys; **Address:** Div Hematology - Level B1, 1500 E Med Ctr Drive, rm 358 Reception B, Ann Arbor, MI 48109-0640; **Phone:** 734-647-8921; **Board Cert:** Internal Medicine 81; Hematology 84; **Med School:** Harvard Med Sch 78; **Resid:** Internal Medicine, Brigham-Womens Hosp 81; **Fellow:** Hematology, Brigham-Womens Hosp 84; **Fac Appt:** Assoc Clin Prof Med, Univ Mich Med Sch

Bukowski, Ronald M MD [Hem] - **Spec Exp:** Kidney Cancer; **Hospital:** Cleveland Clin Fdn (page 92); **Address:** Cleveland Clinic, Taussig Cancer Ctr, 9500 Euclid Ave, Desk R35, Cleveland, OH 44195-0001; **Phone:** 216-444-6825; **Board Cert:** Internal Medicine 74; Medical Oncology 75; Hematology 76; **Med School:** Northwestern Univ 67; **Resid:** Internal Medicine, Cleveland Clin Fdn 69; Internal Medicine, Cleveland Clin Fdn 73; **Fellow:** Hematology, Cleveland Clin Fdn

Flynn, Patrick MD [Hem] - **Spec Exp:** Hematologic Malignancies; **Hospital:** Abbott - Northwestern Hosp; **Address:** 800 E 28th St, Piper Bldg, Ste 405, Minneapolis, MN 55407; **Phone:** 612-863-8585; **Board Cert:** Internal Medicine 78; Medical Oncology 81; Hematology 82; **Med School:** Univ Minn 75; **Resid:** Internal Medicine, Hennepin Co Med Ctr-Univ Minn 78; **Fellow:** Hematology and Oncology, Univ Minnesota Hosp 81; **Fac Appt:** Asst Prof Med, Univ Minn

Gaynor, Ellen MD [Hem] - **Spec Exp:** Lymphoma; **Hospital:** Loyola Univ Med Ctr (page 98); **Address:** Loyola Univ Med Ctr, Dept Hematology, 2160 S First Ave Bldg 112 - rm 108, Maywood, IL 60153; **Phone:** 708-327-3214; **Board Cert:** Internal Medicine 82; Hematology 86; Medical Oncology 85; **Med School:** Univ Wisc 78; **Resid:** Internal Medicine, Loyola Univ Med Ctr 82; **Fellow:** Medical Oncology, Loyola Univ Med Ctr 81; Hematology and Oncology, Univ Chicago Hosp 84; **Fac Appt:** Assoc Prof Med, Loyola Univ-Stritch Sch Med

Gertz, Morie MD [Hem] - **Spec Exp:** Multiple Myeloma; Amyloidosis; Waldenstrom Macroglobulinemia; **Hospital:** Mayo Med Ctr & Clin - Rochester; **Address:** 200 SW 1st St Fl W10, Rochester, MN 55905; **Phone:** 507-284-2511; **Board Cert:** Internal Medicine 79; Hematology 82; Medical Oncology 83; **Med School:** Loyola Univ-Stritch Sch Med 75; **Resid:** Internal Medicine, St Lukes Hosp 79; **Fellow:** Hematology and Oncology, Mayo Clin 82; **Fac Appt:** Prof Med, Mayo Med Sch

Godwin, John MD [Hem] - **Spec Exp:** Thrombotic Disorders; Leukemia-Elderly; **Hospital:** Loyola Univ Med Ctr (page 98); **Address:** Loyola Univ Med Ctr, Dept Hematology, 2160 S 1st Ave Bldg 112 - rm 342, Maywood, IL 60153; **Phone:** 708-327-3180; **Board Cert:** Internal Medicine 81; Hematology 86; **Med School:** Univ Ala 78; **Resid:** Internal Medicine, Baylor Coll Med 81; Internal Medicine, Baylor Coll Med 82; **Fellow:** Hematology, Baylor Coll Med 83; Hematology, North Carolina Meml Hosp 85; **Fac Appt:** Assoc Prof Path, Loyola Univ-Stritch Sch Med

Gordon, Leo I MD [Hem] - **Spec Exp:** Lymphoma, Non-Hodgkin's; Hodgkin's Disease; Bone Marrow Transplant; **Hospital:** Northwestern Meml Hosp; **Address:** 675 N St Clair St, Ste 850, Chicago, IL 60611-3124; **Phone:** 312-695-6180; **Board Cert:** Internal Medicine 76; Hematology 78; Medical Oncology 79; **Med School:** Univ Cincinnati 73; **Resid:** Internal Medicine, Univ Chicago Hosps 76; **Fellow:** Hematology, Univ Minnesota Hosps 78; Hematology and Oncology, Univ Chicago Hosps 79; **Fac Appt:** Prof Med, Northwestern Univ

Gregory, Stephanie A MD [Hem] - **Spec Exp:** Lymphoma; Leukemia; Plasma Cell Disorders; **Hospital:** Rush Univ Med Ctr; **Address:** 1725 W Harrison St, Ste 834, Chicago, IL 60612-3861; **Phone:** 312-563-2320; **Board Cert:** Internal Medicine 72; Hematology 72; **Med School:** Med Coll PA Hahnemann 65; **Resid:** Internal Medicine, Rush/Presby-St Luke's Med Ctr 69; **Fellow:** Hematology, Rush/Presby-St Luke's Med Ctr 72; **Fac Appt:** Prof Med, Rush Med Coll

Greipp, Philip R MD [Hem] - **Spec Exp:** Multiple Myeloma; **Hospital:** Mayo Med Ctr & Clin - Rochester; **Address:** Mayo Clinic, Div Hematology, 200 First St SW Bldg Mayo Fl W-10, Rochester, MN 55905-0001; **Phone:** 507-284-3159; **Board Cert:** Internal Medicine 74; Hematology 94; **Med School:** Georgetown Univ 68; **Resid:** Internal Medicine, Mayo Clinic 73; **Fellow:** Hematology, Mayo Clinic 75; **Fac Appt:** Prof Med, Mayo Med Sch

Habermann, Thomas M MD [Hem] - **Spec Exp:** Lymphoma; Hodgkin's Disease; Leukemia; **Hospital:** Mayo Med Ctr & Clin - Rochester; **Address:** Mayo Clinic, 200 1st St SW, Rochester, MN 55905; **Phone:** 507-284-0923; **Board Cert:** Internal Medicine 82; Hematology 84; **Med School:** Creighton Univ 79; **Resid:** Internal Medicine, Mayo Clinic 82; **Fellow:** Hematology, Mayo Clinic 85; **Fac Appt:** Prof Med, Mayo Med Sch

Larson, Richard A MD [Hem] - **Spec Exp:** Leukemia & Lymphoma; Bone Marrow Transplant; Multiple Myeloma; **Hospital:** Univ of Chicago Hosps; **Address:** Univ Chicago Hospitals, 5841 S Maryland Ave, MC 2115, Chicago, IL 60637; **Phone:** 773-702-6783; **Board Cert:** Internal Medicine 80; Hematology 82; Medical Oncology 83; **Med School:** Stanford Univ 77; **Resid:** Internal Medicine, Univ Chicago Hosps 80; **Fellow:** Hematology, Univ Chicago Hosps 83; Medical Oncology, Univ Chicago Hosps 83; **Fac Appt:** Prof Med, Univ Chicago-Pritzker Sch Med

Laughlin, Mary J MD [Hem] - **Spec Exp:** Bone Marrow Transplant; **Hospital:** Univ Hosps of Cleveland; **Address:** Ireland Cancer Center, 11100 Euclid Ave Fl 6, Cleveland, OH 44106; **Phone:** 216-844-8609; **Board Cert:** Internal Medicine 03; Hematology 94; **Med School:** SUNY Buffalo 88; **Resid:** Internal Medicine, Duke Univ 91; **Fellow:** Hematology and Oncology, Duke Univ 92; Bone Marrow Transplant, Rosewell Park Cancer Inst 94; **Fac Appt:** Assoc Prof Med, Case West Res Univ

Lazarus, Hillard M MD [Hem] - **Spec Exp:** Bone Marrow Transplant; Stem Cell Transplant; Leukemia; **Hospital:** Univ Hosps of Cleveland; **Address:** Univ Hosps of Cleveland, ICC-Bone Marrow Transplant Prog, 11100 Euclid Ave Bldg Wearn - rm 341, Cleveland, OH 44106-5065; **Phone:** 216-844-3629; **Board Cert:** Internal Medicine 77; Medical Oncology 79; Hematology 80; **Med School:** Univ Rochester 74; **Resid:** Internal Medicine, Univ Hosps 77; **Fellow:** Hematology and Oncology, Univ Hosps 79; **Fac Appt:** Prof Med, Case West Res Univ

Litzow, Mark Robert MD [Hem] - **Spec Exp:** Bone Marrow Transplant; Leukemia; **Hospital:** Mayo Med Ctr & Clin - Rochester; **Address:** Mayo Clinic, Div Hematology, 200 First St SW, Rochester, MN 55905; **Phone:** 507-284-5362; **Board Cert:** Internal Medicine 83; Hematology 88; Medical Oncology 89; **Med School:** Univ Chicago-Pritzker Sch Med 80; **Resid:** Internal Medicine, Mayo Clinic 84; **Fellow:** Medical Oncology, Mayo Clinic 90; **Fac Appt:** Asst Prof Med, Mayo Med Sch

Maciejewski, Jaroslow P MD/PhD [Hem] - **Spec Exp:** Anemia-Aplastic; Hematologic Malignancies; Stem Cell Transplant; **Hospital:** Cleveland Clin Fdn (page 92); **Address:** Cleveland Clinic, 9500 Euclid Ave, Desk R40, Cleveland, OH 44195; **Phone:** 216-445-5962; **Board Cert:** Internal Medicine 99; Hematology 01; **Med School:** Germany 87; **Resid:** Internal Medicine, Univ Nevada Med Ctr 97; **Fellow:** Hematology, Natl Inst Hlth 00

McGlave, Philip B MD [Hem] - **Spec Exp:** Leukemia; Bone Marrow Transplant; **Hospital:** Fairview-Univ Med Ctr - Univ Campus; **Address:** Univ Minn, Dept Med - Div Hem/Onc, 420 Delaware St SE, MMC 480, Minneapolis, MN 55455; **Phone:** 612-626-2446; **Board Cert:** Internal Medicine 77; Hematology 80; **Med School:** Univ IL Coll Med 74; **Resid:** Internal Medicine, Univ Minn 77; **Fellow:** Hematology and Oncology, Univ Minn 80; **Fac Appt:** Prof Med, Univ Minn

Nand, Sucha MD [Hem] - **Spec Exp:** Myelodysplastic Syndromes; Myeloproliferative Disorders; Leukemia; **Hospital:** Loyola Univ Med Ctr (page 98); **Address:** Cardinal Bernardin Cancer Ctr, 2160 S First Ave Bldg 112 - rm 342, Maywood, IL 60153-3304; **Phone:** 708-327-3217; **Board Cert:** Internal Medicine 79; Medical Oncology 81; Hematology 82; **Med School:** India 71; **Resid:** Physical Medicine & Rehabilitation, Northwestern Meml Hosp 76; Internal Medicine, North Chicago VA Hosp 78; **Fellow:** Medical Oncology, Northwestern Meml Hosp 81; **Fac Appt:** Prof Med, Loyola Univ-Stritch Sch Med

Singhal, Seema MD [Hem] - **Spec Exp:** Multiple Myeloma; **Hospital:** Northwestern Meml Hosp; **Address:** 675 N St Claire St, Fl 21 - Ste 100, Chicago, IL 60611; **Phone:** 312-695-0990; **Med School:** India ; **Resid:** Internal Medicine, King Edward Meml Hosp; Hematology, King Edward Meml Hosp; **Fellow:** Bone Marrow Transplant, Univ Hosp in Jerusalem; **Fac Appt:** Prof Med, Northwestern Univ

Stiff, Patrick J MD [Hem] - **Spec Exp:** Bone Marrow Transplant; Lymphoma, Non-Hodgkin's; Leukemia; **Hospital:** Loyola Univ Med Ctr (page 98); **Address:** Cardinal Bernadin Cancer Ctr, 2160 S First Ave, Maywood, IL 60153; **Phone:** 708-327-3216; **Board Cert:** Internal Medicine 78; Medical Oncology 81; Hematology 82; **Med School:** Loyola Univ-Stritch Sch Med 75; **Resid:** Internal Medicine, Cleveland Clinic 78; **Fellow:** Hematology and Oncology, Meml Sloan Kettering Cancer Ctr 81; **Fac Appt:** Prof Med, Loyola Univ-Stritch Sch Med

Tallman, Martin S MD [Hem] - **Spec Exp:** Bone Marrow Transplant; Leukemia; Lymphoma; **Hospital:** Northwestern Meml Hosp; **Address:** 676 N St Clair St, Ste 850, Chicago, IL 60611; **Phone:** 312-695-0990; **Board Cert:** Internal Medicine 83; Medical Oncology 87; Hematology 88; **Med School:** Univ Hlth Sci/Chicago Med Sch 80; **Resid:** Internal Medicine, Evanston Hosp 83; **Fellow:** Medical Oncology, Univ Wash Med Ctr 87; **Fac Appt:** Prof Med, Northwestern Univ

van Besien, Koen W MD [Hem] - **Spec Exp:** Lymphoma; Stem Cell Transplant; **Hospital:** Univ of Chicago Hosps; **Address:** Univ Chicago Stem Cell Transplant Program, 5841 S Maryland Ave, MC 2115, Chicago, IL 60637; **Phone:** 773-702-6149; **Board Cert:** Internal Medicine 94; Medical Oncology 95; Hematology 96; **Med School:** Belgium 84; **Resid:** Internal Medicine, U Leuven Med Ctr 87; **Fellow:** Hematology and Oncology, Indiana Univ Med Ctr 90; **Fac Appt:** Assoc Prof Med, Univ Chicago-Pritzker Sch Med

Winter, Jane N MD [Hem] - **Spec Exp:** Lymphoma, Non-Hodgkin's; Hodgkin's Disease; Bone Marrow Transplant; **Hospital:** Northwestern Meml Hosp; **Address:** Northwestern Univ - Div Hematology-Oncology, 675 N St Clair St, Ste 21-600, Chicago, IL 60611; **Phone:** 312-695-4538; **Board Cert:** Internal Medicine 80; Hematology 82; Medical Oncology 83; **Med School:** Univ Pennsylvania 77; **Resid:** Internal Medicine, Univ Chicago Hosps 80; **Fellow:** Hematology and Oncology, Columbia Presby Hosp 81; Hematology and Oncology, Northwestern Meml Hosp 83; **Fac Appt:** Prof Med, Northwestern Univ

Great Plains and Mountains

Vose, Julie M MD [Hem] - **Spec Exp:** Lymphoma; **Hospital:** Nebraska Med Ctr; **Address:** Univ Nebraska Med Assoc, Emile @ 42nd St, Omaha, NE 68198; **Phone:** 402-559-5600; **Board Cert:** Internal Medicine 87; Hematology 00; Medical Oncology 00; **Med School:** Univ Nebr Coll Med 87; **Resid:** Internal Medicine, Univ Nebraska Med Ctr 87; **Fellow:** Hematology and Oncology, Univ Nebraska Med Ctr 90; **Fac Appt:** Assoc Prof Med, Univ Nebr Coll Med

Walters, Theodore MD [Hem] - **Spec Exp:** Bleeding/Coagulation Disorders; Anemia; Breast Cancer; **Hospital:** St. Luke's Reg Med Ctr - Boise; **Address:** 520 S Eagle Rd, Lower Level, Meridian, ID 83642; **Phone:** 208-706-5651; **Board Cert:** Internal Medicine 72; Hematology 76; **Med School:** Oregon Hlth Sci Univ 1963; **Resid:** Internal Medicine, Univ Oregon Med Ctr 70; **Fellow:** Hematology, Univ Oregon Med Ctr 72; **Fac Appt:** Asst Clin Prof, Univ Wash

Southwest

Barlogie, Bartholomew MD/PhD [Hem] - **Spec Exp:** Bone Marrow Transplant; Plasma Cell Disorders; Multiple Myeloma; **Hospital:** UAMS Med Ctr; **Address:** UAMS-Myeloma Inst Rsch & Therapy, 4301 West Markham St, Slot 816, Little Rock, AR 72205; **Phone:** 501-603-1583; **Med School:** Germany 69; **Resid:** Univ Muenster Med Sch; **Fellow:** Medical Oncology, MD Anderson Cancer Ctr-Tumor Inst 76; **Fac Appt:** Prof Med, Univ Ark

Boldt, David H MD [Hem] - **Spec Exp:** Leukemia; **Hospital:** UTSA - Univ Hosp; **Address:** UT Hlth Sci Ctr, Div Hematology, 7703 Floyd Curl Drive, MC 7880, San Antonio, TX 78284; **Phone:** 210-567-4848; **Board Cert:** Internal Medicine 73; Hematology 74; Medical Oncology 75; **Med School:** Tufts Univ 69; **Resid:** Internal Medicine, Barnes Hosp-Wash Univ 71; **Fellow:** Hematology and Oncology, Barnes Hosp 73; **Fac Appt:** Prof Med, Univ Tex, San Antonio

Brenner, Malcolm K MD/PhD [Hem] - **Spec Exp:** Gene Therapy; Bone Marrow Transplant-Adult & Pediatric; **Hospital:** Methodist Hosp - Houston; **Address:** 6565 Fannin St, Houston, TX 77030; **Phone:** 832-824-4671; **Med School:** England 75; **Resid:** Internal Medicine, Cambridge Univ 79; **Fellow:** Immunology, Clinical Research Ctr 84; Hematology and Oncology, Royal Free Hospital 86; **Fac Appt:** Prof Med, Baylor Coll Med

Champlin, Richard E MD [Hem] - **Spec Exp:** Bone Marrow Transplant; Stem Cell Transplant; Leukemia & Lymphoma; **Hospital:** UT MD Anderson Cancer Ctr, The (page 115); **Address:** MD Anderson Cancer Ctr, Div Hematology, 1515 Holcombe Blvd, Box 0423, Houston, TX 77030; **Phone:** 713-792-3618; **Board Cert:** Internal Medicine 78; Hematology 80; Medical Oncology 81; **Med School:** Univ Chicago-Pritzker Sch Med 75; **Resid:** Internal Medicine, LA Co Harbor/UCLA Med Ctr 78; **Fellow:** Hematology and Oncology, LA Co Harbor/UCLA Med Ctr 80; **Fac Appt:** Prof Med, Univ Tex, Houston

Cobos, Everardo MD [Hem] - **Spec Exp:** Bone Marrow Transplant; Bleeding/Coagulation Disorders; **Hospital:** Univ Med Ctr - Lubbock; **Address:** Texas Tech Univ Med Sch, Dept Med, 3601 4th St, Lubbock, TX 79430; **Phone:** 806-743-3155; **Board Cert:** Internal Medicine 85; Medical Oncology 87; Hematology 88; **Med School:** Univ Tex, San Antonio 81; **Resid:** Internal Medicine, Letterman Army Med Ctr 85; **Fellow:** Hematology and Oncology, Letterman Army Med Ctr 88; **Fac Appt:** Prof Med, Texas Tech Univ

Cooper, Barry MD [Hem] - **Spec Exp:** Leukemia; Lymphoma; Bleeding/Coagulation Disorders; **Hospital:** Baylor Univ Medical Ctr (page 86); **Address:** 3535 Worth St, Ste 200, Dallas, TX 75246-2096; **Phone:** 214-370-1002; **Board Cert:** Internal Medicine 74; Medical Oncology 77; Hematology 78; **Med School:** Johns Hopkins Univ 71; **Resid:** Internal Medicine, Johns Hopkins Hosp 73; **Fellow:** Metabolism, Natl Inst of Health 75; Hematology, Peter Bent Brigham Hosp 77; **Fac Appt:** Clin Prof Med, Univ Tex SW, Dallas

Fonseca, Rafael MD [Hem] - **Spec Exp:** Multiple Myeloma; **Hospital:** Mayo Clin Hosp - Scottsdale; **Address:** 13400 E Shea Blvd, JRB-356, Scottsdale, AZ 85259; **Phone:** 480-301-6118; **Board Cert:** Internal Medicine 94; Hematology 98; Medical Oncology 97; **Med School:** Mexico 91; **Resid:** Internal Medicine, Jackson Meml Hosp 94; **Fellow:** Hematology and Oncology, Mayo Clinic 98; **Fac Appt:** Assoc Prof Med, Mayo Med Sch

Kantarjian, Hagop M MD [Hem] - **Spec Exp:** Leukemia; **Hospital:** UT MD Anderson Cancer Ctr, The (page 115); **Address:** 1515 Holcombe Blvd, Unit 428, Houston, TX 77030-4009; **Phone:** 713-792-7026; **Board Cert:** Internal Medicine 80; Medical Oncology 85; **Med School:** Lebanon 79; **Resid:** Internal Medicine, Univ Tex MD Anderson Cancer Ctr 83; **Fellow:** Hematology and Oncology, Univ Tex MD Anderson Cancer Ctr 83; **Fac Appt:** Prof Med, Univ Tex, Houston

Keating, Michael MD [Hem] - **Spec Exp:** Leukemia; Chronic Lymphocytic Leukemia (CLL); **Hospital:** UT MD Anderson Cancer Ctr, The (page 115); **Address:** MD Anderson Cancer Ctr, 1515 Holcombe Blvd, Box 428, Houston, TX 77030; **Phone:** 713-745-2376; **Med School:** Australia 66; **Resid:** Internal Medicine, St Vincents Hosp 73; **Fellow:** Hematology, MD Anderson Cancer Ctr 75; **Fac Appt:** Prof Med, Univ Tex, Houston

Lyons, Roger M MD [Hem] - **Spec Exp:** Infections in Cancer Patients; Immunotherapy; Multiple Myeloma; **Hospital:** SW TX Meth Hosp; **Address:** 4411 Medical Drive, Ste 100, San Antonio, TX 78229-3325; **Phone:** 210-595-5300; **Board Cert:** Internal Medicine 81; Hematology 82; **Med School:** Canada 67; **Resid:** Internal Medicine, Winnipeg Genl Hosp 69; Internal Medicine, Barnes-Wohl Hosps 72; **Fellow:** Hematology, Washington Univ Hosps 75; **Fac Appt:** Clin Prof Med, Univ Tex, San Antonio

Strauss, James F MD [Hem] - **Spec Exp:** Bleeding/Coagulation Disorders; Leukemia; Lymphoma; **Hospital:** Presby Hosp of Dallas; **Address:** Texas Oncology, Professional Bldg 2, 8220 Walnut Hill Ln, Ste 700, Dallas, TX 75231; **Phone:** 214-739-4175; **Board Cert:** Internal Medicine 76; Hematology 78; Medical Oncology 81; **Med School:** NYU Sch Med 72; **Resid:** Internal Medicine, Baylor Univ Medical Ctr 76; **Fellow:** Hematology, Univ Texas SW Medical Ctr 77

West Coast and Pacific

Coutre, Steven E MD **[Hem]** - **Spec Exp:** Leukemia; Multiple Myeloma; Thrombotic Disorders; **Hospital:** Stanford Univ Med Ctr; **Address:** Stanford Univ Med Ctr-Hem Clinic, 875 Blake Wilbur Drive, MC 5821, Stanford, CA 94305; **Phone:** 650-723-9729; **Board Cert:** Internal Medicine 93; Hematology 94; **Med School:** Stanford Univ 86; **Resid:** Internal Medicine, Yale-New Haven Hosp 89; **Fellow:** Hematology, Stanford Univ Med Ctr 92; **Fac Appt:** Assoc Prof Hem, Stanford Univ

Damon, Lloyd E MD **[Hem]** - **Spec Exp:** Multiple Myeloma; Hematologic Malignancies; Stem Cell Transplant; **Hospital:** UCSF Med Ctr; **Address:** UCSF Comprehensive Cancer Ctr, 400 Parnassus Ave, Ste A502, San Francisco, CA 94143; **Phone:** 415-353-2421; **Board Cert:** Internal Medicine 85; Hematology 88; Medical Oncology 87; **Med School:** Univ Mich Med Sch 82; **Resid:** Internal Medicine, UCSF Med Ctr 85; **Fellow:** Hematology and Oncology, UCSF Med Ctr 88; **Fac Appt:** Assoc Clin Prof Med, UCSF

Feinstein, Donald I MD **[Hem]** - **Spec Exp:** Bleeding/Coagulation Disorders; Hematologic Malignancies; **Hospital:** USC Norris Canc Comp Ctr; **Address:** USC Keck Sch Med, Topping Tower, 1441 Eastlake Ave, Ste 3436, Los Angeles, CA 90033-9172; **Phone:** 323-865-3964; **Board Cert:** Internal Medicine 65; Hematology 74; **Med School:** Stanford Univ 58; **Resid:** Internal Medicine, LAC-USC Med Ctr 62; **Fellow:** Hematology, NYU Med Ctr 66; **Fac Appt:** Prof Med, USC Sch Med

Forman, Stephen J MD **[Hem]** - **Spec Exp:** Lymphoma; Leukemia; Bone Marrow Transplant; **Hospital:** City of Hope Natl Med Ctr & Beckman Rsch (page 89); **Address:** City Hope National Medical Ctr, 1500 E Duarte Rd, rm 3002, Duarte, CA 91010-3012; **Phone:** 626-256-4673 x62403; **Board Cert:** Internal Medicine 77; **Med School:** USC Sch Med 74; **Resid:** Internal Medicine, LAC-Harbor-UCLA Med Ctr 76; **Fellow:** Hematology, LAC-USC Med Ctr 78; Hematology, City of Hope Med Ctr 79; **Fac Appt:** Clin Prof Med, USC Sch Med

Heinrich, Michael C MD **[Hem]** - **Spec Exp:** Hematologic Malignancies; Sarcoma; Gastrointestinal Stromal Tumors; **Hospital:** VA Medical Center - Portland; **Address:** 3710 SW Veteran's Hospital Rd Bldg 103 - rm E211, MC RND19, Portland, OR 97239; **Phone:** 503-220-8262; **Board Cert:** Internal Medicine 87; Hematology 00; Medical Oncology 01; **Med School:** Johns Hopkins Univ 84; **Resid:** Internal Medicine, Oreg Hlth Scis Univ 87; **Fellow:** Hematology and Oncology, Oreg Hlth Scis Univ 91; **Fac Appt:** Prof Med, Oregon Hlth Sci Univ

Levine, Alexandra M MD **[Hem]** - **Spec Exp:** Leukemia & Lymphoma; AIDS Related Cancers; Transfusion Free Medicine; **Hospital:** USC Norris Canc Comp Ctr; **Address:** USC Kenneth Norris Jr Cancer Hosp, 1441 Eastlake Ave, rm 3468, Los Angeles, CA 90033; **Phone:** 323-865-3913; **Med School:** USC Sch Med 71; **Resid:** Internal Medicine, LAC-USC Med Ctr 74; **Fellow:** Hematology, Grady Meml Hosp-Emory Univ 75; Hematology, LAC-USC Med Ctr 76; **Fac Appt:** Prof Med, USC Sch Med

Lill, Michael MD **[Hem]** - **Spec Exp:** Lymphoma; Leukemia; Stem Cell Transplant; **Hospital:** Cedars-Sinai Med Ctr (page 88); **Address:** Cedars-Sinai Medical Center- Outpt Cancer Ctr, 8700 Beverly Blvd, Los Angeles, CA 90048; **Phone:** 310-423-1160; **Med School:** Australia 82; **Resid:** Internal Medicine, Sir Charles Gairdner Hospital 85; **Fellow:** Hematology, Royal Perth Hospital 88; **Fac Appt:** Assoc Prof Med, UCLA

Linenberger, Michael MD **[Hem]** - **Spec Exp:** Bone Marrow Transplant; Leukemia & Lymphoma; Multiple Myeloma; **Hospital:** Univ Wash Med Ctr; **Address:** 825 Eastlake Ave E (G6-800), Box 19023, Seattle, WA 98109; **Phone:** 206-288-6202; **Board Cert:** Internal Medicine 85; Hematology 88; **Med School:** Univ Kans 82; **Resid:** Internal Medicine, Rhode Island Hosp 85; **Fellow:** Hematology, Univ Wash Med Ctr 89; **Fac Appt:** Assoc Prof Med, Univ Wash

Linker, Charles A MD [Hem] - **Spec Exp:** Leukemia; Bone Marrow Transplant; Multiple Myeloma; **Hospital:** UCSF Med Ctr; **Address:** 400 Parnassus Ave, Ste A502, San Francisco, CA 94143; **Phone:** 415-353-2421; **Board Cert:** Internal Medicine 78; Hematology 80; Medical Oncology 81; **Med School:** Stanford Univ 74; **Resid:** Internal Medicine, Stanford Univ Hosp 78; **Fellow:** Hematology and Oncology, UCSF Med Ctr 81; **Fac Appt:** Clin Prof Med, UCSF

Maziarz, Richard MD [Hem] - **Spec Exp:** Leukemia & Lymphoma; Immunotherapy; Bone Marrow Transplant; **Hospital:** OR Hlth & Sci Univ; **Address:** OHSU Div of Hematology, 3181 SW Sam Jackson Park Rd, UHN 73C, Portland, OR 97239-3098; **Phone:** 503-494-5058; **Board Cert:** Internal Medicine 82; Hematology 88; Medical Oncology 89; **Med School:** Harvard Med Sch 79; **Resid:** Internal Medicine, Univ Hosp 82; **Fellow:** Hematology and Oncology, Brigham & Womens Hosp 88; **Fac Appt:** Prof Hem, Oregon Hlth Sci Univ

Negrin, Robert S MD [Hem] - **Spec Exp:** Bone Marrow Transplant; **Hospital:** Stanford Univ Med Ctr; **Address:** BMT Program, 300 Pasteur Drive, rm H3249, MC 5623, Stanford, CA 94305; **Phone:** 650-723-0822; **Board Cert:** Internal Medicine 87; Hematology 92; **Med School:** Harvard Med Sch 84; **Resid:** Internal Medicine, Stanford Univ Hosp 87; **Fellow:** Hematology, Stanford Univ Hosp 90; **Fac Appt:** Assoc Prof Med, Stanford Univ

Saven, Alan MD [Hem] - **Spec Exp:** Leukemia; Lymphoma; **Hospital:** Scripps Meml Hosp - La Jolla; **Address:** Scripps Green Hospital, 10666 N Torrey Pines Rd, MS 217, La Jolla, CA 92037; **Phone:** 858-554-9386; **Board Cert:** Internal Medicine 87; Medical Oncology 89; Hematology 90; **Med School:** South Africa 82; **Resid:** Internal Medicine, Albert Einstein Med Ctr 86; **Fellow:** Hematology and Oncology, Scripps Clinic 87

Schiller, Gary John MD [Hem] - **Spec Exp:** Leukemia; **Hospital:** UCLA Med Ctr (page 111); **Address:** UCLA Med Ctr, 10833 Le Conte Ave, rm 42-121 CHS, Los Angeles, CA 90095; **Phone:** 310-825-5513; **Board Cert:** Internal Medicine 87; Hematology 00; Medical Oncology 89; **Med School:** USC Sch Med 84; **Resid:** Internal Medicine, UCLA Med Ctr 87; **Fellow:** Hematology and Oncology, UCLA Med Ctr 90; **Fac Appt:** Assoc Prof Med, UCLA

Snyder, David S MD [Hem] - **Spec Exp:** Leukemia; Bone Marrow Transplant; **Hospital:** City of Hope Natl Med Ctr & Beckman Rsch (page 89); **Address:** 1500 E Duarte Rd, Duarte, CA 91010-3012; **Phone:** 626-256-4673; **Board Cert:** Internal Medicine 80; Hematology 84; **Med School:** Harvard Med Sch 77; **Resid:** Internal Medicine, Beth Israel Hosp 80; **Fellow:** Immunology, Harvard Med Sch 82; Hematology and Oncology, New England Med Ctr 84

MEDICAL ONCOLOGY
New England

Anderson, Kenneth C MD [Onc] - **Spec Exp:** Multiple Myeloma; **Hospital:** Dana-Farber Cancer Inst (page 87); **Address:** Dana Farber Cancer Inst, 44 Binney St, Mayer 557, Boston, MA 02115; **Phone:** 617-632-2144; **Board Cert:** Internal Medicine 80; **Med School:** Johns Hopkins Univ 77; **Resid:** Internal Medicine, Johns Hopkins Hosp 80; **Fellow:** Hematology and Oncology, Dana Farber Cancer Inst 83; **Fac Appt:** Prof Med, Harvard Med Sch

Antin, Joseph Harry MD [Onc] - **Spec Exp:** Bone Marrow Transplant; Stem Cell Transplant; Leukemia; **Hospital:** Brigham & Women's Hosp (page 87); **Address:** 44 Binney St, rm D1B12, Boston, MA 02115-6013; **Phone:** 617-632-3667; **Board Cert:** Internal Medicine 81; Medical Oncology 83; Hematology 84; **Med School:** Cornell Univ-Weill Med Coll 78; **Resid:** Internal Medicine, Peter Bent Brigham Hosp 81; **Fellow:** Hematology and Oncology, Brigham & Womens Hosp/Dana Farber 84; **Fac Appt:** Assoc Prof Med, Harvard Med Sch

Atkins, Michael B MD [Onc] - **Spec Exp:** Melanoma; Kidney Cancer; Immunotherapy; **Hospital:** Beth Israel Deaconess Med Ctr - Boston; **Address:** Beth Israel Deaconess Medical Ctr, Dept Hem/Onc, 330 Brookline Ave, E/KS-153, Boston, MA 02215; **Phone:** 617-667-1930; **Board Cert:** Internal Medicine 83; Medical Oncology 87; **Med School:** Tufts Univ 80; **Resid:** Internal Medicine, New England Med Ctr 83; **Fellow:** Hematology and Oncology, New England Med Ctr 87; **Fac Appt:** Prof Med, Harvard Med Sch

Burstein, Harold J MD [Onc] - **Spec Exp:** Breast Cancer; **Hospital:** Dana-Farber Cancer Inst (page 87); **Address:** Dana Farber Cancer Inst, 44 Binney St, Dana Bldg D1210, Boston, MA 02115; **Phone:** 617-632-3800; **Board Cert:** Internal Medicine 97; Medical Oncology 00; **Med School:** Harvard Med Sch 94; **Resid:** Internal Medicine, Mass Genl Hosp 96; **Fellow:** Medical Oncology, Dana Farber Cancer Inst 99; **Fac Appt:** Asst Prof Med, Harvard Med Sch

Canellos, George P MD [Onc] - **Spec Exp:** Lymphoma; Leukemia; Breast Cancer; **Hospital:** Dana-Farber Cancer Inst (page 87); **Address:** 44 Binney St, Boston, MA 02115; **Phone:** 617-632-3470; **Board Cert:** Internal Medicine 67; Hematology 72; Medical Oncology 73; **Med School:** Columbia P&S 60; **Resid:** Internal Medicine, Mass Genl Hosp 63; Internal Medicine, Mass Genl Hosp 66; **Fellow:** Medical Oncology, Natl Cancer Inst 65; Hematology, Hammersmith Hosp 67; **Fac Appt:** Prof Med, Harvard Med Sch

Chabner, Bruce A. MD [Onc] - **Spec Exp:** Colon & Rectal Cancer; Breast Cancer; **Hospital:** Mass Genl Hosp; **Address:** Mass General Hospital, 55 Fruit St, Bldg Cox - rm 640, Boston, MA 02114; **Phone:** 617-724-3200; **Board Cert:** Internal Medicine 71; Medical Oncology 73; **Med School:** Harvard Med Sch 65; **Resid:** Internal Medicine, Peter Bent Brigham Hosp 67; Internal Medicine, Yale-New Haven Hosp 70; **Fellow:** Medical Oncology, Natl Inst Hlth 69; **Fac Appt:** Prof Med, Harvard Med Sch

Chu, Edward MD [Onc] - **Spec Exp:** Colon & Rectal Cancer; Gastrointestinal Cancer; Clinical Trials; **Hospital:** Yale - New Haven Hosp; **Address:** Yale Cancer Ctr, 333 Cedar St, PO Box 208032, New Haven, CT 06520-8032; **Phone:** 203-785-6879; **Board Cert:** Internal Medicine 86; Medical Oncology 89; **Med School:** Brown Univ 83; **Resid:** Internal Medicine, Roger Williams Hosp 87; **Fellow:** Hematology and Oncology, Natl Cancer Inst 90; Internal Medicine, Natl Cancer Inst 92; **Fac Appt:** Prof Med, Yale Univ

Come, Steven Eliot MD [Onc] - **Spec Exp:** Breast Cancer; Hodgkin's Disease; **Hospital:** Beth Israel Deaconess Med Ctr - Boston; **Address:** 330 Brookline Ave, Boston, MA 02215-5400; **Phone:** 617-667-4599; **Board Cert:** Internal Medicine 75; Medical Oncology 79; **Med School:** Harvard Med Sch 72; **Resid:** Internal Medicine, Beth Israel Hosp 77; **Fellow:** Medical Oncology, Natl Cancer Inst 76; **Fac Appt:** Assoc Prof Med, Harvard Med Sch

De Fusco, Patricia A MD [Onc] - **Spec Exp:** Breast Cancer; **Hospital:** Hartford Hosp; **Address:** 100 Retreat Ave, Ste 605, Hartford, CT 06106-2528; **Phone:** 860-246-6647; **Board Cert:** Internal Medicine 83; Medical Oncology 87; **Med School:** Boston Univ 80; **Resid:** Internal Medicine, Hartford 84; **Fellow:** Medical Oncology, Mayo Clinic 86

De Vita Jr, Vincent T MD [Onc] - **Spec Exp:** Lymphoma; Hodgkin's Disease; **Hospital:** Yale - New Haven Hosp; **Address:** 333 Cedar St, rm WWW-205, Box 208028, New Haven, CT 06520-8028; **Phone:** 203-737-1010; **Board Cert:** Internal Medicine 74; Hematology 72; Medical Oncology 73; **Med School:** Geo Wash Univ 61; **Resid:** Internal Medicine, Geo Wash Hosp 63; Internal Medicine, Yale-New Haven Hosp 66; **Fellow:** Medical Oncology, Natl Cancer Inst 65; **Fac Appt:** Prof Med, Yale Univ

Demetri, George D MD [Onc] - **Spec Exp:** Sarcoma; **Hospital:** Dana-Farber Cancer Inst (page 87); **Address:** Dana Farber Cancer Inst, 44 Binney St, Shields-Warren 530, Boston, MA 02115; **Phone:** 617-632-3985; **Board Cert:** Internal Medicine 86; Medical Oncology 89; **Med School:** Stanford Univ 83; **Resid:** Internal Medicine, Univ Wash Med Ctr 86; **Fellow:** Medical Oncology, Dana Farber Cancer Inst 89; **Fac Appt:** Assoc Prof Med, Harvard Med Sch

Fuchs, Charles S MD [Onc] - **Spec Exp:** Gastrointestinal Cancer; **Hospital:** Dana-Farber Cancer Inst (page 87); **Address:** 44 Binney St, Dana 1220, Boston, MA 02115; **Phone:** 617-632-5840; **Board Cert:** Internal Medicine 89; Medical Oncology 02; Hematology 96; **Med School:** Harvard Med Sch 86; **Resid:** Internal Medicine, Brigham & Womens Hosp 89; **Fellow:** Hematology and Oncology, Dana Farber Cancer Inst 92; **Fac Appt:** Assoc Prof Med, Harvard Med Sch

Garber, Judy E MD [Onc] - **Spec Exp:** Breast Cancer; **Hospital:** Dana-Farber Cancer Inst (page 87); **Address:** Dana Farber Cancer Inst, 44 Binney St, Smith 209, Boston, MA 02115; **Phone:** 617-632-5770; **Board Cert:** Internal Medicine 84; Medical Oncology 87; Hematology 88; **Med School:** Yale Univ 81; **Resid:** Internal Medicine, Brigham & Women's Hosp 84; **Fellow:** Medical Oncology, Dana Farber Canc Inst 88; Epidemiology, Dana Farber Canc Inst 90; **Fac Appt:** Assoc Prof Med, Harvard Med Sch

Garnick, Marc B MD [Onc] - **Spec Exp:** Prostate Cancer; Biotechnology; Urologic Cancer; **Hospital:** Beth Israel Deaconess Med Ctr - Boston; **Address:** Beth Israel Deaconess Medical Ctr, SCC9, 330 Brookline Ave, Boston, MA 02215; **Phone:** 617-667-9187; **Board Cert:** Internal Medicine 76; Medical Oncology 79; **Med School:** Univ Pennsylvania 72; **Resid:** Internal Medicine, Univ Penn Hosp 74; **Fellow:** Research, Natl Inst Hlth 76; Medical Oncology, Dana-Farber Cancer Inst 78; **Fac Appt:** Clin Prof Med, Harvard Med Sch

Grunberg, Steven Marc MD [Onc] - **Spec Exp:** Lung Cancer; **Hospital:** FAHC - UHC Campus; **Address:** FAHC-UHC Campus, St Joseph-3, 1 S Prospect St, Burlington, VT 05401; **Phone:** 802-847-8400; **Board Cert:** Internal Medicine 78; Medical Oncology 83; **Med School:** Cornell Univ-Weill Med Coll 75; **Resid:** Internal Medicine, Mofitt Hosp-U Calif 78; **Fellow:** Medical Oncology, Sidney Farber Cancer Ctr; **Fac Appt:** Prof Med, Univ VT Coll Med

Johnson, Bruce Evan MD [Onc] - **Spec Exp:** Lung Cancer; Thoracic Cancers; **Hospital:** Dana-Farber Cancer Inst (page 87); **Address:** Dana Farber Cancer Inst-Lowe Ctr Thoracic Onc, 44 Binney St, Dana 1234, Boston, MA 02115; **Phone:** 617-632-4790; **Board Cert:** Internal Medicine 82; Medical Oncology 85; **Med School:** Univ Minn 79; **Resid:** Internal Medicine, Univ Chicago Hosps 82; **Fellow:** Medical Oncology, Natl Cancer Inst 85; **Fac Appt:** Assoc Prof Med, Harvard Med Sch

Kaelin, William G MD [Onc] - **Spec Exp:** Drug Discovery & Development; **Hospital:** Dana-Farber Cancer Inst (page 87); **Address:** Dana Farber Cancer Inst, 44 Binney St, rm Mayer 457, Boston, MA 02115; **Phone:** 617-632-4747; **Board Cert:** Internal Medicine 87; Medical Oncology 89; **Med School:** Duke Univ 82; **Resid:** Internal Medicine, Johns Hopkins Hosp 86; **Fellow:** Medical Oncology, Dana Farber Cancer Inst 89; **Fac Appt:** Prof Med, Harvard Med Sch

Kantoff, Philip W MD [Onc] - **Spec Exp:** Genitourinary Cancer; Prostate Cancer; **Hospital:** Dana-Farber Cancer Inst (page 87); **Address:** 44 Binney St, Ste D 1230, Boston, MA 02115; **Phone:** 617-632-3466; **Board Cert:** Internal Medicine 82; Medical Oncology 89; **Med School:** Brown Univ 79; **Resid:** Internal Medicine, NYU/Bellevue Hosp 83; **Fellow:** Gene Therapy Research, NIH 86; **Fac Appt:** Prof Med, Harvard Med Sch

Kaufman, Peter A MD [Onc] - **Spec Exp:** Breast Cancer; Clinical Trials; **Hospital:** Dartmouth - Hitchcock Med Ctr; **Address:** Dartmouth-Hitchcock Med Ctr, Dept Hem/Onc, One Medical Center Drive, Lebanon, NH 03756; **Phone:** 603-650-6700; **Board Cert:** Internal Medicine 86; Medical Oncology 89; **Med School:** NYU Sch Med 83; **Resid:** Internal Medicine, Duke Univ Med Ctr 86; **Fellow:** Hematology and Oncology, Duke Univ Med Ctr 89; **Fac Appt:** Assoc Prof Med, Dartmouth Med Sch

Lynch, Thomas MD [Onc] - **Spec Exp:** Lung Cancer; Thoracic Cancers; **Hospital:** Mass Genl Hosp; **Address:** Mass Genl Hosp, Dept Hem/Onc, 55 Fruit St, Yawkey Bldg - Ste 7B, Boston, MA 02114-2617; **Phone:** 617-724-1136; **Board Cert:** Internal Medicine 89; Medical Oncology 91; **Med School:** Yale Univ 86; **Resid:** Internal Medicine, Mass Genl Hosp 89; **Fellow:** Medical Oncology, Dana-Farber Cancer Inst 91; **Fac Appt:** Asst Prof Med, Harvard Med Sch

Mayer, Robert J MD [Onc] - **Spec Exp:** Colon & Rectal Cancer; Gastrointestinal Cancer; **Hospital:** Dana-Farber Cancer Inst (page 87); **Address:** Dana Farber Cancer Inst, 44 Binney St, rm D1608, Boston, MA 02115-6084; **Phone:** 617-632-3474; **Board Cert:** Internal Medicine 73; Medical Oncology 75; Hematology 76; **Med School:** Harvard Med Sch 69; **Resid:** Internal Medicine, Mt Sinai Hosp 71; Hematology and Oncology, Natl Cancer Inst 74; **Fellow:** Sidney Farber Cancer Inst 76; **Fac Appt:** Prof Med, Harvard Med Sch

Muss, Hyman B MD [Onc] - **Spec Exp:** Breast Cancer; **Hospital:** FAHC - Med Ctr Campus; **Address:** Fletcher Allen Health Care- UNC Campus St., 1 S Prospect St. Joseph 3, Burlington, VT 05401-1429; **Phone:** 802-847-3827; **Board Cert:** Internal Medicine 73; Hematology 74; Medical Oncology 75; **Med School:** SUNY Downstate 68; **Resid:** Internal Medicine, Peter Bent Brigham Hosp 70; **Fellow:** Medical Oncology, Peter Bent Brigham Hosp 74; **Fac Appt:** Prof Med, Univ VT Coll Med

Nadler, Lee M MD [Onc] - **Spec Exp:** Lymphoma; **Hospital:** Dana-Farber Cancer Inst (page 87); **Address:** Dana Farber Cancer Inst, 44 Binney St, Boston, MA 02115; **Phone:** 617-632-3331; **Board Cert:** Internal Medicine 76; **Med School:** Harvard Med Sch 73; **Resid:** Internal Medicine, Columbia-Presby Hosp 75; **Fellow:** Medical Oncology, Natl Cancer Inst 77; Medical Oncology, Dana-Farber Cancer Inst 78; **Fac Appt:** Prof Med, Harvard Med Sch

Posner, Marshall MD [Onc] - **Spec Exp:** Head & Neck Cancer; **Hospital:** Dana-Farber Cancer Inst (page 87); **Address:** Dana-Farber Cancer Inst-H&N Cancer Ctr, 44 Binney St, rm G430, Brookline, MA 02115; **Phone:** 617-632-3090; **Board Cert:** Internal Medicine 78; Medical Oncology 81; **Med School:** Tufts Univ 75; **Resid:** Internal Medicine, Boston City Hosp 78; **Fellow:** Oncology, Dana-Farber Cancer Inst 81; **Fac Appt:** Assoc Prof Med, Harvard Med Sch

Shulman, Lawrence N MD [Onc] - **Spec Exp:** Breast Cancer; Lymphoma; **Hospital:** Dana-Farber Cancer Inst (page 87); **Address:** Dana-Farber Cancer Inst, 44 Binney St, Dana 1608, Boston, MA 02115; **Phone:** 617-632-2277; **Board Cert:** Internal Medicine 78; Medical Oncology 81; Hematology 82; **Med School:** Harvard Med Sch 75; **Resid:** Internal Medicine, Beth Israel Hosp 77; **Fellow:** Hematology and Oncology, Beth Israel Hosp 80; **Fac Appt:** Assoc Prof Med, Harvard Med Sch

Taplin, Mary-Ellen MD [Onc] - **Spec Exp:** Prostate Cancer; Genitourinary Cancer; **Hospital:** Dana-Farber Cancer Inst (page 87); **Address:** Dana Farber Cancer Inst, 44 Binney St, rm D1230, Boston, MA 02115; **Phone:** 617-632-3466; **Board Cert:** Internal Medicine 89; Hematology 96; Medical Oncology 03; **Med School:** Univ Mass Sch Med 86; **Resid:** Internal Medicine, U Mass Med Ctr 90; **Fellow:** Hematology and Oncology, Beth Israel Deaconess Hosp 93; **Fac Appt:** Assoc Prof Med, Univ Mass Sch Med

Weisberg, Tracey MD [Onc] - **Spec Exp:** Breast Cancer; **Hospital:** Maine Med Ctr; **Address:** 100 Campus Drive, Unit 108, Scarborough, ME 04074; **Phone:** 207-885-7600; **Board Cert:** Internal Medicine 87; Medical Oncology 89; **Med School:** SUNY Stony Brook 83; **Resid:** Internal Medicine, Mount Sinai Hosp 85; Internal Medicine, Hartford Hosp 86; **Fellow:** Medical Oncology, Yale Univ Hosp 88

Winer, Eric P MD [Onc] - **Spec Exp:** Breast Cancer; **Hospital:** Dana-Farber Cancer Inst (page 87); **Address:** Dana Farber Cancer Inst, 44 Binney St, Dana 1210, Boston, MA 02115; **Phone:** 617-632-3800; **Board Cert:** Internal Medicine 87; Medical Oncology 89; **Med School:** Yale Univ 83; **Resid:** Internal Medicine, Yale-New Haven Hosp 87; **Fellow:** Hematology and Oncology, Duke Univ 89; **Fac Appt:** Assoc Prof Med, Harvard Med Sch

Mid Atlantic

Abeloff, Martin MD [Onc] - **Spec Exp:** Breast Cancer; **Hospital:** Johns Hopkins Hosp - Baltimore (page 97); **Address:** 401 N Broadway, Ste 1100, Baltimore, MD 21231; **Phone:** 410-955-8822; **Board Cert:** Internal Medicine 73; Medical Oncology 73; **Med School:** Johns Hopkins Univ 66; **Resid:** Internal Medicine, Beth Israel Hosp 70; **Fellow:** Hematology, New England Med Ctr 71; **Fac Appt:** Prof Med, Johns Hopkins Univ

Agarwala, Sanjiv MD [Onc] - **Spec Exp:** Melanoma; Melanoma Clinical Trials; Head & Neck Cancer; **Hospital:** UPMC Shadyside (page 114); **Address:** Univ Pittsburgh Med Ctr - Div Med Oncology, 5150 Centre Ave, Pittsburgh, PA 15232; **Phone:** 412-692-4724; **Board Cert:** Internal Medicine 94; Hematology 96; Medical Oncology 95; **Med School:** India 85; **Resid:** Internal Medicine, Univ Pittsburgh Med Ctr 93; **Fellow:** Hematology and Oncology, Univ Pittsburgh Med Ctr 94; **Fac Appt:** Asst Prof Med, Univ Pittsburgh

Ahlgren, James David MD [Onc] - **Spec Exp:** Gastrointestinal Cancer; **Hospital:** G Washington Univ Hosp; **Address:** Geo Wash Univ Med Ctr, Div. Hem & Onc, 2150 Pennsylvania Ave NW, Ste 3-428, Washington, DC 20037-3201; **Phone:** 202-741-2478; **Board Cert:** Internal Medicine 80; Medical Oncology 89; **Med School:** Georgetown Univ 77; **Resid:** Internal Medicine, Georgetown Univ Hosp 79; **Fellow:** Medical Oncology, Georgetown Univ Hosp 81; **Fac Appt:** Prof Med, Geo Wash Univ

Aisner, Joseph MD [Onc] - **Spec Exp:** Lung Cancer; **Hospital:** Robert Wood Johnson Univ Hosp - New Brunswick (page 106); **Address:** Cancer Inst of New Jersey, 195 Little Albany St, rm 2012, New Brunswick, NJ 08901; **Phone:** 732-235-6777; **Board Cert:** Internal Medicine 73; Medical Oncology 75; **Med School:** Wayne State Univ 70; **Resid:** Internal Medicine, Georgetown Univ Hosp 72; **Fellow:** Medical Oncology, Natl Cancer Inst 75

Algazy, Kenneth M MD [Onc] - **Spec Exp:** Lung Cancer; Mesothelioma; Hematologic Malignancies; **Hospital:** Hosp Univ Penn - UPHS (page 113); **Address:** 51 N 39th St Bldg Medical Arts - Ste 103, Philadelphia, PA 19104-2640; **Phone:** 215-662-8947; **Board Cert:** Internal Medicine 72; Hematology 74; Medical Oncology 79; **Med School:** Temple Univ 69; **Resid:** Internal Medicine, Univ Rochester-Strong Meml Hosp 72; **Fellow:** Hematology and Oncology, Johns Hopkins Med Ctr 74; **Fac Appt:** Assoc Clin Prof Med, Univ Pennsylvania

Ambinder, Richard F MD/PhD [Onc] - **Spec Exp:** Lymphoma; Hodgkin's Disease; AIDS Related Cancers; **Hospital:** Johns Hopkins Hosp - Baltimore (page 97); **Address:** Cancer Research Bldg, 1650 Orleans St, rm 389, Baltimore, MD 21231; **Phone:** 410-955-8964; **Board Cert:** Internal Medicine 82; Medical Oncology 85; **Med School:** Johns Hopkins Univ 79; **Resid:** Internal Medicine, Johns Hopkins Hosp 81; **Fellow:** Internal Medicine, Johns Hopkins Hosp 82; Medical Oncology, Johns Hopkins Hosp 85; **Fac Appt:** Prof Med, Johns Hopkins Univ

Antman, Karen MD [Onc] - **Spec Exp:** Breast Cancer; Sarcoma; **Hospital:** Natl Inst of Hlth - Clin Ctr; **Address:** Natl Cancer Inst, Natl Inst Hlth, 31 Center Drive, MSC 2590 Bldg Bld 31 Fl 11A - rm 1104, Bethesda, MD 20892; **Phone:** 301-496-6511; **Board Cert:** Internal Medicine 77; Medical Oncology 79; **Med School:** Columbia P&S 74; **Resid:** Internal Medicine, Columbia-Presby Med Ctr 77; **Fellow:** Medical Oncology, Dana-Farber Cancer Inst 79

Bashevkin, Michael MD [Onc] - **Spec Exp:** Solid Tumors; Bleeding Disorders; Hematologic Malignancies; **Hospital:** Maimonides Med Ctr (page 99); **Address:** 1660 E 14st St, Ste 501, Brooklyn, NY 11229; **Phone:** 718-382-8500 x501; **Board Cert:** Internal Medicine 76; Hematology 78; Medical Oncology 79; **Med School:** SUNY Downstate 73; **Resid:** Internal Medicine, VA Med Ctr 76; Hematology and Oncology, Maimonides Med Ctr 79

Belani, Chandra MD [Onc] - **Spec Exp:** Lung Cancer; Drug Discovery; Chemoprevention; **Hospital:** UPMC Shadyside (page 114); **Address:** UPMC Cancer Pavilion, 5150 Centre Ave Fl 5, Pittsburgh, PA 15232; **Phone:** 412-648-6619; **Board Cert:** Internal Medicine 86; Medical Oncology 87; **Med School:** India 78; **Resid:** Internal Medicine, SMS Med Hosp 81; Internal Medicine, Good Samaritan/Univ MD Hosp 84; **Fellow:** Hematology and Oncology, Univ MD Hosp 87; **Fac Appt:** Prof Med, Univ Pittsburgh

Bernstein, Zale P MD [Onc] - **Spec Exp:** AIDS Related Cancers; Lymphoma; **Hospital:** Roswell Park Cancer Inst (page 107); **Address:** Roswell Park Cancer Inst, Elm & Carlton Sts, Buffalo, NY 14263; **Phone:** 716-845-1643; **Board Cert:** Internal Medicine 84; Hematology 86; Medical Oncology 87; **Med School:** Geo Wash Univ 80; **Resid:** Internal Medicine, Suny Buffalo Affil Hosp 83; **Fellow:** Hematology and Oncology, SUNY Buffalo Affil Hosp 87; **Fac Appt:** Assoc Clin Prof Med, SUNY Buffalo

Bosl, George MD [Onc] - **Spec Exp:** Testicular Cancer; **Hospital:** Meml Sloan Kettering Cancer Ctr (page 100); **Address:** 1275 York Ave, C1289, New York, NY 10021; **Phone:** 212-639-8473; **Board Cert:** Internal Medicine 76; Medical Oncology 79; **Med School:** Creighton Univ 73; **Resid:** Internal Medicine, New York Hosp 75; Internal Medicine, Memorial Sloan-Kettering Cancer Ctr 77; **Fellow:** Medical Oncology, Univ Minn Hosps 79; **Fac Appt:** Prof Med, Cornell Univ-Weill Med Coll

Brufsky, Adam MD/PhD [Onc] - **Spec Exp:** Breast Cancer; **Hospital:** Magee-Womens Hosp - UPMC (page 114); **Address:** Univ Pittsburgh Cancer Inst/Magee-Women's Hosp, 300 Halleket St, Ste 4628, Pittsburgh, PA 15213; **Phone:** 412-641-4530; **Board Cert:** Internal Medicine 04; Medical Oncology 95; **Med School:** Univ Conn 90; **Resid:** Internal Medicine, Brigham & Women's Hosp 92; **Fellow:** Medical Oncology, Dana Farber Cancer Inst 95; Medical Microbiology, Brigham & Women's Hosp 95; **Fac Appt:** Asst Prof Med, Univ Pittsburgh

Chanan-Khan, Asher A A MD **[Onc]** - **Spec Exp:** Multiple Myeloma; Leukemia; **Hospital:** Roswell Park Cancer Inst (page 107); **Address:** Roswell Park Cancer Inst, Elm & Carlton Sts, Buffalo, NY 14263; **Phone:** 716-845-1643; **Board Cert:** Internal Medicine 97; Medical Oncology 01; **Med School:** Pakistan 93; **Resid:** Internal Medicine, Harlem Hosp Ctr 97; **Fellow:** Hematology and Oncology, New York Univ Hosp 99; **Fac Appt:** Asst Prof Onc, SUNY Buffalo

Chapman, Paul MD **[Onc]** - **Spec Exp:** Melanoma; Immunology; **Hospital:** Meml Sloan Kettering Cancer Ctr (page 100); **Address:** 1275 York Ave, New York, NY 10021; **Phone:** 212-639-5015; **Board Cert:** Internal Medicine 84; Medical Oncology 87; **Med School:** Cornell Univ-Weill Med Coll 81; **Resid:** Internal Medicine, Univ Chicago Hosps 84; **Fellow:** Medical Oncology, Meml Sloan-Kettering Cancer Ctr 87; **Fac Appt:** Assoc Prof Med, Cornell Univ-Weill Med Coll

Cohen, Philip MD **[Onc]** - **Spec Exp:** Breast Cancer; **Hospital:** Georgetown Univ Hosp; **Address:** Georgetown Univ Hosp, Lombardi Cancer Ctr, 3800 Reservoir Rd NW, Washington, DC 20007; **Phone:** 202-444-2198; **Board Cert:** Internal Medicine 73; Medical Oncology 75; Hematology 76; **Med School:** Harvard Med Sch 70; **Resid:** Internal Medicine, Mass Genl Hosp 72; **Fellow:** Medical Oncology, Natl Cancer Inst 74; **Fac Appt:** Assoc Prof Med, Geo Wash Univ

Cohen, Roger MD **[Onc]** - **Spec Exp:** Drug Discovery; Clinical Trials; **Hospital:** Fox Chase Cancer Ctr (page 95); **Address:** Fox Chase Cancer Ctr, 333 Cottman Ave, Ste C307, Philadelphia, PA 19111; **Phone:** 215-214-1676; **Board Cert:** Internal Medicine 84; Medical Oncology 93; Hematology 86; **Med School:** Harvard Med Sch 80; **Resid:** Internal Medicine, Mt Sinai Hosp 82; **Fellow:** Research, Sloan Kettering Cancer Inst 85; Hematology, Mt Sinai Hosp 86

Cohen, Seymour M. MD **[Onc]** - **Spec Exp:** Melanoma; Breast Cancer; Lung Cancer; **Hospital:** Mount Sinai Med Ctr (page 101); **Address:** 1045 5th Ave, New York, NY 10028-0138; **Phone:** 212-249-9141; **Board Cert:** Internal Medicine 71; Medical Oncology 73; **Med School:** Univ Pittsburgh 62; **Resid:** Internal Medicine, Montefiore Med Ctr 64; Internal Medicine, Mount Sinai Med Ctr 65; **Fellow:** Hematology, Mount Sinai Med Ctr 66; Hematology and Oncology, LI Jewish Hosp 68; **Fac Appt:** Assoc Clin Prof Med, Mount Sinai Sch Med

Coleman, Morton MD **[Onc]** - **Spec Exp:** Lymphoma; Multiple Myeloma; Leukemia; **Hospital:** NY-Presby Hosp - NY Weill Cornell Med Ctr (page 103); **Address:** 407 E 70th St, FL 3, New York, NY 10021-5302; **Phone:** 212-517-5900; **Board Cert:** Internal Medicine 71; Hematology 72; Medical Oncology 73; **Med School:** Med Coll VA 63; **Resid:** Internal Medicine, Grady Meml Hosp-Emory 65; Internal Medicine, New York Hosp-Cornell 68; **Fellow:** Hematology and Oncology, New York Hosp-Cornell 70; **Fac Appt:** Clin Prof Med, Cornell Univ-Weill Med Coll

Comis, Robert L MD **[Onc]** - **Spec Exp:** Lung Cancer; **Hospital:** Hahnemann Univ Hosp; **Address:** 1818 Market St, Ste 1100, Philadelphia, PA 19103; **Phone:** 215-789-3609; **Board Cert:** Internal Medicine 75; Medical Oncology 77; **Med School:** SUNY Upstate Med Univ 71; **Resid:** Internal Medicine, SUNY Upstate Med Ctr 75; **Fac Appt:** Prof Med, Drexel Univ Coll Med

Cullen, Kevin MD **[Onc]** - **Spec Exp:** Head & Neck Cancer; **Hospital:** Univ of MD Med Sys; **Address:** Univ Md Greenbaum Cancer Ctr, 22 S Greene St, rm N9E22, Baltimore, MD 21201; **Phone:** 410-328-5506; **Board Cert:** Internal Medicine 86; Medical Oncology 89; **Med School:** Harvard Med Sch 83; **Resid:** Internal Medicine, Beth Israel Hosp 86; Internal Medicine, Hammersmith Hosp; **Fellow:** Medical Oncology, Natl Cancer Inst 88

Czuczman, Myron MD [Onc] - **Spec Exp:** Lymphoma; Multiple Myeloma; Immunotherapy; **Hospital:** Roswell Park Cancer Inst (page 107); **Address:** Elm and Carlton Sts, Buffalo, NY 14201; **Phone:** 716-845-7695; **Board Cert:** Internal Medicine 88; Medical Oncology 91; **Med School:** Penn State Univ-Hershey Med Ctr 85; **Resid:** Internal Medicine, Meml Sloan-Kettering-Cornell Univ 88; **Fellow:** Hematology and Oncology, Meml Sloan-Kettering Cancer Ctr 92; **Fac Appt:** Assoc Prof Med, SUNY Buffalo

Daly, Mary B MD/PhD [Onc] - **Spec Exp:** Breast Cancer; Bone Marrow Transplant; Cancer Prevention/Risk Assessment; **Hospital:** Fox Chase Cancer Ctr (page 95); **Address:** Fox Chase Cancer Ctr, 333 Cottman Ave, P1054, Philadelphia, PA 19111; **Phone:** 215-728-2791; **Board Cert:** Internal Medicine 81; Medical Oncology 83; **Med School:** Univ NC Sch Med 78; **Resid:** Internal Medicine, Univ Texas Hlth Sci Ctr 81; **Fellow:** Medical Oncology, Univ Texas Hlth Sci Ctr 83

Davidson, Nancy E MD [Onc] - **Spec Exp:** Breast Cancer; **Hospital:** Johns Hopkins Hosp - Baltimore (page 97); **Address:** Johns Hopkins Oncology Center, 1650 Orleans St, Bldg CRB - rm 409, Baltimore, MD 21231-1000; **Phone:** 410-955-8964; **Board Cert:** Internal Medicine 82; Medical Oncology 85; **Med School:** Harvard Med Sch 79; **Resid:** Internal Medicine, Johns Hopkins Hosp 82; **Fellow:** Medical Oncology, Natl Cancer Inst 86; **Fac Appt:** Prof Onc, Johns Hopkins Univ

Dawson, Nancy MD [Onc] - **Spec Exp:** Prostate Cancer; Kidney Cancer; Bladder Cancer; **Hospital:** Univ of MD Med Sys; **Address:** Univ Maryland - Greenbaum Canc Ctr, 22 S Greene St, Baltimore, MD 21201; **Phone:** 410-328-2565; **Board Cert:** Internal Medicine 82; Medical Oncology 85; Hematology 84; **Med School:** Georgetown Univ 79; **Resid:** Internal Medicine, Walter Reed AMC 82; **Fellow:** Hematology and Oncology, Walter Reed AMC 85; **Fac Appt:** Prof Med, Univ MD Sch Med

Dickler, Maura N MD [Onc] - **Spec Exp:** Breast Cancer; **Hospital:** Meml Sloan Kettering Cancer Ctr (page 100); **Address:** Meml Sloan Kettering Cancer Ctr, 1275 York Ave, New York, NY 10021; **Phone:** 212-639-5456; **Board Cert:** Internal Medicine 94; Medical Oncology 98; **Med School:** Univ Chicago-Pritzker Sch Med 91; **Resid:** Internal Medicine, Univ Chicago Hosps 94; **Fellow:** Medical Oncology, Meml Sloan Kettering Cancer Ctr 98; **Fac Appt:** Asst Prof Med, Cornell Univ-Weill Med Coll

Donehower, Ross Carl MD [Onc] - **Spec Exp:** Pancreatic Cancer; Colon Cancer; Prostate Cancer; **Hospital:** Johns Hopkins Hosp - Baltimore (page 97); **Address:** Hopkins Kimmel Cancer Ctr, 1650 Orleans St, CRB-187, Baltimore, MD 21231-1000; **Phone:** 410-955-8838; **Board Cert:** Internal Medicine 77; Medical Oncology 79; **Med School:** Univ Minn 74; **Resid:** Internal Medicine, Johns Hopkins Hosp 76; **Fellow:** Medical Oncology, Natl Inst Hlth 80; **Fac Appt:** Prof Med, Johns Hopkins Univ

Doroshow, James H MD [Onc] - **Spec Exp:** Drug Discovery & Development; Colon Cancer; Breast Cancer; **Hospital:** Natl Inst of Hlth - Clin Ctr; **Address:** Natl Cancer Inst, Div Cancer Treatment & Diagnosis, 31 Center, Bldg 31 - rm 3A44, Bethesda, MD 20892; **Phone:** 301-496-4291; **Board Cert:** Internal Medicine 76; Medical Oncology 77; **Med School:** Harvard Med Sch 73; **Resid:** Internal Medicine, Mass Genl Hosp 75; **Fellow:** Medical Oncology, Natl Cancer Inst 78

Eisenberger, Mario MD [Onc] - **Spec Exp:** Prostate Cancer; **Hospital:** Johns Hopkins Hosp - Baltimore (page 97); **Address:** 1650 Orleans St, rm 1M51, Baltimore, MD 21231; **Phone:** 410-614-3511; **Board Cert:** Internal Medicine 76; Medical Oncology 79; **Med School:** Brazil 72; **Resid:** Internal Medicine, Michael Reese Hosp 75; **Fellow:** Hematology, Michael Reese Hosp 76; Medical Oncology, Jackson Meml Hosp/Univ Miami 79; **Fac Appt:** Prof Onc, Johns Hopkins Univ

Ettinger, David Seymour MD [Onc] - **Spec Exp:** Lung Cancer; Sarcoma; Clinical Trials; **Hospital:** Johns Hopkins Hosp - Baltimore (page 97); **Address:** Bunting Blaustein Cancer Rsrch Bldg, 1650 Orleans St, rm G88, Baltimore, MD 21231-1000; **Phone:** 410-955-8847; **Board Cert:** Internal Medicine 76; Medical Oncology 77; **Med School:** Univ Louisville Sch Med 67; **Resid:** Internal Medicine, Mayo Grad Schl 71; **Fellow:** Medical Oncology, Johns Hopkins Hosp 75; **Fac Appt:** Prof Onc, Johns Hopkins Univ

Felix, Carolyn A MD [Onc] - **Spec Exp:** Leukemia; Leukemia in Infants; **Hospital:** Chldns Hosp of Philadelphia, The; **Address:** Childrens Hosp - Div Oncology, 3615 Civic Ctr Blvd, Abramson Cancer Ctr-Rm 902B, Philadelphia, PA 19104; **Phone:** 215-590-2831; **Board Cert:** Pediatrics 87; Pediatric Hematology-Oncology 87; **Med School:** Boston Univ 81; **Resid:** Pediatrics, Chldns Hosp 84; **Fellow:** Pediatric Hematology-Oncology, Natl Cancer Inst-Pediatric Br 87; **Fac Appt:** Assoc Prof Ped, Univ Pennsylvania

Fine, Howard Alan MD [Onc] - **Spec Exp:** Brain Tumors; **Hospital:** Natl Inst of Hlth - Clin Ctr; **Address:** NIH/NCI/NOB, Bloch Building, MSC 8200, 9030 Old Georgetown Rd, Bethesda, MD 20892; **Phone:** 301-402-6298; **Board Cert:** Medical Oncology 89; Internal Medicine 87; **Med School:** Mount Sinai Sch Med 84; **Resid:** Internal Medicine, Hosp U Penn 87; **Fellow:** Oncology, Dana Farber Cancer Ctr

Fisher, Richard I MD [Onc] - **Spec Exp:** Lymphoma; Hodgkin's Disease; **Hospital:** Univ of Rochester Strong Meml Hosp; **Address:** James P. Wilmot Cancer Ctr, 601 Elmwood Ave, Box 704, Rochester, NY 14642; **Phone:** 585-275-5793; **Board Cert:** Internal Medicine 73; Medical Oncology 77; **Med School:** Harvard Med Sch 70; **Resid:** Internal Medicine, Mass Genl Hosp 72; **Fac Appt:** Prof Med, Univ Rochester

Flomenberg, Neal MD [Onc] - **Spec Exp:** Bone Marrow Transplant; Stem Cell Transplant; Leukemia & Lymphoma; **Hospital:** Thomas Jefferson Univ Hosp (page 110); **Address:** Thomas Jefferson Univ Hosp, 125 S 9th St, Ste 801, Philadelphia, PA 19107; **Phone:** 215-955-0356; **Board Cert:** Internal Medicine 79; Medical Oncology 81; Hematology 82; **Med School:** Jefferson Med Coll 76; **Resid:** Internal Medicine, Montefiore Med Ctr 79; **Fellow:** Hematology and Oncology, Meml Sloan Kettering Cancer Ctr 82; **Fac Appt:** Clin Prof Med, Thomas Jefferson Univ

Forastiere, Arlene A MD [Onc] - **Spec Exp:** Esophageal Cancer; Head & Neck Cancer; **Hospital:** Johns Hopkins Hosp - Baltimore (page 97); **Address:** Bunting Blaustein Cancer Research Bldg, 1650 Orleans St, rm G90, Baltimore, MD 21231; **Phone:** 410-955-9818; **Board Cert:** Internal Medicine 78; Medical Oncology 81; **Med School:** NY Med Coll 75; **Resid:** Internal Medicine, Albert Einstein Med Ctr 77; Internal Medicine, Univ Conn Health Ctr 78; **Fellow:** Medical Oncology, Meml Sloan Kettering Cancer Ctr 80; **Fac Appt:** Prof Onc, NY Med Coll

Fox, Kevin R MD [Onc] - **Spec Exp:** Breast Cancer; **Hospital:** Hosp Univ Penn - UPHS (page 113); **Address:** 3400 Spruce St, 16 Penn Tower, Philadelphia, PA 19104; **Phone:** 215-662-7469; **Board Cert:** Internal Medicine 85; Medical Oncology 87; **Med School:** Johns Hopkins Univ 81; **Resid:** Internal Medicine, Johns Hopkins Hosp 84; **Fellow:** Hematology and Oncology, Hosp Univ Penn 87; **Fac Appt:** Assoc Prof Med, Univ Pennsylvania

Gabrilove, Janice MD [Onc] - **Spec Exp:** Myelodysplastic Syndromes; Leukemia; **Hospital:** Mount Sinai Med Ctr (page 101); **Address:** Mount Sinai Med Ctr, Box 1129, One Gustave Levy Pl, New York, NY 10029-6574; **Phone:** 212-241-9650; **Board Cert:** Internal Medicine 80; Medical Oncology 83; **Med School:** Mount Sinai Sch Med 77; **Resid:** Internal Medicine, Columbia-Presby Med Ctr 80; **Fellow:** Hematology and Oncology, Meml Sloan-Kettering Cancer Ctr 83; **Fac Appt:** Prof Med, Mount Sinai Sch Med

Gelmann, Edward P MD [Onc] - **Spec Exp:** Prostate Cancer; Testicular Cancer; **Hospital:** Georgetown Univ Hosp; **Address:** Lombardi Cancer Ctr, Podium A, 3800 Reservoir Rd NW, Washington, DC 20007; **Phone:** 202-444-1587; **Board Cert:** Internal Medicine 79; Medical Oncology 81; **Med School:** Stanford Univ 76; **Resid:** Internal Medicine, Univ Chicago Hosp 78; **Fellow:** Medical Oncology, National Cancer Inst 81; **Fac Appt:** Prof Med, Georgetown Univ

Glick, John H MD [Onc] - **Spec Exp:** Breast Cancer; Hodgkin's Disease; Lymphoma, Non-Hodgkin's; **Hospital:** Hosp Univ Penn - UPHS (page 113); **Address:** Univ Penn Cancer Ctr, 3400 Spruce St, 16 Penn Tower, Philadelphia, PA 19104; **Phone:** 215-662-6334; **Board Cert:** Internal Medicine 73; Medical Oncology 75; **Med School:** Columbia P&S 69; **Resid:** Internal Medicine, Presbyterian Hosp 71; **Fellow:** Medical Oncology, Natl Cancer Inst 73; Medical Oncology, Stanford Univ 74; **Fac Appt:** Prof Med, Univ Pennsylvania

Goldstein, Lori J MD [Onc] - **Spec Exp:** Breast Cancer; **Hospital:** Fox Chase Cancer Ctr (page 95); **Address:** Fox Chase Cancer Ctr, Dept Med Oncology, 333 Cottman Ave, Philadelphia, PA 19111; **Phone:** 215-728-2689; **Board Cert:** Internal Medicine 85; Medical Oncology 02; **Med School:** SUNY Upstate Med Univ 82; **Resid:** Internal Medicine, Presby Univ Hosp 85; **Fellow:** Medical Oncology, Natl Cancer Inst/NIH; **Fac Appt:** Assoc Prof Med, Temple Univ

Grana, Generosa MD [Onc] - **Spec Exp:** Breast Cancer; Cancer Genetics; Cancer Prevention; **Hospital:** Cooper Univ Hosp; **Address:** 900 Centennial Blvd, Ste M-2, Voorhees, NJ 08043; **Phone:** 856-325-6740; **Board Cert:** Internal Medicine 88; Medical Oncology 01; **Med School:** Northwestern Univ 85; **Resid:** Internal Medicine, Temple Univ Hosp 88; **Fellow:** Hematology and Oncology, Fox Chase Cancer Ctr 92; **Fac Appt:** Assoc Prof Med, UMDNJ-RW Johnson Med Sch

Grossbard, Michael L MD [Onc] - **Spec Exp:** Lymphoma; Gastrointestinal Cancer; Breast Cancer; **Hospital:** St Luke's - Roosevelt Hosp Ctr - Roosevelt Div (page 93); **Address:** 1000 10th Ave Fl 11 - Ste C02, New York, NY 10019; **Phone:** 212-523-5419; **Board Cert:** Internal Medicine 89; Medical Oncology 01; **Med School:** Yale Univ 86; **Resid:** Internal Medicine, Mass Genl Hosp 89; **Fellow:** Medical Oncology, Dana Farber Cancer Inst 91; **Fac Appt:** Assoc Clin Prof Med, Columbia P&S

Hait, William MD/PhD [Onc] - **Spec Exp:** Breast Cancer; **Hospital:** Robert Wood Johnson Univ Hosp - New Brunswick (page 106); **Address:** Cancer Inst of NJ, 195 Little Albany St, New Brunswick, NJ 08901-1914; **Phone:** 732-235-8064; **Board Cert:** Internal Medicine 82; Medical Oncology 87; **Med School:** Univ Pennsylvania 78; **Resid:** Internal Medicine, Yale Univ Sch Med 82; **Fellow:** Medical Oncology, Yale Univ Sch Med 83; **Fac Appt:** Prof Med, UMDNJ-RW Johnson Med Sch

Haller, Daniel G MD [Onc] - **Spec Exp:** Gastrointestinal Cancer; Colon & Rectal Cancer; Cancer Prevention; **Hospital:** Hosp Univ Penn - UPHS (page 113); **Address:** Hosp Univ Pennsylvania, Dept Hem-Onc, 3400 Spruce St, 16 Penn Tower, Philadelphia, PA 19104; **Phone:** 215-662-7666; **Board Cert:** Internal Medicine 76; Medical Oncology 79; **Med School:** Univ Pittsburgh 73; **Resid:** Internal Medicine, Georgetown Univ Hosp 76; **Fellow:** Medical Oncology, Georgetown Univ Hosp 78; **Fac Appt:** Prof Med, Univ Pennsylvania

Hesdorffer, Charles MD [Onc] - **Spec Exp:** Bone Marrow Transplant; Stem Cell Transplant; Tumor Immunotherapy; **Hospital:** NY-Presby Hosp - Columbia Presby Med Ctr (page 103); **Address:** 177 Fort Washington Ave, MHB Bldg Fl 6 - rm 435, New York, NY 10032; **Phone:** 212-305-4907; **Board Cert:** Internal Medicine 95; Medical Oncology 97; **Med School:** South Africa 78; **Resid:** Internal Medicine, Univ Wittwatersrand Hosp 84; **Fellow:** Hematology and Oncology, Columbia-Presby Hosp 88; **Fac Appt:** Clin Prof Med, Columbia P&S

Hochster, Howard S MD [Onc] - **Spec Exp:** Gastrointestinal Cancer; Gynecologic Cancer; Colon & Rectal Cancer; **Hospital:** NYU Med Ctr (page 104); **Address:** 160 E 34th St Fl 9, New York, NY 10016; **Phone:** 212-731-5100; **Board Cert:** Internal Medicine 83; Medical Oncology 85; Hematology 86; **Med School:** Yale Univ 80; **Resid:** Internal Medicine, NYU Med Ctr 83; **Fellow:** Hematology and Oncology, NYU Med Ctr 85; Medical Oncology, Jules Bordet Inst 86; **Fac Appt:** Assoc Prof Med, NYU Sch Med

Holland, James F MD [Onc] - **Spec Exp:** Breast Cancer; Metastatic Cancer; Psychiatry in Cancer; **Hospital:** Mount Sinai Med Ctr (page 101); **Address:** Ruttenberg Cancer Ctr, Div Med Oncology, OneL Gustave L Levy Pl, Box 1129, New York, NY 10029-6574; **Phone:** 212-241-4495; **Board Cert:** Internal Medicine 55; **Med School:** Columbia P&S 47; **Resid:** Internal Medicine, Columbia-Presby Hosp 49; **Fellow:** Medical Oncology, Francis Delafield Hosp 53; **Fac Appt:** Prof Med, Mount Sinai Sch Med

Houghton, Alan N MD [Onc] - **Spec Exp:** Melanoma; Immunotherapy; Cancer Vaccines; **Hospital:** Meml Sloan Kettering Cancer Ctr (page 100); **Address:** 1275 York Ave, Box 465, New York, NY 10021; **Phone:** 212-639-7595; **Board Cert:** Medical Oncology 79; Internal Medicine 77; **Med School:** Univ Conn 74; **Resid:** Internal Medicine, Univ Conn Hlth Ctr 77; **Fellow:** Medical Oncology, Mem Sloan Kettering Cancer Ctr 79; **Fac Appt:** Prof Med, Cornell Univ-Weill Med Coll

Hudes, Gary R MD [Onc] - **Spec Exp:** Prostate Cancer; Genitourinary Cancer; Kidney Cancer; **Hospital:** Fox Chase Cancer Ctr (page 95); **Address:** Fox Chase Cancer Ctr, 333 Cottman Ave, rm C307, Philadelphia, PA 19111; **Phone:** 215-728-3889; **Board Cert:** Internal Medicine 82; Hematology 84; Medical Oncology 85; **Med School:** SUNY Downstate 79; **Resid:** Internal Medicine, Graduate Hosp 82; **Fellow:** Hematology and Oncology, Presby-Univ Penn Med Ctr 85

Hudis, Clifford A MD [Onc] - **Spec Exp:** Breast Cancer; **Hospital:** Meml Sloan Kettering Cancer Ctr (page 100); **Address:** Meml Sloan Kettering Cancer Ctr, 1275 York Ave, Box 206, New York, NY 10021-6007; **Phone:** 212-639-5449; **Board Cert:** Internal Medicine 86; Medical Oncology 01; **Med School:** Med Coll PA Hahnemann 83; **Resid:** Internal Medicine, Hosp Med Coll Penn 86; **Fellow:** Medical Oncology, Meml Sloan Kettering Cancer Ctr 91; **Fac Appt:** Assoc Prof Med, Cornell Univ-Weill Med Coll

Isaacs, Claudine J MD [Onc] - **Spec Exp:** Breast Cancer; Breast Cancer Risk Assessment; Breast Cancer-Hereditary; **Hospital:** Georgetown Univ Hosp; **Address:** Lombardi Cancer Ctr, Podium B, 3800 Reservoir Rd NW, Washington, DC 20007; **Phone:** 202-444-2198; **Board Cert:** Internal Medicine 02; Medical Oncology 03; **Med School:** McGill Univ 87; **Resid:** Internal Medicine, Montreal General Hosp 90; Hematology and Oncology, McGill Univ Hosp 92; **Fellow:** Medical Oncology, Georgetown Univ Med Ctr 93; **Fac Appt:** Assoc Prof Med, Georgetown Univ

Jillella, Anand MD [Onc] - **Spec Exp:** Bone Marrow Transplant; Leukemia, Myeloma; Lymphoma; **Hospital:** Temple Univ Hosp; **Address:** Fox-Chase/Temple BMT Program, Jeanes Hosp, 7600 Central Ave, Philadelphia, PA 19111; **Phone:** 215-214-3119; **Board Cert:** Internal Medicine 92; Medical Oncology 97; **Med School:** India 85; **Resid:** Internal Medicine, Med Coll Georgia 92; **Fellow:** Medical Oncology, Yale-New Haven Hosp 96; **Fac Appt:** Assoc Prof Med, Temple Univ

Kelsen, David MD [Onc] - **Spec Exp:** Gastrointestinal Cancer; Neuroendocrine Tumors; Unknown Primary Tumors; **Hospital:** Meml Sloan Kettering Cancer Ctr (page 100); **Address:** Gastrointestinal Oncology Svc, 1275 York Ave Bldg Howard Fl 9 - rm 918, New York, NY 10021; **Phone:** 212-639-8470; **Board Cert:** Internal Medicine 76; Medical Oncology 79; **Med School:** Hahnemann Univ 72; **Resid:** Internal Medicine, Temple U Hosp 76; **Fellow:** Medical Oncology, Meml Sloan Kettering Cancer Ctr 78; **Fac Appt:** Prof Med, Cornell Univ-Weill Med Coll

Kemeny, Nancy MD [Onc] - **Spec Exp:** Colon Cancer; Rectal Cancer; Liver Cancer; **Hospital:** Meml Sloan Kettering Cancer Ctr (page 100); **Address:** Meml Sloan Kettering Cancer Ctr, 1275 York Ave, Howard 916, New York, NY 10021; **Phone:** 212-639-8068; **Board Cert:** Internal Medicine 74; Medical Oncology 81; **Med School:** UMDNJ-NJ Med Sch, Newark 71; **Resid:** Internal Medicine, St Luke's Hosp 74; **Fellow:** Medical Oncology, Mem Sloan Kettering Cancer Ctr 76; **Fac Appt:** Prof Med, Cornell Univ-Weill Med Coll

Kirkwood, John M MD [Onc] - **Spec Exp:** Melanoma; **Hospital:** UPMC Presby, Pittsburgh (page 114); **Address:** 5117 Centre Ave, Ste 1.32, Pittsburgh, PA 15213; **Phone:** 412-623-7707; **Board Cert:** Internal Medicine 76; Medical Oncology 81; **Med School:** Yale Univ 73; **Resid:** Internal Medicine, Yale-New Haven Hosp 76; **Fellow:** Medical Oncology, Dana Farber Cancer Inst/Harvard 79; **Fac Appt:** Prof Med, Univ Pittsburgh

Kris, Mark G MD [Onc] - **Spec Exp:** Lung Cancer; Mediastinal Tumors; Thymoma; **Hospital:** Meml Sloan Kettering Cancer Ctr (page 100); **Address:** 1275 York Ave, Howard H1018, New York, NY 10021; **Phone:** 212-639-7590; **Board Cert:** Internal Medicine 80; Medical Oncology 83; **Med School:** Cornell Univ-Weill Med Coll 77; **Resid:** Internal Medicine, NY Hosp 80; **Fellow:** Medical Oncology, Meml Sloan Kettering Cancer Ctr 83; **Fac Appt:** Prof Med, Cornell Univ-Weill Med Coll

Langer, Corey J MD [Onc] - **Spec Exp:** Lung Cancer; Head & Neck Cancer; Mesothelioma; **Hospital:** Fox Chase Cancer Ctr (page 95); **Address:** Fox Chase Cancer Ctr, 333 Cottman Ave, Philadelphia, PA 19111-2412; **Phone:** 215-728-2985; **Board Cert:** Internal Medicine 84; Hematology 86; Medical Oncology 87; **Med School:** Boston Univ 81; **Resid:** Internal Medicine, Grad Hosp/Univ Penn 84; Hematology and Oncology, Presby Hosp/Univ Penn 86; **Fellow:** Medical Oncology, Fox Chase Cancer Ctr 87; **Fac Appt:** Assoc Prof Med, Temple Univ

Levine, Ellis MD [Onc] - **Spec Exp:** Breast Cancer; Urologic Cancer; **Hospital:** Roswell Park Cancer Inst (page 107); **Address:** Roswell Park Cancer Inst, Elm & Carlton, Buffalo, NY 14263-0001; **Phone:** 716-845-8547; **Board Cert:** Internal Medicine 82; Medical Oncology 85; **Med School:** Univ Pittsburgh 79; **Resid:** Internal Medicine, Univ Minn Hosps 82; **Fellow:** Medical Oncology, Univ Minn Hosps 84; **Fac Appt:** Assoc Prof Med, SUNY Buffalo

Lieberman, Ronald MD [Onc] - **Spec Exp:** Prostate Cancer; Genitourinary Cancer; Chemoprevention; **Hospital:** Natl Inst of Hlth - Clin Ctr; **Address:** Executive Plaza N, rm 2102, 6130 Executive Blvd, MS 7318, Bethesda, MD 20892-7318; **Phone:** 301-594-0456; **Board Cert:** Internal Medicine 77; Hematology 78; Blood Banking 79; Medical Oncology 81; **Med School:** Univ Mich Med Sch 69; **Resid:** Internal Medicine, VA Hosp 72; Hematology and Oncology, UCSF Med Ctr 74; **Fellow:** Hematology, Meml Sloan Kettering Cancer Ctr 76; Clinical Pathology, NIH Clin Ctr 79

Livingston, Philip MD [Onc] - **Spec Exp:** Melanoma; Cancer Immunology; Cancer Vaccines; **Hospital:** Meml Sloan Kettering Cancer Ctr (page 100); **Address:** 1275 York Ave, New York, NY 10021-6007; **Phone:** 212-639-7425; **Board Cert:** Internal Medicine 80; Allergy & Immunology 74; Rheumatology 74; Medical Oncology 81; **Med School:** Harvard Med Sch 69; **Resid:** Internal Medicine, N Shore Hosp-Cornell Med Ctr 71; **Fellow:** Immunology, NYU Med Ctr 73; **Fac Appt:** Prof Onc, Cornell Univ-Weill Med Coll

Lyman, Gary H MD [Onc] - **Spec Exp:** Breast Cancer; **Hospital:** Univ of Rochester Strong Meml Hosp; **Address:** Univ of Rochester Strong Meml Hosp, 601 Elmwood Ave, Box 704, Rochester, NY 14642-8704; **Phone:** 585-275-3335; **Board Cert:** Internal Medicine 87; Medical Oncology 77; Hematology 79; **Med School:** SUNY Buffalo 72; **Resid:** Internal Medicine, Univ North Carolina Hosp 74; **Fellow:** Medical Oncology, Roswell Park Meml Inst 76; Biostatistics, Harvard Med Sch 82; **Fac Appt:** Prof Med, Univ Rochester

Macdonald, John S MD [Onc] - **Spec Exp:** Colon Cancer; Gastrointestinal Cancer; Pancreatic Cancer; **Hospital:** St Vincent Cath Med Ctrs - Manhattan (page 108); **Address:** 325 W 15th St, New York, NY 10011-5903; **Phone:** 212-604-6011; **Board Cert:** Internal Medicine 73; Medical Oncology 75; **Med School:** Harvard Med Sch 69; **Resid:** Internal Medicine, Beth Israel Hosp 71; **Fellow:** Hematology and Oncology, Natl Cancer Inst 74; **Fac Appt:** Prof Med, NY Med Coll

Marks, Stanley M MD [Onc] - **Hospital:** UPMC Shadyside (page 114); **Address:** 5115 Centre Ave, Fl 3, Pittsburgh, PA 15232; **Phone:** 412-235-1020; **Board Cert:** Internal Medicine 76; Hematology 78; **Med School:** Univ Pittsburgh 73; **Resid:** Internal Medicine, Presby Univ Hosp 76; **Fellow:** Hematology, Peter Bent Brigham Hosp 78; **Fac Appt:** Assoc Clin Prof Med, Drexel Univ Coll Med

Marshall, John L MD [Onc] - **Spec Exp:** Gastrointestinal Cancer; Drug Development; **Hospital:** Georgetown Univ Hosp; **Address:** Lombardi Cancer Ctr, Podium A, 3800 Reservoir Rd NW, Washington, DC 20007; **Phone:** 202-444-7064; **Board Cert:** Internal Medicine 01; Medical Oncology 03; **Med School:** Univ Louisville Sch Med 88; **Resid:** Internal Medicine, Georgetown Univ Hosp 91; **Fellow:** Medical Oncology, Georgetown Univ Hosp 93; **Fac Appt:** Assoc Prof Med, Georgetown Univ

Masters, Gregory A MD [Onc] - **Spec Exp:** Lung Cancer; Esophageal Cancer; Thoracic Cancers; **Hospital:** Christiana Hospital; **Address:** Med Onc-Hem Consultants, Graham Cancer Ctr, 4701 Ogletown-Stanton Rd, Ste 2200, Newark, DE 19713; **Phone:** 302-366-1200; **Board Cert:** Internal Medicine 93; Medical Oncology 95; **Med School:** Northwestern Univ 90; **Resid:** Internal Medicine, Hosp Univ Penn 93; **Fellow:** Medical Oncology, Univ Chicago Hosps 95; **Fac Appt:** Asst Prof Med

McGuire III, William P MD [Onc] - **Spec Exp:** Gynecologic Cancer; Ovarian Cancer; Breast Cancer; **Hospital:** Franklin Sqaure Hosp; **Address:** Harry & Jeanette Weinberg Cancer Inst, 9103 Franklin Square Drive, Ste 2200, Baltimore, MD 21287; **Phone:** 443-777-7826; **Board Cert:** Internal Medicine 74; Medical Oncology 81; **Med School:** Baylor Coll Med 71; **Resid:** Internal Medicine, Yale-New Haven Hosp 73

Meropol, Neal J MD [Onc] - **Spec Exp:** Gastrointestinal Cancer; **Hospital:** Fox Chase Cancer Ctr (page 95); **Address:** 333 Cottman Ave, Fox Chase Cancer Ctr, Dept Medical Oncology, Philadelphia, PA 19111; **Phone:** 215-728-2450; **Board Cert:** Internal Medicine 88; Medical Oncology 01; **Med School:** Vanderbilt Univ 85; **Resid:** Internal Medicine, Univ Hosp/Case West Res 88; **Fellow:** Medical Oncology, Hosp Univ Penn 92; **Fac Appt:** Assoc Prof Med, Temple Univ

Mintzer, David M MD [Onc] - **Spec Exp:** Breast Cancer; Gastrointestinal Cancer; Head & Neck Cancer; **Hospital:** Pennsylvania Hosp (page 113); **Address:** 230 W Washington Square Fl 2, Philadelphia, PA 19106; **Phone:** 215-829-6088; **Board Cert:** Internal Medicine 80; Hematology 82; Medical Oncology 83; **Med School:** Jefferson Med Coll 77; **Resid:** Internal Medicine, Pennsylvania Hosp 80; **Fellow:** Hematology, Jefferson Med Coll 82; Medical Oncology, Meml Sloan Kettering Cancer Ctr 84; **Fac Appt:** Assoc Clin Prof Med, Univ Pennsylvania

Moore, Anne MD [Onc] - **Spec Exp:** Breast Cancer; **Hospital:** NY-Presby Hosp - NY Weill Cornell Med Ctr (page 103); **Address:** New York Presbyterian Hosp, 428 E 72nd St, Ste 300, New York, NY 10021-4873; **Phone:** 212-746-2085; **Board Cert:** Internal Medicine 73; Hematology 76; Medical Oncology 77; **Med School:** Columbia P&S 69; **Resid:** Internal Medicine, Cornell Univ Med Ctr 73; **Fellow:** Medical Oncology, Rockefeller Univ 73; **Fac Appt:** Prof Med, Cornell Univ-Weill Med Coll

Motzer, Robert J MD [Onc] - **Spec Exp:** Kidney Cancer; Testicular Cancer; Prostate Cancer; **Hospital:** Meml Sloan Kettering Cancer Ctr (page 100); **Address:** 1275 York Ave, Box 239, New York, NY 10021; **Phone:** 646-422-4312; **Board Cert:** Internal Medicine 84; Medical Oncology 87; **Med School:** Univ Mich Med Sch 81; **Resid:** Internal Medicine, Meml Sloan Kettering Cancer Ctr 84; **Fellow:** Medical Oncology, Meml Sloan Kettering Cancer Ctr 87; **Fac Appt:** Assoc Prof Med, Cornell Univ-Weill Med Coll

Muggia, Franco MD [Onc] - **Spec Exp:** Breast Cancer; Gynecologic Cancer; **Hospital:** NYU Med Ctr (page 104); **Address:** NYU Clinical Cancer Ctr, 160 E 34th St Fl 8, New York, NY 10016; **Phone:** 212-731-5433; **Board Cert:** Internal Medicine 68; Hematology 74; Medical Oncology 73; **Med School:** Cornell Univ-Weill Med Coll 61; **Resid:** Internal Medicine, Hartford Hosp 64; Internal Medicine, Francis A Delafield Hosp 66; **Fac Appt:** Prof Med, NYU Sch Med

Nissenblatt, Michael MD [Onc] - **Spec Exp:** Breast Cancer; Lymphoma & Multiple Myeloma; Colon Cancer; **Hospital:** Robert Wood Johnson Univ Hosp - New Brunswick (page 106); **Address:** 205 Easton Ave, New Brunswick, NJ 08901-1722; **Phone:** 732-828-9570; **Board Cert:** Internal Medicine 76; Medical Oncology 79; **Med School:** Columbia P&S 73; **Resid:** Internal Medicine, Johns Hopkins Hosp 76; **Fellow:** Medical Oncology, Johns Hopkins Hosp 78; **Fac Appt:** Clin Prof Med, Robert W Johnson Med Sch

Norton, Larry MD [Onc] - **Spec Exp:** Breast Cancer; **Hospital:** Meml Sloan Kettering Cancer Ctr (page 100); **Address:** 205 E 64th St, New York, NY 10021; **Phone:** 212-639-5438; **Board Cert:** Internal Medicine 75; Medical Oncology 77; **Med School:** Columbia P&S 72; **Resid:** Internal Medicine, Bronx Muni Hosp 74; **Fac Appt:** Prof Med, Cornell Univ-Weill Med Coll

O'Reilly, Eileen M MD [Onc] - **Spec Exp:** Pancreatic Cancer; Clinical Trials; Hepatobiliary Cancer; **Hospital:** Meml Sloan Kettering Cancer Ctr (page 100); **Address:** 1275 York Ave, Box 324, New York, NY 10021; **Phone:** 212-639-6672; **Med School:** Ireland 89; **Resid:** Internal Medicine, St Vincent's Hosp 94; **Fellow:** Hematology, St Vincent's Hosp 95; Medical Oncology, Memorial-Sloan Kettering Cancer Ctr 97; **Fac Appt:** Asst Prof Med, Cornell Univ-Weill Med Coll

Offit, Kenneth MD [Onc] - **Spec Exp:** Cancer Genetics/Assessment/Prevention; Breast Cancer; Lymphoma; **Hospital:** Meml Sloan Kettering Cancer Ctr (page 100); **Address:** 1275 York Ave, Box 192, New York, NY 10021-6094; **Phone:** 212-434-5149; **Board Cert:** Internal Medicine 85; Medical Oncology 87; **Med School:** Harvard Med Sch 82; **Resid:** Internal Medicine, Lenox Hill Hosp 85; **Fellow:** Hematology and Oncology, Meml Sloan Kettering Cancer Ctr 88; **Fac Appt:** Prof Med, Cornell Univ-Weill Med Coll

Oster, Martin W MD [Onc] - **Spec Exp:** Breast Cancer; Gastrointestinal Cancer; Lung Cancer; **Hospital:** NY-Presby Hosp - Columbia Presby Med Ctr (page 103); **Address:** 161 Fort Washington Ave, New York, NY 10032-3713; **Phone:** 212-305-8231; **Board Cert:** Internal Medicine 74; Medical Oncology 75; **Med School:** Columbia P&S 71; **Resid:** Internal Medicine, Mass Genl Hosp 73; **Fellow:** Medical Oncology, Natl Cancer Inst/NIH 76; **Fac Appt:** Assoc Clin Prof Med, Columbia P&S

Ozols, Robert F MD/PhD [Onc] - **Spec Exp:** Ovarian Cancer; Chemotherapy & Drug Resistance; **Hospital:** Fox Chase Cancer Ctr (page 95); **Address:** Fox Chase Cancer Ctr, 333 Cottman Ave, rm P 2051, Philadelphia, PA 19111; **Phone:** 215-728-2673; **Board Cert:** Internal Medicine 77; Medical Oncology 79; **Med School:** Univ Rochester 74; **Resid:** Internal Medicine, Dartmouth-Hitchcock Hosp 76; **Fellow:** Medical Oncology, National Cancer Inst 79; **Fac Appt:** Prof Med, Temple Univ

Pasmantier, Mark MD [Onc] - **Spec Exp:** Lung Cancer; Ovarian Cancer; **Hospital:** NY-Presby Hosp - NY Weill Cornell Med Ctr (page 103); **Address:** 407 E 70th St, FL 3, New York, NY 10021-5302; **Phone:** 212-517-5900; **Board Cert:** Internal Medicine 72; Hematology 74; Medical Oncology 75; **Med School:** NYU Sch Med 66; **Resid:** Internal Medicine, Harlem Hosp 70; **Fellow:** Hematology, Montefiore Hosp Med Ctr 71; Medical Oncology, New York Hosp 72; **Fac Appt:** Clin Prof Med, Cornell Univ-Weill Med Coll

Petrylak, Daniel P MD [Onc] - **Spec Exp:** Genitourinary Cancer; Prostate Cancer; Bladder Cancer; **Hospital:** NY-Presby Hosp - Columbia Presby Med Ctr (page 103); **Address:** 161 Fort Washington Ave, New York, NY 10032-3713; **Phone:** 212-305-1731; **Board Cert:** Internal Medicine 01; Medical Oncology 93; **Med School:** Case West Res Univ 85; **Resid:** Internal Medicine, Jacobi Med Ctr 88; **Fellow:** Oncology, Meml-Sloan Kettering Cancer Ctr 91; **Fac Appt:** Assoc Prof Med, Columbia P&S

Pfister, David G MD [Onc] - **Spec Exp:** Head & Neck Cancer; Laryngeal Cancer; Thyroid Cancer; **Hospital:** Meml Sloan Kettering Cancer Ctr (page 100); **Address:** Memorial Sloan Kettering Cancer Ctr, 1275 York Ave, Box 188, New York, NY 10021; **Phone:** 212-639-8235; **Board Cert:** Internal Medicine 85; Medical Oncology 89; **Med School:** Univ Pennsylvania 82; **Resid:** Internal Medicine, Hosp Univ Penn 85; **Fellow:** Epidemiology, Yale New Haven Hosp 87; Hematology and Oncology, Meml Sloan Kettering Cancer Ctr 89; **Fac Appt:** Prof Med, Cornell Univ-Weill Med Coll

Reed, Eddie MD [Onc] - **Spec Exp:** Gynecologic Cancer; Prostate Cancer; Drug Discovery; **Hospital:** WV Univ Hosp - Ruby Memorial; **Address:** Robert C Byrd Hlth Scs Ctr-Clinical Trials Resch Unit, PO Box 9260, Morgantown, WV 26506-9260; **Phone:** 304-293-0781; **Board Cert:** Internal Medicine 82; **Med School:** Yale Univ 79; **Resid:** Internal Medicine, Stanford U Hosp 81; **Fellow:** Medical Oncology, Natl Cancer Inst 85; **Fac Appt:** Prof Med, W VA Univ

Saltz, Leonard B MD [Onc] - **Spec Exp:** Colon & Rectal Cancer; Gastrointestinal Cancer/Rare Tumors; Liver Cancer; **Hospital:** Meml Sloan Kettering Cancer Ctr (page 100); **Address:** Memorial Sloan Kettering Cancer Ctr, Howard 917, 1275 York Ave, New York, NY 10021; **Phone:** 212-639-2501; **Board Cert:** Internal Medicine 86; Hematology 88; Medical Oncology 89; **Med School:** Yale Univ 83; **Resid:** Internal Medicine, NY Hosp-Cornell Med Ctr 86; **Fellow:** Hematology and Oncology, NY Hosp-Cornell Med Ctr/Rockefeller Univ 87; **Fac Appt:** Assoc Prof Med, Cornell Univ-Weill Med Coll

Scheinberg, David MD/PhD [Onc] - **Spec Exp:** Leukemia; Immunotherapy; Cancer Vaccines; **Hospital:** Meml Sloan Kettering Cancer Ctr (page 100); **Address:** 1275 York Ave, New York, NY 10021-6007; **Phone:** 212-639-5010; **Board Cert:** Internal Medicine 86; Medical Oncology 95; **Med School:** Johns Hopkins Univ 83; **Resid:** Internal Medicine, New York Hosp/Cornell 85; **Fellow:** Medical Oncology, Meml Sloan Kettering Cancer Ctr 87; **Fac Appt:** Prof Med, Cornell Univ-Weill Med Coll

Scher, Howard MD [Onc] - **Spec Exp:** Genitourinary Cancer; Prostate Cancer; Bladder Cancer; **Hospital:** Meml Sloan Kettering Cancer Ctr (page 100); **Address:** 353 E 68th St, Fl 6, New York, NY 10021; **Phone:** 646-422-4330; **Board Cert:** Internal Medicine 79; Medical Oncology 85; **Med School:** NYU Sch Med 76; **Resid:** Internal Medicine, Bellevue Hosp 80; **Fellow:** Medical Oncology, Meml Sloan Kettering Cancer Ctr 83; **Fac Appt:** Assoc Prof Med, Cornell Univ-Weill Med Coll

Schuchter, Lynn M MD [Onc] - **Spec Exp:** Melanoma; Breast Cancer; Clinical Trials; **Hospital:** Hosp Univ Penn - UPHS (page 113); **Address:** Univ Penn/Abramson Cancer Ctr, 399 S 34th St, Penn Tower Fl 15, Philadelphia, PA 19104; **Phone:** 215-662-7907; **Board Cert:** Internal Medicine 85; Medical Oncology 89; **Med School:** Univ Hlth Sci/Chicago Med Sch 82; **Resid:** Internal Medicine, Michael Reese Hosp 85; **Fellow:** Medical Oncology, Johns Hopkins Hosp 89; **Fac Appt:** Assoc Prof Med, Univ Pennsylvania

Shields, Peter G MD [Onc] - **Spec Exp:** Lung Cancer; Hematologic Malignancies; Hematolgy-Benign; **Hospital:** Georgetown Univ Hosp; **Address:** Lombardi Cancer Ctr, 3800 Reservoir Rd NW, Washington, DC 20007; **Phone:** 202-444-2198; **Board Cert:** Internal Medicine 86; Medical Oncology 89; Hematology 90; **Med School:** Mount Sinai Sch Med 83; **Resid:** Internal Medicine, George Washington Univ Hosp 86; **Fellow:** Hematology and Oncology, George Washington Univ Hosp 90; **Fac Appt:** Prof Med, Georgetown Univ

Sidransky, David MD [Onc] - **Spec Exp:** Head & Neck Cancer; **Hospital:** Johns Hopkins Hosp - Baltimore (page 97); **Address:** Johns Hopkins Hospital, Ross Research Bldg, 720 Rutland Ave, Ste 818, Baltimore, MD 21205; **Phone:** 410-502-5153; **Board Cert:** Internal Medicine 88; Medical Oncology 91; **Med School:** Baylor Coll Med 84; **Resid:** Internal Medicine, Baylor Coll Medicine 88; **Fellow:** Medical Oncology, Johns Hopkins Hosp 92; **Fac Appt:** Prof Oto, Johns Hopkins Univ

Smith, Mitchell R MD/PhD [Onc] - **Spec Exp:** Lymphoma; Leukemia; Multiple Myeloma; **Hospital:** Fox Chase Cancer Ctr (page 95); **Address:** Fox Chase Cancer Center, 333 Cottman Ave, Ste C307, Philadelphia, PA 19111; **Phone:** 215-728-2674; **Board Cert:** Internal Medicine 85; Hematology 88; Medical Oncology 87; **Med School:** Case West Res Univ 79; **Resid:** Pathology, Barnes Jewish Hosp 83; Internal Medicine, Barnes Jewish Hosp 84; **Fellow:** Medical Oncology, Meml Sloan-Ketter Cancer Ctr 88

Speyer, James MD [Onc] - **Spec Exp:** Ovarian Cancer; Breast Cancer; Cardiac Toxicity in Cancer Therapy; **Hospital:** NYU Med Ctr (page 104); **Address:** NYU Clinical Cancer Center, 160 E 34th St, New York, NY 10016-6004; **Phone:** 212-731-5432; **Board Cert:** Internal Medicine 77; Hematology 78; Medical Oncology 79; **Med School:** Johns Hopkins Univ 74; **Resid:** Internal Medicine, Columbia-Presby Med Ctr 76; Hematology, Columbia-Presby Med Ctr 77; **Fellow:** Medical Oncology, Natl Cancer Inst 79; **Fac Appt:** Clin Prof Med, NYU Sch Med

Spriggs, David MD [Onc] - **Spec Exp:** Ovarian Cancer; Drug Development; Head & Neck Cancer; **Hospital:** Meml Sloan Kettering Cancer Ctr (page 100); **Address:** 1275 York Ave, Box 67, New York, NY 10021-6007; **Phone:** 212-639-2203; **Board Cert:** Internal Medicine 81; Medical Oncology 85; **Med School:** Univ Wisc 77; **Resid:** Internal Medicine, Columbia-Presby Hosp 81; **Fellow:** Medical Oncology, Dana-Farber Cancer Inst 85; **Fac Appt:** Prof Med, Cornell Univ-Weill Med Coll

Stadtmauer, Edward A MD [Onc] - **Spec Exp:** Bone Marrow & Stem Cell Transplant; Leukemia; Multiple Myeloma; **Hospital:** Hosp Univ Penn - UPHS (page 113); **Address:** Univ Penn Cancer Ctr, 3400 Spruce St, 16 Penn Tower, Philadelphia, PA 19104; **Phone:** 215-662-7909; **Board Cert:** Internal Medicine 86; Hematology 88; Medical Oncology 89; **Med School:** Univ Pennsylvania 83; **Resid:** Internal Medicine, Bronx Muni Hosp 86; **Fellow:** Hematology and Oncology, Hosp Univ Penn 89; **Fac Appt:** Assoc Prof Med, Univ Pennsylvania

Stoopler, Mark MD [Onc] - **Spec Exp:** Lung Cancer; Esophageal Cancer; **Hospital:** NY-Presby Hosp - Columbia Presby Med Ctr (page 103); **Address:** 161 Fort Washington Ave, Ste 921, New York, NY 10032-3713; **Phone:** 212-305-8230; **Board Cert:** Internal Medicine 78; Medical Oncology 81; **Med School:** Cornell Univ-Weill Med Coll 75; **Resid:** Internal Medicine, North Shore Univ Hosp 78; Internal Medicine, Memorial Hosp 78; **Fellow:** Medical Oncology, Meml-Sloan Kettering Cancer Ctr 80; **Fac Appt:** Assoc Clin Prof Med, Columbia P&S

Straus, David J MD [Onc] - **Spec Exp:** Lymphoma; Multiple Myeloma; **Hospital:** Meml Sloan Kettering Cancer Ctr (page 100); **Address:** 1275 York Ave, Box 406, New York, NY 10021-6094; **Phone:** 212-639-8365; **Board Cert:** Internal Medicine 72; Hematology 76; Medical Oncology 77; **Med School:** Marquette Sch Med 69; **Resid:** Internal Medicine, Montefiore Med Ctr 72; Medical Oncology, Meml Sloan Kettering Cancer Ctr 77; **Fellow:** Hematology, Beth Israel Hosp-Harvard 73; **Fac Appt:** Prof Med, Cornell Univ-Weill Med Coll

Tkaczuk, Katherine H MD [Onc] - **Spec Exp:** Breast Cancer; **Hospital:** Univ of MD Med Sys; **Address:** Univ MD Cancer Ctr, 22 S Greene St, Baltimore, MD 21201; **Phone:** 410-328-7904; **Board Cert:** Infectious Disease 89; Medical Oncology 01; **Med School:** Poland 84; **Resid:** Internal Medicine, St Agnes Hosp 89; **Fellow:** Hematology and Oncology, Univ Maryland Cancer Ctr 92; **Fac Appt:** Assoc Prof Med, Univ MD Sch Med

Treat, Joseph MD [Onc] - **Spec Exp:** Lung Cancer; **Hospital:** Fox Chase Cancer Ctr (page 95); **Address:** Fox Chase Temple Cancer Ctr, 3322 N Broad St, Philadelphia, PA 19140; **Phone:** 215-707-8030; **Board Cert:** Internal Medicine 82; Medical Oncology 85; **Med School:** Temple Univ 79; **Resid:** Internal Medicine, Georgetown Univ Hosp 82; **Fellow:** Medical Oncology, Georgetown Univ Hosp 84; **Fac Appt:** Prof Med, Temple Univ

Trump, Donald MD [Onc] - **Spec Exp:** Prostate Cancer; Genitourinary Cancer; Drug Discovery & Development; **Hospital:** Roswell Park Cancer Inst (page 107); **Address:** Elm & Carlton Sts, Buffalo, NY 14263; **Phone:** 716-845-3499; **Board Cert:** Internal Medicine 73; Medical Oncology 77; **Med School:** Johns Hopkins Univ 70; **Resid:** Internal Medicine, Johns Hopkins Hosp 75; **Fellow:** Medical Oncology, Johns Hopkins Hosp 74

Vogel, Victor G MD [Onc] - **Spec Exp:** Breast Cancer; **Hospital:** Magee-Womens Hosp - UPMC (page 114); **Address:** Magee-Womens Hosp, Breast Cancer Prevention Prog, 300 Halket St, rm 3524, Pittsburgh, PA 15213-3180; **Phone:** 412-641-6500; **Board Cert:** Internal Medicine 84; Medical Oncology 03; Public Health & General Preventive Medicine 93; **Med School:** Temple Univ 78; **Resid:** Internal Medicine, Baltimore City Hosp 81; **Fellow:** Medical Oncology, Johns Hopkins Hosp 86; Epidemiology, Johns Hopkins Hosp 86; **Fac Appt:** Prof Med, Univ Pittsburgh

von Mehren, Margaret MD [Onc] - **Spec Exp:** Sarcoma; Melanoma; Immunotherapy; **Hospital:** Fox Chase Cancer Ctr (page 95); **Address:** Fox Chase Cancer Ctr, Dept Med Oncology, 333 Cottman Ave, Philadelphia, PA 19111; **Phone:** 215-728-2570; **Board Cert:** Internal Medicine 93; Medical Oncology 97; **Med School:** Albany Med Coll 89; **Resid:** Internal Medicine, NYU Med Ctr 93; **Fellow:** Hematology and Oncology, Fox Chase Cancer Ctr 96; **Fac Appt:** Asst Prof Med, Temple Univ

Wadler, Scott MD [Onc] - **Spec Exp:** Gastrointestinal Cancer; Liver Cancer; Colon & Rectal Cancer; **Hospital:** NY-Presby Hosp - NY Weill Cornell Med Ctr (page 103); **Address:** Cornell Med Onc/Solid Tumor Program, 525 E 68th St, Payson 3- Fl 3, New York, NY 10021; **Phone:** 212-746-2844; **Board Cert:** Internal Medicine 84; Medical Oncology 87; **Med School:** NYU Sch Med 80; **Resid:** Internal Medicine, Bellevue Hosp 83; **Fellow:** Medical Oncology, Mount Sinai 84; Medical Oncology, NYU Med Ctr 85; **Fac Appt:** Prof Med, Cornell Univ-Weill Med Coll

Weber, Barbara L MD [Onc] - **Spec Exp:** Breast Cancer; **Hospital:** Hosp Univ Penn - UPHS (page 113); **Address:** Univ Penn Cancer Ctr, 421 Curie Blvd, rm 514, Philadelphia, PA 19104; **Phone:** 215-898-0247; **Board Cert:** Internal Medicine 85; Medical Oncology 87; **Med School:** Univ Wash 82; **Resid:** Internal Medicine, Yale-New Haven Hosp 85; **Fellow:** Medical Oncology, Dana-Farber Cancer Inst 87; **Fac Appt:** Prof Med, Univ Pennsylvania

Weiner, Louis M MD [Onc] - **Spec Exp:** Gastrointestinal Cancer; Immunotherapy; **Hospital:** Fox Chase Cancer Ctr (page 95); **Address:** Fox Chase Cancer Ctr, 333 Cottman Ave, rm C315, Philadelphia, PA 19111; **Phone:** 215-728-2480; **Board Cert:** Internal Medicine 80; Medical Oncology 85; **Med School:** Mount Sinai Sch Med 77; **Resid:** Internal Medicine, Med Ctr Hosp Vermont 80; **Fellow:** Hematology and Oncology, New England Med Ctr - Tufts 82

Wolff, Antonio C MD **[Onc]** - **Spec Exp:** Breast Cancer; Drug Development; **Hospital:** Johns Hopkins Hosp - Baltimore (page 97); **Address:** 1650 Orleans St, rm 189, Baltimore, MD 21231; **Phone:** 410-614-4192; **Board Cert:** Internal Medicine 00; Medical Oncology 00; **Med School:** Brazil 86; **Resid:** Internal Medicine, Mt Sinai Med Ctr 91; **Fellow:** Hematology and Oncology, Washington Univ Med Ctr 92; Medical Oncology, Johns Hopkins Hosp; **Fac Appt:** Asst Prof Med, Johns Hopkins Univ

Zelenetz, Andrew D MD/PhD **[Onc]** - **Spec Exp:** Lymphoma; **Hospital:** Meml Sloan Kettering Cancer Ctr (page 100); **Address:** Meml Sloan-Kettering Cancer Ctr, 1275 York Ave, Box 330, New York, NY 10021; **Phone:** 212-639-2656; **Board Cert:** Internal Medicine 92; Medical Oncology 93; **Med School:** Harvard Med Sch 84; **Resid:** Internal Medicine, Stanford Univ Med Ctr 86; **Fellow:** Medical Oncology, Stanford Univ Med Ctr 91; **Fac Appt:** Asst Prof Med, Cornell Univ-Weill Med Coll

Southeast

Antonia, Scott J MD **[Onc]** - **Spec Exp:** Kidney Cancer; Lung Cancer; **Hospital:** H Lee Moffitt Cancer Ctr & Research Inst; **Address:** H Lee Moffitt Cancer Ctr, 12902 Magnolia Drive, Tampa, FL 33612; **Phone:** 813-979-3883; **Board Cert:** Internal Medicine 02; Medical Oncology 95; **Med School:** Univ Conn 89; **Resid:** Internal Medicine, Yale-New Haven Hosp 91; **Fellow:** Medical Oncology, Yale-New Haven Hosp 94; **Fac Appt:** Assoc Prof Med, Univ S Fla Coll Med

Arteaga, Carlos L MD **[Onc]** - **Spec Exp:** Breast Cancer; **Hospital:** Vanderbilt Univ Med Ctr (page 116); **Address:** Vanderbilt-Ingram Cancer Ctr-Medicine & Cancer Biology, 682 Preston Building, Nashville, TN 37232-6838; **Phone:** 615-936-3524; **Board Cert:** Internal Medicine 84; Medical Oncology 89; **Med School:** Ecuador 80; **Resid:** Internal Medicine, Grady Meml Hosp 84; **Fellow:** Hematology and Oncology, Univ Texas Hlth Sci Ctr 87; **Fac Appt:** Prof Med, Vanderbilt Univ

Balducci, Lodovico MD **[Onc]** - **Spec Exp:** Genitourinary Cancer; Breast Cancer; **Hospital:** H Lee Moffitt Cancer Ctr & Research Inst; **Address:** H Lee Moffitt Cancer Ctr, 12902 Magnolia Drive, rm 3157, Tampa, FL 33612; **Phone:** 813-745-8658; **Board Cert:** Internal Medicine 87; Hematology 78; Medical Oncology 79; **Med School:** Italy 68; **Resid:** Internal Medicine, Univ Miss Med Ctr 76; Hematology and Oncology, Univ Miss Med Ctr 79; **Fellow:** Internal Medicine, A Gemelli Genl Hosp 70; **Fac Appt:** Prof Med, Univ S Fla Coll Med

Berlin, Jordan MD **[Onc]** - **Spec Exp:** Gastrointestinal Cancer; Pancreatic Cancer; Liver Cancer; **Hospital:** Vanderbilt Univ Med Ctr (page 116); **Address:** 777 Preston Research Building, Nashville, TN 37232-6307; **Phone:** 615-343-8422; **Board Cert:** Internal Medicine 02; Medical Oncology 95; **Med School:** Univ IL Coll Med 89; **Resid:** Internal Medicine, Univ Cincinnati 92; **Fellow:** Medical Oncology, Univ Wisc 95; **Fac Appt:** Assoc Prof Med, Vanderbilt Univ

Bernard, Stephen MD **[Onc]** - **Spec Exp:** Gastrointestinal Cancer; Palliative Care; Clinical Trials; **Hospital:** Univ NC Hosps (page 112); **Address:** Univ North Carolina Sch Med, 3009 Old Clinic, CB 7305, Chapel Hill, NC 27599; **Phone:** 919-966-4431; **Board Cert:** Internal Medicine 87; Medical Oncology 79; **Med School:** Univ NC Sch Med 73; **Resid:** Internal Medicine, Columbia-Presby Med Ctr 76; **Fellow:** Hematology and Oncology, Wash Univ Hosps 78; **Fac Appt:** Prof Med, Univ NC Sch Med

Brawley, Otis W MD **[Onc]** - **Spec Exp:** Breast Cancer; Prostate Cancer; **Hospital:** Emory Univ Hosp; **Address:** 1365 Clifton Rd NE, Atlanta, GA 30322; **Phone:** 404-778-1900; **Board Cert:** Internal Medicine 88; Medical Oncology 03; **Med School:** Univ Chicago-Pritzker Sch Med 85; **Resid:** Internal Medicine, Univ Hosp Cleveland 88; **Fellow:** Oncology, Natl Cancer Institute 90; **Fac Appt:** Prof Med, Emory Univ

Brescia, Frank J MD **[Onc]** - **Spec Exp:** Palliative Care; Breast Cancer; Gastrointestinal Cancer; **Hospital:** MUSC Med Ctr; **Address:** MUSC, Div Hem/Onc, 96 Jonathan Lucas St, Ste 903, Box 250635, Charleston, SC 29425; **Phone:** 843-792-4271; **Board Cert:** Internal Medicine 74; Medical Oncology 75; **Med School:** UMDNJ-NJ Med Sch, Newark 75; **Resid:** Internal Medicine, Cornell North Shore Univ Hosp 70; **Fellow:** Medical Oncology, Meml Sloan Kettering Cancer Ctr 74; **Fac Appt:** Prof Med, Med Univ SC

Burris III, Howard A MD **[Onc]** - **Spec Exp:** Drug Development; Drug Discovery; Breast Cancer; **Hospital:** Centennial Med Ctr; **Address:** 250 25th Ave N Bldg Atrium - Ste 100, Nashville, TN 37203; **Phone:** 615-320-5090; **Board Cert:** Internal Medicine 88; Medical Oncology 01; **Med School:** Univ S Ala Coll Med 85; **Resid:** Internal Medicine, Brooke Army Med Ctr 88; **Fellow:** Medical Oncology, Brooke Army Med Ctr 91

Carbone, David MD **[Onc]** - **Spec Exp:** Lung Cancer; **Hospital:** Vanderbilt Univ Med Ctr (page 116); **Address:** Vanderbilt-Ingram Cancer Ctr, 685 Preston Rsch Bldg, 2200 Pierce Ave, Nashville, TN 37232-6838; **Phone:** 615-936-3524; **Board Cert:** Internal Medicine 88; Medical Oncology 01; **Med School:** Johns Hopkins Univ 85; **Resid:** Internal Medicine, Johns Hopkins Hosp 88; **Fellow:** Oncology, Natl Cancer Inst 91; **Fac Appt:** Prof Med, Vanderbilt Univ

Carey, Lisa A MD **[Onc]** - **Spec Exp:** Breast Cancer; **Hospital:** Univ NC Hosps (page 112); **Address:** Univ North Carolina - Div Hem/Onc, Campus Box 7305, 3009 Old Clinic Bldg, Chapel Hill, NC 27599; **Phone:** 919-966-4431; **Board Cert:** Internal Medicine 03; Medical Oncology 03; **Med School:** Johns Hopkins Univ 90; **Resid:** Internal Medicine, Johns Hopkins Hosp 93; **Fellow:** Oncology, Johns Hopkins Hosp 96; **Fac Appt:** Asst Prof Med, Univ NC Sch Med

Carpenter Jr, John MD **[Onc]** - **Spec Exp:** Breast Cancer; **Hospital:** Univ of Ala Hosp at Birmingham; **Address:** 1530 3rd Ave S, Birmingham, AL 35294; **Phone:** 205-934-2084; **Board Cert:** Internal Medicine 72; Hematology 81; Medical Oncology 75; **Med School:** Tulane Univ 68; **Resid:** Internal Medicine, Grady Meml Hosp 71; **Fellow:** Hematology and Oncology, Emory Univ 73; **Fac Appt:** Prof Med, Univ Ala

Chao, Nelson Jen An MD **[Onc]** - **Spec Exp:** Bone Marrow Transplant; Lymphoma; Leukemia; **Hospital:** Duke Univ Med Ctr (page 94); **Address:** Duke Univ Med Ctr, Box 3961, Durham, NC 27710; **Phone:** 919-668-1002; **Board Cert:** Internal Medicine 84; Medical Oncology 87; **Med School:** Yale Univ 81; **Resid:** Internal Medicine, Stanford Univ Med Ctr 84; **Fellow:** Oncology, Stanford Univ Med Ctr 87; **Fac Appt:** Prof Med, Duke Univ

Colon-Otero, Gerardo MD **[Onc]** - **Spec Exp:** Lymphoma; Ovarian Cancer; **Hospital:** Mayo - Jacksonville; **Address:** Mayo Clin Jacksonville, 4500 San Pablo Rd S, Jacksonville, FL 32224-1865; **Phone:** 904-953-2000; **Board Cert:** Internal Medicine 82; Hematology 84; Medical Oncology 85; **Med School:** Puerto Rico 79; **Resid:** Internal Medicine, Mayo Clinic 82; **Fellow:** Hematology, Mayo Clinic 84; Medical Oncology, Univ Va Med Ctr 86; **Fac Appt:** Assoc Prof Med, Mayo Med Sch

Crawford, Jeffrey MD **[Onc]** - **Spec Exp:** Lung Cancer; **Hospital:** Duke Univ Med Ctr (page 94); **Address:** Duke Univ Med Ctr, Box 3476, 2592 Morris Bldg/Trent Drive, Durham, NC 27710-0001; **Phone:** 919-684-5621; **Board Cert:** Internal Medicine 77; Hematology 80; Medical Oncology 81; **Med School:** Ohio State Univ 74; **Resid:** Internal Medicine, Duke Univ Med Ctr 77; **Fellow:** Hematology and Oncology, Duke Univ Med Ctr 81; **Fac Appt:** Prof Med, Duke Univ

Dunphy, Frank R MD [Onc] - **Spec Exp:** Lung Cancer; Head & Neck Cancer; **Hospital:** Duke Univ Med Ctr (page 94); **Address:** Duke Univ, Comprehensive Cancer Ctr, Box 3198, rm 25178, Durham, NC 27710; **Phone:** 919-684-5621; **Board Cert:** Internal Medicine 84; Hematology 86; Medical Oncology 89; **Med School:** Louisiana State Univ 79; **Resid:** Internal Medicine, Lousiana St Univ Hosp 83; **Fellow:** Hematology and Oncology, Louisiana St Univ Hosp 85; **Fac Appt:** Assoc Prof Med, Duke Univ

Fanucchi, Michael P MD [Onc] - **Spec Exp:** Sarcoma; Aerodigestive Tract Disorders; Lung Cancer; **Hospital:** Emory Univ Hosp; **Address:** Winship Cancer Institute of Emory Healthcare, 550 Peachtree St NE, Atlanta, GA 30308; **Phone:** 404-686-8189; **Board Cert:** Internal Medicine 80; Medical Oncology 85; **Med School:** Columbia P&S 77; **Resid:** Internal Medicine, Bronx Muni Hosp Ctr 81; **Fellow:** Medical Oncology, Meml Sloan-Kettering Cancer Ctr 84; **Fac Appt:** Assoc Prof Med, Emory Univ

Gockerman, Jon Paul MD [Onc] - **Spec Exp:** Leukemia; Lymphoma; **Hospital:** Duke Univ Med Ctr (page 94); **Address:** Duke Univ Med Ctr, Box 3872, Durham, NC 27710; **Phone:** 919-684-8964; **Board Cert:** Internal Medicine 72; Hematology 74; Medical Oncology 73; **Med School:** Univ Chicago-Pritzker Sch Med 67; **Resid:** Internal Medicine, Duke Univ Med Ctr 69; **Fellow:** Hematology and Oncology, Duke Univ Med Ctr 71

Goldberg, Richard M MD [Onc] - **Spec Exp:** Stomach Cancer; Esophageal Cancer; Colon & Rectal Cancer; **Hospital:** Univ NC Hosps (page 112); **Address:** Division of Hematology/Oncology, CB 7305, 3009 Old Clinic Bldg SW, Chapel Hill, NC 27599-7305; **Phone:** 919-843-7711; **Board Cert:** Internal Medicine 82; Medical Oncology 85; **Med School:** SUNY Upstate Med Univ 79; **Resid:** Internal Medicine, Emory Univ Med Ctr 82; **Fellow:** Medical Oncology, Georgetown Univ Med Ctr 84; **Fac Appt:** Prof Med, Univ NC Sch Med

Graham, Mark MD [Onc] - **Spec Exp:** Breast Cancer; Breast Cancer Genetics; **Hospital:** WakeMed Cary; **Address:** Univ NC Hlthcare-Cary Oncology, 300 Ashville Ave, Ste 310, Cary, NC 27511; **Phone:** 919-859-6631; **Board Cert:** Internal Medicine 89; **Med School:** Mayo Med Sch 82; **Resid:** Internal Medicine, Duke Univ Med Ctr 85; **Fellow:** Medical Oncology, Univ CO Hlth Sci Ctr 90; **Fac Appt:** Assoc Clin Prof Med, Univ NC Sch Med

Greco, F Anthony MD [Onc] - **Spec Exp:** Lung Cancer; Unknown Primary Tumors; **Hospital:** Centennial Med Ctr; **Address:** Cannon-Pearl Cancer Ctr, 250 25th Ave N, Ste 110, Nashville, TN 37203; **Phone:** 615-986-4300; **Board Cert:** Internal Medicine 75; Medical Oncology 77; **Med School:** W VA Univ 72; **Resid:** Internal Medicine, Univ West Virginia Hosp 74; **Fellow:** Medical Oncology, Natl Cancer Inst 76

Green, Mark MD [Onc] - **Spec Exp:** Lung Cancer; **Hospital:** MUSC Med Ctr; **Address:** Med Univ South Carolina, 96 Jonathan Lucas St, Clinical Sciences Bldg, rm 903, Charleston, SC 29425; **Phone:** 843-792-4271; **Board Cert:** Internal Medicine 73; Medical Oncology 75; **Med School:** Harvard Med Sch 70; **Resid:** Internal Medicine, Beth Israel Hosp 72; Internal Medicine, Stanford Univ Hosp 75; **Fellow:** Medical Oncology, Natl Canc Inst 74; Medical Oncology, Stanford Univ Hosp 76; **Fac Appt:** Prof Med, Univ SC Sch Med

Grosh, William W MD [Onc] - **Spec Exp:** Melanoma & Sarcoma; Liver Cancer; Carcinoid Tumors; **Hospital:** Univ Virginia Med Ctr; **Address:** PO Box 800716, Charlottesville, VA 22908-0716; **Phone:** 434-924-1904; **Board Cert:** Internal Medicine 78; Medical Oncology 85; **Med School:** Columbia P&S 74; **Resid:** Internal Medicine, Vanderbilt Univ Med Ctr 77; **Fellow:** Medical Oncology, Vanderbilt Univ Med Ctr 83

Hande, Kenneth MD [Onc] - **Spec Exp:** Drug Discovery; Sarcoma; Carcinoid Tumors; **Hospital:** Vanderbilt Univ Med Ctr (page 116); **Address:** Vanderbilt Univ Med Ctr, 777 Preston Research Building, Nashville, TN 37232-6307; **Phone:** 615-322-4967; **Board Cert:** Internal Medicine 75; Medical Oncology 77; **Med School:** Johns Hopkins Univ 72; **Resid:** Internal Medicine, Barnes Hosp 74; **Fellow:** Medical Oncology, Natl Cancer Inst 77; **Fac Appt:** Prof Med, Vanderbilt Univ

Horton, John MD [Onc] - **Spec Exp:** Breast Cancer; **Hospital:** H Lee Moffitt Cancer Ctr & Research Inst; **Address:** 12902 Magnolia Dr, Ste 4035, Tampa, FL 33612-9416; **Phone:** 813-972-8373; **Board Cert:** Internal Medicine 68; Medical Oncology 73; **Med School:** England 57; **Resid:** Internal Medicine, Albany Med Ctr Hosp 62; **Fellow:** Medical Oncology, Albany Med Ctr Hosp 63; **Fac Appt:** Prof Med, Univ S Fla Coll Med

Hurd, David MD [Onc] - **Spec Exp:** Lymphoma; Leukemia; Bone Marrow Transplant; **Hospital:** Wake Forest Univ Baptist Med Ctr (page 117); **Address:** Wake Forest Sch Med, Comp Cancer Ctr, Medical Center Boulevard, Winston-Salem, NC 27157-1082; **Phone:** 336-713-5440; **Board Cert:** Internal Medicine 77; Medical Oncology 81; **Med School:** Univ IL Coll Med 74; **Resid:** Internal Medicine, Univ Minn Hosp 77; **Fellow:** Medical Oncology, Univ Minn Hosp 79; **Fac Appt:** Prof Med, Bowman Gray

Johnson, David H MD [Onc] - **Spec Exp:** Lung Cancer; Breast Cancer; **Hospital:** Vanderbilt Univ Med Ctr (page 116); **Address:** Vanderbilt Univ Med Ctr, Div Med Onc, 2220 Pierce Ave, 777 PRB, Nashville, TN 37232; **Phone:** 615-322-6053; **Board Cert:** Internal Medicine 79; Medical Oncology 83; **Med School:** Med Coll GA 76; **Resid:** Internal Medicine, Univ South Alabama Med Ctr 79; Internal Medicine, Med Coll Georgia Hosps 80; **Fellow:** Medical Oncology, Vanderbilt Univ Med Ctr 83; **Fac Appt:** Prof Med, Vanderbilt Univ

Kvols, Larry K MD [Onc] - **Spec Exp:** Gastrointestinal Cancer; Carcinoid Tumors; Neuroendocrine Tumors; **Hospital:** H Lee Moffitt Cancer Ctr & Research Inst; **Address:** H Lee Moffitt Cancer Ctr & Research Inst, MCCGI, 12902 Magnolia Drive, Tampa, FL 33612-9497; **Phone:** 813-972-8324; **Board Cert:** Internal Medicine 76; Medical Oncology 77; **Med School:** Baylor Coll Med 70; **Resid:** Internal Medicine, Johns Hopkins Hosp 72; **Fellow:** Hematology and Oncology, Johns Hopkins Hosp 73; **Fac Appt:** Prof Med, Mayo Med Sch

Lawson, David H MD [Onc] - **Spec Exp:** Melanoma; **Hospital:** Emory Univ Hosp; **Address:** Emory Univ Hosp - Div Medical Oncology, 1365 Clifton Rd NE, Ste B1500, Atlanta, GA 30322; **Phone:** 404-778-1900; **Board Cert:** Internal Medicine 77; Medical Oncology 79; **Med School:** Emory Univ 74; **Resid:** Internal Medicine, Emory Univ Hosps 77; **Fellow:** Medical Oncology, Emory Univ Hosps 79; **Fac Appt:** Assoc Prof Med, Emory Univ

Lesser, Glenn J MD [Onc] - **Spec Exp:** Neuro-Oncology; Brain Tumors; **Hospital:** Wake Forest Univ Baptist Med Ctr (page 117); **Address:** Wake Forest University-Div of Hem/Onc, Medical Center Blvd, Winston-Salem, NC 27157-1082; **Phone:** 336-716-9527; **Board Cert:** Internal Medicine 90; Medical Oncology 93; **Med School:** Penn State Univ-Hershey Med Ctr 87; **Resid:** Internal Medicine, NC Bapt Hosp/Bowman Gray Sch Med 91; **Fellow:** Medical Oncology, Johns Hopkins Oncology Ctr 94

Lossos, Izidore MD [Onc] - **Spec Exp:** Lymphoma; Hodgkin's Disease; **Hospital:** Univ of Miami Hosp & Clins/Sylvester Comp Canc Ctr; **Address:** Univ Miami - Sylvester Comp Cancer Ctr, 1475 NW 12th Ave, (D8-4), Miami, FL 33136; **Phone:** 305-243-4785; **Med School:** Israel 87; **Resid:** Internal Medicine, Hadassah Univ Hosp; **Fellow:** Hematology and Oncology, Hadassah Univ Hosp; Medical Oncology, Stanford Univ 01; **Fac Appt:** Assoc Clin Prof Med, Israel

Lyckholm, Laurel Jean MD [Onc] - **Spec Exp:** Neuro-Oncology; **Hospital:** Med Coll of VA Hosp; **Address:** Med Coll of VA, Div Hem/Onc, PO Box 980230, Richmond, VA 23298; **Phone:** 804-828-9723; **Board Cert:** Internal Medicine 89; Medical Oncology 93; Hematology 94; **Med School:** Creighton Univ 85; **Resid:** Internal Medicine, Creighton Univ 89; **Fellow:** Hematology and Oncology, Univ IA Coll Med 92; **Fac Appt:** Assoc Prof Med, Med Coll VA

Lynch Jr, James W MD [Onc] - **Spec Exp:** Lymphoma; Immunotherapy; Breast Cancer; **Hospital:** Shands Hlthcre at Univ of FL (page 109); **Address:** Shands Hlthcare - Div Hematology/Oncology, PO Box 100277, Gainesville, FL 32610-0277; **Phone:** 352-392-3000; **Board Cert:** Internal Medicine 87; Medical Oncology 01; **Med School:** Eastern VA Med Sch 84; **Resid:** Internal Medicine, Univ Florida 87; **Fellow:** Medical Oncology, Natl Cancer Inst 91; **Fac Appt:** Prof Med, Univ Fla Coll Med

Mitchell, Beverly MD [Onc] - **Spec Exp:** Hematologic Malignancies; Leukemia; Lymphoma; **Hospital:** Univ NC Hosps (page 112); **Address:** Lineberger Comp Cancer Ctr, 102 Mason Farm RD CB#7295, Chapel Hill, NC 27599-7295; **Phone:** 919-843-7710; **Board Cert:** Internal Medicine 73; Hematology 78; **Med School:** Harvard Med Sch 69; **Resid:** Internal Medicine, Univ Washington Med Ctr 72; **Fellow:** Metabolism, Univ Zurich 75; Hematology and Oncology, Univ Michigan 77; **Fac Appt:** Prof Med, Univ NC Sch Med

Moore, Joseph O MD [Onc] - **Spec Exp:** Leukemia; Lymphoma; Sarcoma; **Hospital:** Duke Univ Med Ctr (page 94); **Address:** Duke Univ Med Ctr, Box 3872, Durham, NC 27710; **Phone:** 919-684-8964; **Board Cert:** Internal Medicine 75; Medical Oncology 77; **Med School:** Johns Hopkins Univ 70; **Resid:** Internal Medicine, Johns Hopkins Hosp 75; **Fellow:** Hematology and Oncology, Duke Univ 77; **Fac Appt:** Prof Med, Duke Univ

Perez, Edith A MD [Onc] - **Spec Exp:** Breast Cancer; Breast Cancer Risk Assessment; Clinical Trials; **Hospital:** Mayo - Jacksonville; **Address:** 4500 San Pablo Rd, Davis Bldg, 3N, Jacksonville, FL 32224; **Phone:** 904-953-7283; **Board Cert:** Internal Medicine 83; Hematology 86; Medical Oncology 87; **Med School:** Univ Puerto Rico 79; **Resid:** Internal Medicine, Loma Linda Univ Med Ctr 82; **Fellow:** Hematology and Oncology, Martinez VA Hosp/UC Davis 87; **Fac Appt:** Prof Med, Mayo Med Sch

Powell, Bayard L MD [Onc] - **Spec Exp:** Leukemia; Myelodysplastic Syndromes; **Hospital:** Wake Forest Univ Baptist Med Ctr (page 117); **Address:** Wake Forest Univ Baptist Med Ctr, Med Ctr Blvd-Cancer Center, Winston-Salem, NC 27157; **Phone:** 336-716-2946; **Board Cert:** Medical Oncology 85; Internal Medicine 83; **Med School:** Univ NC Sch Med 80; **Resid:** Internal Medicine, NC Baptist Hospital 83; **Fellow:** Hematology and Oncology, Wake Forest U Sch of Med 86; **Fac Appt:** Prof Hem, Wake Forest Univ

Robert, Nicholas J MD [Onc] - **Spec Exp:** Breast Cancer; Hematologic Malignancies; **Hospital:** Inova Fairfax Hosp; **Address:** 8503 Arlington Blvd, Ste 400, Fairfax, VA 22031; **Phone:** 703-280-5390; **Board Cert:** Internal Medicine 78; Anatomic Pathology 79; Medical Oncology 81; Hematology 84; **Med School:** McGill Univ 74; **Resid:** Internal Medicine, Royal Victoria Hosp 76; Pathology, Mass Genl Hosp 79; **Fellow:** Hematology, Peter Bent Brigham Hosp 84; Medical Oncology, Dana Farber Cancer Inst

Ross, Maureen MD/PhD [Onc] - **Spec Exp:** Bone Marrow Transplant-Adult; Hematologic Malignancies; Breast Cancer; **Hospital:** Univ Virginia Med Ctr; **Address:** Dept Internal Med, Div Hem/Onc, Box 800-130, Charlottesville, VA 22908-0130; **Phone:** 434-924-1693; **Board Cert:** Internal Medicine 88; Medical Oncology 89; Hematology 96; **Med School:** Univ Miami Sch Med 84; **Resid:** Internal Medicine, Duke Univ Med Ctr 87; **Fellow:** Hematology and Oncology, Duke Univ Med Ctr 90; **Fac Appt:** Prof Med, Univ VA Sch Med

Roth, Bruce J MD **[Onc]** - **Spec Exp:** Prostate Cancer; Bladder Cancer; Testicular Cancer; **Hospital:** Vanderbilt Univ Med Ctr (page 116); **Address:** Vanderbilt Ingram Cancer Center, 777 Preston Research Bldg, Nashville, TN 37232-6307; **Phone:** 615-343-4070; **Board Cert:** Internal Medicine 83; Medical Oncology 85; **Med School:** St Louis Univ 80; **Resid:** Internal Medicine, Indiana Univ Med Ctr 83; **Fellow:** Medical Oncology, Indiana Univ Med Ctr 86; **Fac Appt:** Prof Med, Vanderbilt Univ

Rothenberg, Mace MD **[Onc]** - **Spec Exp:** Pancreatic Cancer; Colon & Rectal Cancer; Clinical Trials; **Hospital:** Vanderbilt Univ Med Ctr (page 116); **Address:** Vanderbilt Ingram Cancer Center, 777 Preston Research Bldg, Nashville, TN 37232-6307; **Phone:** 615-322-4967; **Board Cert:** Internal Medicine 85; Medical Oncology 87; **Med School:** NYU Sch Med 82; **Resid:** Internal Medicine, Vanderbilt Univ Med Ctr 85; **Fellow:** Medical Oncology, Natl Cancer Inst 88; **Fac Appt:** Prof Med, Vanderbilt Univ

Sandler, Alan MD **[Onc]** - **Spec Exp:** Lung Cancer; Sarcoma; **Hospital:** Vanderbilt Univ Med Ctr (page 116); **Address:** Vanderbilt Univ Med Ctr-Thoracic Onc, 2220 Pierce Ave, 777Preston Rsch Bldg, Nashville, TN 37232; **Phone:** 615-343-4070; **Med School:** Rush Med Coll 87; **Resid:** Internal Medicine, Yale-New Haven Hosp 90; **Fellow:** Medical Oncology, Yale Univ 93; **Fac Appt:** Assoc Prof Med, Vanderbilt Univ

Schwartz, Michael MD **[Onc]** - **Spec Exp:** Breast Cancer; Lymphoma; Colon Cancer; **Hospital:** Mount Sinai Med Ctr - Miami; **Address:** 4306 Alton Rd, FL 3, Oncology Hematology Assoc, Miami Beach, FL 33140; **Phone:** 305-535-3310; **Board Cert:** Internal Medicine 89; Medical Oncology 91; Hematology 92; **Med School:** UMDNJ-RW Johnson Med Sch 86; **Resid:** Internal Medicine, Mt Sinai Medical Ctr 89; **Fellow:** Hematology and Oncology, Meml Sloan Kettering 92; **Fac Appt:** Asst Clin Prof Onc, Univ Miami Sch Med

Seewaldt, Victoria L MD **[Onc]** - **Spec Exp:** Breast Cancer; Clinical Trials; **Hospital:** Duke Univ Med Ctr (page 94); **Address:** Duke Univ Med Ctr, Box 2628, Rm 221A MSRB, Durham, NC 27710; **Phone:** 919-684-2995; **Board Cert:** Internal Medicine 95; **Med School:** UC Davis 89; **Resid:** Obstetrics & Gynecology, Univ Wash Med Ctr 90; Internal Medicine, Univ Wash Med Ctr 92; **Fellow:** Medical Oncology, Fred Hutchinson Cancer Ctr 95; Breast Cancer, Fred Hutchinson Cancer Ctr 98; **Fac Appt:** Assoc Prof Med, Duke Univ

Serody, Jonathan S MD **[Onc]** - **Spec Exp:** Breast Cancer; Breast Cancer Vaccine Therapy; Clinical Trials; **Hospital:** Univ NC Hosps (page 112); **Address:** Lineberger Comprehensive Cancer Ctr, Univ NC Sch Medicine CB# 7295, Chapel Hill, NC 27599-7295; **Phone:** 919-966-6975; **Board Cert:** Internal Medicine 89; Hematology 96; **Med School:** Univ VA Sch Med 86; **Resid:** Internal Medicine, Univ NC Med Ctr 89; **Fellow:** Hematology, Univ NC Med Ctr 92; Bone Marrow Transplant, Fred Hutchinson Transplant Program; **Fac Appt:** Assoc Prof Med, Univ NC Sch Med

Shea, Thomas MD **[Onc]** - **Spec Exp:** Bone Marrow Transplant; Lymphoma; Leukemia; **Hospital:** Univ NC Hosps (page 112); **Address:** Univ N Carolina, Dept Medicine, 3009 Old Clinic Bldg , Box 7305, Chapel Hill, NC 27599; **Phone:** 919-966-7746; **Board Cert:** Internal Medicine 82; Hematology 84; Medical Oncology 85; **Med School:** Univ NC Sch Med 78; **Resid:** Internal Medicine, Beth Israel Deaconess Med Ctr 82; **Fellow:** Hematology and Oncology, Beth Israel Deaconess Med Ctr 85; Bone Marrow Transplant, Dana Farber Cancer Inst 88; **Fac Appt:** Prof Med, Univ NC Sch Med

Shin, Dong Moon MD **[Onc]** - **Spec Exp:** Head & Neck Cancer; Lung Cancer; Mesothelioma; **Hospital:** Emory Univ Hosp; **Address:** Emory Winship Cancer Inst, 1365C Clifton Rd, Atlanta, GA 30322; **Phone:** 404-778-1900; **Board Cert:** Internal Medicine 85; Medical Oncology 89; **Med School:** South Korea 75; **Resid:** Internal Medicine, Cook Co Hosp 85; **Fellow:** Medical Oncology, Univ Texas MD Anderson Cancer Ctr 86; **Fac Appt:** Prof Med, Emory Univ

Smith, Thomas Joseph MD [Onc] - **Spec Exp:** Breast Cancer; Palliative Care; **Hospital:** Med Coll of VA Hosp; **Address:** 1300 E Marshall St Fl Gr, Richmond, VA 23298; **Phone:** 804-828-9992; **Board Cert:** Internal Medicine 82; Medical Oncology 87; **Med School:** Yale Univ 79; **Resid:** Internal Medicine, Hosp Univ Penn 82; **Fellow:** Medical Oncology, Med Coll Virginia 87; **Fac Appt:** Prof Med, Med Coll VA

Socinski, Mark A MD [Onc] - **Spec Exp:** Lung Cancer; **Hospital:** Univ NC Hosps (page 112); **Address:** UNC Chapel Hill, Div Hem/Onc, 3009 Old Clinic Bldg, Campus Box 7305, Chapel Hill, NC 27599-7305; **Phone:** 919-966-4431; **Board Cert:** Internal Medicine 88; Medical Oncology 91; **Med School:** Univ VT Coll Med 84; **Resid:** Internal Medicine, Beth Israel Hosp 86; **Fellow:** Medical Oncology, Dana-Farber Cancer Inst 89; **Fac Appt:** Assoc Prof Med, Univ NC Sch Med

Sosman, Jeffrey MD [Onc] - **Spec Exp:** Kidney Cancer; Melanoma; Drug Discovery; **Hospital:** Vanderbilt Univ Med Ctr (page 116); **Address:** 1903 Vanderbilt Clinic, 777Preston Research Bldg, Nashville, TN 37232-6307; **Phone:** 615-322-6053; **Board Cert:** Anatomic Pathology 85; Internal Medicine 87; Medical Oncology 89; **Med School:** Albert Einstein Coll Med 81; **Resid:** Anatomic Pathology, Univ Chicago Hosps 85; Internal Medicine, Univ Wisconsin Hosp 86; **Fellow:** Medical Oncology, Univ Wisconsin 89; **Fac Appt:** Clin Prof Med, Vanderbilt Univ

Stone, Joel MD [Onc] - **Spec Exp:** Lung Cancer; Breast Cancer; **Hospital:** St Vincent's Med Ctr - Jacksonville; **Address:** 1801 Barrs St, Ste 800, Jacksonville, FL 32204-4751; **Phone:** 904-388-2619; **Board Cert:** Internal Medicine 77; Medical Oncology 79; **Med School:** Univ VA Sch Med 74; **Resid:** Internal Medicine, Univ KY Med Ctr 77; **Fellow:** Hematology and Oncology, Emory Univ 79

Thigpen, James Tate MD [Onc] - **Spec Exp:** Gynecologic Cancer; Lung Cancer; **Hospital:** Univ Hosps & Clins - Jackson; **Address:** U Miss Med Ctr, 2500 N State St, rm L504, Jackson, MS 39216; **Phone:** 601-984-5590; **Board Cert:** Internal Medicine 72; Hematology 74; Medical Oncology 75; **Med School:** Univ Miss 73; **Resid:** Internal Medicine, Univ Miss Med Ctr 71; **Fellow:** Hematology and Oncology, Univ Miss Med Ctr 73; **Fac Appt:** Prof Med, Univ Miss

Torti, Frank M MD [Onc] - **Spec Exp:** Prostate Cancer; Urologic Cancer; **Hospital:** Wake Forest Univ Baptist Med Ctr (page 117); **Address:** Wake Forest Baptist Med Ctr-Comprehensive Cancer Ctr, Med Center Blvd, Winston-Salem, NC 27157-1082; **Phone:** 336-716-7971; **Board Cert:** Internal Medicine 78; Medical Oncology 79; **Med School:** Harvard Med Sch 74; **Resid:** Internal Medicine, Beth Israel Hosp 76; **Fellow:** Medical Oncology, Stanford Univ Med Ctr 79; **Fac Appt:** Prof Med, Wake Forest Univ

Troner, Michael MD [Onc] - **Spec Exp:** Head & Neck Cancer; **Hospital:** Baptist Hosp of Miami; **Address:** 8940 N Kendall, Ste 300E, Miami, FL 33176-2132; **Phone:** 305-271-6467; **Board Cert:** Internal Medicine 72; Medical Oncology 73; **Med School:** SUNY Downstate 68; **Resid:** Internal Medicine, Univ Maryland Hosp 71; **Fellow:** Medical Oncology, Univ Miami Med Ctr 73; **Fac Appt:** Assoc Clin Prof Med, Univ Miami Sch Med

Vance, Ralph MD [Onc] - **Spec Exp:** Lung Cancer; **Hospital:** Univ Hosps & Clins - Jackson; **Address:** Univ Mississippi Med Ctr-Division of Oncology, 2500 N State St, Jackson, MS 39212; **Phone:** 601-984-5590; **Med School:** Univ Miss 1972; **Resid:** Internal Medicine, Univ Hosp; **Fellow:** Hematology and Oncology, Univ Hosp; **Fac Appt:** Prof Med, Univ Miss

Vaughan, William P MD [Onc] - **Spec Exp:** Bone Marrow Transplant; Breast Cancer; **Hospital:** Univ of Ala Hosp at Birmingham; **Address:** Univ Ala Birmingham, 1900 University Blvd-Tinsley Harrison Tower, rm 541, Birmingham, AL 35294; **Phone:** 205-934-1908; **Board Cert:** Internal Medicine 75; Medical Oncology 79; **Med School:** Univ Conn 72; **Resid:** Internal Medicine, Univ Chicago Hosps 75; **Fellow:** Oncology, Johns Hopkins Hosp 77; **Fac Appt:** Prof Med, Univ Ala

Weiss, Geoffrey R MD [Onc] - **Spec Exp:** Gastrointestinal Cancer; Genitourinary Cancer; Prostate Cancer; **Hospital:** Univ Virginia Med Ctr; **Address:** UVa Hlth System, Div Hem/Onc, PO Box 800716, Charlottesville, VA 22908-0716; **Phone:** 434-924-1693; **Board Cert:** Internal Medicine 77; **Medical Oncology** 81; **Med School:** St Louis Univ 74; **Resid:** Internal Medicine, Temple Univ Hosp 78; **Fellow:** Medical Oncology, Dana-Faber Cancer Inst 82; **Fac Appt:** Prof Med, Univ VA Sch Med

Williams, Michael MD [Onc] - **Spec Exp:** Lymphoma; Multiple Myeloma; Leukemia; **Hospital:** Univ Virginia Med Ctr; **Address:** UVA Hlth System, Div Hem/Onc, PO Box 800716, Charlottesville, VA 22908-0716; **Phone:** 434-924-9637; **Board Cert:** Internal Medicine 82; Medical Oncology 87; Hematology 88; **Med School:** Univ Cincinnati 79; **Resid:** Internal Medicine, Univ Virginia Med Ctr 83; **Fellow:** Hematology and Oncology, Univ Virginia Med Ctr 86; **Fac Appt:** Prof Med, Univ VA Sch Med

Wingard, John R MD [Onc] - **Spec Exp:** Bone Marrow Transplant; Leukemia; Multiple Myeloma; **Hospital:** Shands Hlthcre at Univ of FL (page 109); **Address:** 1600 SW Archer Rd, rm R4-116, Box 100277, Gainesville, FL 32610; **Phone:** 352-846-2814; **Board Cert:** Internal Medicine 77; Medical Oncology 81; **Med School:** Johns Hopkins Univ 73; **Resid:** Internal Medicine, Memphis City Hosps 76; Internal Medicine, VA Hosp 77; **Fellow:** Medical Oncology, Johns Hopkins Hosp 79; **Fac Appt:** Prof Med, Univ Fla Coll Med

Yunus, Furhan MD [Onc] - **Spec Exp:** Multiple Myeloma; Lymphoma; **Hospital:** Meth Healthcare Central - Univ Hosp; **Address:** Univ TN Cancer Inst, 1331 Union Ave, Ste 800, Memphis, TN 38104; **Phone:** 901-722-0561; **Board Cert:** Internal Medicine 93; Medical Oncology 95; **Med School:** Pakistan 86; **Resid:** Internal Medicine, Methodist Hosp 93; **Fellow:** Hematology and Oncology, Univ Ariz Coll Med 95; **Fac Appt:** Asst Prof Med, Univ Tenn Coll Med, Memphis

Midwest

Albain, Kathy MD [Onc] - **Spec Exp:** Breast Cancer; Lung Cancer; **Hospital:** Loyola Univ Med Ctr (page 98); **Address:** Loyola Univ Med Ctr, 2160 S First Ave, Bldg 112 - Ste 109, Maywood, IL 60153-5590; **Phone:** 708-327-3102; **Board Cert:** Internal Medicine 81; Medical Oncology 83; **Med School:** Univ Mich Med Sch 78; **Resid:** Internal Medicine, Univ Illinois Med Ctr 81; **Fellow:** Hematology and Oncology, Univ Chicago Hosps 84; **Fac Appt:** Prof Med, Loyola Univ-Stritch Sch Med

Anderson, Joseph M MD [Onc] - **Spec Exp:** Breast Cancer; Palliative Care; **Hospital:** Henry Ford Hosp; **Address:** 2799 W Grand Blvd, CFP5, Detroit, MI 48202; **Phone:** 313-916-1854; **Board Cert:** Internal Medicine 85; Medical Oncology 89; **Med School:** Univ Mich Med Sch 82; **Resid:** Internal Medicine, Henry Ford Hosp 86; **Fellow:** Medical Oncology, Henry Ford Hosp 88

Baker, Lawrence H DO [Onc] - **Spec Exp:** Sarcoma; **Hospital:** Univ Michigan Hlth Sys; **Address:** 1500 E Med Center Drive, Ste 7216CCGC, Ann Arbor, MI 48109-0999; **Phone:** 734-647-8902; **Board Cert:** Internal Medicine 76; Medical Oncology 77; **Med School:** Univ Osteo Med & Hlth Sci, Des Moines 66; **Resid:** Internal Medicine, Genesys Reg M C-W Flint Campus 67; Internal Medicine, Detroit Osteopathic Hosp 69; **Fellow:** Medical Oncology, Wayne State Univ Affil Hosp 72; **Fac Appt:** Prof Med, Univ Mich Med Sch

Benson III, Al B MD [Onc] - **Spec Exp:** Colon Cancer; Carcinoid Tumors; Pancreatic Cancer; **Hospital:** Northwestern Meml Hosp; **Address:** 675 N St Clair Fl 21 - Ste 100, Chicago, IL 60611; **Phone:** 312-695-0990; **Board Cert:** Internal Medicine 79; Medical Oncology 83; **Med School:** SUNY Buffalo 76; **Resid:** Internal Medicine, Univ Wisc Hosps 79; **Fellow:** Medical Oncology, Univ Wisc Hosps 84; **Fac Appt:** Prof Med, Northwestern Univ

Bitran, Jacob MD **[Onc]** - **Spec Exp:** Breast Cancer; Bone Marrow Transplant; Lung Cancer; **Hospital:** Adv Luth Genl Hosp; **Address:** Lutheran Genl Cancer Care Specialists, 1700 Luther Lane, Park Ridge, IL 60068-1270; **Phone:** 847-268-8200; **Board Cert:** Internal Medicine 74; Hematology 86; Medical Oncology 77; **Med School:** Univ IL Coll Med 71; **Resid:** Pathology, Rush Presby St Luke's Hosp 73; Internal Medicine, Michael Reese Hosp 73; **Fellow:** Hematology and Oncology, Univ Chicago Hosps 77; **Fac Appt:** Prof Med, Univ Hlth Sci/Chicago Med Sch

Bolwell, Brian J MD **[Onc]** - **Spec Exp:** Bone Marrow Transplant; Hematologic Malignancies; **Hospital:** Cleveland Clin Fdn (page 92); **Address:** Cleveland Clinic, R32, 9500 Euclid Ave, Cleveland, OH 44195; **Phone:** 216-444-6922; **Board Cert:** Medical Oncology 87; Internal Medicine 85; **Med School:** Case West Res Univ 81; **Resid:** Internal Medicine, Univ Hosp 84; **Fellow:** Hematology and Oncology, Hosp U Penn 87; **Fac Appt:** Prof Med, Cleveland Cl Coll Med/Case West Res

Bonomi, Philip MD **[Onc]** - **Spec Exp:** Mesothelioma; Thymoma; Lung Cancer; **Hospital:** Rush Univ Med Ctr; **Address:** 1725 W Harrison St, Ste 821, Chicago, IL 60612; **Phone:** 312-942-3312; **Board Cert:** Internal Medicine 75; Medical Oncology 77; **Med School:** Univ IL Coll Med 70; **Resid:** Internal Medicine, Geisinger Med Ctr 72; Internal Medicine, Geisinger Med Ctr 75; **Fellow:** Medical Oncology, Rush Presby-St Luke's Med Ctr 77; **Fac Appt:** Prof Med, Rush Med Coll

Borden, Ernest C MD **[Onc]** - **Spec Exp:** Melanoma; Vaccine Therapy; Sarcoma; **Hospital:** Cleveland Clin Fdn (page 92); **Address:** Cleveland Clinic, Floor R40, 9500 Euclid Ave, Cleveland, OH 44195; **Phone:** 216-444-8183; **Board Cert:** Medical Oncology 75; Internal Medicine 73; **Med School:** Duke Univ 66; **Resid:** Internal Medicine, Hosp U Penn 68; **Fellow:** Medical Oncology, Johns Hopkins Hosp 73; **Fac Appt:** Prof Med, Cleveland Cl Coll Med/Case West Res

Bricker, Leslie J MD **[Onc]** - **Spec Exp:** Hospice Care; Palliative Care; **Hospital:** Henry Ford Hosp; **Address:** Henry Ford Hospital, 2799 W Grand Blvd, CFP 5, Detroit, MI 48202; **Phone:** 313-916-1859; **Board Cert:** Internal Medicine 80; Hematology 82; Medical Oncology 83; **Med School:** Wayne State Univ 77; **Resid:** Internal Medicine, Sinai Hosp 80; **Fellow:** Hematology, Univ Mich Hosp; **Fac Appt:** Assoc Prof Med, Wayne State Univ

Brockstein, Bruce E MD **[Onc]** - **Spec Exp:** Head & Neck Cancer; Sarcoma; Melanoma; **Hospital:** Evanston Hosp; **Address:** Evanston Northwestern Healthcare, Div Hem/Onc, 2650 Ridge Ave, Ste 5134, Evanston, IL 60201; **Phone:** 847-570-2515; **Board Cert:** Internal Medicine 03; Medical Oncology 95; **Med School:** Univ Chicago-Pritzker Sch Med 90; **Resid:** Internal Medicine, Hosp U Penn 93; **Fellow:** Hematology and Oncology, Univ Chicago Hosps 96; **Fac Appt:** Asst Prof Med, Northwestern Univ

Buckner, Jan Craig MD **[Onc]** - **Spec Exp:** Brain Tumors; Neuro-Oncology; **Hospital:** Mayo Med Ctr & Clin - Rochester; **Address:** Mayo Clinic, 200 First St SW, Rochester, MN 55905; **Phone:** 507-284-4320; **Board Cert:** Internal Medicine 83; Medical Oncology 85; **Med School:** Univ NC Sch Med 80; **Resid:** Internal Medicine, Butterworth Hosp 83; **Fellow:** Medical Oncology, Mayo Clinic 85; **Fac Appt:** Prof Onc, Mayo Med Sch

Budd, George Thomas MD **[Onc]** - **Spec Exp:** Breast Cancer; **Hospital:** Cleveland Clin Fdn (page 92); **Address:** Cleveland Clinic, Taussig Cancer Ctr, 9500 Euclid Ave, Desk R35, Cleveland, OH 44195; **Phone:** 216-444-6480; **Board Cert:** Internal Medicine 80; Medical Oncology 83; **Med School:** Univ Kans 76; **Resid:** Internal Medicine, Cleveland Clin Fdn 80; **Fellow:** Hematology and Oncology, Cleveland Clin Fdn 82

Burt, Richard K MD [Onc] - **Spec Exp:** Stem Cell Transplant in Lupus/Crohn's; Stem Cell Transplant in MS/Rhu Arthritis; Autoimmune Diseases; **Hospital:** Northwestern Meml Hosp; **Address:** Northwestern Univ, 750 N Lakeshore Drive Fl 6 - rm 649, Chicago, IL 60611; **Phone:** 312-908-0059; **Board Cert:** Internal Medicine 89; Medical Oncology 93; **Med School:** St Louis Univ 84; **Resid:** Internal Medicine, Baylor Coll Med 88; **Fellow:** Medical Oncology, Natl Inst Hlth Clin Ctr 91; Hematology, Nat Inst Hlth Clin Ctr 93; **Fac Appt:** Assoc Prof Med, Northwestern Univ

Chapman, Robert A MD [Onc] - **Spec Exp:** Lung Cancer; **Hospital:** Henry Ford Hosp; **Address:** 2799 W Grand Blvd, Detroit, MI 48202; **Phone:** 313-916-1841; **Board Cert:** Internal Medicine 85; Medical Oncology 89; **Med School:** Cornell Univ-Weill Med Coll 76; **Resid:** Internal Medicine, Henry Ford Hosp 79; **Fellow:** Medical Oncology, Meml Sloan Kettering Cancer Ctr 81

Chitambar, Christopher R MD [Onc] - **Spec Exp:** Lymphoma; Leukemia; Breast Cancer; **Hospital:** Froedtert Meml Lutheran Hosp; **Address:** Med Coll Wisconsin, Div Neoplastic Diseases, 9200 W Wisconsin Ave, Milwaukee, WI 53226-3512; **Phone:** 414-805-4600; **Board Cert:** Internal Medicine 80; Hematology 82; Medical Oncology 83; **Med School:** India 77; **Resid:** Internal Medicine, Brackenridge Hosp 80; **Fellow:** Hematology and Oncology, Univ Colo Hlth Sci Ctr 83; **Fac Appt:** Prof Med, Med Coll Wisc

Clamon, Gerald MD [Onc] - **Spec Exp:** Lung Cancer; Drug Development; **Hospital:** Univ Iowa Hosp & Clinics; **Address:** Univ Iowa Hosps & Clins, Dept Internal Med, 200 Hawkins Drive, rm 59770 JPP, Iowa City, IA 52242; **Phone:** 319-356-1932; **Board Cert:** Internal Medicine 76; Medical Oncology 79; **Med School:** Washington Univ, St Louis 71; **Resid:** Internal Medicine, Barnes Hosp 76; **Fellow:** Natl Cancer Inst 74; Medical Oncology, Univ Iowa Hosp & Clinics 77; **Fac Appt:** Prof Med, Univ Iowa Coll Med

Clark, Joseph I MD [Onc] - **Spec Exp:** Kidney Cancer; Melanoma; Lung Cancer; **Hospital:** Loyola Univ Med Ctr (page 98); **Address:** Cardinal Bernardin Canc Ctr, Loyola Univ Med Ctr, 2160 S First Ave, rm 343, Maywood, IL 60153; **Phone:** 708-327-3236; **Board Cert:** Internal Medicine 02; Medical Oncology 95; **Med School:** Loyola Univ-Stritch Sch Med 89; **Resid:** Internal Medicine, Loyola Univ Med Ctr/Hines VA Hosp 92; **Fellow:** Hematology and Oncology, Fox Chase Cancer Ctr/Temple Univ Hosp 95; **Fac Appt:** Assoc Prof Med, Loyola Univ-Stritch Sch Med

Cleary, James F MD [Onc] - **Spec Exp:** Palliative Care; Head & Neck Cancer; **Hospital:** Univ WI Hosp & Clins; **Address:** K6/546 CSC, 600 Highland Ave, Madison, WI 53792; **Phone:** 608-263-8090; **Board Cert:** Medical Oncology ; **Med School:** Australia 84; **Resid:** Internal Medicine, Royal Adelaide Hosp 87; **Fellow:** Medical Oncology, Royal Adelaide Hosp 90; **Fac Appt:** Assoc Prof Med, Univ Wisc

Clinton, Steven MD/PhD [Onc] - **Spec Exp:** Genitourinary Cancer; Prostate Cancer; Nutrition & Cancer Prevention/Control; **Hospital:** Ohio St Univ Med Ctr (page 105); **Address:** Ohio State University Medical Ctr, A434 Starling Loving Hall, 320 W 10th Ave, Columbus, OH 43210; **Phone:** 614-293-7560; **Board Cert:** Internal Medicine 87; Medical Oncology 91; **Med School:** Univ IL Coll Med 84; **Resid:** Internal Medicine, Univ Chicago Hosps 87; **Fellow:** Medical Oncology, Dana Farber Cancer Inst/Harvard 91; **Fac Appt:** Assoc Prof Med, Ohio State Univ

Cobleigh, Melody A MD [Onc] - **Spec Exp:** Breast Cancer; **Hospital:** Rush Univ Med Ctr; **Address:** 1725 W Harrison St, Ste 821, Chicago, IL 60612-3828; **Phone:** 312-942-5904; **Board Cert:** Internal Medicine 79; Medical Oncology 81; **Med School:** Rush Med Coll 76; **Resid:** Internal Medicine, Rush Presby-St Lukes Med Ctr 79; **Fellow:** Medical Oncology, Indiana Univ 81; **Fac Appt:** Prof Med, Rush Med Coll

Davis, Mellar MD [Onc] - **Spec Exp:** Palliative Care; **Hospital:** Cleveland Clin Fdn (page 92); **Address:** Cleveland Clin Fdn, 9500 Euclid Ave, MS R35, Cleveland, OH 44195; **Phone:** 216-445-4622; **Board Cert:** Internal Medicine 80; Hematology 82; Medical Oncology 83; **Med School:** Ohio State Univ 77; **Resid:** Internal Medicine, Riverside Meth Hosp 79; **Fellow:** Hematology, Mayo Clinic 81; Medical Oncology, Mayo Clinic

Di Persio, John MD/PhD [Onc] - **Spec Exp:** Bone Marrow Transplant; Hematologic Malignancies; Leukemia; **Hospital:** Barnes-Jewish Hosp (page 85); **Address:** Wash Univ Sch Med, Div Onc, Sect BMT & Leukemia, 660 S Euclid Ave, Box 8007, St Louis, MO 63110; **Phone:** 314-454-8306; **Board Cert:** Internal Medicine 84; Medical Oncology 87; Hematology 88; **Med School:** Univ Rochester 80; **Resid:** Internal Medicine, Parkland Meml Hosp 84; **Fellow:** Hematology and Oncology, UCLA Sch Med 87; **Fac Appt:** Prof Med, Washington Univ, St Louis

Dreicer, Robert MD [Onc] - **Spec Exp:** Breast Cancer; Prostate Cancer; **Hospital:** Cleveland Clin Fdn (page 92); **Address:** Cleveland Clinic, Taussig Cancer Ctr, 9500 Euclid Ave, Desk R35, Cleveland, OH 44195; **Phone:** 216-445-4623; **Board Cert:** Internal Medicine 86; Medical Oncology 89; **Med School:** Univ Tex, Houston 83; **Resid:** Internal Medicine, Ind Univ Med Ctr 86; **Fellow:** Medical Oncology, Univ Wisc Hosp & Clins 89

Einhorn, Lawrence MD [Onc] - **Spec Exp:** Testicular Cancer; Lung Cancer; Urologic Cancer; **Hospital:** Indiana Univ Hosp (page 90); **Address:** 535 Barnhill Drive, rm 473, Indianapolis, IN 46202; **Phone:** 317-274-0920; **Board Cert:** Internal Medicine 72; Medical Oncology 75; **Med School:** UCLA 67; **Resid:** Internal Medicine, Indiana Univ Hosp 69; **Fellow:** Medical Oncology, Indiana Univ Hosp 72; **Fac Appt:** Prof Med, Indiana Univ

Eng, Charis MD [Onc] - **Spec Exp:** Breast Cancer; Ovarian Cancer; Cancer Genetics; **Hospital:** Ohio St Univ Med Ctr (page 105); **Address:** Ohio State Univ Comprehensive Cancer Ctr, 420 W 12 Ave, Medical Research Facility, Columbus, OH 43210; **Phone:** 614-293-6694; **Board Cert:** Internal Medicine 91; Medical Oncology 97; **Med School:** Univ Chicago-Pritzker Sch Med 88; **Resid:** Internal Medicine, Beth Israel Hosp 91; **Fellow:** Medical Oncology, Dana-Farber Cancer Inst 95; **Fac Appt:** Prof Med, Ohio State Univ

Fleming, Gini F MD [Onc] - **Spec Exp:** Breast Cancer; Gynecologic Cancer; **Hospital:** Univ of Chicago Hosps; **Address:** U Chicago Hospitals, 5841 S Maryland MC2115, Chicago, IL 60637-1470; **Phone:** 773-834-7424; **Board Cert:** Internal Medicine 02; Medical Oncology 01; **Med School:** Univ IL Coll Med 85; **Resid:** Internal Medicine, U Chicago-Pritzker Sch Med 88; **Fellow:** Hematology and Oncology, U Chicago-Pritzker Sch Med 92; **Fac Appt:** Assoc Prof Med, Univ Chicago-Pritzker Sch Med

Fracasso, Paula M. MD/PhD [Onc] - **Spec Exp:** Ovarian Cancer; Breast Cancer; Gynecologic Cancer; **Hospital:** Barnes-Jewish Hosp (page 85); **Address:** 660 S Euclid, Box 8056, Washington University Sch Med, St Louis, MO 63110-1002; **Phone:** 314-454-8817; **Board Cert:** Internal Medicine 87; Medical Oncology 93; **Med School:** Yale Univ 84; **Resid:** Internal Medicine, Beth Israel Hosp 87; **Fellow:** Cancer Research, Mass Inst Tech 89; Hematology and Oncology, Tufts-New England Med Ctr 91; **Fac Appt:** Assoc Prof Med, Washington Univ, St Louis

Gerson, Stanton MD [Onc] - **Spec Exp:** Leukemia; Lymphoma, Non-Hodgkin's; Stem Cell Transplant; **Hospital:** Univ Hosps of Cleveland; **Address:** 10900 Euclid Ave, WRB 2133, Cleveland, OH 44106-4937; **Phone:** 216-844-8562; **Board Cert:** Internal Medicine 80; Medical Oncology 83; Hematology 82; **Med School:** Harvard Med Sch 77; **Resid:** Internal Medicine, Hosp of Univ Penn 80; **Fellow:** Hematology and Oncology, Hosp of Univ Penn 83; **Fac Appt:** Prof Hem, Case West Res Univ

Golomb, Harvey MD [Onc] - **Spec Exp:** Lung Cancer; Leukemia; Lymphoma; **Hospital:** Univ of Chicago Hosps; **Address:** 5841 S Maryland Ave, MC-6092, Chicago, IL 60637-1463; **Phone:** 773-702-6115; **Board Cert:** Internal Medicine 75; Medical Oncology 79; **Med School:** Univ Pittsburgh 68; **Resid:** Internal Medicine, Johns Hopkins Hosp 72; Clinical Genetics, Johns Hopkins Hosp 73; **Fellow:** Hematology and Oncology, Univ Chicago Hosps 75; **Fac Appt:** Prof Med, Univ Hlth Sci/Chicago Med Sch

Gradishar, William J MD [Onc] - **Spec Exp:** Breast Cancer; **Hospital:** Northwestern Meml Hosp; **Address:** 676 N St Claire St, Ste 850, Chicago, IL 60611; **Phone:** 312-695-0990; **Board Cert:** Internal Medicine 85; Medical Oncology 89; **Med School:** Univ IL Coll Med 82; **Resid:** Internal Medicine, Michael Reese Hosp 85; **Fellow:** Hematology and Oncology, Univ Chicago Hosps 90; **Fac Appt:** Assoc Prof Med, Northwestern Univ

Gruber, Stephen Bernard MD/PhD [Onc] - **Spec Exp:** Cancer Genetics; Colon & Rectal Cancer; Melanoma; **Hospital:** Univ Michigan Hlth Sys; **Address:** Univ. Michigan-4301 MSRB III, 1150 W Medical Ctr. Dr., Ann Arbor, MI 48109-0638; **Phone:** 734-763-2532; **Board Cert:** Medical Oncology 98; Internal Medicine 95; **Med School:** Univ Pennsylvania 92; **Resid:** Internal Medicine, Univ Penn 94; **Fellow:** Medical Oncology, Johns Hopkins Hosp 97; Clinical Genetics, Univ Michigan Hlth Sys 99; **Fac Appt:** Asst Prof Med, Univ Mich Med Sch

Hartmann, Lynn Carol MD [Onc] - **Spec Exp:** Breast Cancer; Ovarian Cancer; **Hospital:** Mayo Med Ctr & Clin - Rochester; **Address:** Mayo Clinic (E12A), 200 First St SW, Rochester, MN 55905; **Phone:** 507-284-3903; **Board Cert:** Internal Medicine 86; Medical Oncology 89; **Med School:** Northwestern Univ 83; **Resid:** Internal Medicine, Univ Ia Hosps/Clinics 86; **Fellow:** Medical Oncology, Mayo Med Fdn 89

Hayes, Daniel Fleming MD [Onc] - **Spec Exp:** Breast Cancer; **Hospital:** Univ Michigan Hlth Sys; **Address:** Comp Cancer Ctr & Geriatrics Ctr, 1500 E Med Ctr Drive, rm 6312, Box 0942, Ann Arbor, MI 48109-0942; **Phone:** 734-615-6725; **Board Cert:** Internal Medicine 82; Medical Oncology 85; **Med School:** Indiana Univ 79; **Resid:** Internal Medicine, Parkland Meml Hosp 82; **Fellow:** Medical Oncology, Dana Farber Cancer Inst 85; **Fac Appt:** Prof Med, Univ Mich Med Sch

Hoffman, Philip C MD [Onc] - **Spec Exp:** Lung Cancer; Breast Cancer; Esophageal Cancer; **Hospital:** Univ of Chicago Hosps; **Address:** 5841 S Maryland Ave, MC 2115, Chicago, IL 60637-1463; **Phone:** 773-834-7424; **Board Cert:** Internal Medicine 75; Hematology 80; Medical Oncology 81; **Med School:** Jefferson Med Coll 72; **Resid:** Internal Medicine, Hosp Univ Penn 75; **Fellow:** Hematology and Oncology, Univ Chicago Hosps 80; **Fac Appt:** Prof Med, Univ Chicago-Pritzker Sch Med

Hussain, Maha H MD [Onc] - **Spec Exp:** Prostate Cancer; Bladder Cancer; Testicular Cancer; **Hospital:** Univ Michigan Hlth Sys; **Address:** University of Michigan Cancer Ctr, 1500 E Medical Drive, Ann Arbor, MI 48109; **Phone:** 734-936-8906; **Board Cert:** Internal Medicine 86; Medical Oncology 89; **Med School:** Iraq 80; **Resid:** Internal Medicine, Wayne State Univ Affil Hosps 86; **Fellow:** Medical Oncology, Wayne State Univ Affil Hosps 89

Hussein, Mohamad Ahmed MD [Onc] - **Spec Exp:** Multiple Myeloma; Amyloidosis; Plasmacytoma; **Hospital:** Cleveland Clin Fdn (page 92); **Address:** Cleveland Clinic, Taussig Cancer Ctr, 9500 Euclid Ave, Desk R35, Cleveland, OH 44195; **Phone:** 216-445-6830; **Board Cert:** Internal Medicine 86; Medical Oncology 89; **Med School:** Egypt 81; **Resid:** Internal Medicine, Univ Miss Med Ctr 85; Internal Medicine, Cleveland Clin Fdn 86; **Fellow:** Hematology and Oncology, Univ Md Cancer Ctr 89

Ingle, James N MD [Onc] - **Spec Exp:** Breast Cancer; **Hospital:** Rochester Meth Hosp; **Address:** Mayo Clinic, 200 First St SW, 12 East, Rochester, MN 55905; **Phone:** 507-284-8432; **Board Cert:** Internal Medicine 74; Medical Oncology 75; **Med School:** Johns Hopkins Univ 71; **Resid:** Internal Medicine, Johns Hopkins Hosp 76; Medical Oncology, Natl Cancer Inst 75; **Fac Appt:** Prof Med, Mayo Med Sch

Jahanzeb, Mohammad MD [Onc] - **Spec Exp:** Breast Cancer; Lung Cancer; **Hospital:** Meth Healthcare Central - Univ Hosp; **Address:** Univ Tennessee Coll Med, Div Hem/Onc, 1331 Union Ave, Ste 800, Memphis, MN 38104; **Phone:** 901-722-0532; **Board Cert:** Hematology 94; Medical Oncology 03; **Med School:** Pakistan 86; **Resid:** Internal Medicine, New Britain Genl Hosp 90; **Fellow:** Hematology and Oncology, Washington Univ 93; **Fac Appt:** Prof Med, Univ Tenn Coll Med, Memphis

Kalaycio, Matt E MD [Onc] - **Spec Exp:** Leukemia; **Hospital:** Cleveland Clin Fdn (page 92); **Address:** Taussig Cancer Ctr, 9500 Euclid Ave, Desk R35, Cleveland, OH 44195; **Phone:** 216-444-3705; **Board Cert:** Internal Medicine 02; Hematology 94; Medical Oncology 95; **Med School:** W VA Univ 88; **Resid:** Internal Medicine, Mercy Hosp 91; **Fellow:** Hematology and Oncology, Cleveland Clinic 94; **Fac Appt:** Assoc Prof Med, Cleveland Cl Coll Med/Case West Res

Kindler, Hedy Lee MD [Onc] - **Spec Exp:** Mesothelioma; Pancreatic Cancer; Colon & Rectal Cancer; **Hospital:** Univ of Chicago Hosps; **Address:** 5841 S Maryland Ave, Ste MC 2115, Univ Chicago Hospitals, Chicago, IL 60637; **Phone:** 773-702-2036; **Board Cert:** Internal Medicine 02; Medical Oncology 95; **Med School:** SUNY Buffalo 85; **Resid:** Internal Medicine, UCLA Med Ctr; **Fellow:** Medical Oncology, Meml Sloan Kettering Cancer Ctr; **Fac Appt:** Asst Prof Med, Univ Chicago-Pritzker Sch Med

Kosova, Leonard MD [Onc] - **Spec Exp:** Breast Cancer; Lymphoma; Lung Cancer; **Hospital:** Adv Luth Genl Hosp; **Address:** 8915 W Golf Rd, Ste 3, Niles, IL 60714-5825; **Phone:** 847-827-9060; **Board Cert:** Internal Medicine 74; Hematology 72; Medical Oncology 75; **Med School:** Univ IL Coll Med 61; **Resid:** Internal Medicine, Hines VA Hosp 64; **Fellow:** Hematology and Oncology, Hektoen Inst-Cook Cty Hosp 65

Lippman, Marc E MD [Onc] - **Spec Exp:** Breast Cancer; **Hospital:** Univ Michigan Hlth Sys; **Address:** Univ Mich Health Systems, 3101 Taubman Ctr, 1500 E Medical Ctr Dr, Ann Arbor, MI 48109-0368; **Phone:** 734-936-6000; **Board Cert:** Internal Medicine 87; Endocrinology 75; Medical Oncology 77; **Med School:** Yale Univ 68; **Resid:** Internal Medicine, Johns Hopkins Hosp 70; **Fellow:** Medical Oncology, Natl Cancer Inst 73; Endocrinology, Yale-New Haven Hosp 74; **Fac Appt:** Prof Med, Univ Mich Med Sch

Loehrer, Patrick J MD [Onc] - **Spec Exp:** Gastrointestinal Cancer; Thymoma; Genitourinary Cancer; **Hospital:** Indiana Univ Hosp (page 90); **Address:** Indiana Cancer Pavilion, 535 Barnhill Drive, rm 473, Indianapolis, IN 46202; **Phone:** 317-278-7418; **Board Cert:** Internal Medicine 81; Medical Oncology 83; **Med School:** Rush Med Coll 78; **Resid:** Internal Medicine, Rush-Presby-St Lukes Hosp 81; **Fellow:** Medical Oncology, Indiana Univ 83; **Fac Appt:** Prof Med, Indiana Univ

Loprinzi, Charles L MD [Onc] - **Spec Exp:** Melanoma; Breast Cancer; **Hospital:** Mayo Med Ctr & Clin - Rochester; **Address:** Mayo Clinic, Dept Med Onc, 200 First St SW, Rochester, MN 55905-0001; **Phone:** 507-284-4137; **Board Cert:** Internal Medicine 82; Medical Oncology 85; **Med School:** Oregon Hlth Sci Univ 79; **Resid:** Internal Medicine, Maricopa Co Hosp 82; **Fellow:** Medical Oncology, Univ Wisc Med Ctr 84; **Fac Appt:** Prof Onc, Mayo Med Sch

Markowitz, Sanford D MD [Onc] - **Spec Exp:** Colon & Rectal Cancer; Hereditary Cancer; **Hospital:** Univ Hosps of Cleveland; **Address:** WRB 3-127 Case Western Reserve Univ, 10900 Euclid Ave, Cleveland, OH 44106-7285; **Phone:** 216-844-3951; **Board Cert:** Internal Medicine 84; Medical Oncology 87; **Med School:** Yale Univ 80; **Resid:** Internal Medicine, Univ Chicago Hosp 84; **Fellow:** Medical Oncology, Natl Cancer Inst 86; **Fac Appt:** Prof Med, Case West Res Univ

Olopade, Olufunmilayo I F MD [Onc] - **Spec Exp:** Breast Cancer; Hereditary Cancer; Cancer Genetics/Assessment/Prevention; **Hospital:** Univ of Chicago Hosps; **Address:** 5841 S Maryland Ave, MC 2115, Chicago, IL 60637-1470; **Phone:** 773-702-6149; **Board Cert:** Internal Medicine 86; Hematology 01; Medical Oncology 89; **Med School:** Nigeria 80; **Resid:** Internal Medicine, Cook Co Hosp 86; **Fellow:** Hematology and Oncology, Univ Chicago Hosps 91; **Fac Appt:** Prof Med, Univ Chicago-Pritzker Sch Med

Overmoyer, Beth A MD [Onc] - **Spec Exp:** Breast Cancer; **Hospital:** Univ Hosps of Cleveland; **Address:** Ireland Cancer Ctr, UHC-BHC 6th Fl, Cleveland, OH 44106-5055; **Phone:** 216-844-3682; **Board Cert:** Internal Medicine 89; Hematology 96; Medical Oncology 03; **Med School:** Case West Res Univ 86; **Resid:** Internal Medicine, Hosp Univ Penn 89; **Fellow:** Hematology and Oncology, Hosp Univ Penn 93; **Fac Appt:** Asst Prof Med, Case West Res Univ

Perry, Michael MD [Onc] - **Spec Exp:** Lung Cancer; Breast Cancer; **Hospital:** Univ of Missouri Hosp & Clins; **Address:** Ellis Fischel Cancer Ctr, 115 Business Loop 70 W, DC 116.71, rm 524, Columbia, MO 65203-3299; **Phone:** 573-882-4979; **Board Cert:** Internal Medicine 87; Hematology 74; Medical Oncology 75; **Med School:** Wayne State Univ 70; **Resid:** Internal Medicine, Mayo Grad Sch 72; **Fellow:** Hematology and Oncology, Mayo Grad Sch 75; **Fac Appt:** Prof Med, Univ MO-Columbia Sch Med

Peterson, Bruce MD [Onc] - **Spec Exp:** Lymphoma; Leukemia; **Hospital:** Fairview-Univ Med Ctr - Univ Campus; **Address:** Univ Minn, Dept Med, 420 Delaware St SE, MMC 480, Minneapolis, MN 55455; **Phone:** 612-624-5631; **Board Cert:** Internal Medicine 74; Medical Oncology 77; **Med School:** Univ Minn 71; **Resid:** Internal Medicine, Fletcher Allen Hlthcare 73; Internal Medicine, Fairview-Univ Med Ctr 74; **Fellow:** Medical Oncology, Fairview-Univ Med Ctr 77; **Fac Appt:** Prof Med, Univ Minn

Picus, Joel MD [Onc] - **Spec Exp:** Pancreatic Cancer; Prostate Cancer; Colon Cancer; **Hospital:** Barnes-Jewish Hosp (page 85); **Address:** Washington University School of Medicine-Dept Medicine, 660 S Euclid Ave, Box Campus 8056, St Louis, MO 63110; **Phone:** 314-747-1367; **Board Cert:** Internal Medicine 87; Medical Oncology 89; Hematology 90; **Med School:** Harvard Med Sch 84; **Resid:** Internal Medicine, Duke Univ Med Ctr 87; **Fellow:** Hematology and Oncology, UCSF Med Ctr 91; **Fac Appt:** Assoc Prof Med, Washington Univ, St Louis

Piel, Ira MD [Onc] - **Spec Exp:** Breast Cancer; Colon Cancer; Lymphoma; **Hospital:** Lake Forest Hosp; **Address:** 900 N Westmoreland Road, Ste 105, Lake Forest, IL 60045; **Phone:** 847-234-6155; **Board Cert:** Internal Medicine 73; Medical Oncology 75; **Med School:** Univ IL Coll Med 67; **Resid:** Internal Medicine, St Lukes Hosp 72; **Fellow:** Medical Oncology, St Lukes Hosp 74; **Fac Appt:** Asst Prof Med, Rush Med Coll

Pienta, Kenneth J MD [Onc] - **Spec Exp:** Prostate Cancer; **Hospital:** Univ Michigan Hlth Sys; **Address:** Cancer Center/Geriatrics Center, 1500 E Medical Center Drive, rm 7308, Ann Arbor, MI 48109-0946; **Phone:** 734-647-3421; **Board Cert:** Internal Medicine 01; Medical Oncology 01; **Med School:** Johns Hopkins Univ 86; **Resid:** Internal Medicine, Univ Chicago Hosps 88; **Fellow:** Medical Oncology, Johns Hopkins Hosp 91; **Fac Appt:** Prof Med, Univ Mich Med Sch

Raghavan, Derek MD/PhD **[Onc]** - **Spec Exp:** Prostate Cancer; Testicular Cancer; Lung Cancer; **Hospital:** Cleveland Clin Fdn (page 92); **Address:** Cleveland Clinic Taussig Cancer Ctr, 9500 Euclid Ave, MC R35, Cleveland, OH 44195; **Phone:** 216-445-6888; **Med School:** Australia 74; **Resid:** Internal Medicine, Royal Prince Alfred Hosp 77; **Fellow:** Medical Oncology, Royal Prince Alfred Hosp 79; Medical Oncology, Royal Marsden Hosp; **Fac Appt:** Prof Med, Case West Res Univ

Ratain, Mark J MD **[Onc]** - **Spec Exp:** Solid Tumors; Drug Discovery & Development; **Hospital:** Univ of Chicago Hosps; **Address:** 5841 S Maryland Ave, MC 2115, Chicago, IL 60637; **Phone:** 773-702-6149; **Board Cert:** Internal Medicine 83; Hematology 86; Medical Oncology 85; **Med School:** Yale Univ 80; **Resid:** Internal Medicine, Johns Hopkins Hosp 83; **Fellow:** Hematology and Oncology, Univ Chicago 86; **Fac Appt:** Prof Med, Univ Chicago-Pritzker Sch Med

Richards, Jon MD/PhD **[Onc]** - **Spec Exp:** Testicular Cancer; Prostate Cancer; Melanoma; **Hospital:** Adv Luth Genl Hosp; **Address:** Cancer Care Ctr, 1700 Luther Ln, Park Ridge, IL 60068; **Phone:** 847-268-8200; **Board Cert:** Internal Medicine 98; **Med School:** Cornell Univ-Weill Med Coll 83; **Resid:** Internal Medicine, Univ Chicago Hosp 85; **Fellow:** Hematology and Oncology, Univ Chicago Hosp 88; **Fac Appt:** Asst Prof Med, Univ IL Coll Med

Rosen, Steven T MD **[Onc]** - **Spec Exp:** Hematologic Malignancies; Breast Cancer; Lymphoma; **Hospital:** Northwestern Meml Hosp; **Address:** Northwestern Univ, 303 E Chicago Ave, Olsen Pavillion, Ste 8250, Chicago, IL 60611-3013; **Phone:** 312-695-1153; **Board Cert:** Internal Medicine 79; Medical Oncology 81; Hematology 84; **Med School:** Northwestern Univ 76; **Resid:** Internal Medicine, Northwestern Univ Hosp 79; **Fellow:** Medical Oncology, Natl Cancer Inst 81; **Fac Appt:** Prof Med, Northwestern Univ

Ruckdeschel, John C MD **[Onc]** - **Spec Exp:** Lung Cancer; **Hospital:** Harper Univ Hosp; **Address:** Karmanos Cancer Inst-Excutive Offices, 4100 John R Fl 2, Detroit, MI 48201; **Phone:** 800-527-6266; **Board Cert:** Internal Medicine 76; Medical Oncology 77; **Med School:** Albany Med Coll 71; **Resid:** Internal Medicine, Johns Hopkins Hosp 72; Internal Medicine, Beth Israel Hosp 75; **Fellow:** Medical Oncology, Natl Cancer Inst 77; **Fac Appt:** Prof Med, Wayne State Univ

Schiffer, Charles A MD **[Onc]** - **Spec Exp:** Leukemia; Lymphoma; Multiple Myeloma; **Hospital:** Harper Univ Hosp; **Address:** Karmanos Cancer Inst, Div Hem/Onc, 4100 John R, HWCRB Fl 4, Detroit, MI 48201; **Phone:** 313-745-8910; **Board Cert:** Internal Medicine 72; Medical Oncology 73; **Med School:** NYU Sch Med 68; **Resid:** Internal Medicine, Bellevue-NY VA Hosp-NYU 72; **Fac Appt:** Prof Med, Wayne State Univ

Schiller, Joan H MD **[Onc]** - **Spec Exp:** Lung Cancer; **Hospital:** Univ WI Hosp & Clins; **Address:** 600 Highland Ave, rm K4-548 CSC, Madison, WI 53792; **Phone:** 608-263-8090; **Board Cert:** Internal Medicine 83; Medical Oncology 87; **Med School:** Univ IL Coll Med 80; **Resid:** Internal Medicine, Northwestern Meml Hosp 83; **Fellow:** Medical Oncology, Univ Wisconsin Hosp 86; **Fac Appt:** Prof Med, Univ Wisc

Schwartz, Burton S MD **[Onc]** - **Spec Exp:** Lymphoma; Breast Cancer; **Hospital:** Abbott - Northwestern Hosp; **Address:** 800 E 28th St, Piper Bldg, Ste 405, Minneapolis, MN 55417; **Phone:** 612-863-8585; **Board Cert:** Internal Medicine 80; Hematology 76; Medical Oncology 77; **Med School:** Meharry Med Coll 68; **Resid:** Internal Medicine, Michael Reese Hosp 71; **Fellow:** Hematology, Univ Minn Hosp 76; **Fac Appt:** Clin Prof Med, Univ Minn

Shapiro, Charles L MD [Onc] - **Spec Exp:** Breast Cancer; **Hospital:** Arthur G James Cancer Hosp & Research Inst (page 105); **Address:** Starling Loving Hall, rm B405, 320 W 10th Ave, Columbus, OH 43210; **Phone:** 614-293-7530; **Board Cert:** Internal Medicine 87; Medical Oncology 91; **Med School:** SUNY Buffalo 84; **Resid:** Internal Medicine, Temple Univ 87; **Fellow:** Medical Oncology, Brigham & Womens Hosp 90

Silverman, Paula MD [Onc] - **Spec Exp:** Breast Cancer; **Hospital:** Univ Hosps of Cleveland; **Address:** Univ Hosp Cleveland, Ireland Cancer Ctr, 11100 Euclid Ave, Cleveland, OH 44106; **Phone:** 216-844-8510; **Board Cert:** Internal Medicine 84; Medical Oncology 89; **Med School:** Case West Res Univ 81; **Resid:** Internal Medicine, Univ Hosps 84; **Fellow:** Hematology and Oncology, Case Western Reserve Univ 87; **Fac Appt:** Assoc Prof Med, Case West Res Univ

Sledge Jr, George W MD [Onc] - **Spec Exp:** Breast Cancer; **Hospital:** Indiana Univ Hosp (page 90); **Address:** 535 Barnhill Drive, rm 473, Indianapolis, IN 46202; **Phone:** 317-274-0920; **Board Cert:** Internal Medicine 80; Medical Oncology 83; **Med School:** Tulane Univ 77; **Resid:** Internal Medicine, St Louis Univ 80; **Fellow:** Medical Oncology, Univ Texas 83; **Fac Appt:** Prof Med, Indiana Univ

Stadler, Walter M MD [Onc] - **Spec Exp:** Kidney Cancer; Prostate Cancer; **Hospital:** Univ of Chicago Hosps; **Address:** University of Chicago Hospitals, Dept Hematology/Oncology, 5841 S Maryland Ave, MC 2115, Chicago, IL 60637; **Phone:** 773-834-7424; **Board Cert:** Internal Medicine 02; Medical Oncology 03; **Med School:** Yale Univ 88; **Resid:** Internal Medicine, Michael Reese Hosp 91; **Fellow:** Medical Oncology, Univ Chicago Hosps 94; **Fac Appt:** Assoc Prof Med, Univ Chicago-Pritzker Sch Med

Todd III, Robert F MD/PhD [Onc] - **Spec Exp:** Gastrointestinal Cancer; Lung Cancer; **Hospital:** Univ Michigan Hlth Sys; **Address:** Univ Michigan Cancer Ctr, 7216CCGC, 1500 E Med Ctr Dr, Box 0948, Ann Arbor, MI 48109; **Phone:** 734-647-8903; **Board Cert:** Internal Medicine 79; Medical Oncology 81; **Med School:** Duke Univ 76; **Resid:** Internal Medicine, Peter Bent Brigham Hosp 78; **Fellow:** Medical Oncology, Dana Farber Cancer Inst 81; **Fac Appt:** Prof Med, Univ Mich Med Sch

Urba, Susan G MD [Onc] - **Spec Exp:** Head & Neck Cancer; **Hospital:** Univ Michigan Hlth Sys; **Address:** Comp Cancer Ctr & Geriatrics Ctr, 1500 E Med Ctr Drive Bldg 371, Box 0912, Ann Arbor, MI 48109-0922; **Phone:** 734-647-8916; **Board Cert:** Internal Medicine 86; Medical Oncology 91; **Med School:** Univ Mich Med Sch 83; **Resid:** Internal Medicine, Univ Mich Med Ctr 86; **Fellow:** Hematology and Oncology, Univ Mich Med Ctr 88; **Fac Appt:** Assoc Prof Med, Univ Mich Med Sch

Vokes, Everett E MD [Onc] - **Spec Exp:** Lung Cancer; Head & Neck Cancer; Esophageal Cancer; **Hospital:** Univ of Chicago Hosps; **Address:** Univ Chicago Hosps, 5841 S Maryland Ave, Chicago, IL 60637-1470; **Phone:** 773-834-3093; **Board Cert:** Internal Medicine 83; Medical Oncology 85; **Med School:** Germany 80; **Resid:** Internal Medicine, Ravenswood Hosp-Univ Illinois 82; Internal Medicine, USC Med Ctr 83; **Fellow:** Medical Oncology, Univ Chicago 86; **Fac Appt:** Prof Med, Univ Chicago-Pritzker Sch Med

Von Roenn, Jamie H MD [Onc] - **Spec Exp:** Palliative Care; AIDS Related Cancers; Breast Cancer; **Hospital:** Northwestern Meml Hosp; **Address:** Northwestern Meml Hosp, 675 N St Clair Fl 21 - Ste 100, Chicago, IL 60611; **Phone:** 312-695-0990; **Board Cert:** Internal Medicine 83; Medical Oncology 85; **Med School:** Rush Med Coll 80; **Resid:** Internal Medicine, Rush-Presby-St Lukes Hosp 83; **Fellow:** Medical Oncology, Rush-Presby-St Lukes Hosp 85; **Fac Appt:** Prof Med, Northwestern Univ

Wade, James C MD [Onc] - **Spec Exp:** Infections in Cancer Patients; Bone Marrow Transplant; Leukemia; **Hospital:** Froedtert Meml Lutheran Hosp; **Address:** 9200 W Wisconsin Ave, Milwauke, WI 53226; **Phone:** 414-805-6800; **Board Cert:** Internal Medicine 77; Infectious Disease 82; Medical Oncology 81; **Med School:** Univ Utah 74; **Resid:** Internal Medicine, Johns Hopkins Hosp 77; **Fellow:** Medical Oncology, Natl Cancer Inst/NIH 79; Infectious Disease, Univ Wash/Fred Hutchinson Cancer Rsch Ctr 82; **Fac Appt:** Prof Med, Med Coll Wisc

Walsh, T Declan MD [Onc] - **Spec Exp:** Palliative Care; Pain-Cancer; **Hospital:** Cleveland Clin Fdn (page 92); **Address:** 9500 Euclid Ave, M76, Cleveland, OH 44195; **Phone:** 216-444-7793; **Board Cert:** Internal Medicine 86; Medical Oncology 87; **Med School:** Ireland 71; **Resid:** Internal Medicine, Bridgeport Hosp; **Fellow:** Medical Oncology, Meml Sloan Kettering Cancer Ctr 87; St Christophers Hospice

Weiner, George J MD [Onc] - **Spec Exp:** Lymphoma; Leukemia; Immunotherapy; **Hospital:** Univ Iowa Hosp & Clinics; **Address:** Holden Comprehensive Cancer Center, Univ of Iowa, 200 Hawkins Drive Bldg 5970JPP, Iowa City, IA 52242; **Phone:** 319-353-8620; **Board Cert:** Internal Medicine 85; Hematology 88; Medical Oncology 87; **Med School:** Ohio State Univ 81; **Resid:** Medical Oncology, Med Coll Ohio 84; **Fellow:** Hematology and Oncology, Univ Mich Med Ctr 87; **Fac Appt:** Prof Med, Univ Iowa Coll Med

Weissman, David E MD [Onc] - **Spec Exp:** Palliative Care; Pain-Cancer; **Hospital:** Froedtert Meml Lutheran Hosp; **Address:** Med Coll Wisc, Dept Hem/Onc, 9200 W Wisconsin Ave, Milwaukee, WI 53266-3596; **Phone:** 414-805-6800; **Board Cert:** Internal Medicine 83; Medical Oncology 85; **Med School:** UCSD 80; **Resid:** Internal Medicine, UCSD Univ Hosp 83; **Fellow:** Medical Oncology, Johns Hopkins Hosp 85; **Fac Appt:** Prof Med, Univ Wisc

Wicha, Max S MD [Onc] - **Spec Exp:** Breast Cancer; **Hospital:** Univ Michigan Hlth Sys; **Address:** Comp Cancer Ctr & Geriatrics Ctr, 1500 E Med Ctr Dr, rm 6302 CCGC, Box 0942, Ann Arbor, MI 48109-0942; **Phone:** 734-936-1831; **Board Cert:** Internal Medicine 77; Medical Oncology 83; **Med School:** Stanford Univ 74; **Resid:** Internal Medicine, Univ Chicago Hosp 77; **Fellow:** Medical Oncology, Natl Inst Hlth 80; **Fac Appt:** Prof Med, Univ Mich Med Sch

Williams, Stephen D MD [Onc] - **Spec Exp:** Testicular Cancer; Gynecologic Cancer; Genitourinary Cancer; **Hospital:** Indiana Univ Hosp (page 90); **Address:** Indiana University Cancer Ctr, 535 Barnhill Drive, rm RT 455, Inianapolis, IN 46202; **Phone:** 317-278-0070; **Board Cert:** Internal Medicine 76; Medical Oncology 79; **Med School:** Indiana Univ 71; **Resid:** Internal Medicine, Indiana Univ Hosp 75; **Fellow:** Medical Oncology, Indiana Univ Hosp 78; **Fac Appt:** Prof Med, Indiana Univ

Worden, Francis P MD [Onc] - **Spec Exp:** Head & Neck Cancer; Palliative Care; Clinical Trials; **Hospital:** Univ Michigan Hlth Sys; **Address:** Cancer Center & Geriatric Center, 1500 E Medical Center Drive, rm 4214, Ann Arbor, MI 48109; **Phone:** 734-647-8902; **Board Cert:** Internal Medicine 97; Pediatrics 98; Medical Oncology 00; **Med School:** Indiana Univ 93; **Resid:** Internal Medicine & Pediatrics, Detroit Med Ctr 97; **Fellow:** Medical Oncology, Detroit Med Ctr 20; **Fac Appt:** Asst Clin Prof Med, Univ Mich Med Sch

Yee, Douglas MD [Onc] - **Spec Exp:** Breast Cancer; **Hospital:** Fairview-Univ Med Ctr - Univ Campus; **Address:** Univ Minnesota Cancer Ctr, 420 Delaware St SE, Box 806 Mayo, Minneapolis, MN 55455; **Phone:** 612-625-5411; **Board Cert:** Internal Medicine 84; Medical Oncology 87; **Med School:** Univ Chicago-Pritzker Sch Med 81; **Resid:** Internal Medicine, Univ NC Med Ctr; **Fellow:** Medical Oncology, NIH-Clin Ctr; **Fac Appt:** Prof Med, Univ Minn

Great Plains and Mountains

Akerley, Wallace MD [Onc] - **Spec Exp:** Lung Cancer; Clinical Trials; **Hospital:** Univ Utah Hosps and Clins; **Address:** Huntsman Cancer Inst, 2000 Circle of Hope, rm 2165, Salt Lake City, UT 84112; **Phone:** 801-585-3453; **Board Cert:** Internal Medicine 84; Medical Oncology 87; Hematology 88; **Med School:** Brown Univ 81; **Resid:** Internal Medicine, USC Medical Ctr 85; **Fellow:** Medical Oncology, USC Medical Ctr 86; Hematology, Norris Cotton Cancer Ctr/Dartmouth 88; **Fac Appt:** Prof Med, Univ Utah

Armitage, James MD [Onc] - **Spec Exp:** Lymphoma; Bone Marrow Transplant; **Hospital:** Nebraska Med Ctr; **Address:** 987680 Nebraska Medical Center, Omaha, NE 68198-7680; **Phone:** 402-559-7290; **Board Cert:** Internal Medicine 76; Medical Oncology 77; Hematology 84; **Med School:** Univ Nebr Coll Med 73; **Resid:** Internal Medicine, Univ Nebraska Med Ctr 75; **Fellow:** Hematology and Oncology, Univ Iowa Hosp 77; **Fac Appt:** Prof Med, Univ Nebr Coll Med

Beatty, Patrick G MD [Onc] - **Spec Exp:** Hematologic Malignancies; Lymphoma; **Hospital:** St Patrick Hospital - Missoula; **Address:** PO Box 7877, Missoula, MT 59807; **Phone:** 406-728-2539; **Board Cert:** Internal Medicine 80; Medical Oncology 85; **Resid:** Internal Medicine, Vanderbilt U Med Ctr 79; **Fellow:** Oncology, Univ Washington Hosps 82

Bierman, Philip J MD [Onc] - **Spec Exp:** Lymphoma; Bone Marrow Transplant; **Hospital:** Nebraska Med Ctr; **Address:** Nebraska Medical Ctr, Dept Hematology/Oncology, 987680 Nebraska Medical Ctr, Omaha, NE 68198-7680; **Phone:** 402-559-5520; **Board Cert:** Internal Medicine 82; Hematology 86; Medical Oncology 85; **Med School:** Univ MO-Kansas City 79; **Resid:** Internal Medicine, U Nebraska Med Ctr 83; **Fellow:** Medical Oncology, U Nebraska Med Ctr 85; Hematology, City of Hope Natl Med Ctr 86; **Fac Appt:** Assoc Prof Med, Univ Nebr Coll Med

Bunn Jr, Paul MD [Onc] - **Spec Exp:** Lung Cancer; Lymphoma; **Hospital:** Univ Colorado Hosp; **Address:** UCCS At Fitzsimmons, Box 6511, MS 811, 12801 E 17th Ave Bldg RCQ Fl South Tower - rm 8105A, Aurora, CO 80045; **Phone:** 303-724-3155; **Board Cert:** Internal Medicine 74; Medical Oncology 75; **Med School:** Cornell Univ-Weill Med Coll 71; **Resid:** Internal Medicine, Moffitt Hosp/ UCSF Med Ctr 73; **Fellow:** Medical Oncology, Natl Cancer Inst 76; **Fac Appt:** Prof Med, Univ Colorado

Cowan, Kenneth H MD/PhD [Onc] - **Spec Exp:** Breast Cancer; **Hospital:** Nebraska Med Ctr; **Address:** Univ Nebraska Medical Ctr, Eppley Cancer Ctr, 986805 Nebraska Medical Ctr, Omaha, NE 68198-6805; **Phone:** 402-559-4090; **Board Cert:** Internal Medicine 78; Medical Oncology 81; **Med School:** Case West Res Univ 74; **Resid:** Internal Medicine, Parkland Meml Hosp 77

Dakhil, Shaker MD [Onc] - **Spec Exp:** Leukemia; Mesothelioma; Lymphoma; **Hospital:** Univ of Kansas Hosp; **Address:** Cancer Center Kansas, 818 N Emporia, Ste 403, Wichita, KS 67214; **Phone:** 316-262-4467; **Board Cert:** Internal Medicine 78; Medical Oncology 81; **Med School:** Lebanon 76; **Resid:** Internal Medicine, Wayne State Univ Hosp 78; **Fellow:** Hematology and Oncology, Univ Michigan Sch Med 81; **Fac Appt:** Assoc Clin Prof Med, Univ Kans

Ebbert, Larry P MD [Onc] - **Spec Exp:** Breast Cancer; Mesothelioma; **Hospital:** Rapid City Reg Hosp; **Address:** Rapid City Regional Hospital, Dept Medical Oncology, 353 Fairmont Blvd, Rapid City, SD 57701; **Phone:** 605-719-2301; **Board Cert:** Internal Medicine 73; Hematology 74; Medical Oncology 75; **Med School:** Ohio State Univ 69; **Resid:** Internal Medicine, Univ Missouri Med Ctr 71; **Fellow:** Hematology and Oncology, Duke Univ Med Ctr 73; **Fac Appt:** Asst Clin Prof Med, Univ SD Sch Med

Fabian, Carol J MD [Onc] - **Spec Exp:** Breast Cancer; Clinical Trials; **Hospital:** Univ of Kansas Hosp; **Address:** Univ Kansas Med Ctr, Div Clin Onc, 3901 Rainbow Blvd, Ste 1347 Bell, Kansas City, KS 66160-7418; **Phone:** 913-588-7791; **Board Cert:** Internal Medicine 76; Medical Oncology 77; **Med School:** Univ Kans 72; **Resid:** Internal Medicine, Wesley Med Ctr 75; **Fellow:** Medical Oncology, Univ Kansas Med Ctr 77; **Fac Appt:** Prof Med, Univ Kans

Glode, L Michael MD [Onc] - **Spec Exp:** Prostate Cancer; Genitourinary Cancer; **Hospital:** Univ Colorado Hosp; **Address:** U Colo Hlth Scis Ctr, Div Med Onc, PO 6510 F710, Auroa, CO 80045-0510; **Phone:** 720-848-0170; **Board Cert:** Internal Medicine 75; Medical Oncology 81; **Med School:** Washington Univ, St Louis 72; **Resid:** Internal Medicine, Univ Texas SW Med Sch 73; Immunology, Natl Inst Hlth 76; **Fellow:** Medical Oncology, Dana Farber Cancer Inst 78; **Fac Appt:** Prof Med, Univ Colorado

Grem, Jean L MD [Onc] - **Spec Exp:** Colon & Rectal Cancer; Pancreatic Cancer; Stomach & Esophageal Cancer; **Hospital:** Nebraska Med Ctr; **Address:** 987680 Nebraska Medical Ctr, Omaha, NE 68198-7680; **Phone:** 402-559-6210; **Board Cert:** Internal Medicine 83; Medical Oncology 85; **Med School:** Jefferson Med Coll 80; **Resid:** Internal Medicine, Univ Iowa Hosps & Clinics 83; **Fellow:** Medical Oncology, Univ Wisc Clin Cancer Ctr 86; **Fac Appt:** Prof Med, Univ Nebr Coll Med

Kane, Madeleine A MD/PhD [Onc] - **Spec Exp:** Head & Neck Cancer; Gastrointestinal Cancer; Neuroendocrine Tumors; **Hospital:** VA Med Ctr; **Address:** PO Box 6511, MS 8117, Aurora, CO 80045; **Phone:** 303-724-0300; **Board Cert:** Internal Medicine 81; Medical Oncology 83; Hematology 86; **Med School:** Univ Miami Sch Med 78; **Resid:** Internal Medicine, Stanford Med Ctr 81; **Fellow:** Hematology and Oncology, Univ Colo Hlth Sci Ctr 84; **Fac Appt:** Prof Med, Univ Colorado

Kelly, Karen Lee MD [Onc] - **Spec Exp:** Lung Cancer; **Hospital:** Univ Colorado Hosp; **Address:** Univ Colo Cancer Ctr, 1665 N Ursula St, Box F704, Aurora, CO 80010; **Phone:** 720-848-0300; **Board Cert:** Internal Medicine 87; Medical Oncology 93; **Med School:** Univ Kans 84; **Resid:** Internal Medicine, Univ Colo Hlth Sci Ctr; **Fellow:** Medical Oncology, Univ Colo Hlth Sci Ctr; **Fac Appt:** Assoc Prof Onc, Univ Colorado

Samlowski, Wolfram E MD [Onc] - **Spec Exp:** Kidney Cancer; Melanoma; Immunotherapy; **Hospital:** Univ Utah Hosps and Clins; **Address:** Huntsman Cancer Inst, 2000 Circle of Hope Drive, Ste 2100, Salt Lake City, UT 84112; **Phone:** 801-585-0255; **Board Cert:** Internal Medicine 81; Medical Oncology 85; **Med School:** Ohio State Univ 78; **Resid:** Internal Medicine, Wayne State Univ 81; **Fellow:** Hematology and Oncology, Univ Utah 84; **Fac Appt:** Prof Med, Univ Utah

Samuels, Brian L MD [Onc] - **Spec Exp:** Sarcoma; **Hospital:** Kootenai Med Ctr; **Address:** North Idaho Cancer Center, 700 W Ironwood Drive, Ste 103, Coeur D'Alene, ID 83814; **Phone:** 208-666-3800; **Board Cert:** Internal Medicine 84; Medical Oncology 87; **Med School:** Zimbabwe 76; **Resid:** Internal Medicine, Albert Einstein Med Ctr 81; Internal Medicine, Albert Einstein Med Ctr 84; **Fellow:** Hematology and Oncology, Univ Chicago Hosps 88; **Fac Appt:** Assoc Prof Med, Univ IL Coll Med

Ward, John Harris MD [Onc] - **Spec Exp:** Breast Cancer; Gastrointestinal Cancer; **Hospital:** Univ Utah Hosps and Clins; **Address:** Huntsman Cancer Inst, 2000 Circle of Hope, Ste 2100, Salt Lake City, UT 84112-5550; **Phone:** 801-585-0255; **Board Cert:** Internal Medicine 79; Medical Oncology 81; Hematology 82; **Med School:** Univ Utah 76; **Resid:** Internal Medicine, Duke Univ 79; **Fellow:** Hematology and Oncology, Univ Utah 82; **Fac Appt:** Prof Med, Univ Utah

Southwest

Abbruzzese, James L MD **[Onc]** - **Spec Exp:** Gastrointestinal Cancer; Pancreatic Cancer; **Hospital:** UT MD Anderson Cancer Ctr, The (page 115); **Address:** Univ Tex MD Anderson Cancer Ctr, 1515 Holcombe Blvd, Unit 426, Houston, TX 77030-4009; **Phone:** 713-792-2828; **Board Cert:** Internal Medicine 81; Medical Oncology 83; **Med School:** Univ Chicago-Pritzker Sch Med 78; **Resid:** Internal Medicine, Johns Hopkins Hosp 81; **Fellow:** Medical Oncology, Dana-Farber Cancer Inst 83; **Fac Appt:** Assoc Prof Med, Univ Tex, Houston

Ahmann, Frederick R MD **[Onc]** - **Spec Exp:** Prostate Cancer; Testicular Cancer; Bladder Cancer; **Hospital:** Univ Med Ctr - Tucson; **Address:** Arizona Cancer Ctr, 1515 N Campbell Ave, Box 245024, Tucson, AZ 85724; **Phone:** 520-626-2900; **Board Cert:** Internal Medicine 77; Medical Oncology 81; **Med School:** Univ MO-Columbia Sch Med 74; **Resid:** Internal Medicine, Georgetwon Univ Med Ctr 77; **Fellow:** Medical Oncology, Univ Med Ctr 80; **Fac Appt:** Prof Med, Univ Ariz Coll Med

Alberts, David S MD **[Onc]** - **Spec Exp:** Cancer Prevention; **Hospital:** Univ Med Ctr - Tucson; **Address:** Arizona Cancer Center, 1515N Campbell Ave, PO Box 245024, Tucson, AZ 85724; **Phone:** 520-626-7685; **Board Cert:** Internal Medicine 73; Medical Oncology 73; **Med School:** Univ VA Sch Med 66; **Resid:** Medical Oncology, Natl Canc Inst-NIH 69; Internal Medicine, Univ Minn Hosps 71; **Fellow:** Clinical Pharmacology, UC San Francisco 74; **Fac Appt:** Prof Med, Univ Ariz Coll Med

Anthony, Lowell B MD **[Onc]** - **Spec Exp:** Gastrointestinal Cancer; Carcinoid Tumors; Neuroendocrine Tumors; **Hospital:** Louisiana State Univ Hosp; **Address:** LSU-Division Hematology Oncology, 1542 Tulane Ave, Ste 604K, New Orleans, LA 70112; **Phone:** 504-568-5843; **Board Cert:** Internal Medicine 83; Medical Oncology 89; **Med School:** Vanderbilt Univ 79; **Resid:** Internal Medicine, Vanderbilt Univ Med Ctr 82; **Fellow:** Oncology, Vanderbilt Univ Med Ctr 85; **Fac Appt:** Assoc Prof Med, Louisiana State Univ

Arun, Banu K MD **[Onc]** - **Spec Exp:** Breast Cancer; Chemoprevention; Clinical Trials; **Hospital:** UT MD Anderson Cancer Ctr, The (page 115); **Address:** MD Anderson Cancer Ctr, 1515 Holcombe Blvd, Unit 424, Houston, TX 77030; **Phone:** 713-792-2817; **Med School:** Turkey 90; **Resid:** Internal Medicine, Univ Istanbul 94; **Fellow:** Hematology and Oncology, Lombardi Cancer Ctr-Georgetown Univ 97; **Fac Appt:** Assoc Prof Med, Univ Tex, Houston

Benjamin, Robert S MD **[Onc]** - **Spec Exp:** Sarcoma-Soft Tissue; Sarcoma-Bone; **Hospital:** UT MD Anderson Cancer Ctr, The (page 115); **Address:** UT MD Anderson Cancer Ctr, 1515 Holcombe Blvd, Unit 450, Houston, TX 77030; **Phone:** 713-792-3626; **Board Cert:** Internal Medicine 73; Medical Oncology 73; **Med School:** NYU Sch Med 68; **Resid:** Internal Medicine, Bellevue Hosp Ctr-NYU 70; **Fellow:** Medical Oncology, Baltimore Cancer Rsch Ctr 72; **Fac Appt:** Prof Med, Univ Tex, Houston

Bruera, Eduardo MD **[Onc]** - **Spec Exp:** Palliative Care; **Hospital:** UT MD Anderson Cancer Ctr, The (page 115); **Address:** 1515 Holcombe Ave, Unit 8, Houston, TX 77030; **Phone:** 713-792-6085; **Med School:** Argentina ; **Resid:** Internal Medicine, Hospital Privado; **Fellow:** Medical Oncology, Cross Cancer Inst; **Fac Appt:** Prof Med, Univ Tex, Houston

Buzdar, Aman U MD **[Onc]** - **Spec Exp:** Breast Cancer; **Hospital:** UT MD Anderson Cancer Ctr, The (page 115); **Address:** U Texas MD Anderson Cancer Ctr, Dept Breast Med Onc, 1515 Holcombe Blvd, Houston, TX 77030-4009; **Phone:** 713-792-2817; **Board Cert:** Internal Medicine 75; Medical Oncology 79; **Med School:** Pakistan 67; **Resid:** Internal Medicine, Norwalk Hosp 73; Internal Medicine, Lakewood Hosp 71; **Fellow:** Hematology, Norwalk Hosp 74; Oncology, MD Anderson Cancer Ctr 75; **Fac Appt:** Prof Med, Univ Tex, Houston

Fay, Joseph W MD [Onc] - **Spec Exp:** Bone Marrow Transplant; Melanoma (Vaccine Therapy); Leukemia & Lymphoma; **Hospital:** Baylor Univ Medical Ctr (page 86); **Address:** 3409 Worth St, Sammons Tower, Suite 600, Dallas, TX 75246; **Phone:** 214-370-1500; **Board Cert:** Internal Medicine 75; Medical Oncology 77; Hematology 78; **Med School:** Ohio State Univ 72; **Resid:** Internal Medicine, Duke Med Ctr 74; Oncology, Natl Cancer Institute 76; **Fellow:** Hematology, Duke Med Ctr 77; **Fac Appt:** Clin Prof Med, Univ Tex SW, Dallas

Forman, Walter B MD [Onc] - **Spec Exp:** Palliative Care; Pain-Cancer; **Hospital:** Univ NM Hlth & Sci Ctr; **Address:** Univ NM, Palliative Care - MSC11 6020, 1 University New Mexico, Albuquerque, NM 87131-0001; **Phone:** 505-272-4868; **Board Cert:** Internal Medicine 71; Hematology 72; Medical Oncology 75; **Med School:** Wayne State Univ 63; **Resid:** Internal Medicine, Metro Genl Hosp 66; **Fellow:** Pharmacology, Case West Res Univ 71; **Fac Appt:** Prof Med, Univ New Mexico

Fossella, Frank V MD [Onc] - **Spec Exp:** Lung Cancer; **Hospital:** UT MD Anderson Cancer Ctr, The (page 115); **Address:** 1515 Holcombe Blvd, Unit 432, Houston, TX 77030; **Phone:** 713-792-6363; **Board Cert:** Internal Medicine 85; Medical Oncology 87; **Med School:** Baylor Coll Med 82; **Resid:** Internal Medicine, Baylor Coll Med 85; **Fellow:** Medical Oncology, Baylor Coll Med 87; **Fac Appt:** Prof Med, Univ Tex, Houston

Glisson, Bonnie S MD [Onc] - **Spec Exp:** Head & Neck Cancer; Lung Cancer; **Hospital:** UT MD Anderson Cancer Ctr, The (page 115); **Address:** 1515 Holcombe Blvd, Unit 432, Houston, TX 77030; **Phone:** 713-792-6363; **Board Cert:** Internal Medicine 82; Medical Oncology 85; **Med School:** Ohio State Univ 79; **Resid:** Internal Medicine, Univ Va Med Ctr 82; **Fellow:** Medical Oncology, Univ Fla Health Sci Ctr 85; **Fac Appt:** Prof Med, Univ Tex, Houston

Herbst, Roy S MD/PhD [Onc] - **Spec Exp:** Lung Cancer; Head & Neck Cancer; Clinical Trials; **Hospital:** UT MD Anderson Cancer Ctr, The (page 115); **Address:** MD Anderson Cancer Ctr, 1515 Holcombe Blvd, Unit 432, Houston, TX 77030; **Phone:** 713-792-6363; **Board Cert:** Internal Medicine 94; Medical Oncology 97; **Med School:** Cornell Univ-Weill Med Coll 91; **Resid:** Internal Medicine, Brigham & Women's Hosp 94; **Fellow:** Medical Oncology, Dana Farber Cancer Inst 96; **Fac Appt:** Assoc Prof Med, Univ Tex, Houston

Hong, Waun Ki MD [Onc] - **Spec Exp:** Lung Cancer; Head & Neck Cancer; **Hospital:** UT MD Anderson Cancer Ctr, The (page 115); **Address:** 1515 Holcombe Blvd, Unit 421, Houston, TX 77030; **Phone:** 713-745-6791; **Board Cert:** Internal Medicine 76; Medical Oncology 79; **Med School:** South Korea 67; **Resid:** Internal Medicine, Boston VA Hosp 73; **Fellow:** Medical Oncology, Meml Sloan-Kettering Cancer Ctr 75; **Fac Appt:** Prof Onc, Univ Tex, Houston

Hortobagyi, Gabriel N MD [Onc] - **Spec Exp:** Breast Cancer; **Hospital:** UT MD Anderson Cancer Ctr, The (page 115); **Address:** UT MD Anderson Cancer Ctr, Dept Breast Onc, 1515 Holcombe Blvd, Unit 424, Houston, TX 77030; **Phone:** 713-792-2817; **Board Cert:** Internal Medicine 75; Medical Oncology 77; **Med School:** Colombia 70; **Resid:** Internal Medicine, St Lukes Hosp 74; **Fellow:** Medical Oncology, MD Anderson Cancer Ctr 76; **Fac Appt:** Prof Med, Univ Tex, Houston

Hutchins, Laura MD [Onc] - **Spec Exp:** Breast Cancer; Melanoma; **Hospital:** UAMS Med Ctr; **Address:** Univ Arkansas Med Scis, Dept Hem/Onc, 4301 W Markham St, MS 508, Little Rock, AR 72205-7101; **Phone:** 501-686-8511; **Board Cert:** Internal Medicine 80; Hematology 84; Medical Oncology 87; **Med School:** Univ Ark 77; **Resid:** Internal Medicine, Univ Ark Med Scis 80; **Fellow:** Hematology and Oncology, Univ Ark Med Scis 83; **Fac Appt:** Prof Med, Univ Ark

Jones, Stephen E MD [Onc] - **Spec Exp:** Breast Cancer; **Hospital:** Baylor Univ Medical Ctr (page 86); **Address:** Baylor-Sammons Cancer Ctr, 3535 Worth St, Dallas, TX 75246; **Phone:** 214-370-1000; **Board Cert:** Internal Medicine 72; Medical Oncology 73; **Med School:** Case West Res Univ 66; **Resid:** Internal Medicine, Stanford Univ Hosp 68; **Fellow:** Medical Oncology, Stanford Univ 72; **Fac Appt:** Prof Med, Baylor Coll Med

Karp, Daniel David MD [Onc] - **Spec Exp:** Lung Cancer; **Hospital:** UT MD Anderson Cancer Ctr, The (page 115); **Address:** 1515 Holcombe Blvd, Unit 421, Houston, TX 77030; **Phone:** 713-792-6110; **Board Cert:** Internal Medicine 76; Hematology 80; Medical Oncology 81; **Med School:** Duke Univ 73; **Resid:** Internal Medicine, Dartmouth-Hitchcock Med Ctr 76; **Fellow:** Hematology, Dartmouth-Hitchcock Med Ctr 78; Medical Oncology, Dana Farber Inst 79; **Fac Appt:** Prof Med, Univ Tex, Houston

Kies, Merrill S MD [Onc] - **Spec Exp:** Head & Neck Cancer; Lung Cancer; **Hospital:** UT MD Anderson Cancer Ctr, The (page 115); **Address:** Dept Thoracic, Head & Neck Oncology, 1515 Holcombe Unit 432 Blvd, Houston, TX 77030; **Phone:** 713-792-6363; **Board Cert:** Internal Medicine 76; Medical Oncology 79; **Med School:** Loyola Univ-Stritch Sch Med 73; **Resid:** Internal Medicine, Walter Reed AMC 76; **Fellow:** Medical Oncology, Brooke AMC 78; **Fac Appt:** Prof Med, Univ Tex, Houston

Kwak, Larry W MD [Onc] - **Spec Exp:** Lymphoma; Multiple Myeloma; **Hospital:** UT MD Anderson Cancer Ctr, The (page 115); **Address:** M.D. Anderson Cancer Ctr, Dept Lymphoma/Myeloma, 1515 Holcombe Blvd, Ste 429, Houston, TX 77030; **Phone:** 713-745-4244; **Board Cert:** Internal Medicine 87; Medical Oncology 89; **Med School:** Northwestern Univ 82; **Resid:** Internal Medicine, Stanford Univ Hosp 87; **Fellow:** Oncology, Stanford Univ Hosp 89; **Fac Appt:** Prof Med, Univ Tex, Houston

Legha, Sewa Singh MD [Onc] - **Spec Exp:** Melanoma; Breast Cancer; Thyroid & Adrenal Cancers; **Hospital:** St Luke's Episcopal Hosp - Houston; **Address:** 6624 Fannin, Ste 1440, Houston, TX 77030; **Phone:** 713-797-9711; **Board Cert:** Internal Medicine 87; Medical Oncology 77; **Med School:** India 70; **Resid:** Internal Medicine, Milwaukee Co Genl Hosp/Med Coll Wisc 74; Medical Oncology, Natl Cancer Inst 76; **Fellow:** Medical Oncology, MD Anderson Hosp 77; **Fac Appt:** Clin Prof Med, Baylor Coll Med

Lippman, Scott M MD [Onc] - **Spec Exp:** Cancer Prevention; Lung Cancer; Head & Neck Cancer; **Hospital:** UT MD Anderson Cancer Ctr, The (page 115); **Address:** UTMD Anderson Cancer Ctr, Unit 1360, 1515 Holcombe Blvd, P.O.Box 301439, Houston, TX 77230-1439; **Phone:** 713-745-3672; **Board Cert:** Internal Medicine 87; Hematology 88; Medical Microbiology 89; **Med School:** Johns Hopkins Univ 81; **Resid:** Internal Medicine, Harbor-UCLA Med Ctr 83; **Fellow:** Hematology, Stanford Univ Med Ctr 85; Hematology and Oncology, Univ Ariz Hlth Scis Ctr 87; **Fac Appt:** Prof Med, Univ Tex, Houston

Logothetis, Christopher J MD [Onc] - **Spec Exp:** Prostate Cancer; Bladder Cancer; **Hospital:** UT MD Anderson Cancer Ctr, The (page 115); **Address:** UT MD Anderson Cancer Ctr, 1515 Holcombe Blvd, Unit 427, Houston, TX 77030-4009; **Phone:** 713-792-2830; **Board Cert:** Internal Medicine 78; Medical Oncology 81; **Med School:** Greece 74; **Resid:** Internal Medicine, Univ Texas 79; **Fellow:** Hematology and Oncology, Univ Tex-MD Anderson Cancer Ctr 81; **Fac Appt:** Prof Onc, Univ Tex, Houston

Markman, Maurie MD [Onc] - **Spec Exp:** Ovarian Cancer; Gynecologic Cancer; **Hospital:** UT MD Anderson Cancer Ctr, The (page 115); **Address:** Univ Texas MD Anderson Cancer Ctr, 1515 Holcombe Blvd, Box 121, Houston, TX 77030-4009; **Phone:** 713-745-7140; **Board Cert:** Internal Medicine 77; Hematology 82; Medical Oncology 81; **Med School:** NYU Sch Med 74; **Resid:** Internal Medicine, Bellevue Hosp Ctr 78; **Fellow:** Medical Oncology, Johns Hopkins Hosp 80; **Fac Appt:** Prof Med, Univ Tex, Houston

Miller, Thomas P MD [Onc] - **Spec Exp:** Lymphoma; **Hospital:** Univ Med Ctr - Tucson; **Address:** Arizona Cancer Ctr, 1515 N Campbell Ave, PO Box 245024, Tucson, AZ 85724; **Phone:** 520-626-2667; **Board Cert:** Internal Medicine 77; Medical Oncology 81; **Med School:** Univ IL Coll Med 72; **Resid:** Internal Medicine, Univ Illinois Hosps 77; **Fellow:** Hematology and Oncology, Univ Med Ctr 80; **Fac Appt:** Prof Med, Univ Ariz Coll Med

Millikan, Randall MD/PhD [Onc] - **Spec Exp:** Bladder Cancer; Genitourinary Cancer; Clinical Trials; **Hospital:** UT MD Anderson Cancer Ctr, The (page 115); **Address:** 1201 Mulberry Ln, Bellaire, TX 77401; **Phone:** 713-792-2830; **Board Cert:** Internal Medicine 91; Medical Oncology 95; **Med School:** Univ Miami Sch Med 88; **Resid:** Internal Medicine, Mayo Clinic 91; **Fellow:** Medical Oncology, Mayo Clinic 94; **Fac Appt:** Assoc Prof Med, Univ Tex, Houston

Nemunaitis, John G MD [Onc] - **Spec Exp:** Cancer Genetics; Vaccine Therapy; Lung Cancer; **Hospital:** Baylor Univ Medical Ctr (page 86); **Address:** Mary Crowley Med Rsch Ctr, 3535 Worth St, Collins Bldg, Ste 302, Dallas, TX 75246; **Phone:** 214-370-1870; **Board Cert:** Internal Medicine 87; Physical Medicine & Rehabilitation 68; **Med School:** Case West Res Univ 82; **Resid:** Internal Medicine, Boston City Hosp 85; **Fellow:** Hematology and Oncology, Fred Hutchenson Cancer Rsch Ctr

O'Brien, Susan M MD [Onc] - **Spec Exp:** Leukemia; Lymphoma; **Hospital:** UT MD Anderson Cancer Ctr, The (page 115); **Address:** Univ Texas MD Anderson Cancer Ctr, 1515 Holcombe Blvd, Box 428, Houston, TX 77030; **Phone:** 713-792-7305; **Board Cert:** Internal Medicine 83; Medical Oncology 87; **Med School:** UMDNJ-NJ Med Sch, Newark 80; **Resid:** Internal Medicine, UMDNJ Med Ctr 83; **Fellow:** Medical Oncology, Univ TX MD Anderson Med Ctr 87; **Fac Appt:** Prof Med, Univ Tex, Houston

O'Shaughnessy, Joyce A MD [Onc] - **Spec Exp:** Breast Cancer; **Hospital:** Baylor Univ Medical Ctr (page 86); **Address:** US Oncology, 3535 Worth St, Collins 5, Dallas, TX 75246; **Phone:** 214-370-1000; **Board Cert:** Internal Medicine 85; Medical Oncology 87; **Med School:** Yale Univ 82; **Resid:** Internal Medicine, Mass Genl Hosp 85; **Fellow:** Medical Oncology, National Cancer Inst 88

Osborne, Charles K MD [Onc] - **Spec Exp:** Breast Cancer; **Hospital:** Methodist Hosp - Houston; **Address:** 1 Baylor Plaza, BCM 600, Cullen 335A, Houston, TX 77030; **Phone:** 713-798-1641; **Board Cert:** Internal Medicine 75; Medical Oncology 77; **Med School:** Univ MO-Columbia Sch Med 72; **Resid:** Internal Medicine, Johns Hopkins Hosp 74; **Fellow:** Medical Oncology, Natl Cancer Inst 77; **Fac Appt:** Prof Med, Baylor Coll Med

Papadopoulos, Nicholas E MD [Onc] - **Spec Exp:** Melanoma; **Hospital:** UT MD Anderson Cancer Ctr, The (page 115); **Address:** 1515 Holcombe Blvd, rm 11.3004, Houston, TX 77030; **Phone:** 713-792-2821; **Med School:** Greece ; **Resid:** Internal Medicine, Baylor Coll Med 76; **Fellow:** Medical Oncology, MD Anderson Cancer Ctr 78; **Fac Appt:** Assoc Prof Med, Univ Tex, Houston

Patt, Yehuda Z MD [Onc] - **Spec Exp:** Liver Cancer; Biliary Cancer; Colon & Rectal Cancer; **Hospital:** Univ NM Hlth & Sci Ctr; **Address:** Univ New Mexico CRTC, Div Hem/Onc, 900 Camino de Salud NE, MSC 084630, Albuquerque, NM 87131-0001; **Phone:** 505-272-5837; **Board Cert:** Internal Medicine 82; Medical Oncology 87; **Med School:** Israel 67; **Resid:** Internal Medicine, Tel Aviv-Sheba Med Ctr 74; **Fellow:** Medical Oncology, UT MD Anderson Cancer Ctr 77; **Fac Appt:** Prof Med, Univ New Mexico

Pisters, Katherine M W MD [Onc] - **Spec Exp:** Lung Cancer; **Hospital:** UT MD Anderson Cancer Ctr, The (page 115); **Address:** UT MD Anderson Cancer Ctr, PO Box 301402 Unit 432, Houston, TX 77030-1402; **Phone:** 713-792-6363; **Board Cert:** Internal Medicine 88; Medical Oncology 02; **Med School:** Canada 85; **Resid:** Internal Medicine, N Shore Univ Hosp 88; **Fellow:** Medical Oncology, Meml Sloan Kettering Cancer Ctr 91; **Fac Appt:** Assoc Prof Med, Univ Tex, Houston

Saiki, John H MD [Onc] - **Hospital:** Univ NM Hlth & Sci Ctr; **Address:** Univ of New Mexico Cancer Ctr, 900 Camino de Salud NE, MSC 084630, Albuquerque, NM 87131-0001; **Phone:** 505-272-5837; **Board Cert:** Internal Medicine 70; Medical Oncology 73; **Med School:** McGill Univ 61; **Resid:** Internal Medicine, Univ New Mexico 68; Hematology, Univ New Mexico 69; **Fellow:** Medical Oncology, MD Anderson Hosp 70; **Fac Appt:** Prof Med, Univ New Mexico

Salem, Philip Adeeb MD [Onc] - **Spec Exp:** Breast Cancer; Lymphoma; **Hospital:** St Luke's Episcopal Hosp - Houston; **Address:** 6624 Fannin St, Ste 1630, Houston, TX 77030; **Phone:** 713-796-1221; **Med School:** Lebanon 65; **Resid:** Medical Oncology, Meml Sloan Kettering Cancer Ctr 70; **Fellow:** Oncology Research, MD Anderson Cancer Ctr 72; **Fac Appt:** Clin Prof Med, Univ Tex, Houston

Takimoto, Chris H MD/PhD [Onc] - **Spec Exp:** Gastrointestinal Cancer; **Hospital:** UTSA - Univ Hosp; **Address:** Inst for Drug Developmt-Cancer Therapy & Rsch Ctr, 7979 Wurzbach Rd, rm Z414, San Antonio, TX 78229; **Phone:** 210-562-1725; **Board Cert:** Internal Medicine 89; Medical Oncology 93; **Med School:** Yale Univ 86; **Resid:** Internal Medicine, UCSF Med Ctr 89; **Fac Appt:** Assoc Prof Med, Univ Tex, San Antonio

Tripathy, Debasish MD [Onc] - **Spec Exp:** Breast Cancer; Clinical Trials; **Hospital:** UTSW Med Ctr - Dallas; **Address:** Univ Texas SW Med Ctr, 5323 Harry Hines Blvd, Dallas, TX 75390; **Phone:** 214-648-4180; **Board Cert:** Internal Medicine 88; Medical Oncology 01; **Med School:** Duke Univ 85; **Resid:** Internal Medicine, Duke Univ Med Ctr 88; **Fellow:** Hematology and Oncology, USCF Med Ctr 91; **Fac Appt:** Prof Med, Univ Tex SW, Dallas

Valero, Vicente MD [Onc] - **Spec Exp:** Breast Cancer; **Hospital:** UT MD Anderson Cancer Ctr, The (page 115); **Address:** Univ Texas MD Anderson Cancer Ctr, 1515 Holcombe Blvd, Unit 424, Houston, TX 77030; **Phone:** 713-792-2817; **Board Cert:** Internal Medicine 85; Hematology 88; Medical Oncology 87; **Med School:** Mexico 80; **Resid:** Internal Medicine, Univ Cincinnati Med Ctr 85; Hematology and Oncology, Univ Cincinnati Med Ctr 87; **Fellow:** Hematology and Oncology, Univ Texas Med Br 88; **Fac Appt:** Prof Med, Univ Tex, Houston

Verschraegen, Claire F MD [Onc] - **Spec Exp:** Ovarian Cancer; Drug Discovery; **Hospital:** Univ NM Hlth & Sci Ctr; **Address:** UNM Cancer Research & Treatment Ctr, 900 Camino de Salud NE, rm MS C084630, Albuquerque, NM 87131-0001; **Phone:** 505-272-5837; **Board Cert:** Internal Medicine 00; Medical Oncology 00; **Med School:** Belgium 82; **Resid:** Internal Medicine, Bordet 85; Internal Medicine, Univ Texas 90; **Fellow:** Cancer Research, Stehlin Fdn for Cancer Research 88; Oncology, MD Anderson Cancer Ctr 94; **Fac Appt:** Assoc Prof Med, Univ New Mexico

Von Hoff, Daniel D MD [Onc] - **Spec Exp:** Pancreatic Cancer; Breast Cancer; Drug Discovery; **Hospital:** Scottsdale Hlthcare - Shea; **Address:** Translational Genomics Research Institute, 400 N. 5th St. Ste 1600, Phoenix, AZ 85004; **Phone:** 602-343-8492; **Board Cert:** Internal Medicine 76; Medical Oncology 79; **Med School:** Columbia P&S 73; **Resid:** Internal Medicine, UCSF Med Ctr 75; **Fac Appt:** Prof Med, Univ Ariz Coll Med

West Coast and Pacific

Abrams, Donald Ira MD [Onc] - **Spec Exp:** AIDS Related Cancers; **Hospital:** San Francisco Genl Hosp; **Address:** Positive Hlth Program, 995 Potrero Ave, Bldg 80, Ward 84, San Francisco, CA 94110; **Phone:** 415-476-4082 x444; **Board Cert:** Internal Medicine 80; Medical Oncology 83; **Med School:** Stanford Univ 77; **Resid:** Internal Medicine, Kaiser Fdn Hosp 80; **Fellow:** Medical Oncology, UCSF Cancer Rsch 82; **Fac Appt:** Clin Prof Med, UCSF

Appelbaum, Frederick R MD [Onc] - **Spec Exp:** Bone Marrow Transplant; Leukemia; **Hospital:** Univ Wash Med Ctr; **Address:** 1100 Fairview Ave N, PO Box 19024, Seattle, WA 98109; **Phone:** 206-667-5000; **Board Cert:** Internal Medicine 75; Medical Oncology 77; **Med School:** Tufts Univ 72; **Resid:** Internal Medicine, Univ Michigan Med Ctr 74; **Fellow:** Medical Oncology, Natl Cancer Inst 76; **Fac Appt:** Prof Med, Univ Wash

Ball, Edward David MD [Onc] - **Spec Exp:** Bone Marrow & Stem Cell Transplant; Leukemia & Lymphoma; Multiple Myeloma; **Hospital:** UCSD Med Ctr; **Address:** 9500 Gilman Drive, La Jolla, CA 92093-0960; **Phone:** 858-657-7053; **Board Cert:** Internal Medicine 79; Medical Oncology 83; Hematology 00; **Med School:** Case West Res Univ 76; **Resid:** Internal Medicine, Hartford Hosp 79; **Fellow:** Hematology, Univ Hosps Cleveland 81; Hematology and Oncology, Dartmouth-Hitchcock Hosp 82; **Fac Appt:** Prof Med, UCSD

Bensinger, William I MD [Onc] - **Spec Exp:** Multiple Myeloma; Stem Cell Transplant; **Hospital:** Univ Wash Med Ctr; **Address:** Fred Hutchinson Cancer Research Ctr, 1100 Fairview Ave N, D5-390, PO Box 19024, Seattle, WA 98109-1024; **Phone:** 206-288-1024; **Board Cert:** Internal Medicine 78; Medical Oncology 79; **Med School:** Northwestern Univ 73; **Resid:** Internal Medicine, Univ Wash Hosps 78; **Fellow:** Oncology, Univ Wash Hosps 79; **Fac Appt:** Assoc Prof Med, Univ Wash

Blanke, Charles D MD [Onc] - **Spec Exp:** Colon & Rectal Cancer; Gastrointestinal Cancer; **Hospital:** OR Hlth & Sci Univ; **Address:** Oregon Hlth Sci Ctr, 3181 SW Sam Jackson Park Rd, MC L586, Portland, OR 97239; **Phone:** 503-494-8469; **Board Cert:** Internal Medicine 91; Medical Oncology 95; **Med School:** Northwestern Univ 88; **Resid:** Internal Medicine, LaCrosse Lutheran Hosp 91; **Fellow:** Medical Oncology, Clarian-Indiana Univ; **Fac Appt:** Assoc Prof Med, Oregon Hlth Sci Univ

Carlson, Robert Wells MD [Onc] - **Spec Exp:** Breast Cancer; **Hospital:** Stanford Univ Med Ctr; **Address:** Dept Medicine, 875 Blake Wilbur Drive, Stanford, CA 94305; **Phone:** 650-723-7621; **Board Cert:** Internal Medicine 81; Medical Oncology 83; **Med School:** Stanford Univ 78; **Resid:** Internal Medicine, Barnes Hosp Group 80; Internal Medicine, Stanford Univ Hosp 81; **Fellow:** Medical Oncology, Stanford Univ Hosp 83; **Fac Appt:** Prof Med, Stanford Univ

Chap, Linnea MD [Onc] - **Spec Exp:** Breast Cancer; **Hospital:** UCLA Med Ctr (page 111); **Address:** UCLA/ Santa Monica Cancer Ctr, 2336 Santa Monica Blvd, Ste 301, Santa Monica, CA 90404; **Phone:** 310-829-5471; **Board Cert:** Internal Medicine 91; Hematology 94; Medical Oncology 95; **Med School:** Univ Chicago-Pritzker Sch Med 88; **Resid:** Internal Medicine, Northwestern Meml Hosp 91; **Fellow:** Hematology and Oncology, UCLA Med Ctr 92

Chlebowski, Rowan T MD/PhD [Onc] - **Spec Exp:** Breast Cancer; Women's Health; **Hospital:** LAC - Harbor - UCLA Med Ctr; **Address:** 1000 W Carson St Bldg J3, Torrance, CA 90502; **Phone:** 310-222-2218; **Board Cert:** Internal Medicine 80; Medical Oncology 81; **Med School:** Case West Res Univ 74; **Resid:** Internal Medicine, MetroHealth Med Ctr 76; Medical Oncology, LAC-USC Med Ctr 79; **Fac Appt:** Prof Onc, UCLA

Disis, Mary Lenora MD [Onc] - **Spec Exp:** Breast Cancer; Ovarian Cancer; Clinical Trials; **Hospital:** Univ Wash Med Ctr; **Address:** Univ Washington Med Ctr, Div Oncology, 1959 NE Pacific St, Box 356527, Seattle, WA 98195; **Phone:** 206-616-1823; **Board Cert:** Internal Medicine 89; Medical Oncology 97; **Med School:** Univ Nebr Coll Med 86; **Resid:** Internal Medicine, Univ Illinois Med Ctr 90; **Fellow:** Medical Oncology, Fred Hutchinson Cancer Ctr 93; **Fac Appt:** Assoc Prof Med, Univ Wash

Forscher, Charles Adley MD [Onc] - **Spec Exp:** Bone Tumors; Sarcoma-Soft Tissue; **Hospital:** Cedars-Sinai Med Ctr (page 88); **Address:** Cedars Sinai Comprehensive Cancer Ctr, 8700 Beverly Blvd, Los Angeles, CA 90048; **Phone:** 310-423-8045; **Board Cert:** Internal Medicine 81; Hematology 86; Medical Oncology 87; **Med School:** Albert Einstein Coll Med 78; **Resid:** Infectious Disease, Montefiore Med Ctr 81; **Fellow:** Hematology, Montefiore Med Ctr 83; Neoplastic Diseases, Mt Sinai Med Ctr 85; **Fac Appt:** Clin Prof Med, UCLA

Gandara, David R MD [Onc] - **Spec Exp:** Lung Cancer; **Hospital:** UC Davis Med Ctr; **Address:** UC Davis Cancer Ctr, 4501 X St, Ste 3016, Sacramento, CA 95817; **Phone:** 916-734-5959; **Board Cert:** Internal Medicine 76; Medical Oncology 79; **Med School:** Univ Tex Med Br, Galveston 73; **Resid:** Internal Medicine, Madigan Med Ctr 76; **Fellow:** Hematology and Oncology, Letterman AMC 78; **Fac Appt:** Asst Prof Med, UC Davis

Ganz, Patricia Anne MD [Onc] - **Spec Exp:** Breast Cancer; **Hospital:** UCLA Med Ctr (page 111); **Address:** UCLA -Div Canc Prev & Control Rsch, A2-125 CHS, 650 Charles Young Drive S, Box 956900, Los Angeles, CA 90095; **Phone:** 310-206-1404; **Board Cert:** Internal Medicine 76; Medical Oncology 79; **Med School:** UCLA 73; **Resid:** Internal Medicine, UCLA Med Ctr 76; **Fellow:** Hematology, UCLA Med Ctr 78; **Fac Appt:** Prof Med, UCLA

Horning, Sandra J MD [Onc] - **Spec Exp:** Hodgkin's Disease; Bone Marrow & Stem Cell Transplant; Lymphoma; **Hospital:** Stanford Univ Med Ctr; **Address:** Oncology Day Care Ctr, 300 Pasteur Drive, rm H0274, MC 5216, Stanford, CA 94305; **Phone:** 650-725-6456; **Board Cert:** Internal Medicine 78; Medical Oncology 81; **Med School:** Univ Iowa Coll Med 75; **Resid:** Internal Medicine, Strong Meml Hosp 78; **Fellow:** Medical Oncology, Stanford Univ 80; **Fac Appt:** Prof Med, Stanford Univ

Issell, Brian F MD [Onc] - **Spec Exp:** Drug Development; Chemoprevention; **Hospital:** Queen's Med Ctr - Honolulu; **Address:** Cancer Research Ctr Hawaii, 1236 Lauhala St, Honolulu, HI 96813; **Phone:** 808-586-3015; **Board Cert:** Internal Medicine 79; Medical Oncology 81; **Med School:** New Zealand 71; **Resid:** Internal Medicine, Univ Otago-Otago Hosp 75; **Fellow:** Medical Oncology, MD Anderson Hosp 78; **Fac Appt:** Prof Med, Univ Hawaii JA Burns Sch Med

Jacobs, Charlotte D MD [Onc] - **Spec Exp:** Head & Neck Cancer; Sarcoma; **Hospital:** Stanford Univ Med Ctr; **Address:** 875 Blake Wilbur Drive, Stanford, CA 94305; **Phone:** 650-723-7621; **Board Cert:** Internal Medicine 75; Medical Oncology 77; **Med School:** Washington Univ, St Louis 72; **Resid:** Internal Medicine, Barnes Hosp 74; Internal Medicine, UCSF 75; **Fellow:** Medical Oncology, Stanford 77; **Fac Appt:** Prof Med, Stanford Univ

Kaplan, Lawrence D MD [Onc] - **Spec Exp:** AIDS Related Cancers; Lymphoma; **Hospital:** UCSF Med Ctr; **Address:** UCSF Medical Center, 400 Parnassus Ave, rm A502, San Francisco, CA 94143-0324; **Phone:** 415-353-2737; **Board Cert:** Internal Medicine 83; Medical Oncology 85; **Med School:** UCLA 80; **Resid:** Internal Medicine, Boston City Hosp 83; **Fellow:** Hematology and Oncology, UCSF Med Ctr 85; **Fac Appt:** Clin Prof Med, UCSF

Livingston, Robert B MD [Onc] - **Spec Exp:** Bone Marrow Transplant; Breast Cancer; Lung Cancer; **Hospital:** Univ Wash Med Ctr; **Address:** 825 Eastlake Ave E, Seattle, WA 98109-1023; **Phone:** 206-288-2034; **Board Cert:** Internal Medicine 72; Medical Oncology 73; **Med School:** Univ Okla Coll Med 65; **Resid:** Internal Medicine, Univ Oklahoma Med Ctr 71; **Fellow:** Medical Oncology, Univ Texas Cancer Ctr 73; **Fac Appt:** Prof Med, Univ Wash

Margolin, Kim Allyson MD [Onc] - **Spec Exp:** Melanoma; Kidney Cancer; Germ Cell Tumors; **Hospital:** City of Hope Natl Med Ctr & Beckman Rsch (page 89); **Address:** 1500 E Duarte Rd, City of Hope Comprehensive Cancer Ctr, Duarte, CA 91010-3012; **Phone:** 626-359-8111 x62307; **Board Cert:** Internal Medicine 82; Hematology 86; Medical Oncology 85; **Med School:** Stanford Univ 79; **Resid:** Internal Medicine, Yale-New Haven Hosp 82; **Fellow:** Hematology and Oncology, UC San Diego Med Ctr 83; Hematology and Oncology, City of Hope Med Ctr 85

Meyskens, Frank MD [Onc] - **Spec Exp:** Cancer Prevention; Melanoma; Sarcoma; **Hospital:** UC Irvine Med Ctr; **Address:** UC Urvine Cancer Ctr, 101 The City Drive Bldg 56 - rm 215, Orange, CA 92868; **Phone:** 714-456-6310; **Board Cert:** Internal Medicine 75; Medical Oncology 81; **Med School:** UCSF 72; **Resid:** Internal Medicine, Moffit-Calif Hosps 74; **Fellow:** Hematology and Oncology, NCI 77; **Fac Appt:** Prof Med, UC Irvine

Mortimer, Joanne MD [Onc] - **Spec Exp:** Breast Cancer; Clinical Trials; **Hospital:** UCSD Med Ctr; **Address:** Moores UCSD Cancer Ctr, 9500 Gilman Drive, MC 0987, Loyola, CA 92093-0987; **Phone:** 858-657-7029; **Board Cert:** Internal Medicine 80; Medical Oncology 83; **Med School:** Loyola Univ-Stritch Sch Med 77; **Resid:** Internal Medicine, Cleveland Clinic 80; **Fellow:** Medical Oncology, Cleveland Clinic 82; **Fac Appt:** Clin Prof Med, UCSD

Natale, Ronald B MD [Onc] - **Spec Exp:** Lung Cancer; **Hospital:** Cedars-Sinai Med Ctr (page 88); **Address:** Cedars-Sinai Comp Cancer Ctr, 8700 Beverly Blvd, Ste C2000, Los Angeles, CA 90048; **Phone:** 310-423-1101; **Board Cert:** Internal Medicine 77; Medical Oncology 79; **Med School:** Wayne State Univ 74; **Resid:** Internal Medicine, Wayne State Univ 77; **Fellow:** Hematology and Oncology, Meml Sloan Kettering 80; **Fac Appt:** Prof Onc, Univ Mich Med Sch

Nichols, Craig R MD [Onc] - **Spec Exp:** Testicular Cancer; Hodgkin's Disease; Lymphoma; **Hospital:** OR Hlth & Sci Univ; **Address:** Oregon Cancer Center, 3181 SW Sam Jackson Park Rd, MC PZ240, Portland, OR 97239-3098; **Phone:** 503-494-6594; **Board Cert:** Internal Medicine 81; Medical Oncology 85; **Med School:** Oregon Hlth Sci Univ 78; **Resid:** Internal Medicine, Oschner Foundation Hosp 81; **Fellow:** Medical Oncology, Indiana Univ 85; **Fac Appt:** Prof Med, Oregon Hlth Sci Univ

O'Day, Steven J MD [Onc] - **Spec Exp:** Melanoma; Melanoma-Advanced; **Hospital:** St John's Hlth Ctr, Santa Monica; **Address:** Cancer Institute Medical Group, 2001 Santa Monica Blvd, Ste 560-W, Santa Monica, CA 90404; **Phone:** 310-998-3961; **Board Cert:** Medical Oncology 93; Internal Medicine 91; **Med School:** Johns Hopkins Univ 88; **Resid:** Internal Medicine, Johns Hopkins Hosp 91; **Fellow:** Medical Oncology, Dana Farber Cancer Inst 92

Pegram, Mark D MD [Onc] - **Spec Exp:** Breast Cancer; Ovarian Cancer; **Hospital:** UCLA Med Ctr (page 111); **Address:** UCLA Sch Med - Div Hem/Onc 11-934 Factor Bldg, 10833 Le Conte Ave, MC 167817, Los Angeles, CA 90095; **Phone:** 310-829-5471; **Board Cert:** Internal Medicine 89; Hematology 96; Medical Oncology 03; **Med School:** Univ NC Sch Med 86; **Resid:** Internal Medicine, Dallas County Hosp 89; **Fellow:** Hematology and Oncology, UCLA Med Ctr 93; **Fac Appt:** Prof Onc, UCLA

Petersdorf, Stephen MD [Onc] - **Spec Exp:** Lymphoma; Myelodysplastic Syndromes; Leukemia; **Hospital:** Univ Wash Med Ctr; **Address:** Seattle Cancer Care Alliance, 825 Eastlake Ave E, Box 19023, Seattle, WA 98109-1023; **Phone:** 206-288-1024; **Board Cert:** Internal Medicine 86; Hematology 01; Medical Oncology 01; **Med School:** Brown Univ 83; **Resid:** Internal Medicine, Univ Washington Med Ctr 86; **Fellow:** Hematology and Oncology, Univ Washington Med Ctr; **Fac Appt:** Assoc Prof Med, Univ Wash

Pinto, Harlan Andrew MD [Onc] - **Spec Exp:** Head & Neck Cancer; Cancer Clinical Trials; **Hospital:** Stanford Univ Med Ctr; **Address:** Stanford Med Ctr Oncol Div, 875 Blake Wilbur Drive, rm Clinic B, Stanford, CA 94305; **Phone:** 650-723-7621; **Board Cert:** Internal Medicine 86; Medical Oncology 02; **Med School:** Yale Univ 83; **Resid:** Internal Medicine, Mass Genl Hosp 86; **Fellow:** Medical Oncology, Stanford Univ Med Sch 91; **Fac Appt:** Assoc Prof Onc, Stanford Univ

Prados, Michael MD [Onc] - **Spec Exp:** Neuro-Oncology; Brain Tumors; **Hospital:** UCSF Med Ctr; **Address:** UCSF Med Ctr, Div Neuro-Oncology, 400 Parnassus Ave, rm A-808, San Francisco, CA 94143; **Phone:** 415-353-2966; **Board Cert:** Internal Medicine 77; **Med School:** Louisiana State Univ 74; **Resid:** Infectious Disease, Earl K Long Hosp 77; **Fac Appt:** Assoc Prof, UCSF

Press, Oliver William MD/PhD [Onc] - **Spec Exp:** Lymphoma; Bone Marrow Transplant; **Hospital:** Univ Wash Med Ctr; **Address:** 1100 Fairview Ave N, MS D3-190, Seattle, WA 98109; **Phone:** 206-667-1864; **Board Cert:** Internal Medicine 82; Medical Oncology 85; **Med School:** Univ Wash 79; **Resid:** Internal Medicine, Mass Genl Hosp 82; Internal Medicine, Univ Hosp 83; **Fellow:** Medical Oncology, Univ Washington 85; **Fac Appt:** Prof Med, Univ Wash

Quinn, David MD/PhD [Onc] - **Spec Exp:** Testicular Cancer; Prostate Cancer; Kidney Cancer; **Hospital:** USC Norris Canc Comp Ctr; **Address:** 1441 Eastlake Ave, NOR 3453, 9173, Los Angeles, CA 90033; **Phone:** 323-865-3956; **Med School:** Australia 87; **Resid:** Internal Medicine, St Vincent's Hospital 92; **Fellow:** Medical Oncology, St Vincent's Hospital 95; **Fac Appt:** Asst Prof Med, USC Sch Med

Rosen, Peter J MD [Onc] - **Spec Exp:** Lymphoma; Breast Cancer; Colon Cancer; **Hospital:** UCLA Med Ctr (page 111); **Address:** 10945 Le Conte Ave, Ste 2333, Los Angeles, CA 90095; **Phone:** 310-794-1092; **Board Cert:** Internal Medicine 72; Hematology 74; Medical Oncology 75; **Med School:** USC Sch Med 66; **Resid:** Internal Medicine, Johns Hopkins Hosp 68; **Fellow:** Hematology, USC Med Ctr 72; Medical Oncology, USC Med Ctr 74; **Fac Appt:** Prof Med, UCLA

Rugo, Hope S MD [Onc] - **Spec Exp:** Breast Cancer; Complementary Cancer Therapies; **Hospital:** UCSF Med Ctr; **Address:** UCSF Breast Care Ctr, Box 1710, San Francisco, CA 94143-1710; **Phone:** 415-353-7070; **Board Cert:** Internal Medicine 87; Medical Oncology 89; **Med School:** Univ Pennsylvania 84; **Resid:** Internal Medicine, UCSF Med Ctr 87; **Fellow:** Hematology and Oncology, UCSF Med Ctr 89; **Fac Appt:** Assoc Clin Prof Med, UCSF

Small, Eric Jay MD [Onc] - **Spec Exp:** Prostate Cancer; Genitourinary Cancer; **Hospital:** UCSF Med Ctr; **Address:** UCSF Urologic Oncology Practice, Box 1711, San Francisco, CA 94143-1711; **Phone:** 415-353-7171; **Board Cert:** Internal Medicine 88; Hematology 90; Medical Oncology 91; **Med School:** Case West Res Univ 85; **Resid:** Internal Medicine, Beth Israel Hosp 88; **Fellow:** Hematology and Oncology, Cancer Research Inst/UCSF 91; **Fac Appt:** Assoc Prof Med, UCSF

Stockdale, Frank E MD/PhD [Onc] - **Spec Exp:** Breast Cancer; **Hospital:** Stanford Univ Med Ctr; **Address:** Stanford University Medical Ctr, 300 Pasteur Drive, Stanford, CA 94305; **Phone:** 650-725-6449; **Med School:** Univ Pennsylvania ; **Resid:** Internal Medicine, Cleveland Clinic; **Fellow:** Hematology and Oncology, NIH; **Fac Appt:** Prof Emeritus Med, Stanford Univ

Tempero, Margaret MD [Onc] - **Spec Exp:** Pancreatic Cancer; Gastrointestinal Cancer; **Hospital:** UCSF Med Ctr; **Address:** UCSF, Box 1705, San Francisco, CA 94143-1705; **Phone:** 415-353-9888; **Board Cert:** Internal Medicine 80; Hematology 84; Medical Oncology 83; **Med School:** Univ Nebr Coll Med 77; **Resid:** Internal Medicine, Univ Nebraska Hosp 80; **Fellow:** Medical Oncology, Univ Nebraska 82

Urba, Walter J MD [Onc] - **Spec Exp:** Breast Cancer; **Hospital:** Providence Portland Med Ctr; **Address:** Oregon Clinic, Div of Medical Oncology, 5050 NE Hoyt, Ste 611, Portland, OR 97213; **Phone:** 503-215-5696; **Board Cert:** Internal Medicine 85; Medical Oncology 87; **Med School:** Univ Miami Sch Med 81; **Resid:** Internal Medicine, Morristown Meml Hosp 83; **Fellow:** Medical Oncology, Natl Cancer Inst 86; **Fac Appt:** Assoc Clin Prof Med, Oregon Hlth Sci Univ

Venook, Alan P MD [Onc] - **Spec Exp:** Gastrointestinal Cancer; Colon & Rectal Cancer; Liver Cancer; **Hospital:** UCSF Med Ctr; **Address:** UCSF Comprehensive Cancer Ctr, Multi Disciplinary Practice, Box 1705, San Francisco, CA 94143-1705; **Phone:** 415-353-9888; **Board Cert:** Internal Medicine 85; Medical Oncology 87; Hematology 88; **Med School:** UCSF 80; **Resid:** Internal Medicine, UC Davis Med Ctr 85; **Fellow:** Hematology and Oncology, UCSF Med Ctr 87; **Fac Appt:** Prof Med, UCSF

Vescio, Robert A MD [Onc] - **Spec Exp:** Multiple Myeloma; Amyloidosis; **Hospital:** Cedars-Sinai Med Ctr (page 88); **Address:** 8700 Beverly Blvd, Cedars Sinai Medical Ctr, Dept Hematology & Oncology, Los Angeles, CA 90048; **Phone:** 310-423-1825; **Board Cert:** Internal Medicine 89; Hematology 94; Medical Oncology 03; **Med School:** UCSD 86; **Resid:** Internal Medicine, UCSD Med Ctr 89; **Fellow:** Hematology and Oncology, UCLA Med Ctr 93; **Fac Appt:** Assoc Prof Med, UCLA

Vogelzang, Nicholas MD [Onc] - **Spec Exp:** Prostate Cancer; Testicular Cancer; Kidney Cancer; **Hospital:** Univ Med Ctr - Las Vegas; **Address:** 10000 W Charleston Blvd, Ste 260, Las Vegas, NV 89135; **Phone:** 702-821-0013; **Board Cert:** Internal Medicine 78; Medical Oncology 81; **Med School:** Univ IL Coll Med 74; **Resid:** Internal Medicine, Rush-Presby St Luke's Med Ctr 78; **Fellow:** Medical Oncology, Univ Minn Med Ctr 81; **Fac Appt:** Prof Med, Univ Nevada

Volberding, Paul Arthur MD [Onc] - **Spec Exp:** AIDS Related Cancers; **Hospital:** UCSF Med Ctr; **Address:** 4150 Clemens St, VAMC 111, San Francisco, CA 94121; **Phone:** 415-750-2203; **Board Cert:** Internal Medicine 78; Medical Oncology 81; **Med School:** Univ Minn 75; **Resid:** Internal Medicine, Univ Utah Med Ctr 78; **Fellow:** Medical Oncology, UCSF Med Ctr 81; **Fac Appt:** Prof Med, UCSF

Weber, Jeffrey S MD/PhD [Onc] - **Spec Exp:** Kidney Cancer; Melanoma; Breast Cancer; **Hospital:** USC Norris Canc Comp Ctr; **Address:** USC/ Norris Cancer Ctr, 1441 Eastlake Ave, NOR 6428, 9173, Ste 3440, Los Angeles, CA 90032-1048; **Phone:** 323-865-3962; **Board Cert:** Internal Medicine 83; Medical Oncology 87; **Med School:** NYU Sch Med 80; **Resid:** Internal Medicine, UCSD Med Ctr 83; **Fellow:** Medical Oncology, Natl Cancer Inst 90; **Fac Appt:** Assoc Prof Med, USC Sch Med

Yen, Yun MD [Onc] - **Spec Exp:** Liver Cancer; Gallbladder Cancer; **Hospital:** City of Hope Natl Med Ctr & Beckman Rsch (page 89); **Address:** City of Hope Comprehensive Cancer Ctr, 1500 E Duarte Rd, San Diego, CA 91010; **Phone:** 626-359-8111 x62307; **Board Cert:** Internal Medicine 90; Medical Oncology 03; **Med School:** Taiwan 82; **Resid:** Internal Medicine, St Luke's Hosp 90; **Fellow:** Hematology and Oncology, Yale-New Haven Hosp 93; **Fac Appt:** Prof Med, USC Sch Med

NEUROLOGICAL SURGERY

A *neurological surgeon provides the operative and non-operative management (i.e., prevention, diagnosis, evaluation, treatment, critical care and rehabilitation) of disorders of the central, peripheral and autonomic nervous systems, including their supporting structures and vascular supply; the evaluation and treatment of pathological processes which modify function or activity of the nervous system; and the operative and non-operative management of pain. A neurological surgeon treats patients with disorders of the nervous system; disorders of the brain, meninges, skull and their blood supply, including the extracranial carotid and vertebral arteries; disorders of the pituitary gland; disorders of the spinal cord, meninges and vertebral column, including those which may require treatment by spinal fusion or instrumentation; and disorders of the cranial and spinal nerves throughout their distribution.*

Training required: *Seven years (including general surgery)*

PHYSICIAN LISTINGS

253

PEDIATRIC NEUROLOGICAL SURGERY: *The American Board of Pediatric Neurological Surgery (ABPNS) is not a recognized ABMS subspecialty. However, this designation has been included because the certification process is meaningful and rigorous. It is awarded to those doctors who hold a current ABMS certification in Neurological Surgery, have completed a fully accredited one year, post-graduate fellowship in pediatric neurological surgery, and have submitted surgical logs indicating a practice of pediatric neurological surgery for one year, followed by a written examination.*

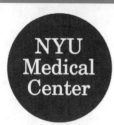

NYU Medical Center

550 First Avenue (at 31st Street)
New York, NY 10016
Physician Referral:
1 888 7-NYU-MED
www.nyumc.org

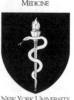

SCHOOL OF MEDICINE

NEW YORK UNIVERSITY

NEUROSURGERY

The Department of Neurosurgery at NYU Medical Center offers the most advanced surgical procedures available anywhere in the world, along with compassionate care and supportive services for patients and their families. In an environment of leading-edge research and medical education, the department's interdisciplinary team of physicians, nurses, and allied health professionals are world-renowned for their highly specialized training and their down-to-earth approach to clinical care. The department also is home to some of the most sophisticated equipment in the region.

Because neurosurgery encompasses the surgical treatment of disorders of the entire nervous system and its coverings – the brain, spinal cord, skull, scalp, and vertebral column – many physicians subspecialize in a particular aspect of the field. At NYU Medical Center, neurosurgeons treat a broad range of conditions, including tumors, vascular disorders, Parkinson's disease, and epilepsy, among others.

THE CENTER FOR THE STUDY AND TREATMENT OF MOVEMENT DISORDERS

The Center for Study and Treatment of Movement Disorders provides surgical care for patients with Parkinson's disease and other movement disorders. Its highly focused surgeons perform pallidotomy surgery when a patient suffers from severe stiffness, rigidity, and movement difficulties; and thalamotomy for those with disabling tremor. One of the center's most innovative treatments is deep brain stimulation, used to relieve the disabling symptoms of Parkinson's disease. NYU's neurosurgeons perform these procedures using the latest computer technology in conjunction with electrophysiologic monitoring.

THE GAMMA KNIFE

In the recent past, patients with brain abnormalities considered too deep or too delicate to reach with a scalpel had little reason for hope. But with the Gamma Knife, neurosurgeons at NYU Medical Center can now remove deep-seated tumors, vascular malformations, and other sites of dysfunction with outstanding results. The Leksell Gamma Knife® – a revolutionary tool developed in Sweden for performing stereotactic radiosurgery – is the latest such technology in the New York and New England regions. Aided by three-dimensional MRI technology that pinpoints the problem area, the neurosurgeon uses the Gamma Knife to bombard its target with precise doses of radiation.

The Tumor Surgery Program at NYU Medical Center treats patients referred from all over the world. The program is committed to the development and application of minimally invasive methods for the complete removal of brain tumors. With an emphasis on noninvasive brain mapping via magnetoencephalo-tomography (MEG) and functional MRI, NYU's neurosurgeons are able to plan a surgical approach that minimizes risk and ensures the best possible outcome. Stereotactic volumetric resection, a method developed by Patrick J. Kelly, MD – Professor and Chairman of Neurosurgery – assures exceptionally thorough surgical removal of the tumor.

PHYSICIAN REFERRAL
1-888-7-NYU-MED
(1-888-769-8633)
www.nyumc.org

Kimmel Cancer Center at Jefferson
THOMAS JEFFERSON UNIVERSITY HOSPITALS

111 S. 11th Street
Philadelphia, PA 19107-5098
Tel. 215-955-6000
www.JeffersonHospital.org

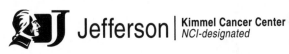

Network Affiliation: Thomas Jefferson University Hospitals, an academic medical center, and a member of the Jefferson Health System

NEUROSURGICAL AND RADIATION ONCOLOGY EXPERTS TREATING BRAIN CANCER

Thomas Jefferson University Hospital's Kimmel Cancer Center houses outstanding cancer experts, state-of-the-art technology and treatment options. Cancer specialists combine breakthrough treatment for brain tumors with compassionate care and support. The center is recognized as a National Cancer Institute (NCI)-designated clinical cancer center for excellence in cancer research and treatment. In fact, Thomas Jefferson University Hospital's doctors have been cited as among the nation's best for cancer treatment by "Best Doctors in America." Our oncologists contribute to leading scientific journals such as Cancer, Cell and the Journal of Clinical Oncology. Our five radiation oncology satellites located throughout the community make this expertise conveniently accessible. At Jefferson Hospital for Neuroscience, our neurosurgeons published a landmark paper in the journal, The Lancet, on the radiosurgical management of intracranial metastases, which now defines how this disease is treated worldwide.

AT THE FOREFRONT OF BRAIN TUMOR TREATMENT

Neurosurgeons at Jefferson Hospital for Neuroscience offer innovative therapies and clinical trials for brain tumors. Comprehensive care includes diagnosis, highly promising leading-edge treatments not widely available elsewhere, and educational and powerful emotional support.

- A history of leadership—Achieving international prominence, Jefferson neurosurgeons and radiation oncologists pioneered a non-surgical procedure considered to be one of the most significant advances in treating brain tumors in the last decade. Stereotactic radiosurgery attacks malignant and nonmalignant brain tumors with precisely targeted doses of radiation while sparing normal tissue. Jeff neurosurgeons demonstrated that radiosurgery, now the standard of care for brain lesions, can destroy benign tumors that may cause blindness and improve quality of life for others with cancers that have spread to the brain.

- Jefferson was the first hospital in the world to dedicate a linear accelerator for radiosurgery in 1994. Recently Jeff neurosurgeons and radiation oncologists refined the technique with a Novalis shaped beam stereotactic radiosurgery unit.

- Jeff continues to treat more patients with brain tumors than any other hospital in the country. A national leader in clinical trials as well, Jefferson is laying the groundwork for a multidisciplinary Brain Tumor Center focused on research. Studying the disease at the molecular level will enable physicians to develop superior methodologies for care while bridging basic research and clinical care.

- Jefferson scientists are also exploring therapeutic drugs that could be infused directly in the brain.

- The Kimmel Cancer Center at Jefferson and Thomas Jefferson University have partnered with area community hospitals to operate the Jefferson Cancer Network (JCN), a network of hospitals in the region dedicated to the furthering of clinical research and education in the prevention, diagnosis and treatment of cancer. Through JCN, community cancer programs are able to provide their patients access to hundreds of state-of-the-art cancer prevention and therapeutic clinical research protocols.

Access to any of these programs, materials or treatment centers is simplified by calling 1-800-JEFF-NOW or visiting www.JeffersonHospital.org/cancer

NEUROLOGICAL SURGERY

New England

Black, Peter MD/PhD [NS] - **Spec Exp:** Brain Tumors; Pituitary Tumors; Seizure Disorders Surgery; **Hospital:** Brigham & Women's Hosp (page 87); **Address:** Brigham & Women's Hosp, Dept Neurosurg, 75 Francis St, Boston, MA 02115; **Phone:** 617-732-6810; **Board Cert:** Neurological Surgery 84; **Med School:** McGill Univ 70; **Resid:** Surgery, Mass Genl Hosp 72; Neurological Surgery, Mass Genl Hosp 80; **Fellow:** Neurological Oncology, Mass Genl Hosp 76; **Fac Appt:** Prof NS, Harvard Med Sch

Borges, Lawrence F MD [NS] - **Spec Exp:** Spinal Surgery; Spinal Tumors; **Hospital:** Mass Genl Hosp; **Address:** Mass Genl Hosp, Div Neurosurg, 32 Fruit St, Boston, MA 02114-2620; **Phone:** 617-726-6156; **Board Cert:** Neurological Surgery 86; **Med School:** Johns Hopkins Univ 77; **Resid:** Neurological Surgery, Mass Genl Hosp 83; **Fac Appt:** Assoc Prof S, Harvard Med Sch

Chapman, Paul H MD [NS] - **Spec Exp:** Pediatric Neurosurgery; Brain & Spinal Tumors-Pediatric; Congenital Anomalies; **Hospital:** Mass Genl Hosp; **Address:** 55 Fruit St, MGH Gray 5, rm GRB-502, Boston, MA 02114-2622; **Phone:** 617-726-3887; **Board Cert:** Neurological Surgery 76; Pediatric Neurological Surgery ; **Med School:** Harvard Med Sch 64; **Resid:** Surgery, Mass Genl Hosp 66; Neurological Surgery, Mass Genl Hosp 72; **Fellow:** Neurological Surgery, Hosp Sick Chldn; **Fac Appt:** Prof S, Harvard Med Sch

Cosgrove, G. Rees MD [NS] - **Spec Exp:** Epilepsy/Seizure Disorders; Brain Tumors; **Hospital:** Lahey Clin; **Address:** Lahey Clinic, 41 Mall Rd, Burlington, MA 01805; **Phone:** 781-744-1990; **Board Cert:** Neurological Surgery 89; **Med School:** Queens Univ 80; **Resid:** Neurological Surgery, Montreal Neur Inst 86; **Fac Appt:** Assoc Prof S, Harvard Med Sch

David, Carlos MD [NS] - **Spec Exp:** Cerebrovascular Surgery; Skull Base Tumors & Surgery; **Hospital:** Lahey Clin; **Address:** Lahey Clinic, Dept Neurosurgery, 41 Mall Rd, Burlington, MA 01805; **Phone:** 781-744-8643; **Board Cert:** Neurological Surgery 01; **Med School:** Univ Miami Sch Med 90; **Resid:** Neurological Surgery, Jackson Memorial Hosp 95; **Fellow:** Cerebrovascular & Skull Base Surgery, Borrou Neuro Inst 97; **Fac Appt:** Assoc Clin Prof NS, Tufts Univ

Day, Arthur L MD [NS] - **Spec Exp:** Cerebrovascular Surgery; Cranial/Orbital Tumors; Carotid Artery Surgery; **Hospital:** Brigham & Women's Hosp (page 87); **Address:** Brigham & Women's Hospital, Dept Neurosurgery, 75 Francis St, Boston, MA 02115; **Phone:** 617-732-6846; **Board Cert:** Neurological Surgery 80; **Med School:** Louisiana State Univ 72; **Resid:** Neurological Surgery, Shands-Univ Florida Hosp 77; **Fellow:** Neurological Pathology, Shands-Univ Florida Hosp 78; **Fac Appt:** Prof NS, Harvard Med Sch

Goumnerova, Liliana MD [NS] - **Spec Exp:** Pediatric Neurosurgery; Brain Tumors; Ventriculoscopy; **Hospital:** Children's Hospital - Boston; **Address:** Chldns Hosp, 300 Longwood Ave, Bader Fl 3, Boston, MA 02115; **Phone:** 617-355-6364; **Board Cert:** Neurological Surgery 92; Pediatric Neurological Surgery 97; **Med School:** Canada 80; **Resid:** Neurological Surgery, Univ Ottawa 86; **Fellow:** Pediatric Neurological Surgery, Hosp for Sick Chldn 88; Neurological Science, Univ Penn 90; **Fac Appt:** Asst Prof S, Harvard Med Sch

Martuza, Robert L MD [NS] - **Spec Exp:** Brain Tumors; Acoustic Nerve Tumors; Skull Base Surgery; **Hospital:** Mass Genl Hosp; **Address:** Mass General Hosp, 55 Fruit St, White Bldg, rm 502, Boston, MA 02114; **Phone:** 617-726-8581; **Board Cert:** Neurological Surgery 83; **Med School:** Harvard Med Sch 73; **Resid:** Neurological Surgery, Mass Genl Hosp 80; **Fac Appt:** Prof NS, Harvard Med Sch

Piepmeier, Joseph MD **[NS]** - **Spec Exp:** Neuro-Oncology; Brain & Spinal Cord Tumors; **Hospital:** Yale - New Haven Hosp; **Address:** Yale Sch Med, Dept Neurosurgery, 333 Cedar St, TMP-410, New Haven, CT 06520; **Phone:** 203-785-2791; **Board Cert:** Neurological Surgery 84; **Med School:** Univ Tenn Coll Med, Memphis 75; **Resid:** Neurological Surgery, Yale-New Haven Hosp 82; **Fac Appt:** Prof NS, Yale Univ

Scott, R Michael MD **[NS]** - **Spec Exp:** Brain Tumors-Pediatric; Stroke (Moya Moya & AVM); Brain & Spinal Malformations-Pediatric; **Hospital:** Children's Hospital - Boston; **Address:** Chldns Hosp, Dept Neurosurg, 300 Longwood Ave,   Bldg Bader - rm 319, Boston, MA 02115-5724; **Phone:** 617-355-6011; **Board Cert:** Neurological Surgery 76; Pediatric Neurological Surgery 96; **Med School:** Temple Univ 66; **Resid:** Neurological Surgery, Mass Genl Hosp 73; **Fac Appt:** Prof S, Harvard Med Sch

Mid Atlantic

Albright, A Leland MD **[NS]** - **Spec Exp:** Pediatric Neurosurgery; Spasticity & Movement Disorders; Brain Tumors; **Hospital:** Chldns Hosp of Pittsburgh - UPMC (page 114); **Address:** Chldns Hosp-Pittsburgh, Dept Neurosurgery, 3705 5th Ave, Ste 3705, Pittsburgh, PA 15213-2524; **Phone:** 412-692-8142; **Board Cert:** Neurological Surgery 81; Pediatric Neurological Surgery 96; **Med School:** Louisiana State Univ 69; **Resid:** Surgery, Wash Hosps 71; Neurological Surgery, Univ Pittsburgh Med Ctr 78; **Fellow:** Neurological Surgery, Natl Inst Hlth 74; Immunopathology, Univ Pittsburgh Med Ctr; **Fac Appt:** Prof NS, Univ Pittsburgh

Andrews, David MD **[NS]** - **Spec Exp:** Brain Tumors; Neuro-Endoscopy; Stereotactic Radiosurgery; **Hospital:** Thomas Jefferson Univ Hosp (page 110); **Address:** Thom Jefferson Univ Hosp, Dept Neurosurg, 909 Walnut St Fl 3, Philadelphia, PA 19107-5109; **Phone:** 215-503-7005; **Board Cert:** Neurological Surgery 92; **Med School:** Univ Colorado 83; **Resid:** Neurological Surgery, NY Presby Hos-Cornell Med Ctr 89; **Fellow:** Neurological Oncology, Meml Sloan Kettering Cancer Ctr 87; **Fac Appt:** Prof NS, Thomas Jefferson Univ

Bilsky, Mark H MD **[NS]** - **Spec Exp:** Spinal Tumors & Reconstruction; Skull Base Tumors; Brain Tumors; **Hospital:** Meml Sloan Kettering Cancer Ctr (page 100); **Address:** Memorial Sloan Kettering Cancer Ctr, 1275 York Ave, rm C705, New York, NY 10021; **Phone:** 212-639-8526; **Board Cert:** Neurological Surgery 99; **Med School:** Emory Univ 88; **Resid:** Neurological Surgery, NY Hosp-Cornell Med Ctr 94; **Fellow:** Neurological Oncology, Louisville Univ Med Ctr 95

Brem, Henry MD **[NS]** - **Spec Exp:** Brain & Spinal Cord Tumors; Skull Base Tumors; Pituitary Tumors; **Hospital:** Johns Hopkins Hosp - Baltimore (page 97); **Address:** Johns Hopkins Med Ctr-Dept NeuroSurg, 600 N Wolfe St Bldg Meyer 7-113, Baltimore, MD 21287; **Phone:** 410-955-2248; **Board Cert:** Neurological Surgery 86; **Med School:** Harvard Med Sch 78; **Resid:** Neurological Surgery, Columbia-Presby Ctr 84; **Fellow:** Neurological Surgery, Johns Hopkins Hosp 80; **Fac Appt:** Prof NS, Johns Hopkins Univ

Bruce, Jeffrey MD **[NS]** - **Spec Exp:** Brain Tumors; Pituitary Tumors; Skull Base Surgery; **Hospital:** NY-Presby Hosp - Columbia Presby Med Ctr (page 103); **Address:** 710 W 168 St Bldg N1 Fl 4 - rm 434, New York Presbyterian Hospital, Dept Neurosurgery, New York, NY 10032-2603; **Phone:** 212-305-7346; **Board Cert:** Neurological Surgery 93; **Med School:** UMDNJ-RW Johnson Med Sch 83; **Resid:** Neurological Surgery, Columbia-Presby Med Ctr 90; **Fellow:** Neurological Surgery, Nat Inst Health 85; **Fac Appt:** Prof NS, Columbia P&S

Camins, Martin B MD [NS] - **Spec Exp:** Spinal Surgery; Brain Tumors; Microsurgery; **Hospital:** Mount Sinai Med Ctr (page 101); **Address:** 205 E 68th St, Ste T1C, New York, NY 10021-5735; **Phone:** 212-570-0100; **Board Cert:** Neurological Surgery 80; **Med School:** Univ Hlth Sci/Chicago Med Sch 69; **Resid:** Neurology, Neuro Inst-Columbia-Presby Med Ctr 71; Neurological Surgery, Neuro Inst-Columbia Presb Med Ctry 75; **Fellow:** Neurological Surgery, National Hosp; Neurological Surgery, NYU Med Ctr 77; **Fac Appt:** Clin Prof NS, Mount Sinai Sch Med

Carmel, Peter MD [NS] - **Spec Exp:** Brain Tumors-Pediatric; Skull Base Surgery; **Hospital:** UMDNJ-Univ Hosp-Newark; **Address:** 90 Bergen St, Ste 8100, Newark, NJ 07103; **Phone:** 973-972-2323; **Board Cert:** Neurological Surgery 69; **Med School:** NYU Sch Med 60; **Resid:** Neurological Surgery, Neuro Inst/Columbia Presby Med Ctr 67; **Fac Appt:** Prof NS, UMDNJ-NJ Med Sch, Newark

Carson, Benjamin S MD [NS] - **Spec Exp:** Brain Injury; Brain & Spinal Cord Tumors; Pediatric Neurosurgery; **Hospital:** Johns Hopkins Hosp - Baltimore (page 97); **Address:** 600 N Wolfe St, Harvey 811, Baltimore, MD 21287-8811; **Phone:** 410-955-7888; **Board Cert:** Neurological Surgery 88; Pediatric Neurological Surgery ; **Med School:** Univ Mich Med Sch 77; **Resid:** Neurological Surgery, Johns Hopkins Hosp 83; **Fellow:** Pediatric Neurological Surgery, Queen Elizabeth II Med Ctr 84; **Fac Appt:** Assoc Prof NS, Johns Hopkins Univ

DiGiacinto, George V MD [NS] - **Spec Exp:** Spinal Surgery; Brain Tumors; Pain Management; **Hospital:** St Luke's - Roosevelt Hosp Ctr - Roosevelt Div (page 93); **Address:** 425 W 59th St, Ste 4E, New York, NY 10019; **Phone:** 212-523-8500; **Board Cert:** Neurological Surgery 81; **Med School:** Harvard Med Sch 70; **Resid:** Surgery, Roosevelt Hosp 72; Neurological Surgery, Columbia-Presby Hosp 78

Eisenberg, Howard M MD [NS] - **Spec Exp:** Acoustic Nerve Tumors; Parkinson's Disease/Movement Disorders; Epilepsy/Seizure Disorders; **Hospital:** Univ of MD Med Sys; **Address:** Univ MD Sch Med, Dept Neurosurg, 22 S Greene St, Ste S-12-D, Baltimore, MD 21201-1544; **Phone:** 410-328-3514; **Board Cert:** Neurological Surgery 73; **Med School:** SUNY Downstate 64; **Resid:** Surgery, New York Hosp 66; Neurological Surgery, Peter Bent Brigham Hosp/Chldns Hosp 70; **Fellow:** Harvard Univ 70; **Fac Appt:** Prof NS, Univ MD Sch Med

Flamm, Eugene MD [NS] - **Spec Exp:** Aneurysm-Cerebral; Spinal Cord Lesions; Vascular Brain/Spine Problems; **Hospital:** Montefiore Med Ctr; **Address:** 3316 Rochambeau Ave, Bronx, NY 10467; **Phone:** 718-920-7476; **Board Cert:** Neurological Surgery 73; **Med School:** SUNY Buffalo 62; **Resid:** Surgery, New York Hosp 64; Neurological Surgery, NYU Med Ctr 70; **Fellow:** Neurological Surgery, Univ Zurich 71; **Fac Appt:** Prof NS, Albert Einstein Coll Med

Germano, Isabelle M MD [NS] - **Spec Exp:** Brain Tumors; Movement Disorders; Epilepsy; **Hospital:** Mount Sinai Med Ctr (page 101); **Address:** 5 E 98th St, Box 1136, New York, NY 10029-6504; **Phone:** 212-241-9638; **Board Cert:** Neurological Surgery 95; **Med School:** Italy 84; **Resid:** Neurological Surgery, UCSF Med Ctr 90; Neurological Surgery, Albert Einstein Coll Med 93; **Fac Appt:** Assoc Prof NS, Mount Sinai Sch Med

Goodrich, James T MD [NS] - **Spec Exp:** Craniofacial Surgery; Spina Bifida; Brain Tumors-Pediatric; **Hospital:** Montefiore Med Ctr; **Address:** Montefiore Med Ctr, Dept Ped Neurosurgery, 111 E 210th St, Bronx, NY 10467-2401; **Phone:** 718-920-4197; **Board Cert:** Neurological Surgery 89; Pediatric Neurological Surgery 96; **Med School:** Columbia P&S 80; **Resid:** Neurological Surgery, NY Neurological Inst 86; **Fac Appt:** Prof NS, Albert Einstein Coll Med

Gutin, Philip MD [NS] - **Spec Exp:** Brain Tumors; Meningioma; Acoustic Nerve Tumors; **Hospital:** Meml Sloan Kettering Cancer Ctr (page 100); **Address:** Meml Sloan Kettering Cancer Ctr, Dept Neuro Surg, 1275 York Ave, New York, NY 10021-6007; **Phone:** 212-639-8556; **Board Cert:** Neurological Surgery 81; **Med School:** Univ Pennsylvania 71; **Resid:** Neurological Surgery, UCSF Med Ctr 79; **Fellow:** Natl Cancer Inst 76; **Fac Appt:** Prof NS, Cornell Univ-Weill Med Coll

Judy, Kevin MD [NS] - **Spec Exp:** Brain Tumors; **Hospital:** Hosp Univ Penn - UPHS (page 113); **Address:** Hosp Univ Penn - Dept Neurosurg, 3400 Spruce St, 3 Silverstein, Philadelphia, PA 19104; **Phone:** 215-662-7854; **Board Cert:** Neurological Surgery 97; **Med School:** Univ Pittsburgh 84; **Resid:** Surgery, Mercy Hosp 86; Neurological Surgery, Johns Hopkins Hosp 92; **Fellow:** Neurological Surgery, Johns Hopkins Hosp 91; **Fac Appt:** Assoc Prof NS, Univ Pennsylvania

Kassam, Amin MD [NS] - **Spec Exp:** Skull Base Tumors & Surgery; Cranial Nerve Disorders; Cerebrovascular Surgery; **Hospital:** UPMC Presby, Pittsburgh (page 114); **Address:** University of Pittsburgh Medical Ctr, Dept Neurosurgery, 200 othrop St, Ste B400, Pittburgh, PA 15213; **Phone:** 412-647-6358; **Board Cert:** Neurological Surgery 90; **Med School:** Univ Toronto 84; **Resid:** Neurological Surgery, Univ Ottawa Med Ctr 88; **Fellow:** Skull Base Surgery, Univ Ottawa Med Ctr 90; Epidemiology, Univ Ottawa Med Ctr; **Fac Appt:** Assoc Prof NS, Univ Pennsylvania

Kelly, Patrick J MD [NS] - **Spec Exp:** Brain Tumors; Movement Disorders; Gliomas; **Hospital:** NYU Med Ctr (page 104); **Address:** NYU Med Ctr, Dept Neurological Surgery, 530 1st Ave, Ste 8R, New York, NY 10016; **Phone:** 212-263-8002; **Board Cert:** Neurological Surgery 78; **Med School:** SUNY Buffalo 66; **Resid:** Neurological Surgery, Northwestern Univ Hosp 72; Neurological Surgery, Univ Texas Med Br Hosp 74; **Fellow:** Neurological Surgery, St Anne Hosp; **Fac Appt:** Prof NS, NYU Sch Med

Kobrine, Arthur MD/PhD [NS] - **Spec Exp:** Spinal Cord Surgery; Brain & Spinal Cord Tumors; **Hospital:** Sibley Mem Hosp; **Address:** 2440 M St NW, Ste 315, Washington, DC 20037-1404; **Phone:** 202-293-7136; **Board Cert:** Neurological Surgery 76; **Med School:** Northwestern Univ 68; **Resid:** Neurological Surgery, Northwestern Univ Hosp 70; Neurological Surgery, Walter Reed Army Hosp 73; **Fellow:** Physiology, Geo Wash Univ; **Fac Appt:** Clin Prof NS, Georgetown Univ

Kondziolka, Douglas MD [NS] - **Spec Exp:** Brain Tumors-Adult & Pediatric; Movement Disorders; Gamma Knife Surgery; **Hospital:** UPMC Presby, Pittsburgh (page 114); **Address:** Univ Pittsburgh Med Ctr-Dept of Neurological Surg, 200 Lothrop St, Ste B400, Pittsburgh, PA 15213; **Phone:** 412-647-9990; **Board Cert:** Neurological Surgery 94; **Med School:** Univ Toronto 85; **Resid:** Neurological Surgery, Univ Toronto 91; **Fellow:** Stereo Neurological Surgery, UPMC Presby 91; **Fac Appt:** Prof NS, Univ Pittsburgh

Lavyne, Michael H MD [NS] - **Spec Exp:** Spinal Surgery; Skull Base Surgery; Acoustic Nerve Tumors; **Hospital:** NY-Presby Hosp - NY Weill Cornell Med Ctr (page 103); **Address:** 523 E 72nd St, New York, NY 10021-4099; **Phone:** 212-717-0200; **Board Cert:** Neurological Surgery 82; **Med School:** Cornell Univ-Weill Med Coll 72; **Resid:** Neurological Surgery, Mass Genl Hosp 79; **Fellow:** Neurology, Beth Israel Hosp 74; **Fac Appt:** Assoc Clin Prof S, Cornell Univ-Weill Med Coll

Loftus, Christopher M MD [NS] - **Spec Exp:** Cerebrovascular Surgery; Brain Tumors; Spinal Disorders-Cervical; **Hospital:** Temple Univ Hosp; **Address:** Temple Univ Sch Med, Parkinson Pavilion # 580, 3401 N Broad St, Philadelphia, PA 19140; **Phone:** 215-707-9790; **Board Cert:** Neurological Surgery 87; **Med School:** SUNY Downstate 79; **Resid:** Neurological Surgery, Columbia-Presby Med Ctr 85; **Fac Appt:** Prof NS, Temple Univ

Long, Donlin M MD/PhD **[NS]** - **Spec Exp:** Skull Base Tumors; Acoustic Nerve Tumors; Spinal Disorders; **Hospital:** Johns Hopkins Hosp - Baltimore (page 97); **Address:** 600 N Wolfe St, Carnegie , rm 466, Baltimore, MD 21287; **Phone:** 410-614-3536; **Board Cert:** Neurological Surgery 68; **Med School:** Univ MO-Columbia Sch Med 59; **Resid:** Neurological Surgery, Univ Minnesota Hosp 64; Peter Bent Brigham Hosp; **Fac Appt:** Prof NS, Johns Hopkins Univ

Lunsford, L Dade MD **[NS]** - **Spec Exp:** Brain Tumors; Stereotactic Radiosurgery; Movement Disorders; **Hospital:** UPMC Presby, Pittsburgh (page 114); **Address:** UPMC Presbyterian Hosp, 200 Lothrop St, Ste B400, Pittsburgh, PA 15213; **Phone:** 412-647-3685; **Board Cert:** Neurological Surgery 83; **Med School:** Columbia P&S 74; **Resid:** Neurological Surgery, Univ Pittsburgh Med Ctr 80; **Fellow:** Stereo Neurological Surgery, Karolinska Hospital 81; **Fac Appt:** Prof NS, Univ Pittsburgh

McCormick, Paul C MD **[NS]** - **Spec Exp:** Spinal Surgery; Spinal Tumors; Spinal Microsurgery; **Hospital:** NY-Presby Hosp - Columbia Presby Med Ctr (page 103); **Address:** 710 W 168th St, Ste 406, New York, NY 10032-2603; **Phone:** 212-305-7976; **Board Cert:** Neurological Surgery 93; **Med School:** Columbia P&S 82; **Resid:** Neurological Surgery, Columbia Presby Med Ctr 89; **Fellow:** Neurological Surgery, Natl Inst Hlth 84; Spinal Surgery, Med Coll Wisconsin 90; **Fac Appt:** Prof NS, Columbia P&S

O'Rourke, Donald MD **[NS]** - **Spec Exp:** Neuro-Oncology; Brain Tumors; Spinal Disorders-Cervical; **Hospital:** Hosp Univ Penn - UPHS (page 113); **Address:** Hosp Univ Penn - Dept Neurosurg, 3400 Spruce St, 3 Silverstein, Philadelphia, PA 19104; **Phone:** 215-662-3483; **Board Cert:** Neurological Surgery 98; **Med School:** Univ Pennsylvania 87; **Resid:** Neurological Surgery, Hosp Univ Penn 94; **Fac Appt:** Assoc Prof NS, Univ Pennsylvania

Pollack, Ian MD **[NS]** - **Spec Exp:** Pediatric Neurosurgery; Brain Tumors; Craniofacial Surgery; **Hospital:** Chldns Hosp of Pittsburgh - UPMC (page 114); **Address:** Chldns Hosp Pittsburgh, Dept Neurosurg, 3705 Fifth Ave, Ste 3670A, Pittsburgh, PA 15213-2524; **Phone:** 412-692-5881; **Board Cert:** Neurological Surgery 96; Pediatric Neurological Surgery 97; **Med School:** Johns Hopkins Univ 84; **Resid:** Neurological Surgery, Univ Pittsburgh Med Ctr 91; **Fellow:** Pediatric Neurological Surgery, Hosp Sick Chldn 92; **Fac Appt:** Prof NS, Univ Pittsburgh

Post, Kalmon MD **[NS]** - **Spec Exp:** Pituitary Surgery; Acoustic Nerve Tumors; Meningioma; **Hospital:** Mount Sinai Med Ctr (page 101); **Address:** 5 E 98th St, Fl 7, New York, NY 10029-6501; **Phone:** 212-241-0933; **Board Cert:** Neurological Surgery 78; **Med School:** NYU Sch Med 67; **Resid:** Surgery, Bellevue Hosp 69; Neurological Surgery, Bellevue Hosp-NYU 75; **Fac Appt:** Prof NS, Mount Sinai Sch Med

Rosenwasser, Robert H MD **[NS]** - **Spec Exp:** Aneurysm-Cerebral; Cerebrovascular Surgery; Neuro-Oncology/Stereotactic Radiosurgery; **Hospital:** Thomas Jefferson Univ Hosp (page 110); **Address:** Thomas Jefferson University Hospital, 909 Walnut St Fl 2, Philadelphia, PA 19107; **Phone:** 215-955-7000; **Board Cert:** Neurological Surgery 87; **Med School:** Louisiana State Univ ; **Resid:** Neurological Surgery, Temple Univ Hosp 84; **Fellow:** Neurological Vascular Surgery, Univ West Ontarion; Interventional Neuroradiology, NYU Med Ctr; **Fac Appt:** Prof NS, Thomas Jefferson Univ

Sen, Chandranath MD **[NS]** - **Spec Exp:** Brain Tumors; Skull Base Tumors & Surgery; **Hospital:** St Luke's - Roosevelt Hosp Ctr - Roosevelt Div (page 93); **Address:** St Lukes Roosevelt Hosp Ctr, Dept Neurosurgery, 1000 10th Ave, Ste 5G-80, New York, NY 10019; **Phone:** 212-523-6720; **Board Cert:** Neurological Surgery 89; **Med School:** India 76; **Resid:** Surgery, Univ Wisconsin Hosps 80; Neurological Surgery, Univ Wisconsin Hosps 85; **Fellow:** Microsurgery, Univ Pittsburgh 86

Stieg, Philip E MD/PhD **[NS]** - **Spec Exp:** Cerebrovascular Surgery; Acoustic Nerve Tumors; Skull Base Surgery; **Hospital:** NY-Presby Hosp - NY Weill Cornell Med Ctr (page 103); **Address:** 525 E 68th St, STARR 651, New York, NY 10021-9800; **Phone:** 212-746-4684; **Board Cert:** Neurological Surgery 92; **Med School:** Med Coll Wisc 83; **Resid:** Neurological Surgery, Dallas Chldns Hosp/Parkland Meml Hosp 88; **Fellow:** Neurological Biology, Karolinska Inst 88; **Fac Appt:** Prof NS, Cornell Univ-Weill Med Coll

Sutton, Leslie N MD **[NS]** - **Spec Exp:** Brain Tumors; Fetal Neurosurgery; Hydrocephalus; **Hospital:** Chldns Hosp of Philadelphia, The; **Address:** Childrens Hosp of Phila -Div Neurosurgery, 34th St & Civic Ctr Blvd, Wood 6, Philadelphia, PA 19104; **Phone:** 215-590-2780; **Board Cert:** Neurological Surgery 84; Pediatric Neurological Surgery 96; **Med School:** Univ Pennsylvania 75; **Resid:** Neurological Surgery, Hosp Univ Penn 81; **Fac Appt:** Prof NS, Univ Pennsylvania

Wisoff, Jeffrey H MD **[NS]** - **Spec Exp:** Pediatric Neurosurgery; Brain Tumors-Pediatric; Hydrocephalus; **Hospital:** NYU Med Ctr (page 104); **Address:** 317 E 34th St, Ste 1002, New York, NY 10016-4974; **Phone:** 212-263-6419; **Board Cert:** Neurological Surgery 90; Pediatric Neurological Surgery 96; **Med School:** Geo Wash Univ 78; **Resid:** Neurological Surgery, NYU Med Ctr/Bellevue Hosp 84; **Fellow:** Pediatric Neurological Surgery, NYU Med Ctr 85; **Fac Appt:** Assoc Prof NS, NYU Sch Med

Southeast

Boop, Frederick A MD **[NS]** - **Spec Exp:** Pediatric Neurosurgery; Epilepsy; Brain Tumors; **Hospital:** Le Bonheur Chldns Med Ctr; **Address:** Semmes Murphy Clinic, 1211 Union Ave, Ste 200, Memphis, TN 38104-3562; **Phone:** 901-259-5340; **Board Cert:** Neurological Surgery 93; Pediatric Neurological Surgery ; **Med School:** Univ Ark 83; **Resid:** Neurological Surgery, Univ Tex Hlth Sci Ctr 89; Neurological Surgery, Inst Neur/Hosp Sick Chldn 87; **Fellow:** Epilepsy, Univ Minn; Pediatric Neurological Surgery, Ark Chldns Hosp; **Fac Appt:** Assoc Prof NS, Univ Tenn Coll Med, Memphis

Brem, Steven MD **[NS]** - **Spec Exp:** Brain Tumors; Pituitary Tumors; Clinical Trials; **Hospital:** H Lee Moffitt Cancer Ctr & Research Inst; **Address:** H. Lee Moffitt Cancer Ctr/ Neuro, 12902 Magnolia Drive, Tampa, FL 33612-9497; **Phone:** 813-979-3063; **Board Cert:** Neurological Surgery 83; **Med School:** Harvard Med Sch 72; **Resid:** Neurological Surgery, Massachusetts Genl Hosp 81; **Fellow:** Oncology, Natl Cancer Inst 76; **Fac Appt:** Prof NS, Univ S Fla Coll Med

Ewend, Matthew MD **[NS]** - **Spec Exp:** Brain Tumors; Pituitary Tumors; Pediactric Neurosurgery; **Hospital:** Univ NC Hosps (page 112); **Address:** U of North Carolina Neurosurgery, 2160 Bioinformatics Bldg CB#7060, Chapel Hill, NC 27599; **Phone:** 919-966-1374; **Board Cert:** Neurological Surgery 01; **Med School:** Johns Hopkins Univ 90; **Resid:** Neurological Surgery, Johns Hopkins Hospital 94; **Fellow:** Neurological Oncology, National Institutes of Health 96; **Fac Appt:** Asst Prof NS, Univ NC Sch Med

Ferraz, Francisco M MD **[NS]** - **Spec Exp:** Brain Tumors; Spinal Surgery-Cervical; **Hospital:** Virginia Hosp Ctr - Arlington; **Address:** 611 S Carlin Springs Rd, Ste 105, Arlington, VA 22204; **Phone:** 703-845-1552; **Board Cert:** Neurological Surgery 87; **Med School:** Brazil 75; **Resid:** Neurological Surgery, Georgetown Univ Affil Hosp 82

Friedman, Allan H MD **[NS]** - **Spec Exp:** Brain Tumors; Skull Base Tumors; Cerebrovascular Surgery; **Hospital:** Duke Univ Med Ctr (page 94); **Address:** Brain Tumor Ctr at Duke Univ Med Ctr, Baker House, Rm 047 - DUMC Box 3624, Durham, NC 27710; **Phone:** 919-681-6421; **Board Cert:** Neurological Surgery 83; **Med School:** Univ IL Coll Med 74; **Resid:** Neurological Surgery, Duke Univ Med Ctr 80; **Fellow:** Vascular Surgery, Univ Western Ontario 81; **Fac Appt:** Prof S, Duke Univ

Fuchs, Herbert E MD/PhD [NS] - **Spec Exp:** Pediatric Neurosurgery; Brain Tumors-Pediatric; **Hospital:** Duke Univ Med Ctr (page 94); **Address:** Duke Univ Med Ctr, Box 3272, Durham, NC 27710; **Phone:** 919-681-0894; **Board Cert:** Neurological Surgery 95; Pediatric Neurological Surgery 97; **Med School:** Duke Univ 84; **Resid:** Neurological Surgery, Duke Univ Med Ctr 91; **Fellow:** Pediatric Neurological Surgery, Chldns Meml Hosp 92; **Fac Appt:** Assoc Prof S, Duke Univ

Heros, Roberto MD [NS] - **Spec Exp:** Cerebrovascular Surgery; Skull Base Surgery; Brain Tumors; **Hospital:** Jackson Meml Hosp; **Address:** Univ Miami, Dept Neurosurgery, 1095 NW 14th Terr, Pope Life Ctr D46, Miami, FL 33136; **Phone:** 305-243-4572; **Board Cert:** Neurological Surgery 79; **Med School:** Univ Tenn Coll Med, Memphis 68; **Resid:** Surgery, Mass Genl Hosp 70; Neurological Surgery, Mass Genl Hosp 76; **Fac Appt:** Prof NS, Univ Miami Sch Med

Laws Jr., Edward R MD [NS] - **Spec Exp:** Pituitary Surgery; Epilepsy/Seizure Disorders; Brain Tumors; **Hospital:** Univ Virginia Med Ctr; **Address:** Univ VA Hlth Scis Ctr, Dept Neurosurgery, Box 800212, Charlottesville, VA 22908-0212; **Phone:** 434-924-2650; **Board Cert:** Neurological Surgery 74; **Med School:** Johns Hopkins Univ 63; **Resid:** Neurological Surgery, Johns Hopkins Hosp 71; **Fac Appt:** Prof NS, Univ VA Sch Med

Morrison, Glenn MD [NS] - **Spec Exp:** Pediatric Neurosurgery-Brain Tumors; Epilepsy; Craniofacial Surgery; **Hospital:** Miami Children's Hosp; **Address:** Medical Arts Bldg, 3200 SW 60th Ct, Ste 301, Miami, FL 33155-4071; **Phone:** 305-662-8386; **Board Cert:** Neurological Surgery 76; Pediatric Neurological Surgery 96; **Med School:** Case West Res Univ 67; **Resid:** Neurological Surgery, Case Western Univ Hosp 74; **Fac Appt:** Prof NS, Univ Miami Sch Med

Parent, Andrew D MD [NS] - **Spec Exp:** Pediatric Neurosurgery; Neuro-Endocrinology; Pituitary Tumors; **Hospital:** Univ Hosps & Clins - Jackson; **Address:** Univ Miss Med Ctr- Dept Neurosurgery, 2500 N State St, Jackson, MS 39216-4500; **Phone:** 601-984-5703; **Board Cert:** Neurological Surgery 81; Pediatric Neurological Surgery ; **Med School:** Univ VT Coll Med 70; **Resid:** Neurological Surgery, Emory Univ 78; **Fellow:** Neurological Surgery, Univ Tex Med Br 74; **Fac Appt:** Prof NS, Univ Miss

Sampson, John H MD/PhD [NS] - **Spec Exp:** Brain Tumors; Clinical Trials; **Hospital:** Duke Univ Med Ctr (page 94); **Address:** Duke Univ Med Ctr, Box 3050, Durham, NC 27710; **Phone:** 919-684-9041; **Board Cert:** Neurological Surgery 02; **Med School:** Univ Manitoba 90; **Resid:** Neurological Surgery, Duke Univ Med Ctr 98; **Fellow:** Neurological Intensive Care, Duke Univ Med Ctr; **Fac Appt:** Assoc Prof S, Duke Univ

Tatter, Stephen MD/PhD [NS] - **Spec Exp:** Brain & Pituitary Tumors; Stereotactic Radiosurgery; Parkinson's Disease; **Hospital:** Wake Forest Univ Baptist Med Ctr (page 117); **Address:** Wake Forest Univ Sch Med, Dept Neurosurg, Medical Center Blvd, Winston-Salem, NC 27157-1029; **Phone:** 336-716-4047; **Board Cert:** Neurological Surgery ; **Med School:** Cornell Univ-Weill Med Coll 90; **Resid:** Neurological Surgery, Mass Genl Hosp 96; **Fellow:** Mass Genl Hosp 97; **Fac Appt:** Asst Prof NS, Wake Forest Univ

Wharen Jr, Robert E MD [NS] - **Spec Exp:** Parkinson's Disease; Brain Tumors; Epilepsy; **Hospital:** St Luke's Hosp - Jacksonville; **Address:** Mayo Clinic, Dept Neurosurgery, 4500 San Pablo Rd, Jacksonville, FL 32224-1865; **Phone:** 904-953-2103; **Board Cert:** Neurological Surgery 88; **Med School:** Penn State Univ-Hershey Med Ctr 79; **Resid:** Neurological Surgery, Mayo Clinic 85; **Fac Appt:** Assoc Prof NS, Mayo Med Sch

Young, A Byron MD [NS] - **Spec Exp:** Brain Tumors; Stereotactic Radiosurgery; Parkinson's Disease; **Hospital:** Univ Kentucky Med Ctr; **Address:** University of Kentucky Medical Ctr, MS 101, Div Neurosurgery, 00 Rose St, Lexington, KY 40536-0298; **Phone:** 859-323-5861; **Board Cert:** Neurological Surgery 74; **Med School:** Univ KY Coll Med 65; **Resid:** Surgery, Vanderbilt Hosp 67; Neurological Surgery, Vanderbilt Hosp 71; **Fac Appt:** Prof S, Univ KY Coll Med

Midwest

Badie, Behnam MD [NS] - **Spec Exp:** Brain Tumors; **Hospital:** Univ WI Hosp & Clins; **Address:** Univ Wisconsin, Dept Neurosurgery, 600 Highland Ave, K4 8, Madison, WI 53792; **Phone:** 608-263-1411; **Board Cert:** Neurological Surgery 98; **Med School:** UCLA 89; **Resid:** Neurological Surgery, UCLA Med Ctr 96; **Fac Appt:** Assoc Prof NS, Univ Wisc

Bakay, Roy A. E. MD [NS] - **Spec Exp:** Parkinson's Disease/Movement Disorders; Epilepsy; Brain Tumors; **Hospital:** Rush Univ Med Ctr; **Address:** Rush Presby-St Luke's Med Ctr, Inst Neurosurgery, 1725 W Harrison St, Ste 970, Chicago, IL 60612; **Phone:** 312-942-6644; **Board Cert:** Neurological Surgery 85; **Med School:** Northwestern Univ 75; **Resid:** Neurological Surgery, Univ Washington Sch Med 81; **Fellow:** Neuronal Plasticity, Natl Inst Hlth 82; **Fac Appt:** Prof NS, Rush Med Coll

Barnett, Gene H MD [NS] - **Spec Exp:** Brain Tumors; Stereotactic Radiosurgery; **Hospital:** Cleveland Clin Fdn (page 92); **Address:** Cleveland Clinic Brain Tumor Inst, 9500 Euclid Ave, Cleveland, OH 44195-0001; **Phone:** 216-444-5381; **Board Cert:** Neurological Surgery 90; **Med School:** Case West Res Univ 80; **Resid:** Neurological Surgery, Cleveland Clinic 86; **Fellow:** Neurology, Cleveland Clinic 82; Research, Mass Genl Hosp-Harvard 87

Bauer, Jerry MD [NS] - **Spec Exp:** Pain-Back & Neck; Brain Tumors; Spinal Surgery; **Hospital:** Adv Luth Genl Hosp; **Address:** Ctr Brain & Spine Surg-Parkside Ctr, 1875 Dempster St, Ste 605, Park Ridge, IL 60068; **Phone:** 847-698-1088; **Board Cert:** Neurological Surgery 82; **Med School:** Univ IL Coll Med 74; **Resid:** Neurological Surgery, Univ Illinios Med Ctr 79; **Fac Appt:** Asst Clin Prof NS, Univ IL Coll Med

Chandler, William F MD [NS] - **Spec Exp:** Pituitary Surgery; Brain Tumors; **Hospital:** Univ Michigan Hlth Sys; **Address:** 1500 E Med Center Drive, Ste 3470, Tauban Center, Ann Arbor, MI 48109; **Phone:** 734-936-5020; **Board Cert:** Neurological Surgery 80; **Med School:** Univ Mich Med Sch 71; **Resid:** Neurological Surgery, Michigan Hosp 77; **Fac Appt:** Prof NS, Univ Mich Med Sch

Cohen, Alan MD [NS] - **Spec Exp:** Pediatric Neurosurgery; Brain & Spinal Tumors-Pediatric; Minimally Invasive Neurosurgery; **Hospital:** Rainbow Babies & Chldns Hosp; **Address:** Rainbow Babies & Chldns Hosp, 11100 Euclid Ave S, Ste B501, Cleveland, OH 44106; **Phone:** 216-844-5741; **Board Cert:** Neurological Surgery 91; Pediatric Neurological Surgery 97; **Med School:** Cornell Univ-Weill Med Coll 78; **Resid:** Surgery, NYU Medical Ctr 80; Neurological Surgery, NYU Medical Ctr 87; **Fellow:** Neurology, Natl Hosp Queen's Square; **Fac Appt:** Prof NS, Case West Res Univ

Dacey Jr, Ralph G MD [NS] - **Spec Exp:** Cerebrovascular Surgery; Aneurysm-Cerebral; Brain Tumors; **Hospital:** Barnes-Jewish Hosp (page 85); **Address:** Wash Univ Sch Med, Dept Neurosurgery, 660 S Euclid Ave, Box 8057, St. Louis, MO 63110; **Phone:** 314-362-3577; **Board Cert:** Internal Medicine 78; Neurological Surgery 85; **Med School:** Univ VA Sch Med 74; **Resid:** Internal Medicine, Strong Meml Hosp 77; Neurological Surgery, Univ Virginia Med Ctr 83; **Fac Appt:** Prof NS, Washington Univ, St Louis

Frim, David M MD/PhD **[NS]** - **Spec Exp:** Pediatric Neurosurgery; Hydrocephalus & Congenital Anomalies; Brain & Spinal Tumors; **Hospital:** Univ of Chicago Hosps; **Address:** Univ of Chicago Hosps-Chief, Pediatric Neurosurg, 5841 S Maryland Ave, MC 4066, Chicago, IL 60637-1463; **Phone:** 773-702-2475; **Board Cert:** Neurological Surgery 98; Pediatric Neurological Surgery 98; **Med School:** Harvard Med Sch 88; **Resid:** Neurological Surgery, Mass Genl Hosp 95; **Fellow:** Pediatric Neurological Surgery, Children's Hosp 96; **Fac Appt:** Assoc Prof S, Univ Chicago-Pritzker Sch Med

Grubb Jr, Robert L MD **[NS]** - **Spec Exp:** Brain & Skull Base Tumors; Acoustic Nerve Tumors; Trigeminal Neuralgia; **Hospital:** Barnes-Jewish Hosp (page 85); **Address:** Wash Univ Sch Med, Dept Neurosurgery, 660 S Euclid Ave, Box 8057, St Louis, MO 63110; **Phone:** 314-362-3577; **Board Cert:** Neurological Surgery 76; **Med School:** Univ NC Sch Med 65; **Resid:** Surgery, Barnes Jewish Hosp 67; Neurological Surgery, Barnes Jewish Hosp 73; **Fellow:** Neurological Surgery, National Inst Health 69; **Fac Appt:** Prof NS, Washington Univ, St Louis

Gutierrez, Francisco A MD **[NS]** - **Spec Exp:** Brain Tumors; Cerebrovascular Surgery; Spinal Surgery; **Hospital:** Northwestern Meml Hosp; **Address:** 201 E Huron St, Ste 9-160, Chicago, IL 60611; **Phone:** 312-926-3490; **Board Cert:** Neurological Surgery 76; **Med School:** Colombia 65; **Resid:** Neurological Surgery, San Juan de Dios Hosp 67; Neurological Surgery, Northwestern Meml Hosp 73; **Fac Appt:** Assoc Prof NS, Northwestern Univ

Hekmatpanah, Javad MD **[NS]** - **Spec Exp:** Brain Tumors; Spinal Surgery; Chiari's Deformity; **Hospital:** Univ of Chicago Hosps; **Address:** Univ Chicago Hosp, Dept Neurosurg, 5841 S Maryland Ave, MC 3026, Chicago, IL 60637; **Phone:** 773-702-6157; **Board Cert:** Neurological Surgery 66; Neurology 67; **Med School:** Iran 56; **Resid:** Neurology, Wisconsin Genl Hosp 61; Neurological Surgery, Univ Chicago Hosps 64; **Fac Appt:** Prof NS, Univ Chicago-Pritzker Sch Med

Kranzler, Leonard I MD **[NS]** - **Spec Exp:** Brain Tumors; **Hospital:** Adv Illinois Masonic Med Ctr; **Address:** 3000 N Halstead St, Ste 701, Chicago, IL 60657; **Phone:** 773-296-6666; **Board Cert:** Neurological Surgery 74; **Med School:** Northwestern Univ 63; **Resid:** Neurological Surgery, Northwestern Univ 69; Neurological Surgery, Chldns Meml Hosp 67; **Fellow:** Neurological Surgery; **Fac Appt:** Assoc Clin Prof NS, Univ Chicago-Pritzker Sch Med

Levy, Robert M MD/PhD **[NS]** - **Spec Exp:** Stereotactic Radiosurgery; Brain Tumors; Pain-Chronic; **Hospital:** Northwestern Meml Hosp; **Address:** 676 N Saint Clair St, Ste 2210, Chicago, IL 60611; **Phone:** 312-695-8143; **Board Cert:** Neurological Surgery 91; **Med School:** Stanford Univ 81; **Resid:** Neurological Surgery, UCSF Med Ctr 87; **Fellow:** Neurological Surgery, UCSF Med Ctr 86; **Fac Appt:** Prof NS, Northwestern Univ

Link, Michael J MD **[NS]** - **Spec Exp:** Skull Base Tumors; Brain Tumors; Cerebrovascular Surgery; **Hospital:** Mayo Med Ctr & Clin - Rochester; **Address:** Mayo Clinic, Dept Neurosurgery, 200 First St SW, Rochester, MN 55905; **Phone:** 507-284-4871; **Board Cert:** Neurological Surgery 00; **Med School:** Mayo Med Sch 90; **Resid:** Neurological Surgery, Mayo Clinic 96; **Fellow:** Cerebrovascular & Skull Base Surgery, Univ Cincinnati/Mayfield Clinic 98; **Fac Appt:** Asst Prof NS, Mayo Med Sch

Macdonald, R Loch MD/PhD **[NS]** - **Spec Exp:** Cerebrovascular Surgery; Brain & Spinal Cord Tumors; Spinal Surgery; **Hospital:** Univ of Chicago Hosps; **Address:** University of Chicago Hospitals, 5841 S Maryland Ave, MC 3026, Chicago, IL 60637; **Phone:** 773-702-2123; **Board Cert:** Neurological Surgery 95; **Med School:** Canada 85; **Resid:** Neurological Surgery, Univ of Toronto Med Ctr 93; **Fac Appt:** Prof S, Univ Chicago-Pritzker Sch Med

Malik, Ghaus MD [NS] - **Spec Exp:** Trigeminal Neuralgia; Cerebrovascular Surgery; Brain & Spinal Cord Tumors; **Hospital:** Henry Ford Hosp; **Address:** Henry Ford Hosp, Dept Neurosurg, 2799 W Grand Blvd, Detroit, MI 48202; **Phone:** 313-916-1093; **Board Cert:** Neurological Surgery 78; **Med School:** Pakistan 68; **Resid:** Surgery, Henry Ford Hosp 71; Neurological Surgery, Henry Ford Hosp 75

Mikkelsen, Tom MD [NS] - **Spec Exp:** Brain Tumors; Glioblastomas; **Hospital:** Henry Ford Hosp; **Address:** Henry Ford Hospital, Dept Neurology/Neurosurgery, 2799 W Grand Blvd, Detroit, MI 48202; **Phone:** 313-916-8641; **Board Cert:** Neurology 98; **Med School:** Univ Calgary 83; **Resid:** Internal Medicine, Calgary General Hosp 85; Neurology, Montreal Neurological Inst 88; **Fac Appt:** Assoc Prof N, Case West Res Univ

Origitano, Thomas MD/PhD [NS] - **Spec Exp:** Skull Base Tumors & Surgery; Cerebrovascular Surgery; Brain Tumors; **Hospital:** Loyola Univ Med Ctr (page 98); **Address:** Loyola University Medical Ctr, Dept Neurosurgery, 2160 S First Ave Bldg 105 - rm 1900, Maywood, IL 60153-3304; **Phone:** 708-216-8920; **Board Cert:** Neurological Surgery 95; **Med School:** Loyola Univ-Stritch Sch Med 84; **Resid:** Neurological Surgery, Loyola Univ Med Ctr 90; **Fac Appt:** Prof NS, Loyola Univ-Stritch Sch Med

Park, Tae Sung MD [NS] - **Spec Exp:** Pediatric Neurosurgery & Neuro-Oncology; Cerebral Palsy-Select Dorsal Rhizotomy; Chiari's Deformity; **Hospital:** St Louis Chldns Hosp; **Address:** St Louis Children's Hospital, 1 Children's Place, Ste 4-S20, St Louis, MO 63110; **Phone:** 314-454-4629; **Board Cert:** Neurological Surgery 85; Pediatric Neurological Surgery 88; **Med School:** Korea 71; **Resid:** Neurological Surgery, Univ Virginia Hosp 80; **Fellow:** Neuropathology, Mass General; Pediatric Neurological Surgery, Hospital for Sick Children; **Fac Appt:** Prof NS, St Louis Univ

Raffel, Corey MD/PhD [NS] - **Spec Exp:** Pediatric Neurosurgery; Brain Tumors; Medulloblastoma; **Hospital:** Mayo Med Ctr & Clin - Rochester; **Address:** Mayo Clinic, Dept Neurosurgery, 200 1st St SW, Rochester, MN 55905; **Phone:** 507-284-8008; **Board Cert:** Neurological Surgery 90; Pediatric Neurological Surgery 96; **Med School:** UCSD 80; **Resid:** Neurological Surgery, UCSF Med Ctr 86; **Fellow:** Pediatric Neurological Surgery, Hosp Sick Chldn 88; **Fac Appt:** Prof NS, Mayo Med Sch

Rich, Keith M MD [NS] - **Spec Exp:** Brain Tumors; Neurovascular Disorders; Stereotactic Radiosurgery; **Hospital:** Barnes-Jewish Hosp (page 85); **Address:** Washington University School of Medicine, 660 S Euclid Ave, Box 8057, St Louis, MO 63110; **Phone:** 314-362-3577; **Board Cert:** Neurological Surgery 87; **Med School:** Indiana Univ 77; **Resid:** Neurological Surgery, Barnes Jewish Hosp 82; **Fellow:** Neurological Pharmacology, Barnes Jewish Hosp 84; **Fac Appt:** Assoc Prof NS, Washington Univ, St Louis

Rock, Jack P MD [NS] - **Spec Exp:** Neuro-Oncology; Pituitary Surgery; Skull Base Surgery; **Hospital:** Henry Ford Hosp; **Address:** Henry Ford Hosp, Dept Neurosurg, 2799 W Grand Blvd, Detroit, MI 48202; **Phone:** 313-916-2241; **Board Cert:** Neurological Surgery 89; **Med School:** Univ Miami Sch Med 79; **Resid:** Neurological Surgery, NY Hosp-Cornell Med Ctr 85; **Fellow:** Univ Maryland 86

Rosenblum, Mark L MD [NS] - **Spec Exp:** Brain Tumors; Spinal Surgery; Infections of Nervous System; **Hospital:** Henry Ford Hosp; **Address:** Henry Ford Hospital, K11, 2799 W Grand Blvd, Detroit, MI 48202; **Phone:** 313-916-1340; **Board Cert:** Neurological Surgery 82; **Med School:** NY Med Coll 69; **Resid:** Surgery, UCLA Med Ctr 73; Neurological Surgery, UCSF Med Ctr 79; **Fellow:** Neurological Oncology, Natl Cancer Inst 72; **Fac Appt:** Prof NS, Case West Res Univ

Ruge, John MD [NS] - **Spec Exp:** Pediatric Neurosurgery; Brain Tumors; Hydrocephalus; **Hospital:** Adv Luth Genl Hosp; **Address:** 1875 Dempster St, Ste 605, Park Ridge, IL 60068; **Phone:** 847-698-1088; **Board Cert:** Neurological Surgery 93; **Med School:** Northwestern Univ 83; **Resid:** Neurological Surgery, Northwestern Meml Hosp 89; **Fellow:** Pediatric Neurological Surgery, Children's Hosp 90; **Fac Appt:** Asst Prof S, Univ IL Coll Med

Shapiro, Scott A MD **[NS]** - **Spec Exp:** Brain & Pituitary Tumors; Aneyrysm-Cerebral; Spinal Cord Injury; **Hospital:** Indiana Univ Hosp (page 90); **Address:** Inidiana University, Wishard Memorial Hospital, 1001 W 10th St, rm 323E, Indianapolis, IN 46202; **Phone:** 317-630-7635; **Board Cert:** Neurological Surgery 90; **Med School:** Indiana Univ 81; **Resid:** Neurological Surgery, Indiana Univ Med Ctr 87; **Fac Appt:** Prof NS, Indiana Univ

Thompson, B Gregory MD **[NS]** - **Spec Exp:** Acoustic Neuromas; Neurovascular Surgery; Skull Base Tumors & Surgery; **Hospital:** Univ Michigan Hlth Sys; **Address:** Univ Michigan, Dept Neurosurgery, 2128 Taubman, 1500 E Medical Center Drive, Ann Arbor, MI 48109; **Phone:** 734-936-7493; **Board Cert:** Neurological Surgery 98; **Med School:** Univ Kans 86; **Resid:** Neurological Surgery, Univ Pittsburgh 93; **Fellow:** Research, Natl Inst Hlth 92; Neurological Surgery, Barrow Neuro Inst 94; **Fac Appt:** Assoc Prof NS, Univ Mich Med Sch

Tomita, Tadanori MD **[NS]** - **Spec Exp:** Brain Tumors-Pediatric; Hydrocephalus; Pediatric Neurosurgery; **Hospital:** Children's Mem Hosp; **Address:** Chldns Meml Hosp, Div Ped Neurosurg, 2300 Children's Plaza, Box 28, Chicago, IL 60614-3318; **Phone:** 773-880-4373; **Board Cert:** Neurological Surgery 84; **Med School:** Japan 70; **Resid:** Neurological Surgery, Kobe Univ 74; Neurological Surgery, Northwestern Meml Hosp 80; **Fellow:** Surgery, Meml Sloan Kettering Canc Ctr 81; **Fac Appt:** Prof NS, Northwestern Univ

Warnick, Ronald E MD **[NS]** - **Spec Exp:** Neuro-Oncology; Brain Tumors; **Hospital:** Univ Hosp - Cincinnati; **Address:** 222 Piedmont Ave, Ste 3100, Cincinnati, OH 45219; **Phone:** 513-475-8629; **Board Cert:** Neurological Surgery 95; **Med School:** Univ Rochester 82; **Resid:** Neurological Surgery, New York-Cornell Med Ctr 89; **Fellow:** Neurological Oncology, UCSF Med Ctr 91; **Fac Appt:** Prof NS, Univ Cincinnati

Great Plains and Mountains

Couldwell, William MD/PhD **[NS]** - **Spec Exp:** Brain & Pituitary Tumors; Epilepsy/Movement Disorder; Parkinson's Disease; **Hospital:** Univ Utah Hosps and Clins; **Address:** 30 North 1900 East, Ste 3B409, Salt Lake City, UT 84132-2303; **Phone:** 801-581-6908; **Board Cert:** Neurological Surgery 94; **Med School:** McGill Univ 84; **Resid:** Neurological Surgery, LAC/USC Med Ctr 89; **Fellow:** Neurological Immunology, Montreal Neur Inst/McGill Univ 91; Neurological Surgery, CHUV; **Fac Appt:** Prof NS, Univ Utah

Johnson, Stephen D MD **[NS]** - **Spec Exp:** Skull Base Tumors & Surgery; **Hospital:** Presby - St Luke's Med Ctr; **Address:** Western Neurological Group, 1601 E 19th Ave, Ste 4400, Denver, CO 80218; **Phone:** 303-861-2266; **Board Cert:** Neurological Surgery 88; **Med School:** Univ Tenn Coll Med, Memphis 74; **Fac Appt:** Assoc Prof NS, Univ Colorado

Lillehei, Kevin O MD **[NS]** - **Spec Exp:** Neuro-Oncology; Pituitary Tumors; Peripheral Nerve Surgery; **Hospital:** Univ Colorado Hosp; **Address:** Univ Colo Hlth Sci Ctr, Div Neurosurg, 4200 E 9th Ave, Campus Box C-307, Denver, CO 80262; **Phone:** 303-315-5651; **Board Cert:** Neurological Surgery 89; **Med School:** Univ Minn 79; **Resid:** Neurological Surgery, Univ Mich Med Ctr 85; **Fac Appt:** Prof NS, Univ Colorado

Southwest

Al-Mefty, Ossama MD **[NS]** - **Spec Exp:** Skull Base Surgery; Brain Tumors; Cerebrovascular Surgery; **Hospital:** UAMS Med Ctr; **Address:** Univ Hosp of Arkansas for Med Scis, 4301 W Markham Slot 507, Little Rock, AR 72205; **Phone:** 501-686-8757; **Board Cert:** Neurological Surgery 80; **Med School:** Syria 72; **Resid:** Surgery, Med Coll Ohio 74; Neurological Surgery, West Va Med Ctr 78; **Fac Appt:** Prof NS, Univ Ark

Awasthi, Deepak MD [NS] - **Spec Exp:** Spinal Surgery; Skull Base Tumors & Surgery; **Hospital:** Louisiana State Univ Hosp; **Address:** LSU Health Scis Ctr, Dept Neurosurgery, 1542 Tulane Ave, Box T 7-3, New Orleans, LA 70112; **Phone:** 504-568-6125; **Board Cert:** Neurological Surgery 96; **Med School:** NYU Sch Med 86; **Resid:** Neurological Surgery, LSU Med Ctr 93; **Fellow:** Skull Base Surgery, LSU Med Ctr 88; **Fac Appt:** Assoc Prof NS, Louisiana State Univ

De Monte, Franco MD [NS] - **Spec Exp:** Skull Base Tumors & Surgery; **Hospital:** UT MD Anderson Cancer Ctr, The (page 115); **Address:** UT MD Anderson Cancer Ctr, Dept Neurosurgery, 1515 Holcombe Blvd, Ste 442, Houston, TX 77030; **Phone:** 713-792-2400; **Board Cert:** Neurological Surgery 95; **Med School:** Canada 85; **Resid:** Neurological Surgery, Univ Western Ontario 91; **Fellow:** Skull Base Surgery, Loyola Univ-Stritch Sch Med 92; **Fac Appt:** Assoc Prof NS, Baylor Coll Med

Hankinson, Hal L MD [NS] - **Spec Exp:** Brain Tumors; **Hospital:** Presbyterian Hospital - Albuquerque; **Address:** New Mexico Neurosurgery, 522 Lomas Blvd NE, Albuquerque, NM 87102-2454; **Phone:** 505-247-4253; **Board Cert:** Neurological Surgery 77; **Med School:** Tulane Univ 67; **Resid:** Neurological Surgery, UCSF Med Ctr 75; **Fac Appt:** Clin Prof NS, Univ New Mexico

Hassenbusch, Samuel J MD/PhD [NS] - **Spec Exp:** Pain Management; Stereotactic Radiosurgery; Intratumoral Chemotherapy; **Hospital:** UT MD Anderson Cancer Ctr, The (page 115); **Address:** 1515 Holcombe Blvd, Box 442, Houston, TX 77030; **Phone:** 713-792-2400; **Board Cert:** Neurological Surgery 92; **Med School:** Johns Hopkins Univ 78; **Resid:** Surgery, Johns Hopkins Univ 80; Neurological Surgery, Johns Hopkins Univ 88; **Fellow:** Research, Keck Fdn-UCSF 86; **Fac Appt:** Prof NS, Univ Tex, Houston

Lang Jr, Frederick F MD [NS] - **Spec Exp:** Brain & Spinal Tumors; Neuro-Oncology; **Hospital:** UT MD Anderson Cancer Ctr, The (page 115); **Address:** Univ Texas MD Anderson Cancer Ctr, 1515 Holcombe Blvd, Box 0442, Houston, TX 77030; **Phone:** 713-792-2400; **Board Cert:** Neurological Surgery 00; **Med School:** Yale Univ 88; **Resid:** Neurological Surgery, NYU Med Ctr 95; **Fellow:** Neurological Oncology, MD Anderson Cancer Ctr 96; **Fac Appt:** Assoc Prof NS, Univ Tex, Houston

Sawaya, Raymond MD [NS] - **Spec Exp:** Brain Tumors; **Hospital:** UT MD Anderson Cancer Ctr, The (page 115); **Address:** MD Anderson Cancer Ctr, 1515 Holcombe Blvd, Unit 442, Houston, TX 77030; **Phone:** 713-792-6500; **Board Cert:** Neurological Surgery 85; **Med School:** Lebanon 74; **Resid:** Neurological Surgery, Univ Cincinnati Med Ctr 80; Neurological Surgery, Johns Hopkins Med Ctr 81; **Fellow:** Neurological Oncology, Natl Inst Hlth 82; **Fac Appt:** Prof NS, Univ Tex, Houston

Spetzler, Robert MD [NS] - **Spec Exp:** Skull Base Tumors & Surgery; Cerebrovascular Surgery; **Hospital:** St Joseph's Hosp & Med Ctr - Phoenix; **Address:** Barrow Neurosurgical Assocs, 2910 N Third Ave, Phoenix, AZ 85013; **Phone:** 602-406-3489; **Board Cert:** Neurological Surgery 79; **Med School:** Northwestern Univ 71; **Resid:** Neurological Surgery, UCSF Med Ctr 76; **Fac Appt:** Prof S, Univ Ariz Coll Med

West Coast and Pacific

Adler Jr, John R MD [NS] - **Spec Exp:** Stereotactic Radiosurgery; Brain Tumors; Acoustic Nerve Tumors; **Hospital:** Stanford Univ Med Ctr; **Address:** Stanford Univ Med Ctr, Dept Neurosurg-R 205, 300 Pasteur Drive, Stanford, CA 94305-5327; **Phone:** 650-723-5573; **Board Cert:** Neurological Surgery 90; **Med School:** Harvard Med Sch 80; **Resid:** Neurological Surgery, Chldns Hosp 87; Neurological Surgery, Mass Genl Hosp 85; **Fellow:** Cerebrovascular Disease, Karolinska Inst 86; **Fac Appt:** Prof NS, Stanford Univ

Apuzzo, Michael L J MD [NS] - **Spec Exp:** Brain Tumors; Epilepsy/Seizure Disorders; Stereotactic Radiosurgery; **Hospital:** LAC & USC Med Ctr; **Address:** 1200 N State St, Ste 5046, Los Angeles, CA 90033-1029; **Phone:** 323-226-7421; **Board Cert:** Neurological Surgery 75; **Med School:** Boston Univ 65; **Resid:** Neurological Surgery, Hartford Hosp; Neurological Surgery, Hartford Hosp 73; **Fellow:** Neurological Physiology, Yale Univ Hosp; **Fac Appt:** Prof NS, USC Sch Med

Batzdorf, Ulrich MD [NS] - **Spec Exp:** Chiari's Deformity; Syringomyelia; Spinal Cord Tumors; **Hospital:** UCLA Med Ctr (page 111); **Address:** UCLA Med Ctr, Box 956901, Los Angeles, CA 90095-6901; **Phone:** 310-825-5079; **Board Cert:** Neurological Surgery 68; **Med School:** NY Med Coll 55; **Resid:** Surgery, Univ Maryland Hosp 60; Neurological Surgery, UCLA Ctr Hlth Sci 65; **Fellow:** Neurological Pathology, UCSF-Moffit Hosp 62; **Fac Appt:** Prof NS, UCLA

Berger, Mitchel S MD [NS] - **Spec Exp:** Brain & Spinal Cord Tumors; Pituitary Tumors; Neuro-Oncology, Adult & Pediatric; **Hospital:** UCSF Med Ctr; **Address:** UCSF Med Ctr, Dept Neurosurgery, 505 Parnassus Avenue, M-786, San Francisco, CA 94143-0112; **Phone:** 415-502-7673; **Board Cert:** Neurological Surgery 91; **Med School:** Univ Miami Sch Med 79; **Resid:** Neurological Surgery, UCSF Med Ctr 84; **Fellow:** Neurological Oncology, UCSF Med Ctr 85; Pediatric Neurological Surgery, Hosp Sick Chldn 86; **Fac Appt:** Prof NS, UCSF

Black, Keith L MD [NS] - **Spec Exp:** Brain Tumors; Pituitary Surgery; Trigeminal Neuralgia; **Hospital:** Cedars-Sinai Med Ctr (page 88); **Address:** Cedars Sinai Medical Ctr, Dept Neurosurgery, 8631 W 3rd St, Ste 800E, Los Angeles, CA 90048; **Phone:** 310-423-7900; **Board Cert:** Neurological Surgery 90; **Med School:** Univ Mich Med Sch 81; **Resid:** Neurological Surgery, Univ Michigan Med Ctr 87; **Fac Appt:** Prof NS, UCLA

Boggan, James E MD [NS] - **Spec Exp:** Skull Base Tumors & Surgery; **Hospital:** UC Davis Med Ctr; **Address:** University of California, Davis, Dept Neurological Surgery, 4860 Y St, Ste 3740, Sacramento, CA 95817; **Phone:** 916-734-2371; **Board Cert:** Neurological Surgery 85; **Med School:** Univ Chicago-Pritzker Sch Med 76; **Resid:** Neurological Surgery, UCSF Med Ctr 82; **Fac Appt:** Prof NS, UC Davis

Delashaw Jr, Johnny B MD [NS] - **Spec Exp:** Skull Base Tumors & Surgery; Aneurysm-Cerebral; Neuro-Oncology; **Hospital:** OR Hlth & Sci Univ; **Address:** Oregon Hlth & Sci Univ, Dept Neurosurgery, 3181 SW Sam Jackson Park Rd, Ste L472, Portland, OR 97239; **Phone:** 503-494-4314; **Board Cert:** Neurological Surgery 93; **Med School:** Univ Wash 83; **Resid:** Neurological Surgery, Univ Virginia Medical Ctr 90; **Fac Appt:** Prof NS, Oregon Hlth Sci Univ

Ellenbogen, Richard MD [NS] - **Spec Exp:** Pediatric Neurosurgery; Chiari's Deformity; Brain Tumors; **Hospital:** Chldns Hosp and Regl Med Ctr - Seattle; **Address:** 4800 Sand Point Way NE, MS G0035, Seattle, WA 98105; **Phone:** 206-987-2544; **Board Cert:** Neurological Surgery 92; Pediatric Neurological Surgery ; **Med School:** Brown Univ 83; **Resid:** Neurological Surgery, Brigham Womens Hosp/Childrens Hosp 89; **Fac Appt:** Assoc Prof NS, Univ Wash

Giannotta, Steven L MD [NS] - **Spec Exp:** Aneurysm-Cerebral; Skull Base Tumors; Acoustic Nerve Tumors; **Hospital:** USC Univ Hosp - R K Eamer Med Plz; **Address:** 1200 N State St, rm 5046, Los Angeles, CA 90033; **Phone:** 323-442-5720; **Board Cert:** Neurological Surgery 80; **Med School:** Univ Mich Med Sch 72; **Resid:** Neurological Surgery, Univ Michigan Med Ctr 78; **Fac Appt:** Prof NS, USC Sch Med

Greene Jr, Clarence S MD [NS] - **Spec Exp:** Pediatric Neurosurgery; Congenital Nervous System Malformations; Brain Tumors; **Hospital:** Long Beach Meml Med Ctr; **Address:** 2865 Atlantic Ave, Ste 202, Long Beach, CA 90806; **Phone:** 562-426-4121; **Board Cert:** Neurological Surgery 84; Pediatric Neurological Surgery ; **Med School:** Howard Univ 74; **Resid:** Neurological Surgery, Chldns Hosp 81; Neurological Surgery, Peter Bent Brigham Hosp 81; **Fellow:** Pediatric Neurological Surgery, Chldns Hosp 85; **Fac Appt:** Assoc Clin Prof NS, UC Irvine

Harsh IV, Griffith MD [NS] - **Spec Exp:** Brain & Spinal Tumors; Skull Base Tumors; Acoustic Neuromas & Pituitary Tumors; **Hospital:** Stanford Univ Med Ctr; **Address:** Stanford Cancer Ctr, Dept Neurosurgery, 875 Blake Wilbur Drive, MC 5826, Stanford, CA 94305; **Phone:** 650-725-8430; **Board Cert:** Neurological Surgery 89; **Med School:** Harvard Med Sch 80; **Resid:** Neurological Surgery, UCSF Med Ctr 86; **Fellow:** Neurological Oncology, UCSF Med Ctr 87; **Fac Appt:** Prof NS, Stanford Univ

Liau, Linda MD/PhD [NS] - **Spec Exp:** Neuro-Oncology; Brain Tumors; **Hospital:** UCLA Med Ctr (page 111); **Address:** CHS 74-145, Box 956901, 10833 Le Conte Ave, Los Angeles, CA 90095-6901; **Phone:** 310-267-2621; **Board Cert:** Neurological Surgery 02; **Med School:** Stanford Univ 91; **Resid:** Neurological Surgery, UCLA Med Ctr 98; **Fellow:** Neurological Oncology, UCLA Med Ctr; **Fac Appt:** Assoc Prof NS, UCLA

Mamelak, Adam N MD [NS] - **Spec Exp:** Brain & Spinal Tumors; Epilepsy; Spinal Tumors; **Hospital:** City of Hope Natl Med Ctr & Beckman Rsch (page 89); **Address:** City of Hope Cancer Ctr, Dept Neurosurgery, 1500 E Duarte Rd, Duarte, CA 91105; **Phone:** 626-359-8111 x64516; **Board Cert:** Neurological Surgery 00; **Med School:** Harvard Med Sch 90; **Resid:** Neurological Surgery, UCSF Med Ctr 94; **Fellow:** Epilepsy, UCSF Epilepsy Research Lab 95

Mayberg, Marc MD [NS] - **Spec Exp:** Pituitary Surgery; Stroke/Cerebrovascular Disease; Skull Base Tumors; **Hospital:** Swedish Med Ctr Providence Campus; **Address:** Seattle Neuroscience Inst, 1600 E Jefferson St, Ste #620, Seattle, WA 98122; **Phone:** 206-320-2800; **Board Cert:** Neurological Surgery 88; **Med School:** Mayo Med Sch 78; **Resid:** Neurological Surgery, Mass Genl Hosp 84; **Fellow:** Neurological Surgery, Natl Hosp for Nervous Dis

Neuwelt, Edward A. MD [NS] - **Spec Exp:** Neuro-Oncology; Brain Tumors; **Hospital:** OR Hlth & Sci Univ; **Address:** Oregon Hlth Sci Univ, Dept NS, 3181 SW Sam Jackson Pk Rd, MC-L603, Portland, OR 97239; **Phone:** 503-494-5626; **Board Cert:** Neurological Surgery 80; **Med School:** Univ Colorado 72; **Resid:** Neurological Surgery, Univ Tex SW Med Sch 78; **Fac Appt:** Prof NS, Oregon Hlth Sci Univ

Ott, Kenneth H MD [NS] - **Spec Exp:** Brain Tumors & Disorders; Gamma Knife Surgery; **Hospital:** Scripps Meml Hosp - La Jolla; **Address:** Neurosurgical Medical Clinic, 501 Washington St, Ste 700, San Diego, CA 92103-2231; **Phone:** 619-297-4481; **Board Cert:** Neurological Surgery 80; **Med School:** UCSF 70; **Resid:** Surgery, Mass Genl Hosp 72; Neurological Surgery, Mass Genl Hosp 76; **Fac Appt:** Assoc Clin Prof S, UCSD

Pitts, Lawrence H MD [NS] - **Spec Exp:** Acoustic Nerve Tumors; Skull Base Surgery; Spinal Surgery; **Hospital:** UCSF Med Ctr; **Address:** 400 Parnassus Ave, Ste A808, San Francisco, CA 94143-0350; **Phone:** 415-353-7500; **Board Cert:** Neurological Surgery 78; **Med School:** Case West Res Univ 69; **Resid:** Neurological Surgery, UCSF Med Ctr 75; **Fac Appt:** Prof NS, UCSF

Silbergeld, Daniel MD [NS] - **Spec Exp:** Brain Tumors; **Hospital:** Univ Wash Med Ctr; **Address:** Univ Wash Med Ctr, Dept Neurosurg, 1959 NE Pacific, Box 356470, Seattle, WA 98195; **Phone:** 206-598-5637; **Board Cert:** Neurological Surgery 95; **Med School:** Univ Cincinnati 84; **Resid:** Neurological Surgery, Univ Wash Med Ctr 90; Research, Univ Wash Med Ctr 88; **Fellow:** Neurological Oncology, Univ Wash Med Ctr; Epilepsy, Univ Wash Med Ctr; **Fac Appt:** Assoc Prof NS, Univ Wash

Weiss, Martin Harvey MD [NS] - **Spec Exp:** Brain Tumors; Spinal Cord Tumors; Pituitary Tumors; **Hospital:** USC Univ Hosp - R K Eamer Med Plz; **Address:** LAC-USC Med Ctr, 1200 N State St, Ste 5046, Los Angeles, CA 90033-1029; **Phone:** 323-442-5720; **Board Cert:** Neurological Surgery 72; **Med School:** Cornell Univ-Weill Med Coll 63; **Resid:** Surgery, US Army Hosp 66; Neurological Surgery, Univ Hosp 70; **Fellow:** Neurological Surgery, NIH-Univ Hosp 70; **Fac Appt:** Prof NS, USC Sch Med

Yu, John S MD [NS] - **Spec Exp:** Brain Tumors; Spinal Tumors; Clinical Trials; **Hospital:** Cedars-Sinai Med Ctr (page 88); **Address:** Cedars Sinai Med Ctr, Comp Brain Tumor Prog, 8631 W 3rd St, Ste 800E, Los Angeles, CA 90048; **Phone:** 310-423-7900; **Board Cert:** Neurological Surgery 02; **Med School:** Harvard Med Sch 90; **Resid:** Neurological Surgery, Mass General Hosp 97

NEUROLOGY

A neurologist specializes in the diagnosis and treatment of all types of disease or impaired function of the brain, spinal cord, peripheral nerves, muscles and autonomic nervous system, as well as the blood vessels that relate to these structures.

Training required: *Four years*

Certification in the following subspecialty requires additional training and examination

CHILD NEUROLOGY: *A neurologist with special qualifications in child neurology has special skills in the diagnosis and management of neurologic disorders of the neonatal period, infancy, early childhood and adolescence.*

Training required: *Four years*

SPINAL CORD INJURY MEDICINE:

A physician who addresses the prevention, diagnosis, treatment and management of traumatic spinal cord injury and non-traumatic etiologies of spinal cord dysfunction by working in an interdisciplinary manner. Care is provided to patients of all ages on a lifelong basis and covers related medical, physical, psychological and vocational disabilities and complications.

PHYSICIAN LISTINGS

Neurology:

Child Neurolgy:

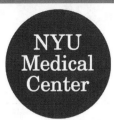
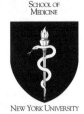
NEUROLOGY

Dedicated to exceptional patient care, advanced scientific research, and high-quality graduate education, the Department of Neurology at NYU Medical Center evaluates and treats children and adults with a broad spectrum of neurological diseases. Specialty groups within the department deliver integrated care to patients with behavioral disorders and dementia, brain tumors, genetic and degenerative diseases, headache and pain sydromes, movement disorders including Parkinson's disease, multiple sclerosis, neuromuscular diseases, and diseases of children. NYU Medical Center is home to the largest multiple sclerosis program in New York.

The clinical mission especially benefits from a 30-bed neurorehabilitation unit, a state-of-the-art neurophysiology laboratory, and neurogenetics testing facility, each conducted under departmental auspices.

NYU COMPREHENSIVE EPILEPSY CENTER

Among the department's core programs is the NYU Comprehensive Epilepsy Center – the largest epilepsy program in the Eastern United States. The center offers testing, evaluation, treatment, drug trials, alternative therapies, and surgical intervention for patients with all forms of epilepsy. Beyond control of seizures, the center aims to improve quality of life by addressing problems of social isolation and helping patients achieve gratification at school, at work, at home, and in their communities.

At present, medications adequately control about 75 percent of those who suffer from recurrent epileptic seizures. But when medications fail to bring these debilitating seizures under control, a patient may be a candidate for surgery.

In the past two decades, enormous strides in understanding, technology, and surgical techniques have made surgery a safe and effective option for patients with intractable seizure disorders. Key to surgical success is functional mapping, which involves testing the brain to make sure it is safe to remove the tissues that are responsible for the seizures. Using a variety of imaging technologies, including MRI, PET, and SPECT, NYU's epileptologists are able to visualize abnormal anatomy and physiology and define a surgical target. Video-EEG recording is the most important test of all for characterizing and localizing seizures.

The most common surgical procedure for epilepsy is temporal lobe resection, often involving the removal of the deepest temporal structures. A low incidence of permanent complications makes this surgery a safe and attractive option when appropriate. At NYU, temporal lobe resection is performed without removing the patient's hair, using computer-assisted navigation and microscopic techniques. Patients are normally able to leave the hospital in 4 to 5 days. Vagus nerve stimulation (VNS), a reversible technique that was approved by the FDA in 1997, is just one of several additional surgical options for patients with particular types of seizures.

Brain diseases can cause intellectual impairments of profound complexity. The diagnosis and management of the cognitive disabilities accompanying traumatic brain injury or such diseases as stroke, Alzheimer's disease, epilepsy, and systemic illness often require an integrated approach. The Cognitive Neurology Program is an outpatient specialty clinic that serves adults with brain-based memory, perceptual, cognitive, or emotional impairments. Its specialists work closely with other branches of the Department of Neurology, and have close ties with Rusk Institute for Rehabilitation Medicine, where patients receive cognitive rehabilitation and speech therapy.

PHYSICIAN REFERRAL
1-888-7-NYU-MED
(1-888-769-8633)
www.nyumc.org

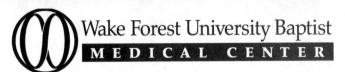

Wake Forest University Baptist
MEDICAL CENTER

BRAIN TUMOR CENTER OF EXCELLENCE
COMPREHENSIVE CANCER CENTER
Medical Center Boulevard • Winston-Salem, NC 27157
Health On-Call® (Patient Access) 1-800-446-2255
PAL® (Physician-to-physician calls) 1-800-277-7654
www.wfubmc.edu/cancer

OVERVIEW

The Brain Tumor Center of Excellence of Wake Forest University was formed in June 2003. With the goal of being a national leader in patient care and research, the Center has built its program with three basic components: an excellent group of clinicians, a world-renowned researcher to direct the Center, and a mission to grow the clinical and basic research programs to a magnitude that would place Wake Forest among the top six brain tumor centers in the United States.

RESEARCH

The Brain Tumor Center of Excellence has three areas of research focus:

- Novel therapeutics – identifying innovative treatments that will improve outcome.
- Bioanatomic imaging – identifying the unique signatures of a cancer through non-invasive imaging of tumor biology, chemistry and physiology, thus allowing individual treatment planning.
- Radiation-induced brain injury – understanding the mechanisms of injury and ways to prevent and treat side effects of brain tumor therapy.

Laboratory researchers are exploring new therapies such as novel chemotherapy drugs, cytotoxins, gene therapy, and radiosensitizers, translating these unique approaches into clinical trials for patients. In addition to studies written and conducted by Comprehensive Cancer Center doctors, clinical trials are also offered from several national Cooperative Groups as well as the pharmaceutical industry. Wake Forest Baptist is one of only ten centers in the country that is part of the New Approaches to Brain Tumor Therapy (NABTT) consortium. In addition, the clinicians and researchers have one of the most extensive laboratory and clinical research programs in the world for the diagnosis, prevention, and treatment of brain injury resulting from a brain tumor and its treatments, particularly radiation therapy.

MULTIDISCIPLINARY CARE

Offering the region's only multidisciplinary clinic for brain tumor treatment, patients are evaluated by a medical oncologist, neurosurgeon, radiation oncologist and other specialists as needed. Weekly, the entire clinical neuro-oncology team meets to discuss all patients seen in the prior week, as well as cases sent in from around the region, southeast, and nationally/internationally. Recommendations for multidisciplinary care are made and communicated to referring physicians and patients.

For patients who receive their brain tumor care at Wake Forest Baptist, the most sophisticated tools in the world are available for diagnosis and treatment. Imaging brain tumor and normal brain anatomy using modalities such as magnetic resonance (MR) imaging, MR spectroscopy, functional MR, and positron emission tomography, helps the team plan surgical and radiotherapeutic treatments that have the best chance of cure. Image guided surgery, cortical mapping, awake craniotomy, Leksell® Gamma Knife stereotactic radiosurgery, Gliadel® wafer chemotherapy, convection enhanced drug delivery, and GliaSite® brachytherapy are just some of the leading-edge approaches used for brain tumor patients.

a world of difference in the world of medicine ™

To make an appointment or find a specialist at Wake Forest University Baptist Medical Center, call

HEALTH ON-CALL®
1-800-446-2255

NEUROLOGY

Mid Atlantic

De Angelis, Lisa MD [N] - **Spec Exp:** Neuro-Oncology; **Hospital:** Meml Sloan Kettering Cancer Ctr (page 100); **Address:** 1275 York Ave, New York, NY 10021-6007; **Phone:** 212-639-7123; **Board Cert:** Neurology 86; **Med School:** Columbia P&S 80; **Resid:** Neurology, Neuro Inst - Presby Hosp 84; **Fellow:** Neurological Oncology, Neuro Inst - Presby Hosp 85; Neurological Oncology, Meml Sloan-Kettering Cancer Ctr 86; **Fac Appt:** Prof N, Cornell Univ-Weill Med Coll

Hiesiger, Emile MD [N] - **Spec Exp:** Pain Management; Neuro-Oncology; **Hospital:** NYU Med Ctr (page 104); **Address:** 530 1st Ave, Ste A5, New York, NY 10016-6402; **Phone:** 212-263-6123; **Board Cert:** Neurology 83; **Med School:** NY Med Coll 78; **Resid:** Neurology, NYU Med Ctr 82; **Fellow:** Neurology, Meml Sloan-Kettering Cancer Ctr 84; **Fac Appt:** Assoc Clin Prof N, NYU Sch Med

Laterra, John J MD/PhD [N] - **Spec Exp:** Neuro-Oncology; Brain Tumors; **Hospital:** Johns Hopkins Hosp - Baltimore (page 97); **Address:** Johns Hopkins Hosp, Phipps 115, 600 N Wolfe St, Baltimore, MD 21287; **Phone:** 410-614-3853; **Board Cert:** Neurology 90; **Med School:** Case West Res Univ 84; **Resid:** Neurology, Univ Mich Hosps 88; **Fellow:** Research, Johns Hopkins Hosp 89; **Fac Appt:** Prof N, Johns Hopkins Univ

Posner, Jerome MD [N] - **Spec Exp:** Neuro-Oncology; Brain Tumors; **Hospital:** Meml Sloan Kettering Cancer Ctr (page 100); **Address:** 1275 York Ave, rm C731, New York, NY 10021-6007; **Phone:** 212-639-7047; **Board Cert:** Neurology 62; **Med School:** Univ Wash 55; **Resid:** Neurology, Univ WA Affil Hosp 59; **Fellow:** Biochemistry, Univ WA Affil Hosp 63; **Fac Appt:** Prof N, Cornell Univ-Weill Med Coll

Rosenfeld, Myrna MD/PhD [N] - **Spec Exp:** Neuro-Oncology; **Hospital:** Hosp Univ Penn - UPHS (page 113); **Address:** Hosp Univ Penn, Dept Neurology, 3400 Spruce St, 3W Gates, Philadelphia, PA 19104; **Phone:** 215-746-4707; **Board Cert:** Neurology 90; **Med School:** Northwestern Univ 85; **Resid:** Neurology, Northwestern Univ Hosp 87; Neurology, Univ Hosp Cleveland 89; **Fellow:** Neurological Oncology, Meml Sloan Kettering Cancer Ctr; **Fac Appt:** Assoc Prof N, Univ Pennsylvania

Southeast

Janss, Anna J MD/PhD [N] - **Spec Exp:** Brain Tumors-Pediatric; Clinical Trials; Cancer Survivors-Late Effects of Therapy; **Hospital:** Chldns Hlthcare Atlanta - Egleston; **Address:** Chldns Hlthcare Atlanta - Egleston, 1405 Clifton Rd NE, Div Neuro-Oncology, Atlanta, GA 30322; **Phone:** 404-785-1200; **Board Cert:** Neurology 93; **Med School:** Univ Iowa Coll Med 88; **Resid:** Neurology, Hosp Univ Penn 92; **Fellow:** Pediatric Neuro-Oncology, Chldns Hosp 96; **Fac Appt:** Assoc Prof N, Emory Univ

Patchell, Roy MD [N] - **Spec Exp:** Neuro-Oncology; Brain Tumors; **Hospital:** Univ Kentucky Med Ctr; **Address:** Univ Kentucky-Chandler Med Ctr, 800 Rose St, MS 105, Lexington, KY 40536; **Phone:** 859-323-5672; **Board Cert:** Neurology 84; **Med School:** Univ KY Coll Med 79; **Resid:** Neurology, Johns Hopkins Hosp 83; **Fellow:** Neurological Oncology, Meml Sloan-Kettering Canc Ctr 85; **Fac Appt:** Assoc Prof N, Univ KY Coll Med

Rosenfeld, Steven S MD [N] - **Spec Exp:** Brain Tumors; Gliomas; Neuro-Oncology; **Hospital:** Univ of Ala Hosp at Birmingham; **Address:** 510 20th St S, FOT rm 1020, Birmingham, AL 35294; **Phone:** 205-934-1432; **Board Cert:** Neurology 94; **Med School:** Northwestern Univ 85; **Resid:** Neurology, Duke University Med Ctr 89; **Fellow:** Neurological Oncology, Duke University Med Ctr 90; **Fac Appt:** Assoc Prof N, Univ Ala

Schiff, David MD [N] - **Spec Exp:** Brain Tumors; **Hospital:** Univ Virginia Med Ctr; **Address:** Univ VA, Div of Neuro-Oncology, PO Box 800432, Charlottesville, VA 22908; **Phone:** 434-982-4415; **Board Cert:** Neurology 94; **Med School:** Harvard Med Sch 88; **Resid:** Harvard Longwood 92; **Fellow:** Meml Sloan Kettering 93; Mayo Clinic 94; **Fac Appt:** Assoc Prof NS, Univ VA Sch Med

Schold Jr, S Clifford MD [N] - **Spec Exp:** Brain Tumors; Neuro-Oncology; **Hospital:** H Lee Moffitt Cancer Ctr & Research Inst; **Address:** H Lee Moffitt Cancer Ctr, 12902 Magnolia Dr, MCC VP Admin, Tampa, FL 33612; **Phone:** 813-745-7426; **Board Cert:** Neurology 80; **Med School:** Univ Ariz Coll Med 73; **Resid:** Neurology, Colorado Med Ctr 77; **Fellow:** Neurological Oncology, Sloan-Kettering Cancer Ctr 78; **Fac Appt:** Prof N, Univ S Fla Coll Med

Midwest

Cascino, Terrence L MD [N] - **Spec Exp:** Neuro-Oncology; **Hospital:** Mayo Med Ctr & Clin - Rochester; **Address:** Mayo Clinic, 200 1st St SW, Rocherster, MN 55905-0001; **Phone:** 507-284-2576; **Board Cert:** Neurology 84; **Med School:** Loyola Univ-Stritch Sch Med 72; **Resid:** Neurology, Mayo Clinic 80; **Fellow:** Neurological Oncology, Meml Sloan Kettering Cancer Ctr; **Fac Appt:** Assoc Prof N, Mayo Med Sch

Greenberg, Harry S. MD [N] - **Spec Exp:** Neuro-Oncology; Brain Tumors; **Hospital:** Univ Michigan Hlth Sys; **Address:** Taubman Ctr 1914-0316, 1500 E Med Ctr Dr, Ann Arbor, MI 48109-0316; **Phone:** 734-936-9055; **Board Cert:** Neurology 80; **Med School:** SUNY Upstate Med Univ 73; **Resid:** Neurology, Stanford Univ Hosp 77; **Fellow:** Neurological Oncology, Sloan Kettering Cancer Ctr; **Fac Appt:** Prof N, Univ Mich Med Sch

Newton, Herbert B MD [N] - **Spec Exp:** Neuro-Oncology; Brain & Spinal Tumors; **Hospital:** Ohio St Univ Med Ctr (page 105); **Address:** 1654 Upham Dr., 465 Means Hall 4th Fl, Columbus, OH 43210; **Phone:** 614-293-8930; **Board Cert:** Neurology 89; **Med School:** SUNY Buffalo 84; **Resid:** Neurology, Univ Michigan 88; **Fellow:** Neurological Oncology, Meml Sloan-Kettering Cancer Ctr 90; **Fac Appt:** Prof N, Ohio State Univ

Rogers, Lisa R DO [N] - **Spec Exp:** Neuro-Oncology; Brain Tumors; Spinal Tumors; **Hospital:** Henry Ford Hosp; **Address:** Henry Ford Hosp, Dept Neur, 2799 W Grand Blvd Fl K-11, Detroit, MI 48202-2608; **Phone:** 313-916-8662; **Board Cert:** Neurology 82; **Med School:** Kirksville Coll Osteo Med 76; **Resid:** Neurology, Cleveland Clinic Fdn 80; **Fellow:** Neurological Oncology, Meml-Sloan Kettering Cancer Ctr 82; **Fac Appt:** Prof N, Wayne State Univ

Sagar, Stephen M MD [N] - **Spec Exp:** Neuro-Oncology; **Hospital:** Univ Hosps of Cleveland; **Address:** Univ Hosp Cleveland, Hanna House, 11100 Euclid Ave Fl 5, Cleveland, OH 44106; **Phone:** 216-844-7510; **Board Cert:** Internal Medicine 76; Neurology 79; **Med School:** Harvard Med Sch 72; **Resid:** Internal Medicine, Peter Bent Brigham Hosp 74; Neurology, Mass Genl Hosp 77; **Fellow:** Neurology, Chldns Hosp Med Ctr 79; **Fac Appt:** Prof N, Case West Res Univ

Vick, Nicholas A MD [N] - **Spec Exp:** Brain Tumors; Neuro-Oncology; **Hospital:** Evanston Hosp; **Address:** Evanston Hosp, Div Neurology, 2650 Ridge Ave, Bldg Burch - rm 309, Evanston, IL 60201-1718; **Phone:** 847-570-2570 x11; **Board Cert:** Neurology 71; **Med School:** Univ Chicago-Pritzker Sch Med 65; **Resid:** Neurology, Univ Chicago Hosps 68; **Fellow:** Neurology, Natl Inst Hlth 70; **Fac Appt:** Prof N, Northwestern Univ

Great Plains and Mountains

Blumenthal, Deborah T MD **[N]** - **Spec Exp:** Brain Tumors; Spinal Tumors; Clinical Trials; **Hospital:** Univ Utah Hosps and Clins; **Address:** Huntsman Cancer Inst, 2000 Circle of Hope, Ste 2152, Salt Lake City, UT 84112; **Phone:** 801-585-0211; **Board Cert:** Neurology 97; **Med School:** Med Coll GA 90; **Resid:** Neurology, W Virginia Univ Hosps 96; **Fellow:** Neurological Oncology, Meml Sloan-Kettering Cancer Ctr 98; **Fac Appt:** Asst Prof N, Univ Utah

Southwest

Gilbert, Mark MD **[N]** - **Spec Exp:** Brain Tumors; Neuro-Oncology; **Hospital:** UT MD Anderson Cancer Ctr, The (page 115); **Address:** Univ Tex MD Anderson Cancer Ctr, 1515 Holcombe Blvd, Unit 431, Houston, TX 77030; **Phone:** 713-792-6600; **Board Cert:** Internal Medicine 85; Neurology 90; **Med School:** Johns Hopkins Univ 82; **Resid:** Internal Medicine, Johns Hopkins Hosp 85; Neurology, Johns Hopkins Hosp 88; **Fellow:** Neurology, Johns Hopkins Hosp; **Fac Appt:** Assoc Prof N, Univ Tex, Houston

Levin, Victor A MD **[N]** - **Spec Exp:** Brain Tumors; Neuro-Oncology; **Hospital:** UT MD Anderson Cancer Ctr, The (page 115); **Address:** 1515 Holcombe Blvd, Unit #431, Houston, TX 77030-4009; **Phone:** 713-792-8297; **Board Cert:** Neurology 76; **Med School:** Univ Wisc 66; **Resid:** Neurology, Mass Genl Hosp 72; **Fac Appt:** Prof N, Univ Tex, Houston

Shapiro, William R. MD **[N]** - **Spec Exp:** Neuro-Oncology; **Hospital:** St Joseph's Hosp & Med Ctr - Phoenix; **Address:** Barrow Neurology Clinics, 500 W Thomas Rd, Ste 300, Phoenix, AZ 85013; **Phone:** 602-406-6208; **Board Cert:** Neurology 69; **Med School:** UCSF 61; **Resid:** Internal Medicine, Univ Wash Hosp 63; Neurology, NY Hosp-Cornell Med Ctr 66; **Fellow:** Neurological Oncology, Natl Inst Hlth 69; **Fac Appt:** Prof N, Univ Ariz Coll Med

Yung, Wai-Kwan MD **[N]** - **Spec Exp:** Neuro-Oncology; Brain Tumors; **Hospital:** UT MD Anderson Cancer Ctr, The (page 115); **Address:** 1515 Holcombe Blvd, Unit 0431, Houston, TX 77030; **Phone:** 713-794-1285; **Board Cert:** Neurology 80; **Med School:** Univ Chicago-Pritzker Sch Med 75; **Resid:** Neurology, UCSD Med Ctr 78; **Fellow:** Neurological Oncology, Meml Sloan Kettering Cancer Ctr 81; **Fac Appt:** Prof N, Univ Tex, Houston

West Coast and Pacific

Cloughesy, Timothy F MD **[N]** - **Spec Exp:** Neuro-Oncology; Seizure Disorders; Brain Tumors; **Hospital:** UCLA Med Ctr (page 111); **Address:** UCLA Neurological Services, 710 Westwood Plaza, Ste I-230, Los Angeles, CA 90095; **Phone:** 310-825-5321; **Board Cert:** Neurology 93; **Med School:** Tulane Univ 87; **Resid:** Neurology, UCLA Med Ctr 91; **Fellow:** Neurological Oncology, Meml Sloan-Kettering Canc Ctr; **Fac Appt:** Clin Prof N, UCLA

Fisher, Paul G MD **[N]** - **Spec Exp:** Neuro-Oncology; **Hospital:** Lucile Packard Chldns Hosp/Stanford Univ Med Ctr; **Address:** Stanford Cancer Ctr-Dept Neurology, 300 Pasteur Drive, rm A343, Stanford, CA 94303; **Phone:** 650-725-8630; **Board Cert:** Pediatrics 95; Child Neurology 98; **Med School:** UCSF 89; **Resid:** Pediatrics, Johns Hopkins Univ Hosp 91; Neurology, Johns Hopkins Univ Hosp 94; **Fellow:** Neurological Oncology, Children's Hosp; **Fac Appt:** Assoc Prof Ped, Stanford Univ

Spence, Alexander Morton MD **[N]** - **Spec Exp:** Neuro-Oncology; **Hospital:** Univ Wash Med Ctr; **Address:** Univ Wash, Dept Neur, 1959 NE Pacific St, MC 356465, Seattle, WA 98195-0001; **Phone:** 206-543-0252; **Board Cert:** Neurology 71; **Med School:** Univ Chicago-Pritzker Sch Med 65; **Resid:** Neurology, Chldns Hosp 69; Neuropathology, Stanford Univ Med Ctr 74; **Fac Appt:** Prof N, Univ Wash

CHILD NEUROLOGY
New England

Mandelbaum, David E MD/PhD **[ChiN]** - **Spec Exp:** Epilepsy/Seizure Disorders; Brain Tumors-Pediatric; Neurodevelopmental Disabilities; **Hospital:** Rhode Island Hosp; **Address:** Physician Office Bldg, 110 Lockwood St, Ste 342, MC 0, Providence, RI 02903; **Phone:** 401-444-4345; **Board Cert:** Neurology 87; Pediatrics 87; Clinical Neurophysiology 03; Neurodevelopmental Disabilities 01; **Med School:** Columbia P&S 80; **Resid:** Pediatrics, Yale-New Haven Hosp 82; Neurology, Neuro Inst-Columbia 83; **Fellow:** Child Neurology, Neuro Inst-Columbia 85; **Fac Appt:** Prof N, Brown Univ

Mid Atlantic

Duffner, Patricia Kressel MD **[ChiN]** - **Spec Exp:** Seizure Disorders; Cancer Survivors-Late Effects of Therapy; **Hospital:** Women's & Chldn's Hosp of Buffalo, The; **Address:** Womwn & Children's Hospital, Dept Neurology, 219 Bryant St, Buffalo, NY 14222; **Phone:** 716-878-7848; **Board Cert:** Pediatrics 77; Child Neurology 79; **Med School:** SUNY Buffalo 72; **Resid:** Pediatrics, Buffalo Chldns Hosp 75; **Fellow:** Child Neurology, Buffalo Chldns Hosp 78; **Fac Appt:** Prof N, SUNY Buffalo

Packer, Roger MD **[ChiN]** - **Spec Exp:** Brain Tumors; Neurofibromatosis; **Hospital:** Chldns Natl Med Ctr; **Address:** Childrens Natl Med Ctr, Dept Neurology, 111 Michigan Ave NW, Washington, DC 20010-2978; **Phone:** 202-884-2120; **Board Cert:** Child Neurology 82; Pediatrics 82; **Med School:** Northwestern Univ 76; **Resid:** Pediatrics, Chldns Med Ctr 78; Neurology, Chldns Hosp-Univ Penn 81; **Fac Appt:** Prof N, Geo Wash Univ

Phillips, Peter C MD **[ChiN]** - **Spec Exp:** Brain Tumors; Neuro-Oncology; **Hospital:** Chldns Hosp of Philadelphia, The; **Address:** Childrens Hosp Philadelphia, 34th St & Civic Center Blvd, Philadelphia, PA 19104; **Phone:** 215-590-5188; **Board Cert:** Pediatrics 85; Child Neurology 86; **Med School:** Univ Conn 78; **Resid:** Pediatrics, Chldns Hosp 80; Pediatric Neurology, Neuro Inst 83; **Fellow:** Neurological Oncology, Meml Sloan Kettering Hosp 86; **Fac Appt:** Prof N, Univ Pennsylvania

Midwest

Cohen, Bruce H MD **[ChiN]** - **Spec Exp:** Brain Tumors; Pediatric Neurology; **Hospital:** Cleveland Clin Fdn (page 92); **Address:** Cleveland Clinic, 9500 Euclid Ave, Desk S71, Cleveland, OH 44195; **Phone:** 216-444-9182; **Board Cert:** Pediatrics 04; Child Neurology 90; **Med School:** Albert Einstein Coll Med 82; **Resid:** Pediatrics, Chldns Hosp 84; Child Neurology, Neurology Inst-Columbia 87; **Fellow:** Pediatric Neuro-Oncology, Chldns Hosp 89

Kovnar, Edward H MD **[ChiN]** - **Spec Exp:** Epilepsy; Neuro-Oncology; Developmental Delay; **Hospital:** Chldns Hosp - Wisconsin; **Address:** Advanced Healthcare, SC, 3003 W Good Hope Rd, Milwaukee, WI 53209-0996; **Phone:** 414-352-3100; **Board Cert:** Pediatrics 84; Child Neurology 84; Clinical Neurophysiology 94; **Med School:** Washington Univ, St Louis 77; **Resid:** Pediatrics, Chldns Hosp 79; Neurology, Barnes Hosp 80; **Fellow:** Pediatric Neurology, Chldns Hosp 82; **Fac Appt:** Assoc Prof Ped, Univ Wisc

OBSTETRICS & GYNECOLOGY

*A*n obstetrician/gynecologist possesses special knowledge, skills and professional capability in the medical and surgical care of the female reproductive system and associated disorders. This physician serves as a consultant to other physicians and as a primary physician for women.

Training required: *Four years plus two years in clinical practice before certification is complete.*

GYNECOLOGIC ONCOLOGY

An obstetrician/gynecologist who provides consultation and comprehensive management of patients with gynecologic cancer, including those diagnostic and therapeutic procedures necessary for the total care of the patient with gynecologic cancer and resulting complications.

Training required: *Four years plus two years in clinical practice before certification in obstetrics and gynecology is complete plus additional training and examination in gynecologic oncology.*

PHYSICIAN LISTINGS:

Gynecologic Oncology

REPRODUCTIVE ENDOCRINOLOGY

An obstetrician/gynecologist who is capable of managing complex problems relating to reproductive endocrinology and infertility.

Training required: Four years plus two years in clinical practice before certification in obstetrics and gynecology is complete plus additional training and examination in reproductive endocrinology.

PHYSICIAN LISTINGS:

Obstetrics / Gynecology

Reproductive Endocrinology

DANA-FARBER/BRIGHAM AND WOMEN'S
CANCER CENTER
GILLETTE CENTER FOR WOMEN'S CANCERS

75 FRANCIS STREET • 44 BINNEY STREET
BOSTON, MA 02115
1-877-DFCI-BWH • WWW.DFBWCANCER.ORG

Trusted Expertise

The Gillette Center for Women's Cancers brings together the world's leading experts in gynecologic and breast cancers to provide women with the latest, most promising treatments, including therapies that are available only through clinical research trials. The Gillette Center is part of Dana-Farber/Brigham and Women's Cancer Center—a collaboration of Dana-Farber Cancer Institute, one of the nation's leading cancer institutes, with Brigham and Women's Hospital, one of the nation's leading teaching hospitals. Dana-Farber Cancer Institute and Brigham and Women's Hospital are teaching affiliates of Harvard Medical School.

Diseases Treated

Serving thousands of patients each year, the Gillette Center offers advanced treatment for a wide range of women's cancers, including cervical, ovarian, endometrial, breast, choriocarcinoma, parametrium, tubal, uterine, vaginal, and vulvar cancers, as well as gestational trophoblastic tumors and molar pregnancies.

Comprehensive & Coordinated Care

Diagnosis and treatment is provided by a team of renowned cancer specialists who are dedicated to providing the most advanced care for women with gynecologic or breast cancers. A multidisciplinary team—including surgeons, gynecologic oncologists, medical oncologists, radiation oncologists, radiologists, pathologists, reproductive medicine specialists, plastic surgeons, psychiatrists, social workers, nurses, genetic counselors, physical therapists, and dietitians –works closely together to ensure that each patient's care plan offers the best possible outcomes.

Advanced Treatment

The most advanced surgical, radiation, and medical oncology treatments are provided at the Center, including innovative clinical trials. Specialized centers include the Familial Ovarian Cancer Center, the New England Trophoblastic Disease Center, the Pap Smear Evaluation Center, and the Breast Oncology Center. These Centers work closely with advanced research programs, including the Gynecologic Oncology Laboratory at Dana-Farber/Brigham and Women's Cancer Center, to ensure that patients receive the latest diagnostic tests and treatments available, as well as access to the most up-to-date research information.

Innovative Clinical Trials

In addition to providing comprehensive, compassionate care to patients, the Center's physicians are deeply committed to conducting an active program of clinical research that may benefit current patients, as well as future generations of women. Patients have access to innovative clinical trials through Dana-Farber/Harvard Cancer Center, a National Cancer Institute-designated Comprehensive Cancer Center.

Comprehensive Support Services

Dana-Farber/Brigham and Women's Cancer Center also provides a wide array of support services and complementary therapies for patients with gynecologic and breast cancers, including counseling and support groups, services for international patients, interpreter services, hospitality, and housing.

Call **1-877-DFCI-BWH** for more information, or to make an appointment with a specialist at Dana-Farber/Brigham and Women's Cancer Center.

DANA-FARBER / PARTNERS CANCERCARE

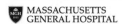 MASSACHUSETTS GENERAL HOSPITAL

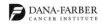 DANA-FARBER CANCER INSTITUTE

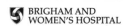 BRIGHAM AND WOMEN'S HOSPITAL

THE UNIVERSITY OF TEXAS
MD ANDERSON
CANCER CENTER

Making Cancer History™

1515 Holcombe Blvd.
Houston, Texas 77030-4095
Tel. 713-792-6161
Toll Free 800-392-1611
www.mdanderson.org

GYNECOLOGIC ONCOLOGY

Over 1,200 new patients come from around the world each year to M. D. Anderson's Gynecologic Oncology Center which specializes in diagnosis, early detection, prevention and treatment of cancers of the vagina, cervix, uterus, ovaries, vulva and fallopian tubes.

Our multidisciplinary team of specialists in pathology, diagnostic imaging, gynecologic oncology, radiation oncology, medical oncology, blood and marrow transplantation, provide patients with a wide range of treatment options that include standard care and clinical treatment studies.

Standard treatment available from our Gynecologic Oncologists include:

- Radical and ultraradical operative procedures for gynecologic cancers
- Minimally invasive surgery, including pelvic mass evaluation
- Surgical procedures performed and chemotherapy prescribed by specialists
- Treatment of such uncommon malignancies as germ cell tumors of the ovary, gestational trophoblastic disease, sarcomas, and vulvar and vaginal cancers.

CLINICAL TRIALS

The Gynecologic Oncology Center offers an extensive array of clinical trials. A clinical trial is one of the most advanced stages of a long careful research process. Clinical trials are designed to test the effectiveness of new treatment, including novel drugs, surgical procedures, or combinations of therapy.

New and innovative therapies generally are available at M. D. Anderson several years before they become standard in the community. Our clinical trials incorporate state-of-the-art patient care, while evaluating the most recent developments in cancer medicine. They also offer treatment opportunities for difficult or aggressive tumors.

Examples of innovative research conducted by the Gynecologic Oncology specialists include:

- Incorporation of high-dose chemotherapy with stem cell transplant in the primary treatment of ovarian cancer.
- Drug development studies in multiple disease sites using agents such as Gleevec, TLK286, Xeloda, RU-486, PEG Intron, and IL12.
- Combination chemotherapy and radiation studies for the treatment of advanced cervical cancer.
- Minimally invasive surgical procedures, including lymphatic mapping with sentinel node identification and laparoscopic surgery for endometrial and cervical cancer.
- Evaluation of patients and families for hereditary cancers of the ovary and uterus.

M. D. Anderson is one of the largest cancer centers in the world. We've been working to eliminate cancer for more than six decades. Our depth of experience informs every aspect of your care.

We focus exclusively on cancer and have seen cases of every kind. Our doctors treat more rare cancers in a single day than most physicians see in a lifetime. That means you receive expert care no matter what your diagnosis.

We are the top-ranked cancer hospital in the United States according to the 2004 *U.S. News and World Report* annual survey of hospitals.

M. D. Anderson ranks first in the number and amount of research grants awarded by the National Cancer Institute. By studying how cancer begins and responds to various treatments, we can help patients overcome disease and prevent recurrence.

At M. D. Anderson, we understand that cancer is not just a physical disease. To help you cope with every aspect of cancer, we provide a number of support programs.

GYNECOLOGIC ONCOLOGY

New England

Beecham, Jackson B MD [GO] - **Spec Exp:** Gynecologic Cancer; Ovarian Cancer; **Hospital:** Dartmouth - Hitchcock Med Ctr; **Address:** Dartmouth Hitchcock Medical Ctr, 1 Medical Center Drive, Lebanon, NH 03756; **Phone:** 603-653-3525; **Board Cert:** Obstetrics & Gynecology 76; Gynecologic Oncology 80; **Med School:** Temple Univ 69; **Resid:** Obstetrics & Gynecology, Medical Ctr Hosp 74; **Fellow:** Gynecologic Oncology, Norwegian Radium Hosp 75; Gynecologic Oncology, New England Med Ctr 77; **Fac Appt:** Assoc Prof ObG, Dartmouth Med Sch

Fuller, Arlan F MD [GO] - **Spec Exp:** Ovarian Cancer; Cervical Cancer; **Hospital:** Mass Genl Hosp; **Address:** 55 Fruit St, Yawkey 9, Boston, MA 02114; **Phone:** 617-724-6880; **Board Cert:** Obstetrics & Gynecology 79; Gynecologic Oncology 82; **Med School:** Harvard Med Sch 71; **Resid:** Surgery, Mass Genl Hosp 74; Obstetrics & Gynecology, Brigham & Womens Hosp 77; **Fellow:** Gynecologic Oncology, Meml Sloan Kettering Cancer Ctr 79; **Fac Appt:** Assoc Prof ObG, Harvard Med Sch

Goodman, Annekathryn MD [GO] - **Spec Exp:** Gynecologic Cancer; Gynecologic Surgery-Complex; Acupuncture for Symptom Relief; **Hospital:** Mass Genl Hosp; **Address:** 55 Fruit St, Yawkey 9, Boston, MA 02114; **Phone:** 617-724-4800; **Board Cert:** Obstetrics & Gynecology 03; Gynecologic Oncology 03; **Med School:** Tufts Univ 83; **Resid:** Obstetrics & Gynecology, Tufts New England Med Ctr 87; **Fellow:** Gynecologic Oncology, Mass Genl Hosp 90; **Fac Appt:** Assoc Prof ObG, Harvard Med Sch

Niloff, Jonathan M MD [GO] - **Spec Exp:** Ovarian Cancer; Gynecologic Surgery-Complex; Uterine Cancer; **Hospital:** Beth Israel Deaconess Med Ctr - Boston; **Address:** Beth Israel Deaconess Medical Ctr, 330 Brookline Ave, rm KS-330, Boston, MA 02215-5400; **Phone:** 617-667-4040; **Board Cert:** Obstetrics & Gynecology 87; Gynecologic Oncology 87; **Med School:** McGill Univ 78; **Resid:** Obstetrics & Gynecology, Brigham & Women's Hosp 82; **Fellow:** Gynecologic Oncology, Brigham & Women's Hosp 84; **Fac Appt:** Assoc Prof ObG, Harvard Med Sch

Rutherford, Thomas MD [GO] - **Spec Exp:** Ovarian Cancer; Uterine Cancer; **Hospital:** Yale - New Haven Hosp; **Address:** Yale Univ Sch Med Dept Ob-Gyn, 333 Cedar St, Box 208063, New Haven, CT 06520; **Phone:** 203-785-6301; **Board Cert:** Obstetrics & Gynecology 97; Gynecologic Oncology 00; **Med School:** Med Coll OH 89; **Resid:** Obstetrics & Gynecology, Cooper Hosp MC-UMDNJ 93; **Fellow:** Gynecologic Oncology, Yale U Sch Med 95; **Fac Appt:** Assoc Prof ObG, Yale Univ

Schwartz, Peter E MD [GO] - **Spec Exp:** Ovarian Cancer; Uterine Cancer; Gynecologic Surgery; **Hospital:** Yale - New Haven Hosp; **Address:** Yale Univ Sch Med, Dept Ob/Gyn, 333 Cedar St, rm FMB-316, New Haven, CT 06510-3289; **Phone:** 203-785-4014; **Board Cert:** Obstetrics & Gynecology 73; Gynecologic Oncology 79; **Med School:** Albert Einstein Coll Med 66; **Resid:** Obstetrics & Gynecology, Yale-New Haven Hosp 70; **Fellow:** Gynecologic Oncology, MD Anderson Cancer Ctr 75; **Fac Appt:** Prof ObG, Yale Univ

Tarraza, Hector MD [GO] - **Hospital:** Maine Med Ctr; **Address:** 887 Congress St, Ste 100, Portland, ME 04102; **Phone:** 207-761-0125; **Board Cert:** Gynecologic Oncology 98; Obstetrics & Gynecology 98; **Med School:** Harvard Med Sch 81; **Resid:** Obstetrics & Gynecology, Mass Genl Hosp 85; **Fellow:** Gynecologic Oncology, Mass Genl Hosp 87; **Fac Appt:** Asst Prof ObG, Univ VT Coll Med

Mid Atlantic

Barakat, Richard MD [GO] - **Spec Exp:** Laparoscopic Surgery; Ovarian Cancer; Uterine Cancer; **Hospital:** Meml Sloan Kettering Cancer Ctr (page 100); **Address:** Memorial Sloan Kettering Cancer Ctr, 1275 York Ave, rm C1091, New York, NY 10021; **Phone:** 212-639-2453; **Board Cert:** Obstetrics & Gynecology 92; Gynecologic Oncology 94; **Med School:** SUNY Hlth Sci Ctr 85; **Resid:** Obstetrics & Gynecology, Bellevue Hosp 89; **Fellow:** Gynecologic Oncology, Mem Sloan Kettering Cancer Ctr 91; **Fac Appt:** Assoc Prof ObG, Cornell Univ-Weill Med Coll

Barnes, Willard MD [GO] - **Spec Exp:** Pelvic Tumors; Gynecologic Cancer; **Hospital:** Georgetown Univ Hosp; **Address:** GUMC - Lombardi Cancer Center, Dept Gyn Onc, 3800 Reservoir Rd NW Fl 2, Washington, DC 20007-2194; **Phone:** 202-444-2114; **Board Cert:** Obstetrics & Gynecology 97; Gynecologic Oncology 97; **Med School:** Univ Miss 79; **Resid:** Obstetrics & Gynecology, Univ Miss Med Ctr 83; **Fellow:** Gynecologic Oncology, Georgetown Univ Med Ctr 85; **Fac Appt:** Assoc Prof ObG, Georgetown Univ

Barter, James MD [GO] - **Spec Exp:** Laparoscopic Surgery; Ovarian Cancer; Gynecologic Cancer; **Hospital:** Suburban Hosp - Bethesda; **Address:** 6301 Executive Blvd, Rockville, MD 20852; **Phone:** 301-770-4967; **Board Cert:** Obstetrics & Gynecology 97; Gynecologic Oncology 97; **Med School:** Univ VA Sch Med 77; **Resid:** Internal Medicine, Univ of KY 79; Obstetrics & Gynecology, Duke Univ 83; **Fellow:** Gynecologic Oncology, Univ of Alabama 86; **Fac Appt:** Clin Prof GO, Georgetown Univ

Bristow, Robert E MD [GO] - **Spec Exp:** Ovarian Cancer; Cervical Cancer; Uterine Cancer; **Hospital:** Johns Hopkins Hosp - Baltimore (page 97); **Address:** Johns Hopkins Hosp, 600 N Wolfe St, Phipps 281, Baltimore, MD 21287; **Phone:** 410-955-8240; **Board Cert:** Obstetrics & Gynecology 99; Gynecologic Oncology 03; **Med School:** USC Sch Med 91; **Resid:** Obstetrics & Gynecology, Johns Hopkins Hosp 95; **Fellow:** Gynecologic Oncology, UCLA Med Ctr 98; **Fac Appt:** Assoc Prof ObG, Johns Hopkins Univ

Caputo, Thomas A MD [GO] - **Spec Exp:** Cervical Cancer; Ovarian Cancer; Uterine Cancer; **Hospital:** NY-Presby Hosp - NY Weill Cornell Med Ctr (page 103); **Address:** 525 E 68th St, Ste J130, New York, NY 10021; **Phone:** 212-746-3179; **Board Cert:** Obstetrics & Gynecology 93; Gynecologic Oncology 77; **Med School:** UMDNJ-NJ Med Sch, Newark 65; **Resid:** Obstetrics & Gynecology, Martland Hosp 69; **Fellow:** Gynecologic Oncology, Emory Univ Hosp 74; **Fac Appt:** Clin Prof ObG, Cornell Univ-Weill Med Coll

Carlson, John MD [GO] - **Spec Exp:** Gynecologic Cancer; Ovarian Cancer; Gynecologic Surgery; **Hospital:** Hahnemann Univ Hosp; **Address:** Hahnemann Univ Hosp, South Tower, Broad & Vine Sts, Fl 15, Philadelphia, PA 19102; **Phone:** 215-762-2640; **Board Cert:** Obstetrics & Gynecology 81; Gynecologic Oncology 82; **Med School:** Georgetown Univ 74; **Resid:** Obstetrics & Gynecology, Hartford Hosp 75; Obstetrics & Gynecology, Hosp Univ Penn 78; **Fellow:** Gynecologic Oncology, MD Anderson Hosp 80; **Fac Appt:** Prof ObG, Drexel Univ Coll Med

Chalas, Eva MD [GO] - **Spec Exp:** Gynecologic Cancer; **Hospital:** Stony Brook Univ Hosp; **Address:** 994 W Jericho Tpke, Ste 103, Smithtown, NY 11787; **Phone:** 631-864-5440; **Board Cert:** Obstetrics & Gynecology 98; Gynecologic Oncology 90; **Med School:** SUNY Stony Brook 81; **Resid:** Obstetrics & Gynecology, Univ Hosp 85; **Fellow:** Gynecologic Oncology, Meml Sloan Kettering Cancer Ctr 87; **Fac Appt:** Assoc Prof ObG, SUNY Stony Brook

Cohen, Carmel MD **[GO]** - **Spec Exp:** Ovarian Cancer; Cervical Cancer; Pelvic Cancer-Laparoscopic Surgery; **Hospital:** NY-Presby Hosp - Columbia Presby Med Ctr (page 103); **Address:** Mt Sinai Hosp, 5 E 98th St, Fl 2, New York, NY 10029-6501; **Phone:** 212-427-9898; **Board Cert:** Obstetrics & Gynecology 03; Gynecologic Oncology 03; **Med School:** Tulane Univ 58; **Resid:** Obstetrics & Gynecology, Mount Sinai Hosp 64; **Fellow:** Gynecologic Oncology, Mount Sinai Hosp 65; **Fac Appt:** Prof ObG, Columbia P&S

Curtin, John P MD **[GO]** - **Spec Exp:** Uterine Cancer; Ovarian Cancer; Laparoscopic Surgery; **Hospital:** NYU Med Ctr (page 104); **Address:** NYU Sch Med, Dept Gyn/Onc, 160 S 34th St Fl 4, New York, NY 10016-6402; **Phone:** 212-731-5345; **Board Cert:** Obstetrics & Gynecology 96; Gynecologic Oncology 96; **Med School:** Creighton Univ 79; **Resid:** Obstetrics & Gynecology, Univ Minn Med Ctr 84; **Fellow:** Gynecologic Oncology, Meml Sloan-Kettering Cancer Ctr 88; **Fac Appt:** Prof GO, NYU Sch Med

Dottino, Peter MD **[GO]** - **Spec Exp:** Laparoscopic Surgery; **Hospital:** Mount Sinai Med Ctr (page 101); **Address:** 800A 5th Ave, Ste 405, New York, NY 10021-7215; **Phone:** 212-888-8439; **Board Cert:** Obstetrics & Gynecology 96; Gynecologic Oncology 96; **Med School:** Georgetown Univ 79; **Resid:** Obstetrics & Gynecology, SUNY Downstate Med Ctr; **Fellow:** Gynecologic Oncology, Mount Sinai Hosp

Dunton, Charles J MD **[GO]** - **Spec Exp:** Ovarian Cancer; Uterine Cancer; Cervical Cancer; **Hospital:** Lankenau Hosp; **Address:** 100 Lancaster Ave, Med Office Bldg East, Ste 661, Wynnewood, PA 19096; **Phone:** 610-649-8085; **Board Cert:** Obstetrics & Gynecology 96; Gynecologic Oncology 96; **Med School:** Jefferson Med Coll 80; **Resid:** Obstetrics & Gynecology, Lankenau Hosp 84; **Fellow:** Gynecologic Oncology, Hosp Univ Penn 89; **Fac Appt:** Prof ObG, Jefferson Med Coll

Fishman, David A MD **[GO]** - **Spec Exp:** Ovarian Cancer; Ovarian Cancer-Early Detection; Gynecologic Cancer; **Hospital:** NYU Med Ctr (page 104); **Address:** NYU Clinical Cancer Ctr, 160 E 34 St Fl 4, New York, NY 10016; **Phone:** 212-731-5345; **Board Cert:** Obstetrics & Gynecology 95; Gynecologic Oncology 98; **Med School:** Texas Tech Univ 88; **Resid:** Obstetrics & Gynecology, Yale-New Haven Hosp 92; **Fellow:** Gynecologic Oncology, Yale-New Haven Hosp 94; **Fac Appt:** Prof ObG, NYU Sch Med

Kelley II, Joseph L MD **[GO]** - **Spec Exp:** Breast Cancer; Gynecologic Cancer; **Hospital:** Magee-Womens Hosp - UPMC (page 114); **Address:** Magee-Womens Hosp Dept. OB/GYN, 300 Halket St, Pittsburgh, PA 15213; **Phone:** 412-641-1153; **Board Cert:** Obstetrics & Gynecology 03; Gynecologic Oncology 03; **Med School:** St Louis Univ 85; **Resid:** Obstetrics & Gynecology, Magee-Womens Hosp 88; **Fellow:** Gynecologic Oncology, MD Anderson Cancer Ctr 91; **Fac Appt:** Assoc Prof ObG, Univ Pittsburgh

Koulos, John MD **[GO]** - **Spec Exp:** Cervical Cancer; Uterine Cancer; Ovarian Cancer; **Hospital:** St Vincent Cath Med Ctrs - Manhattan (page 108); **Address:** 325 W 15th St, New York, NY 10011; **Phone:** 212-604-2070; **Board Cert:** Obstetrics & Gynecology 95; Gynecologic Oncology 95; **Med School:** Northwestern Univ 78; **Resid:** Obstetrics & Gynecology, Northwestern Univ Med Sch 82; **Fellow:** Gynecologic Oncology, Meml Sloan Kettering Cancer Ctr 84; **Fac Appt:** Assoc Prof ObG, NY Med Coll

Kwon, Tae MD **[GO]** - **Spec Exp:** Uterine Cancer; Cervical Cancer; Ovarian Cancer; **Hospital:** Our Lady of Mercy Med Ctr; **Address:** 33 W Main St, Ste 304, Elmsford, NY 10523; **Phone:** 914-592-3811; **Board Cert:** Obstetrics & Gynecology 78; Gynecologic Oncology 81; **Med School:** South Korea 65; **Resid:** Obstetrics & Gynecology, Lenox Hill Hosp 74; Gynecologic Oncology, Lenox Hill Hosp 76; **Fellow:** Gynecologic Oncology, Univ Mississippi Hosp 78; **Fac Appt:** Assoc Prof ObG, NY Med Coll

GYNECOLOGIC ONCOLOGY

Morgan, Mark A MD [GO] - **Spec Exp:** Laparoscopic Surgery; Gynecologic Surgery-Complex; Urogynecology; **Hospital:** Hosp Univ Penn - UPHS (page 113); **Address:** Hosp Univ Penn - Div Gyn Oncology, 3400 Spruce St, 1000 Courtyard Bldg, Philadelphia, PA 19104; **Phone:** 215-662-3318; **Board Cert:** Obstetrics & Gynecology 02; Gynecologic Oncology 02; **Med School:** SUNY Downstate 82; **Resid:** Obstetrics & Gynecology, Hosp Univ Penn 86; **Fellow:** Gynecologic Oncology, Hosp Univ Penn 88; **Fac Appt:** Assoc Prof ObG, Univ Pennsylvania

Rosenblum, Norman G MD/PhD [GO] - **Spec Exp:** Ovarian Cancer; Endometrial Cancer; Vulvar Cancer; **Hospital:** Thomas Jefferson Univ Hosp (page 110); **Address:** 111 S 11th St, Ste 6200, Philadelphia, PA 19107; **Phone:** 215-955-6200; **Board Cert:** Obstetrics & Gynecology 96; Gynecologic Oncology 96; **Med School:** Jefferson Med Coll 78; **Resid:** Obstetrics & Gynecology, Hosp Univ Penn 82; **Fellow:** Gynecologic Oncology, Hosp Univ Penn 84; **Fac Appt:** Clin Prof ObG, Jefferson Med Coll

Rubin, Stephen C MD [GO] - **Spec Exp:** Gynecologic Cancer; Ovarian Cancer; Cervical Cancer; **Hospital:** Hosp Univ Penn - UPHS (page 113); **Address:** Hosp Univ Penn - Gyn Oncology, 3400 Spruce St, 1000 Courtyard Bldg, Philadelphia, PA 19104-4283; **Phone:** 215-662-3318; **Board Cert:** Obstetrics & Gynecology 93; Gynecologic Oncology 84; **Med School:** Univ Pennsylvania 76; **Resid:** Obstetrics & Gynecology, Hosp Univ Penn 80; **Fellow:** Gynecologic Oncology, Hosp Univ Penn 82; **Fac Appt:** Prof ObG, Univ Pennsylvania

Smith, Daniel MD [GO] - **Spec Exp:** Ovarian Cancer; **Hospital:** Hackensack Univ Med Ctr (page 96); **Address:** 20 Prospect Ave, Ste 703, Hackensack, NJ 07601; **Phone:** 201-996-5373; **Board Cert:** Obstetrics & Gynecology 94; Gynecologic Oncology 83; Surgery 01; **Med School:** Harvard Med Sch 72; **Resid:** Surgery, Mass Genl Hosp 79; Obstetrics & Gynecology, LAC-USC Med Ctr 78; **Fellow:** Gynecologic Oncology, Mem Sloan Kettering Cancer Ctr 81; **Fac Appt:** Assoc Prof ObG, UMDNJ-NJ Med Sch, Newark

Wallach, Robert C MD [GO] - **Spec Exp:** Vulvar & Vaginal Cancer & Pre-Cancer; Ovarian, Tubal & Uterine Cancer; Cervical Cancer & Dysplasia; **Hospital:** NYU Med Ctr (page 104); **Address:** NYU Clinical Cancer Ctr, 160 E 34th St, New York, NY 10016; **Phone:** 212-735-5345; **Board Cert:** Obstetrics & Gynecology 67; Gynecologic Oncology 74; **Med School:** Yale Univ 60; **Resid:** Obstetrics & Gynecology, Beth Israel Med Ctr 65; **Fellow:** Gynecologic Oncology, SUNY Downstate Med Ctr 66; **Fac Appt:** Clin Prof ObG, NYU Sch Med

Southeast

Alleyn, James MD [GO] - **Spec Exp:** Cervical Cancer & Dysplasia; **Hospital:** Mercy Hosp - Miami; **Address:** 3661 S Miami Ave, Ste 308, Miami, FL 33133-4232; **Phone:** 305-854-3603; **Board Cert:** Obstetrics & Gynecology 78; **Med School:** Indiana Univ 72; **Resid:** Obstetrics & Gynecology, Miami-Jackson Meml Hosp 76; **Fellow:** Gynecologic Oncology, Miami-Jackson Meml Hosp 78; **Fac Appt:** Asst Clin Prof ObG, Univ Miami Sch Med

Alvarez, Ronald D MD [GO] - **Spec Exp:** Gynecologic Cancer; Ovarian Cancer; **Hospital:** Univ of Ala Hosp at Birmingham; **Address:** University of Alabama at Birmingham, Div Gynecologic Oncology, 619 19th St S Bldg OHB - rm 538, Birmingham, AL 35249-7333; **Phone:** 205-934-4986; **Board Cert:** Obstetrics & Gynecology 01; Gynecologic Oncology 92; **Med School:** Louisiana State Univ 83; **Resid:** Obstetrics & Gynecology, Univ of Alabama Hosp 87; **Fellow:** Gynecologic Oncology, Univ of Alabama Hosp 90; **Fac Appt:** Assoc Prof ObG, Univ Ala

Berchuck, Andrew MD [GO] - **Spec Exp:** Ovarian Cancer-Hereditary; Uterine Cancer; **Hospital:** Duke Univ Med Ctr (page 94); **Address:** Duke Univ Med Center, Box 3079, Durham, NC 27710; **Phone:** 919-684-3765; **Board Cert:** Obstetrics & Gynecology 98; Gynecologic Oncology 98; **Med School:** Case West Res Univ 80; **Resid:** Obstetrics & Gynecology, Case Western Resrv 84; **Fellow:** Gynecology, UT Southwestern 85; Gynecologic Oncology, Meml Sloan-Kettering 87; **Fac Appt:** Prof ObG, Duke Univ

Clarke-Pearson, Daniel L MD [GO] - **Spec Exp:** Pelvic Reconstruction; Gynecologic Surgery-Complex; Gynecologic Cancer; **Hospital:** Duke Univ Med Ctr (page 94); **Address:** Duke Univ Med Ctr, Box 3079, Durham, NC 27710-0001; **Phone:** 919-684-3765; **Board Cert:** Obstetrics & Gynecology 00; Gynecologic Oncology 00; **Med School:** Case West Res Univ 75; **Resid:** Obstetrics & Gynecology, Duke Univ Med Ctr 79; **Fellow:** Gynecologic Oncology, Duke Univ Med Ctr 81; **Fac Appt:** Prof ObG, Duke Univ

Creasman, William T MD [GO] - **Spec Exp:** Uterine Cancer; Ovarian Cancer; Cervical & Vulvar Cancer; **Hospital:** MUSC Med Ctr; **Address:** Med U SC-Dept ObG, Charleston, SC 29425; **Phone:** 843-792-4509; **Board Cert:** Obstetrics & Gynecology 91; Gynecologic Oncology 74; **Med School:** Baylor Coll Med 60; **Resid:** Obstetrics & Gynecology, Rochester Med Ctr 67; **Fellow:** Gynecologic Oncology, Anderson Hosp Tumor Inst 69; **Fac Appt:** Prof ObG, Med Univ SC

Currie, John L MD [GO] - **Spec Exp:** Gynecologic Cancer; Pelvic Reconstruction; Gynecological Problems of Obese Patients; **Hospital:** Vanderbilt Univ Med Ctr (page 116); **Address:** Vanderbilt Univ Hosp, Dept Gyn Oncology, B-1100 Medical Center N, Nashville, TN 37232-2519; **Phone:** 615-322-2114; **Board Cert:** Obstetrics & Gynecology 91; Gynecologic Oncology 82; **Med School:** Univ NC Sch Med 67; **Resid:** Gynecologic Oncology, Hosp Univ Penn 72; **Fellow:** Gynecologic Oncology, Duke Univ Med Ctr 80; **Fac Appt:** Prof ObG, Vanderbilt Univ

Fiorica, James V MD [GO] - **Spec Exp:** Gynecologic Cancer; Breast Cancer; Cervical Cancer; **Hospital:** Sarasota Meml Hosp; **Address:** 1921 Waldemere St, Ste 613, Sarasota, FL 34239; **Phone:** 941-917-8383; **Board Cert:** Obstetrics & Gynecology 03; Gynecologic Oncology 03; **Med School:** Tufts Univ 82; **Resid:** Obstetrics & Gynecology, Univ South Fla Affil Hosp 86; **Fellow:** Gynecologic Oncology, Univ South Fla Affil Hosp 89; Breast Disease, Tufts Univ

Fowler Jr, Wesley C MD [GO] - **Spec Exp:** Vulvar Disease/Cancer; DES-Exposed Females; **Hospital:** Univ NC Hosps (page 112); **Address:** U NC Chapel Hill, Div of Ob/Gyn, Campus Box 7570, Chapel Hill, NC 27599-7570; **Phone:** 919-966-1196; **Board Cert:** Obstetrics & Gynecology 91; Gynecologic Oncology 79; **Med School:** Univ NC Sch Med 66; **Resid:** Obstetrics & Gynecology, NC Memorial Hosp 71; **Fac Appt:** Prof ObG, Univ NC Sch Med

Horowitz, Ira MD [GO] - **Hospital:** Emory Univ Hosp; **Address:** Emory Clinic, 1365 Clifton Rd NE, Atlanta, GA 30322; **Phone:** 404-778-4416; **Board Cert:** Obstetrics & Gynecology 97; Gynecologic Oncology 97; **Med School:** Baylor Coll Med 80; **Resid:** Obstetrics & Gynecology, Baylor Coll Med 84; **Fellow:** Gynecologic Oncology, Johns Hopkins Hosp 87; **Fac Appt:** Prof ObG, Emory Univ

Hoskins, William MD [GO] - **Spec Exp:** Ovarian Cancer; **Hospital:** Meml Med Ctr - Savannah; **Address:** Anderson Cancer Inst, Meml Hlth Univ Med Ctr, 4700 Waters Ave, Savannah, GA 31404; **Phone:** 912-350-8337; **Board Cert:** Obstetrics & Gynecology 93; Gynecologic Oncology 79; **Med School:** Univ Tenn Coll Med, Memphis 65; **Resid:** Obstetrics & Gynecology, Naval Med Ctr 71; **Fellow:** Gynecologic Oncology, Univ Miami Hosp 75; **Fac Appt:** Prof ObG, Mercer Univ Sch Med

Jones III, Howard Wilbur MD [GO] - **Hospital:** Vanderbilt Univ Med Ctr (page 116); **Address:** Vanderbilt Univ Med Ctr, Medical Center North, rm B1100, Nashville, TN 37232-2519; **Phone:** 615-322-2114; **Board Cert:** Obstetrics & Gynecology 99; Gynecologic Oncology 99; **Med School:** Duke Univ 68; **Resid:** Obstetrics & Gynecology, Univ Colo Med Ctr 72; **Fellow:** Gynecologic Oncology, Univ Tex-MD Anderson Hosp 74; **Fac Appt:** Prof ObG, Vanderbilt Univ

Kohler, Matthew MD [GO] - **Hospital:** MUSC Med Ctr; **Address:** MUSC Med Ctr- Women's Hlth Ob/Gyn, 96 Jonathan Lucas St, Ste 634, Box 250619, Charleston, SC 29425; **Phone:** 843-792-8176; **Board Cert:** Obstetrics & Gynecology 95; Gynecologic Oncology 97; **Med School:** Duke Univ 87; **Resid:** Obstetrics & Gynecology, Duke University Med Ctr 91; **Fellow:** Gynecologic Oncology, Duke University Med Ctr 93; **Fac Appt:** Assoc Prof ObG, Med Univ SC

Lentz, Samuel S MD [GO] - **Spec Exp:** Gynecologic Cancer; Pelvic Reconstruction; **Hospital:** Pitt Cty Mem Hosp - Univ Med Ctr East Carolina; **Address:** ECU Brody Sch Med-Brody Bldg, 600 Moye Blvd, rm 25-12, Greenville, NC 27858; **Phone:** 252-744-3587; **Board Cert:** Obstetrics & Gynecology 04; Gynecologic Oncology 04; **Med School:** Wake Forest Univ ; **Resid:** Obstetrics & Gynecology, NC Baptist Hosp 82; **Fellow:** Gynecologic Oncology, Mayo Clinic 89; **Fac Appt:** Prof ObG, E Carolina Univ

Parham, Groesbeck P MD [GO] - **Spec Exp:** Cervical Cancer; **Hospital:** Univ of Ala Hosp at Birmingham; **Address:** Univ Alabama at Birmingham, 619 19th St S, OHB 538, Birmingham, AL 35249-7337; **Phone:** 205-934-4986; **Board Cert:** Obstetrics & Gynecology 99; Gynecologic Oncology 99; **Med School:** Univ Ala 81; **Resid:** Obstetrics & Gynecology, Univ Ala Hosp 85; **Fellow:** Gynecologic Oncology, UC Irvine Med Ctr 88; **Fac Appt:** Prof ObG, Univ Ala

Partridge, Edward E MD [GO] - **Spec Exp:** Ovarian Cancer; **Hospital:** Univ of Ala Hosp at Birmingham; **Address:** Univ Ala Hosp at Birmingham, Div Gyn Oncology, 619 19th St S, OHB 538, Birmingham, AL 35249-7333; **Phone:** 205-934-4986; **Board Cert:** Obstetrics & Gynecology 93; Gynecologic Oncology 81; **Med School:** Univ Ala 73; **Resid:** Obstetrics & Gynecology, Univ Alabama Hosp 77; **Fellow:** Gynecologic Oncology, Univ Alabama Hosp 79; **Fac Appt:** Prof ObG, Univ Ala

Penalver, Manuel A MD [GO] - **Spec Exp:** Gynecologic Cancer; Cervical Cancer; Pelvic Tumors; **Hospital:** Doctors' Hosp; **Address:** South Florida Gyn Oncology, 5000 University Drive, Ste 3300, Coral Gables, FL 33146; **Phone:** 305-663-7001; **Board Cert:** Obstetrics & Gynecology 97; Gynecologic Oncology 97; **Med School:** Univ Miami Sch Med 77; **Resid:** Obstetrics & Gynecology, Univ Miami/Jackson Meml Hosp 82; **Fellow:** Gynecologic Oncology, Univ Miami/Jackson Meml Hosp 84

Poliakoff, Steven MD [GO] - **Spec Exp:** Ovarian Cancer; Minimally Invasive Surgery; Genetic Testing; **Hospital:** Mount Sinai Med Ctr - Miami; **Address:** 6280 Sunset Dr, Ste 502, South Miami, FL 33143-4870; **Phone:** 305-596-0870; **Board Cert:** Obstetrics & Gynecology 83; **Med School:** Univ NC Sch Med 75; **Resid:** Obstetrics & Gynecology, Johns Hopkins Hosp 79; **Fellow:** Gynecologic Oncology, Jackson Meml Hosp/Univ Miami 81

Sevin, Bernd-Uwe MD [GO] - **Spec Exp:** Ovarian Cancer; Pelvic Reconstruction; Pelvic Surgery; **Hospital:** St Luke's Hosp - Jacksonville; **Address:** 4500 San Pablo Rd, Dept Gynecology, Jacksonville, FL 32224; **Phone:** 904-953-0612; **Board Cert:** Obstetrics & Gynecology 80; Gynecologic Oncology 81; **Med School:** Germany ; **Resid:** Obstetrics & Gynecology, Stanford U Med Ctr 77; **Fellow:** Gynecologic Oncology, U Miami 79; **Fac Appt:** Prof ObG, Mayo Med Sch

Taylor Jr, Peyton T MD **[GO]** - **Spec Exp:** Gynecologic Surgery-Complex; Gynecologic Cancer; **Hospital:** Univ Virginia Med Ctr; **Address:** Univ VA Hlth Sys, Dept Ob/Gyn, PO Box 800712, Charlottesville, VA 22908; **Phone:** 434-924-9933; **Board Cert:** Obstetrics & Gynecology 94; Gynecologic Oncology 81; **Med School:** Univ Ala 68; **Resid:** Obstetrics & Gynecology, Univ VA Hosp 70; Obstetrics & Gynecology, Univ VA Hosp 75; **Fellow:** Surgical Oncology, Natl Cancer Inst 72; Gynecologic Oncology, Univ Va Hosp 77; **Fac Appt:** Prof ObG, Univ VA Sch Med

Van Nagell Jr, John R MD **[GO]** - **Spec Exp:** Ovarian Cancer; Cervical Cancer; **Hospital:** Univ Kentucky Med Ctr; **Address:** Dept Ob/Gyn, 800 Rose St Bldg Whitney-Hendrickson Fl 3 - rm 331E1, Lexington, KY 40536-0001; **Phone:** 859-323-5553; **Board Cert:** Obstetrics & Gynecology 73; Gynecologic Oncology 76; **Med School:** Univ Pennsylvania 67; **Resid:** Obstetrics & Gynecology, Kentucky Med Ctr 71; **Fac Appt:** Prof ObG, Univ KY Coll Med

Midwest

Belinson, Jerome Leslie MD **[GO]** - **Spec Exp:** Ovarian Cancer; Cervical Cancer & Dysplasia; **Hospital:** Cleveland Clin Fdn (page 92); **Address:** 9500 Euclid Ave, Desk A81, Cleveland, OH 44195; **Phone:** 216-444-7933; **Board Cert:** Obstetrics & Gynecology 98; Gynecologic Oncology 80; **Med School:** Univ MO-Columbia Sch Med 68; **Resid:** Obstetrics & Gynecology, Columbia Presby Med Ctr 73; **Fellow:** Gynecologic Oncology, Jackson Meml Hosp 77; **Fac Appt:** Prof ObG, Ohio State Univ

Copeland, Larry J MD **[GO]** - **Spec Exp:** Ovarian Cancer; Uterine Cancer; Gynecologic Cancer; **Hospital:** Arthur G James Cancer Hosp & Research Inst (page 105); **Address:** 1654 Upham Drive, Ste 505, Columbus, OH 43210-1250; **Phone:** 614-293-8697; **Board Cert:** Obstetrics & Gynecology 91; Gynecologic Oncology 81; **Med School:** Canada 73; **Resid:** Obstetrics & Gynecology, McMaster Univ Affil Hosps 77; **Fellow:** Gynecologic Oncology, MD Anderson Cancer Ctr-Univ Tex 79; **Fac Appt:** Prof ObG, Ohio State Univ

De Geest, Koen MD **[GO]** - **Spec Exp:** Ovarian Cancer; Cervical Cancer; Clinical Trials; **Hospital:** Univ Iowa Hosp & Clinics; **Address:** Univ Iowa, Div Gynecological Oncology, 200 Hawkins Drive, rm 4630 JCP, Iowa City, IA 52242; **Phone:** 319-356-2015; **Board Cert:** Gynecologic Oncology 97; Obstetrics & Gynecology 97; **Med School:** Belgium 77; **Resid:** Obstetrics & Gynecology, Univ Ghent 82; **Fellow:** Gynecologic Oncology, Penn State/Hershey Med Ctr 90; **Fac Appt:** Prof ObG, Univ Iowa Coll Med

Fowler, Jeffrey M MD **[GO]** - **Spec Exp:** Laparoscopic Surgery; Gynecologic Cancer; **Hospital:** Ohio St Univ Med Ctr (page 105); **Address:** Ohio State Univ, Div Gynecologic Oncology, 320 W Tenth Ave, M-210 SLH, Columbus, OH 43210; **Phone:** 614-293-8737; **Board Cert:** Obstetrics & Gynecology 02; Gynecologic Oncology 02; **Med School:** Northwestern Univ 85; **Resid:** Obstetrics & Gynecology, Ohio State Univ Hosp 89; **Fellow:** Gynecologic Oncology, Cedars-Sinai Med Ctr 91; **Fac Appt:** Prof ObG, Ohio State Univ

Herbst, Arthur MD **[GO]** - **Spec Exp:** Ovarian Cancer; DES-Exposed Females; Cervical Cancer; **Hospital:** Univ of Chicago Hosps; **Address:** 5841 S Maryland Ave, MC 2050, Chicago, IL 60637; **Phone:** 773-834-2882; **Board Cert:** Obstetrics & Gynecology 83; Gynecologic Oncology 74; **Med School:** Harvard Med Sch 59; **Resid:** Surgery, Mass Genl Hosp 62; Obstetrics & Gynecology, Womens Hosp 65; **Fac Appt:** Prof ObG, Univ Chicago-Pritzker Sch Med

Johnston, Carolyn Marie MD **[GO]** - **Spec Exp:** Gynecologic Surgery-Complex; **Hospital:** Univ Michigan Hlth Sys; **Address:** Womens Hosp-Div Gyn Onc, 1500 E Med Ctr Drive, rm L4510, Ann Arbor, MI 48109-0276; **Phone:** 734-647-8906; **Board Cert:** Obstetrics & Gynecology 00; Gynecologic Oncology 00; **Med School:** Yale Univ 84; **Resid:** Obstetrics & Gynecology, Univ Chicago Hosp 88; **Fellow:** Gynecologic Oncology, Mt Sinai Hosp 90; **Fac Appt:** Assoc Clin Prof ObG, Univ Mich Med Sch

Kim, Woo Shin MD [GO] - **Spec Exp:** Ovarian Cancer; Uterine Cancer; Gestational Trophoblastic Disease; **Hospital:** Henry Ford Hosp; **Address:** 2799 W Grand Blvd, Detroit, MI 48202-2608; **Phone:** 313-916-2465; **Board Cert:** Obstetrics & Gynecology 77; Gynecologic Oncology 79; **Med School:** South Korea 66; **Resid:** Obstetrics & Gynecology, Boston City Hosp 73; **Fellow:** Gynecologic Oncology, Meml Sloan-Kettering Cancer Ctr 76; **Fac Appt:** Assoc Clin Prof ObG, Wayne State Univ

Look, Katherine MD [GO] - **Spec Exp:** Ovarian Cancer; **Hospital:** Indiana Univ Hosp (page 90); **Address:** 535 Barnhill Drive, Ste 434, Indianapolis, IN 46202; **Phone:** 317-274-8987; **Board Cert:** Obstetrics & Gynecology 96; Gynecologic Oncology 96; **Med School:** Univ Mich Med Sch 79; **Resid:** Obstetrics & Gynecology, Univ Illinois 83; **Fellow:** Gynecologic Oncology, Meml Sloan Kettering Cancer Ctr 86; **Fac Appt:** Prof ObG, Indiana Univ

Lurain, John R MD [GO] - **Spec Exp:** Gestational Trophoblastic Disease; Uterine Cancer; Ovarian Cancer; **Hospital:** Northwestern Meml Hosp; **Address:** Northwestern Univ Feinberg Sch Med, 333 E Superior St, Chicago, IL 60611-3056; **Phone:** 312-926-7365; **Board Cert:** Obstetrics & Gynecology 77; Gynecologic Oncology 81; **Med School:** Univ NC Sch Med 72; **Resid:** Obstetrics & Gynecology, Univ Pittsburgh 75; **Fellow:** Gynecologic Oncology, Roswell Park Cancer Ctr 79; **Fac Appt:** Prof ObG, Northwestern Univ

Moore, David H MD [GO] - **Spec Exp:** Cervical Cancer; Ovarian Cancer; **Hospital:** Indiana Univ Hosp (page 90); **Address:** 535 Barnhill Drive, Ste 433, Indianapolis, IN 46202; **Phone:** 317-274-2422; **Board Cert:** Obstetrics & Gynecology 03; Gynecologic Oncology 03; **Med School:** Indiana Univ 82; **Resid:** Obstetrics & Gynecology, Indiana Univ 86; **Fellow:** Gynecologic Oncology, Univ North Carolina 88; **Fac Appt:** Clin Prof ObG, Indiana Univ

Mutch, David MD [GO] - **Spec Exp:** Gynecologic Cancer; Pelvic Reconstruction; **Hospital:** Barnes-Jewish Hosp (page 85); **Address:** 4911 Barnes Hospital Plaza, Maternity Bldg-Fl 3, St. Louis, MO 63110; **Phone:** 314-362-3181; **Board Cert:** Obstetrics & Gynecology 01; Gynecologic Oncology 01; **Med School:** Washington Univ, St Louis 80; **Resid:** Obstetrics & Gynecology, Barnes Hosp-Wash Univ 84; **Fellow:** Gynecologic Oncology, Duke Univ Med Ctr 87; **Fac Appt:** Prof ObG, Washington Univ, St Louis

Podratz, Karl C MD/PhD [GO] - **Spec Exp:** Pelvic Cancer; Pelvic Reconstruction; **Hospital:** Mayo Med Ctr & Clin - Rochester; **Address:** 200 1st St SW, Rochester, MN 55905-0001; **Phone:** 507-266-7712; **Board Cert:** Obstetrics & Gynecology 93; Gynecologic Oncology 93; **Med School:** St Louis Univ 74; **Resid:** Obstetrics & Gynecology, Univ Chicago Hosps 77; **Fellow:** Gynecologic Oncology, Mayo Clinic 79; **Fac Appt:** Prof ObG, Mayo Med Sch

Potkul, Ronald MD [GO] - **Spec Exp:** Ovarian Cancer; Cervical Cancer; **Hospital:** Loyola Univ Med Ctr (page 98); **Address:** 2160 S First Ave, Bldg 112 - rm 267, Maywood, IL 60153; **Phone:** 708-327-3500; **Board Cert:** Obstetrics & Gynecology 97; Gynecologic Oncology 97; **Med School:** Univ Chicago-Pritzker Sch Med 81; **Resid:** Obstetrics & Gynecology, Univ Chicago Hosps 85; **Fellow:** Gynecologic Oncology, Georgetown Univ 88; **Fac Appt:** Prof ObG, Loyola Univ-Stritch Sch Med

Reynolds, R Kevin MD [GO] - **Hospital:** Univ Michigan Hlth Sys; **Address:** Women's Hosp, Div Gyn Onc, 1500 E Med Ctr Drive, rm L4510, Ann Arbor, MI 48109-0276; **Phone:** 734-764-9106; **Board Cert:** Obstetrics & Gynecology 98; Gynecologic Oncology 94; **Med School:** Univ New Mexico 82; **Resid:** Obstetrics & Gynecology, Univ Vt Hosp 86; **Fellow:** Gynecologic Oncology, Univ Mich Med Ctr 91; **Fac Appt:** Asst Prof ObG, Univ Mich Med Sch

Rose, Peter G MD [GO] - **Spec Exp:** Cervical Cancer; Ovarian Cancer; **Hospital:** Cleveland Clin Fdn (page 92); **Address:** Cleveland Clinic Fdn, 9500 Euclid Ave, MS A81, Cleveland, OH 44195; **Phone:** 216-444-1712; **Board Cert:** Obstetrics & Gynecology 99; Gynecologic Oncology 90; **Med School:** Boston Univ 81; **Resid:** Surgery, Vanderbilt Med Ctr 83; Obstetrics & Gynecology, Ohio State Univ Med Ctr 86; **Fellow:** Gynecologic Oncology, Roswell Park Med Ctr 88; **Fac Appt:** Prof ObG, Case West Res Univ

Rotmensch, Jacob MD [GO] - **Spec Exp:** Gynecologic Cancer; Ovarian Cancer; Cervical Cancer; **Hospital:** Rush Univ Med Ctr; **Address:** Gyn Oncology Assocs, 1725 W Harrison St, Ste 842, MC 2050, Chicago, IL 60612; **Phone:** 312-942-6300; **Board Cert:** Obstetrics & Gynecology 86; Gynecologic Oncology 90; **Med School:** Meharry Med Coll 77; **Resid:** Obstetrics & Gynecology, Johns Hopkins Hosp 81; **Fellow:** Gynecologic Oncology, Johns Hopkins Hosp 84; **Fac Appt:** Prof ObG, Rush Med Coll

Schink, Julian C MD [GO] - **Spec Exp:** Ovarian Cancer; **Hospital:** Northwestern Meml Hosp; **Address:** 675 N St Clair St, Fl 21 - Ste 100, Chicago, IL 60611; **Phone:** 312-695-0990; **Board Cert:** Obstetrics & Gynecology 00; Gynecologic Oncology 00; **Med School:** Univ Tex, San Antonio 82; **Resid:** Obstetrics & Gynecology, Northwestern Univ Med Sch 86; **Fellow:** Gynecologic Oncology, UCLA Med Ctr 88; **Fac Appt:** Prof ObG, Northwestern Univ

Smith, Donna Marie MD [GO] - **Spec Exp:** Cervical Cancer; Ovarian Cancer; **Hospital:** Loyola Univ Med Ctr (page 98); **Address:** 2160 S First Ave Bldg 112 - rm 244, Maywood, IL 60153; **Phone:** 708-327-3500; **Board Cert:** Obstetrics & Gynecology 97; Gynecologic Oncology 97; **Med School:** Univ MO-Kansas City 80; **Resid:** Obstetrics & Gynecology, Emory Univ Hosp 84; **Fellow:** Gynecologic Oncology, Georgetown Univ Med Ctr 87; **Fac Appt:** Assoc Prof ObG, Loyola Univ-Stritch Sch Med

Stehman, Frederick B MD [GO] - **Spec Exp:** Clinical Trials; Gynecologic Cancer; **Hospital:** Indiana Univ Hosp (page 90); **Address:** Indiana Univ Hosp, Dept ObGyn, 550 N University Blvd, rm 2440, Indianapolis, IN 46202; **Phone:** 317-274-8609; **Board Cert:** Obstetrics & Gynecology 04; Gynecologic Oncology 04; **Med School:** Univ Mich Med Sch 72; **Resid:** Obstetrics & Gynecology, Univ Kansas Medical Ctr 75; Surgery, Univ Kansas Medical Ctr 77; **Fellow:** Gynecologic Oncology, UCLA Medical Ctr 79; **Fac Appt:** Prof ObG, Indiana Univ

Waggoner, Steven MD [GO] - **Spec Exp:** Ovarian Cancer; Cervical Cancer; Uterine Cancer; **Hospital:** Univ Hosps of Cleveland; **Address:** Dept Ob/Gyn, Div Gyn Oncology, 111000 Euclid Ave, MAC 5034, Cleveland, OH 44106; **Phone:** 216-844-3954; **Board Cert:** Obstetrics & Gynecology 02; Gynecologic Oncology 02; **Med School:** Univ Wash 84; **Resid:** Obstetrics & Gynecology, Univ Chicago Hosps 88; **Fellow:** Gynecologic Oncology, Georgetown Univ 91; **Fac Appt:** Prof ObG, Case West Res Univ

Great Plains and Mountains

Davidson, Susan MD [GO] - **Spec Exp:** Gynecologic Cancer; **Hospital:** Univ Colorado Hosp; **Address:** University of Colorado Hospital, Dept OB/GYN, 4200 E Ninth Ave, Box B198, Denver, CO 80262; **Phone:** 303-315-7897; **Board Cert:** Obstetrics & Gynecology 03; Gynecologic Oncology 03; **Med School:** Univ Tex, San Antonio 84; **Resid:** Obstetrics & Gynecology, Univ Texas Med Ctr 88; **Fellow:** Gynecologic Oncology, Meml Sloan Kettering Cancer Ctr 90; **Fac Appt:** Assoc Prof GO, Univ Colorado

Soisson, Andrew MD [GO] - **Spec Exp:** Cervical Cancer; **Hospital:** LDS Hosp; **Address:** Univ Utah, Div Gyn Onc, 30 N 1900 E, Ste 2B200, Salt Lake City, UT 84132; **Phone:** 801-585-0100; **Board Cert:** Obstetrics & Gynecology 02; Gynecologic Oncology 02; **Med School:** Georgetown Univ 1981; **Resid:** Obstetrics & Gynecology, Madigan AMC 85; **Fellow:** Gynecologic Oncology, Duke Univ Med Ctr 90; **Fac Appt:** Assoc Prof ObG, W VA Univ

Southwest

Brewer, Molly A MD [GO] - **Spec Exp:** Ovarian Cancer; **Hospital:** Univ Med Ctr - Tucson; **Address:** Arizona Cancer Ctr-Rm 1968G, 1515 N Campbell Ave, Box 245024, Tucson, AZ 85724; **Phone:** 520-626-9283; **Board Cert:** Obstetrics & Gynecology 99; Gynecologic Oncology 01; **Med School:** SUNY Upstate Med Univ 91; **Resid:** Obstetrics & Gynecology, Oregon Health Sciences Univ Hosp 95; **Fellow:** Gynecologic Oncology, MD Anderson Cancer Ctr 97

Finan, Michael A MD [GO] - **Spec Exp:** Ovarian Cancer; Cervical Cancer; Uterine Cancer; **Hospital:** Ochsner Fdn Hosp; **Address:** Ochsner Clin, Div Gyn Oncology, 1514 Jefferson Hwy, New Orleans, LA 70121-2429; **Phone:** 504-842-4165; **Board Cert:** Obstetrics & Gynecology 04; Gynecologic Oncology 04; **Med School:** Louisiana State Univ 86; **Resid:** Obstetrics & Gynecology, Univ South Fla Affil Hosps 90; **Fellow:** Gynecologic Oncology, H Lee Moffitt Cancer Ctr 92

Follen-Mitchell, Michele MD/PhD [GO] - **Spec Exp:** Gynecologic Cancer Prevention; Clinical Trials; **Hospital:** UT MD Anderson Cancer Ctr, The (page 115); **Address:** MD Anderson Cancer Ctr, 1515 Holcombe Blvd, rm 193, Houston, TX 77030; **Phone:** 713-745-2564; **Board Cert:** Obstetrics & Gynecology 99; Gynecologic Oncology 99; **Med School:** Univ Mich Med Sch 80; **Resid:** Obstetrics & Gynecology, Columbia-Presby Med Ctr 83; **Fellow:** Gynecologic Oncology, MD Anderson Cancer Ctr 86; **Fac Appt:** Prof ObG, Univ Tex, Houston

Freedman, Ralph S MD [GO] - **Spec Exp:** Immune Deficiency; Ovarian Cancer; **Hospital:** UT MD Anderson Cancer Ctr, The (page 115); **Address:** UT MD Anderson Cancer Ctr, Dept Gynecologic Oncology, 1515 Holcombe Blvd, Unit 440, Houston, TX 77030; **Phone:** 713-792-2764; **Board Cert:** Obstetrics & Gynecology 80; **Med School:** South Africa 65; **Resid:** Obstetrics & Gynecology, Queen Victoria-Johannesburg-Baragwanath Hosps 71; **Fellow:** Gynecologic Oncology, Univ Tex MD Anderson Canc Ctr; **Fac Appt:** Prof GO, Univ Tex, Houston

Fromm, Geri Lynn MD [GO] - **Hospital:** St Luke's Episcopal Hosp - Houston; **Address:** 2223 Dorrington St, Houston, TX 77030; **Phone:** 713-665-0404; **Board Cert:** Obstetrics & Gynecology 04; Gynecologic Oncology 04; **Med School:** Northwestern Univ 81; **Resid:** Obstetrics & Gynecology, Magee Womens-Univ Pittsburgh 85; **Fellow:** Gynecologic Oncology, MD Anderson-Univ Texas 87; **Fac Appt:** Assoc Clin Prof ObG, Baylor Coll Med

Gershenson, David M MD [GO] - **Spec Exp:** Ovarian Cancer & Borderline Tumors; Peritoneal Cancer; Fertility Preservation; **Hospital:** UT MD Anderson Cancer Ctr, The (page 115); **Address:** Univ Tex MD Anderson Cancer Ctr, 1515 Holcombe Blvd, Unit 440, Houston, TX 77030; **Phone:** 713-745-2565; **Board Cert:** Obstetrics & Gynecology 91; Gynecologic Oncology 81; **Med School:** Vanderbilt Univ 71; **Resid:** Obstetrics & Gynecology, Yale-New Haven Hosp 75; **Fellow:** Gynecologic Oncology, MD Anderson Cancer Ctr 79; **Fac Appt:** Prof ObG, Univ Tex, Houston

Levenback, Charles MD [GO] - **Spec Exp:** Vulvar Cancer; Cervical Cancer; **Hospital:** UT MD Anderson Cancer Ctr, The (page 115); **Address:** 1515 Holcombe Blvd , Box 440, Houston, TX 77030; **Phone:** 713-745-2563; **Board Cert:** Obstetrics & Gynecology 03; Gynecologic Oncology 03; **Med School:** Mount Sinai Sch Med 83; **Resid:** Obstetrics & Gynecology, Albert Einstein Coll Med 87; **Fellow:** Gynecologic Oncology, Meml Sloan Kettering Cancer Ctr 89; **Fac Appt:** Prof ObG, Univ Tex, Houston

Roman-Lopez, Juan J MD [GO] - **Spec Exp:** Vulvar Disease/Cancer; Bladder Problems Post-Hysterectomy; Gynecologic Cancer; **Hospital:** UAMS Med Ctr; **Address:** 4301 W Markham St, Slot 793, Little Rock, AR 72205-7199; **Phone:** 501-296-1099; **Board Cert:** Obstetrics & Gynecology 71; **Med School:** Univ Puerto Rico 63; **Resid:** Obstetrics & Gynecology, San Juan City Hosp 67; Obstetrics & Gynecology, Tulane-Charity Hosp 69; **Fellow:** Gynecologic Oncology, Tulane-LSU Med Ctr 70; **Fac Appt:** Assoc Clin Prof ObG, Univ Ark

West Coast and Pacific

Berek, Jonathan S MD **[GO]** - **Spec Exp:** Ovarian Cancer; Uterine Cancer; Cervical Cancer; **Hospital:** UCLA Med Ctr (page 111); **Address:** 200 UCLA Med Plaza, Ste 430, Los Angeles, CA 90095-6928; **Phone:** 310-794-7274; **Board Cert:** Obstetrics & Gynecology 91; Gynecologic Oncology 01; **Med School:** Johns Hopkins Univ 75; **Resid:** Obstetrics & Gynecology, Brigham & Woman's Hosp/Harvard 79; **Fellow:** Gynecologic Oncology, UCLA Sch Med 81; **Fac Appt:** Prof ObG, UCLA

Berman, Michael L MD **[GO]** - **Spec Exp:** Gynecologic Cancer; **Hospital:** UC Irvine Med Ctr; **Address:** UCI Med Ctr, Div Gyn/Onc, 101 The City Drive S Bldg 56 - Ste 260, Orange, CA 92868-3201; **Phone:** 714-456-8020; **Board Cert:** Obstetrics & Gynecology 00; Gynecologic Oncology 00; **Med School:** Geo Wash Univ 67; **Resid:** Obstetrics & Gynecology, GW Univ Hosp 69; Obstetrics & Gynecology, Los Angeles Co-Harbor 74; **Fellow:** Gynecologic Oncology, UCLA Med Ctr 76; **Fac Appt:** Prof ObG, UC Irvine

Cain, Joanna MD **[GO]** - **Spec Exp:** Ovarian Cancer; Breast/Ovarian Cancer Risk Assessment; Uterine Cancer; **Hospital:** OR Hlth & Sci Univ; **Address:** 3181 SW Sam Jackson Park Rd, MC L-466, Portland, OR 97239; **Phone:** 503-494-2999; **Board Cert:** Obstetrics & Gynecology 03; Gynecologic Oncology 04; **Med School:** Creighton Univ 78; **Resid:** Obstetrics & Gynecology, Univ Washington Med Ctr 81; **Fellow:** Gynecologic Oncology, Meml Sloan Kettering Cancer Ctr 83; **Fac Appt:** Prof ObG, Oregon Hlth Sci Univ

Di Saia, Philip J MD **[GO]** - **Spec Exp:** Ovarian Cancer; Gynecologic Cancer; Cervical Cancer; **Hospital:** UC Irvine Med Ctr; **Address:** UC Irvine Cancer Ctr, 101 The City Drive South, Bldg 26, Orange, CA 92668; **Phone:** 714-456-8000; **Board Cert:** Obstetrics & Gynecology 83; Gynecologic Oncology 74; **Med School:** Tufts Univ 63; **Resid:** Obstetrics & Gynecology, Yale-New Haven Hosp 67; **Fellow:** Gynecologic Oncology, MD Anderson Hosp 71; **Fac Appt:** Prof ObG, UC Irvine

Goff, Barbara MD **[GO]** - **Spec Exp:** Ovarian Cancer; Uterine Cancer; Cervical Cancer; **Hospital:** Univ Wash Med Ctr; **Address:** Univ Wash Dept ObGynec, Box 356460, Seattle, WA 98195; **Phone:** 206-543-3669; **Board Cert:** Obstetrics & Gynecology 94; Gynecologic Oncology 96; **Med School:** Univ Pennsylvania 86; **Resid:** Obstetrics & Gynecology, Mass Genl Hosp/Brigham & Womens Hosp 90; **Fellow:** Gynecologic Oncology, Mass Genl Hosp 93; **Fac Appt:** Assoc Prof ObG, Univ Wash

Greer, Benjamin MD **[GO]** - **Spec Exp:** Gynecologic Cancer; **Hospital:** Univ Wash Med Ctr; **Address:** Univ Wash, Dept OB/GYN, 1959 NE Pacific St, Box 356460, Seattle, WA 98195; **Phone:** 206-685-2463; **Board Cert:** Obstetrics & Gynecology 01; Gynecologic Oncology 83; **Med School:** Univ Pennsylvania 66; **Resid:** Obstetrics & Gynecology, Univ Colorado Med Ctr 70; **Fac Appt:** Prof ObG, Univ Wash

Karlan, Beth Young MD **[GO]** - **Spec Exp:** Ovarian Cancer; **Hospital:** Cedars-Sinai Med Ctr (page 88); **Address:** 8700 Beverly Blvd, Ste 160 West, Los Angeles, CA 90048; **Phone:** 310-423-3302; **Board Cert:** Obstetrics & Gynecology 98; Gynecologic Oncology 98; **Med School:** Harvard Med Sch 82; **Resid:** Obstetrics & Gynecology, Yale-New Haven Hosp 86; **Fellow:** Gynecologic Oncology, UCLA Med Sch 89; **Fac Appt:** Prof ObG, UCLA

Lagasse, Leo D MD **[GO]** - **Spec Exp:** Ovarian Cancer; **Hospital:** Cedars-Sinai Med Ctr (page 88); **Address:** Cedars-Sinai Med Ctr, 8700 Beverly Blvd Ste 160W, Los Angeles, CA 90048-1804; **Phone:** 310-423-0701; **Board Cert:** Obstetrics & Gynecology 67; Gynecologic Oncology 74; **Med School:** Univ VA Sch Med 59; **Resid:** Obstetrics & Gynecology, UCLA Med Ctr 64; **Fac Appt:** Prof ObG, UCLA

Morrow, Charles P MD **[GO]** - **Spec Exp:** Gestational Trophoblastic Disease; **Hospital:** USC Norris Canc Comp Ctr; **Address:** USC K Norris Jr Cancer Hosp, 1441 Eastlake Ave, Ste 7419, Los Angeles, CA 90033; **Phone:** 323-865-3922; **Board Cert:** Obstetrics & Gynecology 70; Gynecologic Oncology 74; **Med School:** Loyola Univ-Stritch Sch Med 62; **Resid:** Obstetrics & Gynecology, Little Co Mary Hosp 66; Obstetrics & Gynecology, Chicago Mercy Hosp 68; **Fellow:** Gynecologic Oncology, MD Anderson Hosp 70; **Fac Appt:** Prof ObG, UCLA

Muntz, Howard G MD **[GO]** - **Spec Exp:** Gynecologic Cancer; **Hospital:** Virginia Mason Med Ctr; **Address:** Virginia Mason Medical Ctr, 1100 9th Ave, MS X8-GYO, Seattle, WA 89111; **Phone:** 206-223-6191; **Board Cert:** Obstetrics & Gynecology 03; Gynecologic Oncology 03; **Med School:** Harvard Med Sch 84; **Resid:** Obstetrics & Gynecology, Brigham & Women's Hosp 88; **Fellow:** Gynecologic Oncology, Mass General Hosp 91; **Fac Appt:** Assoc Clin Prof ObG, Univ Wash

Smith, Lloyd H MD **[GO]** - **Spec Exp:** Ovarian Cancer; Uterine Cancer; Vaginal & Vulvar Cancer; **Hospital:** UC Davis Med Ctr; **Address:** UC Davis Med Ctr, Dept Ob/Gyn, 4860 Y St, Ste 2500, Sacramento, CA 95817; **Phone:** 916-734-6946; **Board Cert:** Obstetrics & Gynecology 98; Gynecologic Oncology 98; **Med School:** UC Davis 81; **Resid:** Obstetrics & Gynecology, UC Davis Med Ctr 85; **Fellow:** Gynecologic Oncology, Stanford Univ Hosp 88; **Fac Appt:** Prof ObG, UC Davis

Spirtos, Nicola Michael MD **[GO]** - **Spec Exp:** Pelvic Cancer-Laparoscopic Surgery; Ovarian Cancer; **Hospital:** Good Samaritan Hosp - San Jose; **Address:** 815 Pollard Rd, Los Gatos, CA 95032; **Phone:** 650-326-6500; **Board Cert:** Obstetrics & Gynecology 98; Gynecologic Oncology 98; **Med School:** Northwestern Univ 80; **Resid:** Obstetrics & Gynecology, Women's Hosp LA Co/USC Med Ctr 84; **Fellow:** Gynecologic Oncology, Stanford Univ 87; **Fac Appt:** Assoc Prof ObG, Stanford Univ

Stern, Jeffrey L MD **[GO]** - **Hospital:** Alta Bates Summit Med Ctr - Ashby Campus; **Address:** Womens Cancer Ctr Northern Calif, 2100 Webster St, Ste 300, San Francisco, CA 94115; **Phone:** 510-215-8712; **Board Cert:** Obstetrics & Gynecology 83; Gynecologic Oncology 84; **Med School:** SUNY Upstate Med Univ 76; **Resid:** Obstetrics & Gynecology, Johns Hopkins Hosp 80; **Fellow:** Gynecologic Oncology, USC Med Ctr 82; **Fac Appt:** Assoc Prof ObG, UCSF

Teng, Nelson NH MD/PhD **[GO]** - **Hospital:** Stanford Univ Med Ctr; **Address:** Stanford Univ Sch Med, Dept Gyn Onc, 300 Pasteur Drive, rm HH333, Stanford, CA 94305-5317; **Phone:** 650-498-8080; **Board Cert:** Obstetrics & Gynecology 85; Gynecologic Oncology 87; **Med School:** Univ Miami Sch Med 77; **Resid:** Obstetrics & Gynecology, UCLA Med Ctr 81; **Fellow:** Gynecologic Oncology, Stanford Univ Sch Med; **Fac Appt:** Assoc Prof ObG, Stanford Univ

OBSTETRICS & GYNECOLOGY

New England

Cramer, Daniel W MD [ObG] - **Spec Exp:** Ovarian Cancer; Ovarian Cancer-Familial; **Hospital:** Brigham & Women's Hosp (page 87); **Address:** Brigham-Womens Hosp Ob/Gyn Epidemiology Ctr, 221 Longwood Ave, Boston, MA 02115; **Phone:** 617-732-4895; **Board Cert:** Obstetrics & Gynecology 79; **Med School:** Univ Colorado 70; **Resid:** Obstetrics & Gynecology, Boston Hosp-Women 76; **Fellow:** Public Health, Harvard Med Sch 82; **Fac Appt:** Prof ObG, Harvard Med Sch

Harper, Diane L MD [ObG] - **Spec Exp:** Cervical Cancer Screening; Human Papillomavirus (HPV); Vaccine Therapy; **Hospital:** Dartmouth - Hitchcock Med Ctr; **Address:** Dartmouth Hitchcock Med Ctr, Norris Cancer Ctr, One Medical Center Drive, Hb 7999, Lebanon, NH 03756; **Phone:** 603-653-9310; **Board Cert:** Family Medicine 02; **Med School:** Univ Kans 86; **Resid:** Obstetrics & Gynecology, Univ Kansas Sch Med 97; Family Medicine, Univ Kansas 90; **Fellow:** Inter-Insts Genetics Clin-NIH 94; Stanford Univ 94; **Fac Appt:** Assoc Prof FMed, Dartmouth Med Sch

Noller, Kenneth L MD [ObG] - **Spec Exp:** DES-Exposed Females; Gynecology Only; **Hospital:** Tufts-New England Med Ctr; **Address:** New England Med Ctr, 750 Washington St, Box 324, Boston, MA 02111; **Phone:** 617-636-2382; **Board Cert:** Obstetrics & Gynecology 91; **Med School:** Creighton Univ 70; **Resid:** Obstetrics & Gynecology, Mayo Clinic 74; **Fac Appt:** Prof ObG, Univ Mass Sch Med

Southeast

Morgan, Linda S MD [ObG] - **Spec Exp:** Gynecologic Cancer; Women's Health; **Hospital:** Shands Hlthcre at Univ of FL (page 109); **Address:** 2000 SW Archer Rd, Women's Health Clinic PO Box 100383, Gainesville, FL 32610-0383; **Phone:** 352-392-4161; **Board Cert:** Obstetrics & Gynecology 82; Gynecologic Oncology 83; **Med School:** Med Coll PA Hahnemann 75; **Resid:** Obstetrics & Gynecology, Shands Hosp 79; **Fellow:** Gynecologic Oncology, Mass Genl Hosp 81; **Fac Appt:** Prof ObG, Univ Fla Coll Med

Midwest

Galask, Rudolph P MD [ObG] - **Spec Exp:** Vulvar Disease/Cancer; Infectious Disease; Gynecologic Surgery; **Hospital:** Univ Iowa Hosp & Clinics; **Address:** Univ Iowa Hosp & Clinics, Dept Ob/Gyn, 200 Hawkins Drive Fl 2nd - rm BT-2004, Iowa City, IA 52242; **Phone:** 319-353-6323; **Board Cert:** Obstetrics & Gynecology 72; **Med School:** Univ Iowa Coll Med 64; **Resid:** Obstetrics & Gynecology, Univ Iowa Hosp 70; **Fac Appt:** Prof ObG, Univ Iowa Coll Med

Shulman, Lee MD [ObG] - **Spec Exp:** Prenatal Diagnosis; Breast Cancer Genetics; Ovarian Cancer Genetics; **Hospital:** Northwestern Meml Hosp; **Address:** Northwestern Univ, Dept Ob/Gyn, 333 Superior St, Ste 484, Chicago, IL 60611; **Phone:** 312-926-6627; **Board Cert:** Obstetrics & Gynecology 99; Clinical Genetics 90; **Med School:** Cornell Univ-Weill Med Coll 83; **Resid:** Obstetrics & Gynecology, North Shore Univ Hosp 87; **Fellow:** Reproductive Genetics, Univ Tenn Med Ctr 89; **Fac Appt:** Prof ObG, Northwestern Univ

Southwest

Kaufman, Raymond H MD [ObG] - **Spec Exp:** DES-Exposed Females; Vulvar Disease/Cancer; **Hospital:** Methodist Hosp - Houston; **Address:** St Luke's Med Twr, 6624 Fannin St, Ste 1800, Houston, TX 77030; **Phone:** 713-798-7523; **Board Cert:** Obstetrics & Gynecology 00; **Med School:** Univ MD Sch Med 48; **Resid:** Obstetrics & Gynecology, Beth Israel Med Ctr 53; **Fellow:** Pathology, Methodist Hosp 57; **Fac Appt:** Prof ObG, Baylor Coll Med

Smith, Harriet Olivia MD [ObG] - **Spec Exp:** Uterine Cancer; Pelvic Reconstruction; Ovarian Cancer; **Hospital:** Univ NM Hlth & Sci Ctr; **Address:** 2211 Lomas NE, Albuquerque, NM 87106-2745; **Phone:** 505-272-0185; **Board Cert:** Obstetrics & Gynecology 95; Gynecologic Oncology 96; **Med School:** Med Coll GA 1980; **Resid:** Obstetrics & Gynecology, Med Coll Georgia 85; Gynecologic Oncology, MD Anderson; **Fellow:** Gynecologic Oncology, Albert Einstein Coll Med; Reconstructive Pelvic Surgery, Emory Univ Hosp; **Fac Appt:** Assoc Prof ObG, Univ New Mexico

REPRODUCTIVE ENDOCRINOLOGY

New England

Crowley, William F MD [RE] - **Spec Exp:** Gonadotropin Deficiency; Kallmann Syndrome; Fertility Preservation in Cancer; **Hospital:** Mass Genl Hosp; **Address:** Mass Genl Hosp, Reproductive Science Ctr, 55 Fruit St, Bartlett Hall-Exten 5, Boston, MA 02114; **Phone:** 617-726-5390; **Board Cert:** Internal Medicine 74; Endocrinology 77; **Med School:** Tufts Univ 69; **Resid:** Internal Medicine, Mass Genl Hosp 71; Internal Medicine, Mass Genl Hosp 74; **Fellow:** Endocrinology, Mass Genl Hosp 76; **Fac Appt:** Prof Med, Harvard Med Sch

Ginsburg, Elizabeth MD [RE] - **Spec Exp:** Infertility-IVF; Fertility Preservation in Cancer; **Hospital:** Brigham & Women's Hosp (page 87); **Address:** Brigham & Women's Hosp - Ctr Reproductive Med, 75 Francis St, Boston, MA 02115; **Phone:** 617-732-4222; **Board Cert:** Obstetrics & Gynecology 03; Reproductive Endocrinology 03; **Med School:** Mount Sinai Sch Med 85; **Resid:** Obstetrics & Gynecology, Brigham & Women's Hosp 89; **Fellow:** Reproductive Endocrinology, Brigham & Women's Hosp 91

Patrizio, Pasquale MD [RE] - **Spec Exp:** Infertility-Male & Female; Infertility-IVF/ICSI/PGD; Fertility Preservation in Cancer; **Hospital:** Yale - New Haven Hosp; **Address:** Yale Fertility Ctr, Dept OB/GYN, 150 Sargent Drive, New Haven, CT 06511; **Phone:** 203-785-4708; **Board Cert:** Obstetrics & Gynecology 97; Reproductive Endocrinology 99; **Med School:** Italy 83; **Resid:** Obstetrics & Gynecology, Univ Naples 87; Univ Pisa 90; **Fellow:** Infertility, UC Irvine 95; **Fac Appt:** Prof ObG, Yale Univ

Mid Atlantic

Coutifaris, Christos MD/PhD [RE] - **Spec Exp:** Infertility-IVF; Fertility Preservation in Cancer; **Hospital:** Hosp Univ Penn - UPHS (page 113); **Address:** 3701 Market St Fl 8, Philadelphia, PA 19104; **Phone:** 215-662-6100; **Board Cert:** Obstetrics & Gynecology 98; Reproductive Endocrinology 98; **Med School:** Univ Pennsylvania 82; **Resid:** Obstetrics & Gynecology, Hosp Univ Penn 86; **Fellow:** Reproductive Endocrinology, Univ Penn 87; **Fac Appt:** Assoc Prof ObG, Univ Pennsylvania

Licciardi, Frederick L MD [RE] - **Spec Exp:** Infertility-IVF; Infertility-Female; Fertility Preservation; **Hospital:** NYU Med Ctr (page 104); **Address:** NYU Medical Ctr, 660 First Ave, 5th Fl, New York, NY 10016; **Phone:** 212-263-7754; **Board Cert:** Obstetrics & Gynecology 03; Reproductive Endocrinology 03; **Med School:** Rutgers Univ 86; **Resid:** Obstetrics & Gynecology, St Barnabas Med Ctr 90; **Fellow:** Reproductive Endocrinology, NY Hosp-Cornell Med Ctr 92; **Fac Appt:** Assoc Prof ObG, NYU Sch Med

Noyes, Nicole MD [RE] - **Spec Exp:** Infertlity-IVF; Fertility Preservation; **Hospital:** NYU Med Ctr (page 104); **Address:** NYU Medical Ctr, 660 First Ave, 5th FL, New York, NY 10016; **Phone:** 212-263-7981; **Board Cert:** Obstetrics & Gynecology 03; Reproductive Endocrinology 03; **Med School:** Univ VT Coll Med 86; **Resid:** Obstetrics & Gynecology, NY Hosp-Cornell Med Ctr 90; **Fellow:** Reproductive Endocrinology, NY Hosp-Cornell Med Ctr 92; **Fac Appt:** Assoc Prof ObG, NYU Sch Med

Rosenwaks, Zev MD [RE] - **Spec Exp:** Infertility-IVF; Genetic Disorders; Fertility Preservation; **Hospital:** NY-Presby Hosp - NY Weill Cornell Med Ctr (page 103); **Address:** Ctr For Reproductive Medicine & Infertility, 505 E 70th St, Ste 340, New York, NY 10021-4872; **Phone:** 212-746-1743; **Board Cert:** Obstetrics & Gynecology 78; Reproductive Endocrinology 81; **Med School:** SUNY Downstate 72; **Resid:** Obstetrics & Gynecology, LI Jewish Med Ctr 76; **Fellow:** Reproductive Endocrinology, Johns Hopkins Hosp 78; **Fac Appt:** Prof ObG, Cornell Univ-Weill Med Coll

Midwest

Wood Molo, Mary MD [RE] - **Spec Exp:** Infertility; Uterine Fibroids; Fertility Preservation in Cancer; **Hospital:** Rush Univ Med Ctr; **Address:** 1725 W Harrison St, 408E, Chicago, IL 60612; **Phone:** 312-997-2229; **Board Cert:** Obstetrics & Gynecology 04; Reproductive Endocrinology 04; **Med School:** Southern IL Univ 82; **Resid:** Obstetrics & Gynecology, Southern Illinois Affil Hosps 84; Obstetrics & Gynecology, Rush Presby St Lukes Hosp 87; **Fellow:** Reproductive Endocrinology, Rush Presby St Lukes Hosp 89; **Fac Appt:** Asst Prof ObG, Rush Med Coll

OPHTHALMOLOGY

*A*n ophthalmologist has the knowledge and professional skills needed to provide eye and vision care. Ophthalmologists are medically trained to diagnose, monitor and medically or surgically treat all ocular and visual disorders. This includes problems affecting the eye and its component structures, the eyelids, the orbit and the visual pathways. In so doing, an ophthalmologist prescribes vision services, including glasses and contact lenses.

Training required: Four years

PHYSICIAN LISTINGS

307

THE NEW YORK EYE & EAR INFIRMARY

310 East 14th Street • New York, NY 10003
Tel. (212) 979-4000 • Fax. (212) 228-0664
www.nyee.edu
Information and Referral Line: (800) 449-HOPE (4673)

OPHTHALMOLOGY

Ocular Tumor Service: The Infirmary is a major referral center within the Collaborative Ocular Melanoma Study of the National Eye Institute/NIH. New and innovative treatments include radioactive plaques for intraocular tumors and chemotherapy for conjunctival neoplasia. Patients with tumors of the iris, retina, choroid and optic nerve are also treated here.

Oculoplastic, Orbital & Reconstructive Surgery: A leading service in this country and abroad for the treatment of orbital and eyelid cancer, these specialists also commonly see systemic diseases affecting the eye socket, including thyroid disease and lymphoproliferative disorders. A multidisciplinary Ocular Tumor Board meets monthly to discuss the most difficult cases and formulate therapeutic options.

OTOLARYNGOLOGY/ HEAD & NECK SURGERY

Head & Neck Oncology: A team comprised of board-certified surgeons, medical & radiation oncologists, nutritionists and rehabilitation specialists ensure rapid recovery from complex, life saving surgical procedures and return to daily activities.

Thyroid Center: A unique center concentrates on streamlining the diagnosis and treatment of thyroid diseases and cancers with a highly skilled team of surgeons, endocrinologists and radiologists. An area of expertise is cancer resulting from radiation exposure such as Chernobyl.

Facial Plastics and Reconstructive Surgery: Treatment of facial tumors, both benign and cancerous, frequently requires expert reconstruction. Designed to restore the function and appearance of the face, these procedures may be required after appropriate treatment of skin cancers or deep tumors.

Otology–Neuro-otology: These rare cancers can be treated by our highly skilled team of surgeons which includes a neuro-otologist and a neurosurgeon.

Center for the Voice: The Center is cooperatively staffed by a team of specialists able to diagnose cancer of the vocal cords early and rehabilitate the voice after surgical and radiation treatment.

PATHOLOGY & LABORATORY MEDICINE

The laboratory of the Ocular Pathology Service is utilized by ophthalmologists throughout the entire Northeast. The Infirmary is the site of promising studies into diseases and cancers of the eye, ear, nose and throat. Research includes cellular markers of oral cancer risk, non-invasive detection of thyroid cancer, basic cell biology of the growth of ocular melanoma cells, and persistence of biomaterials for repair in plastic and reconstructive surgery.

ABOUT NYEEI

Established in 1820, the Infirmary is the oldest continuously operating specialty hospital in the nation and one of the most experienced in terms of the number of patients it treats and complexity of cases.

Each year the Ophthalmology Department performs more than 16,000 surgeries and sees more than 80,000 visits from outpatients. The Otolaryngology Department performs more than 6,000 surgeries and has some 60,000 outpatient visits. A third clinical department, the Department of Plastic and Reconstructive Surgery, is a natural complement to the Infirmary's other services and annually treats more than 1,000 patients who seek reconstructive surgery as a result of accident, birth defect or cancer, and those who elect cosmetic surgery.

NYEEI is a teaching affiliate of New York Medical College and a member of Continuum Health Partners, Inc.

OPHTHALMOLOGY

Mid Atlantic

Abramson, David H MD **[Oph]** - **Spec Exp:** Eye Tumors/Cancer; Orbital Tumors; Retinoblastoma/Ocular Melanoma; **Hospital:** Meml Sloan Kettering Cancer Ctr (page 100); **Address:** 70 E 66th St, New York, NY 10021; **Phone:** 212-744-1700; **Board Cert:** Ophthalmology 75; **Med School:** Albert Einstein Coll Med 69; **Resid:** Ophthalmology, Harkness Eye Inst 74; **Fellow:** Ocular Oncology, Columbia-Presby Med Ctr 75; **Fac Appt:** Clin Prof Oph, Cornell Univ-Weill Med Coll

Della Rocca, Robert MD **[Oph]** - **Spec Exp:** Orbital Tumors/Cancer; Eyelid Cancer & Reconstruction; Thyroid Eye Disease; **Hospital:** New York Eye & Ear Infirm (page 102); **Address:** 310 E 14th St, South Bldg, rm 319, New York, NY 10003; **Phone:** 212-979-4575; **Board Cert:** Ophthalmology 75; **Med School:** Creighton Univ 67; **Resid:** Ophthalmology, NY Eye & Ear Infirm 73; **Fellow:** Oculoplastic Surgery, Albany Med Ctr

Finger, Paul T MD **[Oph]** - **Spec Exp:** Eye Tumors/Cancer; Macular Disease/Degeneration; **Hospital:** New York Eye & Ear Infirm (page 102); **Address:** 115 E 61st St, New York, NY 10021-8183; **Phone:** 212-832-8170; **Board Cert:** Ophthalmology 90; **Med School:** Tulane Univ 82; **Resid:** Ophthalmology, Manhattan EET Hosp 86; **Fellow:** Ocular Oncology, N Shore Univ Hosp-Cornell 87; **Fac Appt:** Clin Prof Oph, NYU Sch Med

Shields, Carol L MD **[Oph]** - **Spec Exp:** Orbital Tumors/Cancer; Melanoma; Retinoblastoma; **Hospital:** Wills Eye Hosp; **Address:** Wills Eye Hosp, Ocular Oncology Service, 840 Walnut St, Phildelphia, PA 19107; **Phone:** 215-928-3105; **Board Cert:** Ophthalmology 89; **Med School:** Univ Pittsburgh 83; **Resid:** Ophthalmology, Willis Eye Hosp 88; **Fellow:** Ophthalmic Oncololgy, Willis Eye Hosp 89; Ophthalmic Pathology, Willis Eye Hosp 88; **Fac Appt:** Prof Oph, Jefferson Med Coll

Shields, Jerry MD **[Oph]** - **Spec Exp:** Eye Tumors/Cancer; Pediatric Ophthalmology; Retinoblastoma; **Hospital:** Wills Eye Hosp; **Address:** 840 Walnut St Fl 14 - Ste 1440, Philadelphia, PA 19107; **Phone:** 215-928-3105; **Board Cert:** Ophthalmology 72; **Med School:** Univ Mich Med Sch 64; **Resid:** Ophthalmology, Wills Eye Hosp 70; **Fellow:** Ophthalmology, Wills Eye Hosp 72; **Fac Appt:** Prof Oph, Thomas Jefferson Univ

Southeast

Dutton, Jonathan J MD/PhD **[Oph]** - **Spec Exp:** Oculoplastic Surgery; Eye Tumors/Cancer; Melanoma-Choroidal (eye); **Hospital:** Univ NC Hosps (page 112); **Address:** Univ North Carolina - Dept Ophthalmology, 130 Mason Farm Rd, 5110 Bioinformatics, CB 7040, Chapel Hill, NC 27599-7040; **Phone:** 919-966-5296; **Board Cert:** Ophthalmology 83; **Med School:** Washington Univ, St Louis 77; **Resid:** Ophthalmology, Washington Univ Med Ctr 82; **Fellow:** Oculoplastic Surgery, Univ Iowa Med Ctr 83; **Fac Appt:** Clin Prof Oph, Univ NC Sch Med

Grossniklaus, Hans E MD **[Oph]** - **Spec Exp:** Ophthalmic Pathology; Melanoma-Choroidal (eye); Macular Disease/Degeneration; **Hospital:** Emory Univ Hosp; **Address:** Emory Eye Center, 1365-B Clifton Rd NE, rm BT428, Atlanta, GA 30322; **Phone:** 404-778-4611; **Board Cert:** Ophthalmology 85; Anatomic Pathology 87; **Med School:** Ohio State Univ 80; **Resid:** Ophthalmology, Case West Res Univ Hosp 84; Pathology, Case West Res Univ Hosp 87; **Fellow:** Ophthalmological Pathology, Johns Hopkins Hosp 85; **Fac Appt:** Prof Oph, Emory Univ

Haik, Barrett MD [Oph] - **Spec Exp:** Eye Tumors/Cancer; **Hospital:** St Jude Children's Research Hosp; **Address:** Univ Tenn Med Group, 920 Madison Ave, Ste 915, Memphis, TN 38103; **Phone:** 901-448-6650; **Board Cert:** Ophthalmology 81; **Med School:** Louisiana State Univ 76; **Resid:** Ophthalmology, Columbia-Presby/Harkness Eye Inst 80; **Fac Appt:** Prof Oph, Univ Tenn Coll Med, Memphis

Murray, Timothy MD [Oph] - **Spec Exp:** Retinal Disease; Eye Tumors/Cancer; **Hospital:** Bascom Palmer Eye Inst.; **Address:** 900 NW 17th St, Rm 254, Miami, FL 33136-1119; **Phone:** 305-326-6166; **Board Cert:** Ophthalmology 90; **Med School:** Johns Hopkins Univ 85; **Resid:** Ophthalmology, UCSF Med Ctr 89; **Fellow:** Ophthalmology, UCSF 99; Ophthalmology, Med Coll Wisconsin 91; **Fac Appt:** Prof Oph, Univ Miami Sch Med

Sternberg Jr, Paul MD [Oph] - **Spec Exp:** Retina/Vitreous Surgery; Macular Disease/Degeneration; Eye Tumors/Cancer; **Hospital:** Vanderbilt Univ Med Ctr (page 116); **Address:** Vanderbilt Eye Institute, 8000 Medical Center E, Nashville, TN 37232-8808; **Phone:** 615-936-1453; **Board Cert:** Ophthalmology 85; **Med School:** Univ Chicago-Pritzker Sch Med 79; **Resid:** Ophthalmology, Johns Hopkins Hosp 83; **Fellow:** Vitreoretinal Surgery, Duke Univ Med Ctr 84; **Fac Appt:** Prof Oph, Vanderbilt Univ

Tse, David MD [Oph] - **Spec Exp:** Oculoplastic & Orbital Surgery; Orbital Tumors/Cancer; Lacrimal Gland Disorders; **Hospital:** Bascom Palmer Eye Inst.; **Address:** Bascom Palmer Eye Inst, 900 NW 17th St, Miami, FL 33136-1119; **Phone:** 305-326-6086; **Board Cert:** Ophthalmology 02; **Med School:** Univ Miami Sch Med 76; **Resid:** Ophthalmology, LAC/USC Med Ctr 81; **Fellow:** Oculoplastic Surgery, Univ Iowa Hosps 82; **Fac Appt:** Prof Oph, Univ Miami Sch Med

Wilson, Matthew MD [Oph] - **Spec Exp:** Eye Tumors/Cancer; Retinoblastoma; Melanoma-Choroidal (eye); **Hospital:** St Jude Children's Research Hosp; **Address:** Univ Tennessee - Ophthalmology, 920 Madison Ave, Ste 915, Memphis, TN 38103; **Phone:** 901-448-6650; **Board Cert:** Ophthalmology 96; **Med School:** Emory Univ 90; **Resid:** Ophthalmology, Emory Univ 94; **Fellow:** Ophthalmological Pathology, Emory Univ 95; Ocular Oncology, Moorfields Eye Hosp 96; **Fac Appt:** Assoc Prof Oph, Univ Tenn Coll Med, Memphis

Midwest

Albert, Daniel M MD [Oph] - **Spec Exp:** Eye Tumors/Cancer; Ophthalmic Pathology; **Hospital:** Univ WI Hosp & Clins; **Address:** Univ Wisconsin, Dept Ophthalmology/VisualSci, 600 Highland Ave, CSC Bldg - Ste F4-344 Fl 2, Madison, WI 53792; **Phone:** 608-263-7171; **Board Cert:** Ophthalmology 69; **Med School:** Univ Pennsylvania 62; **Resid:** Ophthalmology, Hosp Univ Penn 66; Neurological Ophthalmology, Natl Inst Hlth 68; **Fellow:** Pathology, Armed Forces Inst Path 69; **Fac Appt:** Prof Oph, Univ Wisc

Augsburger, James MD [Oph] - **Spec Exp:** Eye Tumors/Cancer; **Hospital:** Univ Hosp - Cincinnati; **Address:** University Cincinnati Coll Med-Dept Oph, 3223 Eden Ave Bldg Hlth Professions - Ste 350, Cincinnati, OH 45267; **Phone:** 513-558-5151; **Board Cert:** Ophthalmology 79; **Med School:** Univ Cincinnati ; **Resid:** Ophthalmology, Univ Hosp-Cincinnati 78; **Fellow:** Wills Eye Hosp 80

Blair, Norman P MD [Oph] - **Spec Exp:** Eye Tumors/Cancer; Melanoma-Choroidal (eye); Retinal Disorders & Injury; **Hospital:** Univ of IL Med Ctr at Chicago; **Address:** 1905 W Taylor St Bldg L120, University of Illinois Eye Ctr, Chicago, IL 60612-7245; **Phone:** 312-996-6660; **Board Cert:** Ophthalmology 78; **Med School:** Indiana Univ 70; **Resid:** Ophthalmology, Massachusetts Eye & Ear Infirmary 77; **Fellow:** Retina/Vitreous, Massachusetts Eye & Ear Infirmary 79; Ophthalmic Pathology, Univ Illinois Eye & Ear Infirmary 81; **Fac Appt:** Prof Oph, Univ IL Coll Med

Harbour, James W MD **[Oph]** - **Spec Exp:** Eye Tumors/Cancer; Melanoma-Choroidal (eye); **Hospital:** Barnes-Jewish Hosp (page 85); **Address:** Washington Univ Sch Med, Dept Ophthalmology, 660 S Euclid Ave, Box 8096, St Louis, MO 63110; **Phone:** 314-367-1181; **Board Cert:** Ophthalmology 96; **Med School:** Johns Hopkins Univ 90; **Resid:** Ophthalmology, Wills Eye Hosp 94; **Fellow:** Retina/Vitreous, Bascom Palmer Eye Inst 95; Ocular Oncology, UCSF Med Ctr 96; **Fac Appt:** Asst Prof Oph, Washington Univ, St Louis

Lueder, Gregg T MD **[Oph]** - **Spec Exp:** Retinoblastoma; Eye Tumors-Pediatric; Pediatric Ophthalmology; **Hospital:** St Louis Chldns Hosp; **Address:** St Louis Children's Hospital, One Children's Pl, rm 2S89, St Louis, MO 63110; **Phone:** 314-454-6026; **Board Cert:** Pediatrics 89; Ophthalmology 03; **Med School:** Univ Iowa Coll Med 85; **Resid:** Pediatrics, St Louis Children's Hosp 88; Ophthalmology, Univ Iowa Med Ctr 91; **Fellow:** Pediatric Ophthalmology, Hosp for Sick Children 93; **Fac Appt:** Assoc Prof Oph, Washington Univ, St Louis

Mieler, William F MD **[Oph]** - **Spec Exp:** Eye Tumors/Cancer; Retina/Vitreous Surgery; **Hospital:** Univ of Chicago Hosps; **Address:** Dept of Opthalmology & Visual Science Univ of Chicago, 5841 S Maryland, rm F209, MC 2114, Chicago, IL 60637; **Phone:** 773-702-3838; **Board Cert:** Ophthalmology 84; **Med School:** Univ Wisc 79; **Resid:** Ophthalmology, Bascom-Palmer Eye Inst 83; **Fellow:** Vitreoretinal Surgery & Disease, Med Ctr Wisc Eye Inst 84; Oculoplastic Surgery, Wills Eye Hosp 86; **Fac Appt:** Prof Oph, Univ Chicago-Pritzker Sch Med

Weingeist, Thomas A MD/PhD **[Oph]** - **Spec Exp:** Retinal Disorders & Surgery; Eye Tumors/Cancer; **Hospital:** Univ Iowa Hosp & Clinics; **Address:** Univ Iowa, Dept Ophthalmology, 200 Hawkins Drive, Iowa City, IA 52242; **Phone:** 319-356-2864; **Board Cert:** Ophthalmology 76; **Med School:** Univ Iowa Coll Med 72; **Resid:** Ophthalmology, Univ Iowa Hosp 75; **Fellow:** Vitreoretinal Surgery, Univ Iowa 76; **Fac Appt:** Prof Oph, Univ Iowa Coll Med

Great Plains and Mountains

Anderson, Richard L MD **[Oph]** - **Spec Exp:** Orbital & Eyelid Tumors/Cancer; Eyelid Problems/Blepharospasm/Ptosis; Eyelid & Facial Cosmetic Surgery; **Hospital:** Salt Lake Regional Med Ctr; **Address:** 1002 E South Temple, Ste 308, Salt Lake City, UT 84102-1525; **Phone:** 801-363-3355; **Board Cert:** Ophthalmology 76; **Med School:** Univ Iowa Coll Med 71; **Resid:** Ophthalmology, U Ia Hosps-Clins 75; **Fellow:** Albany Med Ctr; UCSF Med Ctr; **Fac Appt:** Prof PlS, Univ Utah

Gigantelli, James W MD **[Oph]** - **Spec Exp:** Orbital Surgery & Cancer; Eyelid Cancer; Lymphoma-Ocular (eye); **Hospital:** Nebraska Med Ctr; **Address:** 985540 Nebraska Medical Ctr, Omaha, NE 68198-5540; **Phone:** 402-559-4276; **Board Cert:** Ophthalmology 91; **Med School:** Vanderbilt Univ 85; **Resid:** Ophthalmology, Baylor Coll Med 89; **Fellow:** Oculoplastic Surgery, Duke Unv Med Ctr 90; **Fac Appt:** Assoc Prof Oph, Univ Nebr Coll Med

Southwest

Boniuk, Milton MD **[Oph]** - **Spec Exp:** Oculoplastic Surgery; Eye Tumors/Cancer; **Hospital:** Methodist Hosp - Houston; **Address:** 6550 Fannin St, Smith Twr, Ste 1501, Houston, TX 77030; **Phone:** 713-798-6100; **Board Cert:** Ophthalmology 60; **Med School:** Dalhousie Univ 56; **Resid:** Ophthalmology, Wills Eye Hosp 59; **Fellow:** Ophthalmological Pathology, AFIP 61; **Fac Appt:** Prof Oph, Baylor Coll Med

Piest, Kenneth L MD [Oph] - **Spec Exp:** Eyelid Cosmetic & Reconstructive Surgery; Pediatric Eye Reconstructive Surgery; Orbital Surgery & Cancer; **Hospital:** Metro Methodist Hosp; **Address:** Texas Ophthalmic Plastic Surg, 225 E Sonterra Blvd, Ste 201, San Antonio, TX 78258; **Phone:** 210-494-8859; **Board Cert:** Ophthalmology 91; **Med School:** Univ IL Coll Med 84; **Resid:** Ophthalmology, Univ Tex Hlth Scis Ctr 89; **Fellow:** Ophthalmic Plastic Surgery, Chldns Hosp/Sheie Eye Inst/Univ Penn 90; Craniofacial Ophthalmic Plastic Surgery, Chldns Hosp/Univ Penn 91; **Fac Appt:** Assoc Clin Prof Oph, Univ Tex, San Antonio

West Coast and Pacific

Boxrud, Cynthia Ann MD [Oph] - **Spec Exp:** Oculoplastic Surgery; Eye Tumors/Cancer; Orbital Diseases; **Hospital:** UCLA Med Ctr (page 111); **Address:** 2021 Santa Monica Blvd, Ste 700E, Santa Monica, CA 90404-2208; **Phone:** 310-829-9060; **Board Cert:** Ophthalmology 97; **Med School:** Case West Res Univ 86; **Resid:** Ophthalmology, NYU-Bellevue Hosp Ctr 90; **Fellow:** Ophthalmic Oncololgy, New York Hosp-Cornell Med Ctr 92; Ophthalmic Plastic Surgery, UCLA - Jules Stein Eye Inst 93; **Fac Appt:** Asst Prof Oph, UCLA

Char, Devron H MD [Oph] - **Spec Exp:** Eye Tumors/Cancer; Thyroid Eye Disease; **Hospital:** CA Pacific Med Ctr - Pacific Campus; **Address:** 45 Castro St, Ste 309, San Francisco, CA 94114; **Phone:** 415-522-0700; **Board Cert:** Ophthalmology 78; **Med School:** Univ Minn 70; **Resid:** Internal Medicine, Mass Genl Hosp 72; Ophthalmology, UCSF Med Ctr 77; **Fellow:** Medical Oncology, Natl Cancer Inst 74; Ophthalmology, UCSF Med Ctr 78; **Fac Appt:** Prof Oph, Stanford Univ

Cockerham, Kimberly P MD [Oph] - **Spec Exp:** Meningioma-Orbital (eye); Orbital Tumors; Eyelid Cancer; **Hospital:** UCSF Med Ctr; **Address:** UCSF Medical Ctr, ACC Bldg, Dept Ophthalmology, 500 Parnassus Ave Fl 7, San Francisco, CA 94143; **Phone:** 415-476-3705; **Board Cert:** Ophthalmology 04; **Med School:** Geo Wash Univ 87; **Resid:** Ophthalmology, Walter Reed Army Med Ctr 92; **Fellow:** Neurological Ophthalmology, Walter Reed Army Med Ctr 93; Neurological Ophthalmology, Alleghany General Hosp 95; **Fac Appt:** Assoc Prof Oph, UCSF

Murphree, A Linn MD [Oph] - **Spec Exp:** Pediatric Ophthalmology; Eye Diseases-Hereditary; Retinoblastoma & Orbital Tumors; **Hospital:** Chldns Hosp - Los Angeles; **Address:** Chldns Hosp, Div Oph, 4650 W Sunset Blvd, MS 88, Los Angeles, CA 90027-6016; **Phone:** 323-669-2299; **Board Cert:** Ophthalmology 78; **Med School:** Baylor Coll Med 72; **Resid:** Clinical Genetics, Baylor Heed 73; Ophthalmology, Baylor Coll Med 76; **Fellow:** Ophthalmology, Wilmer Inst/Johns Hopkins 77; **Fac Appt:** Prof Oph, USC Sch Med

O'Brien, Joan M MD [Oph] - **Spec Exp:** Eye Tumors/Cancer; Retinoblastoma; **Hospital:** UCSF Med Ctr; **Address:** UCSF, Dept Ophthalmology, 8 Kirkham St, Box 0730, San Francisco, CA 94143; **Phone:** 415-502-3206; **Board Cert:** Ophthalmology 96; **Med School:** Dartmouth Med Sch 86; **Resid:** Ophthalmology, Mass Eye & Ear Infirm 92; **Fellow:** Ophthalmic Pathology, Mass Eye & Ear Infirm 89; UCSF Med Ctr 93; **Fac Appt:** Prof Oph, UCSF

Seiff, Stuart R MD [Oph] - **Spec Exp:** Oculoplastic & Reconstructive Surgery; Orbital Tumors/Cancer; **Hospital:** UCSF Med Ctr; **Address:** 400 Parnassus Ave, Fl 7 - rm A750, San Francisco, CA 94143; **Phone:** 415-535-2142; **Board Cert:** Ophthalmology 86; **Med School:** UCSF 80; **Resid:** Ophthalmology, UCSF Med Ctr 84; **Fellow:** Ophthalmic Plastic & Reconstructive Surgery, UCLA Med Ctr 85; Oculoplastic Surgery, Moorfield's Eye Hosp; **Fac Appt:** Prof Oph, UCSF

Stout, J Timothy MD/PhD [Oph] - **Spec Exp:** Retinal Disorders-Pediatric; Retinoblastoma; Retinopathy of Prematurity; **Hospital:** OR Hlth & Sci Univ; **Address:** 3375 SW Terwilliger Blvd, Portland, OR 97239; **Phone:** 503-494-2435; **Board Cert:** Ophthalmology 99; **Med School:** Baylor Coll Med 89; **Resid:** Ophthalmology, Doheny Eye Inst 93; **Fellow:** Ophthalmology, Moorfields Eye Hosp 94; Retinal Surgery, Doheny Eye Inst 95; **Fac Appt:** Assoc Clin Prof Oph, Oregon Hlth Sci Univ

ORTHOPAEDIC SURGERY

*A*n orthopaedic surgeon is trained in the preservation, investigation and restoration of the form and function of the extremities, spine and associated structures by medical, surgical and physical means.

An orthopaedic surgeon is involved with the care of patients whose musculoskeletal problems include congenital deformities, trauma, infections, tumors, metabolic disturbances of the musculoskeletal system, deformities, injuries and degenerative diseases of the spine, hands, feet, knee, hip, shoulder and elbow in children and adults. An orthopaedic surgeon is also concerned with primary and secondary muscular problems and the effects of central or peripheral nervous system lesions of the musculoskeletal system.

Training required: *Five years (including general surgery training) plus two years in clinical practice before final certification is achieved.*

HAND SURGERY

A specialist trained in the investigation, preservation and restoration by medical, surgical and rehabilitative means of all structures of the upper extremity directly affecting the form and function of the hand and wrist.

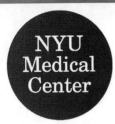

NYU Medical Center

NYU MEDICAL CENTER
550 First Avenue (at 31st St.)
New York, NY 10016
Physician Referral:
1-888-7-NYU-MED
www.nyumc.org

HOSPITAL FOR JOINT DISEASES
301 East 17th Street (at 2nd Ave.), New York, NY 10003
Physician Referral: 1-888-HJD-DOCS 1-888-453-3627
www.hjd.org

SCHOOL OF MEDICINE

NEW YORK UNIVERSITY

NYU-HOSPITAL FOR JOINT DISEASES ORTHOPAEDIC SERVICES

LEADERS IN THE TREATMENT OF ADULT AND CHILDREN'S BONE AND JOINT DISORDERS.

The NYU-Hospital for Joint Diseases Department of Orthopaedic Surgery Offers the Following Services and Treatments:

- Hip and Knee Replacement Center
- The Spine Center
- Arthroscopic Surgery
- Pediatric Orthopaedics
- Sports Medicine
- Bone Tumor Service
- Foot and Ankle Surgery
- Hand Surgery
- Limb Lengthening and Bone Growth
- Occupational and Industrial Orthopaedic Care
- Shoulder Institute
- Center for Neuromuscular and Developmental Disorders
- The Geriatric Hip Fracture Program
- The Scoliosis Program
- The Harkness Center for Dance Injuries
- Immediate Orthopaedic Care Center

NYU-Hospital for Joint Diseases Orthopaedics provides care at NYU Tisch Hospital, Hospital for Joint Diseases, Manhattan VA, Jamaica Hospital, and Bellevue Hospital Center, where more than 15,000 surgical procedures are performed each year. The orthopaedic faculty maintains offices in all five boroughs as well as in Rockland County and New Jersey.

The NYU-Hospital for Joint Diseases Department of Orthopaedic Surgery is the largest and most accomplished in the region for the diagnosis and treatment of musculoskeletal disorders as well as in research and education. The clinical expertise of the faculty represents all subspecialty areas of orthopaedic surgery, including spine, total joint replacement, sports medicine and arthroscopy, pediatric orthopaedics, shoulder, hand, and foot-and-ankle.

PHYSICIAN REFERRAL
1-888-7-NYU-MED
(1-888-769-8633)
www.nyumc.org

ORTHOPAEDIC SURGERY

New England

Friedlaender, Gary E MD [OrS] - **Spec Exp:** Bone & Soft Tissue Tumors; Reconstructive Limb Surgery; Fractures-Non Union; **Hospital:** Yale - New Haven Hosp; **Address:** Yale Univ Sch Med, Dept Orthopedic Surgery, 800 Howard Ave Bldg YPB - rm 133, Box 208071, New Haven, CT 06520-8071; **Phone:** 203-737-5656; **Board Cert:** Orthopaedic Surgery 75; **Med School:** Univ Mich Med Sch 69; **Resid:** Surgery, Michigan Med Ctr 71; Orthopaedic Surgery, Yale-New Haven Hosp 74; **Fellow:** Musculoskeletal Oncology, Mass Genl Hosp; **Fac Appt:** Prof OrS, Yale Univ

Gebhardt, Mark MD [OrS] - **Spec Exp:** Musculoskeletal Tumors; Bone Tumors; **Hospital:** Beth Israel Deaconess Med Ctr - Boston; **Address:** 330 Brookline Ave, Boston, MA 02215; **Phone:** 617-667-2181; **Board Cert:** Orthopaedic Surgery 92; **Med School:** Univ Cincinnati 75; **Resid:** Surgery, Univ Pittsburg Med Ctr 77; Orthopaedic Surgery, Harvard 82; **Fellow:** Pediatric Orthopaedic Surgery, Boston Chldns Hosp 83; Orthopedic Oncology, Mass Genl Hosp 83; **Fac Appt:** Clin Prof OrS, Harvard Med Sch

Ready, John E MD [OrS] - **Spec Exp:** Bone Cancer; Sarcoma; Trauma; **Hospital:** Brigham & Women's Hosp (page 87); **Address:** Brigham & Women's Hospital, Dept Orthopaedics, 75 Francis St, Boston, MA 02115; **Phone:** 617-732-5368; **Board Cert:** Orthopaedic Surgery 02; **Med School:** Dalhousie Univ 82; **Resid:** Orthopaedic Surgery, Dalhousie Univ Hosp 87; **Fellow:** Orthopedic Oncology, St Michael's Hosp 88

Mid Atlantic

Benevenia, Joseph MD [OrS] - **Spec Exp:** Limb Sparing Surgery; Bone Cancer & Transplant; Musculoskeletal Tumors; **Hospital:** UMDNJ-Univ Hosp-Newark; **Address:** 90 Bergen St, Ste 1200, Newark, NJ 07103; **Phone:** 973-972-2150; **Board Cert:** Orthopaedic Surgery 03; **Med School:** UMDNJ-NJ Med Sch, Newark 84; **Resid:** Orthopaedic Surgery, UMDNJ-NJ Med Sch Hosp 88; **Fellow:** Orthopedic Oncology, Case Western Reserve Univ 91; **Fac Appt:** Assoc Prof OrS, UMDNJ-NJ Med Sch, Newark

Dormans, John P MD [OrS] - **Spec Exp:** Tumor Surgery-Pediatric; Spinal Surgery-Pediatric; **Hospital:** Chldns Hosp of Philadelphia, The; **Address:** Childrens Hosp Philadelphia, 34 St & Civic Center Blvd, Wood Bldg Fl 2-rm 2315, Philadelphia, PA 19104; **Phone:** 215-590-1534; **Board Cert:** Orthopaedic Surgery 02; **Med School:** Indiana Univ 83; **Resid:** Orthopaedic Surgery, Michigan State Univ Hosps 88; **Fellow:** Pediatric Orthopaedic Surgery, Hosp Sick Chldn 89; **Fac Appt:** Prof OrS, Univ Pennsylvania

Frassica, Frank John MD [OrS] - **Spec Exp:** Bone Cancer; **Hospital:** Johns Hopkins Hosp - Baltimore (page 97); **Address:** 601 N Caroline St, rm 5210, Baltimore, MD 21287-0882; **Phone:** 410-955-9300; **Board Cert:** Orthopaedic Surgery 01; **Med School:** Univ SC Sch Med 82; **Resid:** Orthopaedic Surgery, Mayo Clinic 87; **Fellow:** Orthopedic Oncology, Mayo Clinic 88; **Fac Appt:** Prof OrS, Johns Hopkins Univ

Healey, John H MD [OrS] - **Spec Exp:** Bone Tumors & Soft Tissue Sarcomas; Knee Replacement in Bone Tumors; Prosthetic Reconstruction; **Hospital:** Meml Sloan Kettering Cancer Ctr (page 100); **Address:** 1275 York Ave, Ste A-342, New York, NY 10021-6007; **Phone:** 212-639-7610; **Board Cert:** Orthopaedic Surgery 97; **Med School:** Univ VT Coll Med 78; **Resid:** Orthopaedic Surgery, Hosp Special Surg 83; **Fellow:** Orthopedic Oncology, Meml Sloan Kettering Cancer Ctr 84; Orthopaedic Surgery, Hosp Special Surgery 84; **Fac Appt:** Assoc Prof OrS, Cornell Univ-Weill Med Coll

Kenan, Samuel MD [OrS] - **Spec Exp:** Bone Tumors; Joint Replacement; **Hospital:** Hosp For Joint Diseases; **Address:** 317 E 34th St, Fl 9, New York, NY 10016; **Phone:** 212-684-5511; **Med School:** Israel 76; **Resid:** Orthopaedic Surgery, Hadassah Univ Hosp 84; **Fellow:** Orthopaedic Pathology, Hosp for Joint Diseases 87; **Fac Appt:** Prof OrS, NYU Sch Med

Lackman, Richard D MD [OrS] - **Spec Exp:** Bone Cancer; Sarcoma; Limb Salvage; **Hospital:** Hosp Univ Penn - UPHS (page 113); **Address:** Hosp Univ Penn - Dept Orthopaedic Surg, 3400 Spruce St, Silverstein Pavilion Fl 2, Philadelphia, PA 19104; **Phone:** 215-662-3340; **Board Cert:** Orthopaedic Surgery 85; **Med School:** Univ Pennsylvania 77; **Resid:** Orthopaedic Surgery, Hosp Univ Penn 82; **Fellow:** Orthopedic Oncology, Mayo Clinic 83; **Fac Appt:** Assoc Prof OrS, Univ Pennsylvania

Lane, Joseph MD [OrS] - **Spec Exp:** Metabolic Bone Disease; Osteoporosis-Kyphoplasty Procedure; Bone Cancer; **Hospital:** Hosp For Special Surgery; **Address:** Hosp for Special Surgery, 535 E 70th St, New York, NY 10021; **Phone:** 212-606-1172; **Board Cert:** Orthopaedic Surgery 98; **Med School:** Harvard Med Sch 65; **Resid:** Surgery, Hosp Univ Penn 67; Orthopaedic Surgery, Hosp Univ Penn 73; **Fac Appt:** Prof OrS, Cornell Univ-Weill Med Coll

Malawer, Martin MD [OrS] - **Spec Exp:** Bone Tumors & Soft Tissue Sarcomas; Limb Sparing Surgery; Pediatric Orthopaedic Surgery; **Hospital:** Washington Hosp Ctr; **Address:** Washington Cancer Institute, 110 Irving St NW, #C2173, Washington, DC 20010; **Phone:** 202-877-3970; **Board Cert:** Orthopaedic Surgery 76; **Med School:** NYU Sch Med 69; **Resid:** Surgery, Bronx Muni Hosp-Albert Einstein 72; Orthopaedic Surgery, Bellevue Hosp Ctr-NYU 75; **Fellow:** Orthopaedic Pathology, Shands Hosp-Univ Florida 78; **Fac Appt:** Prof OrS, Geo Wash Univ

Springfield, Dempsey MD [OrS] - **Spec Exp:** Bone Tumors & Metastices; Soft Tissue Tumors; **Hospital:** Mount Sinai Med Ctr (page 101); **Address:** 5 E 98th St Fl 9, Box 1188, New York, NY 10029-6501; **Phone:** 212-241-8311; **Board Cert:** Orthopaedic Surgery 92; **Med School:** Univ Fla Coll Med 71; **Resid:** Orthopaedic Surgery, Univ Florida/Shands 76; **Fellow:** Orthopaedic Surgery, Univ Florida/Shands 79; **Fac Appt:** Prof OrS, Mount Sinai Sch Med

Southeast

Scarborough, Mark MD [OrS] - **Spec Exp:** Bone Tumors; Sarcoma; **Hospital:** Shands Hlthcre at Univ of FL (page 109); **Address:** Shands Hlthcare Univ FL, 1600 SW Archer Rd, Box 112727, Gainesville, FL 32611; **Phone:** 352-273-7000; **Board Cert:** Orthopaedic Surgery 03; **Med School:** Univ Fla Coll Med 85; **Resid:** Orthopaedic Surgery, UT Med Ctr 90; **Fellow:** Orthopaedic Surgery, Mass Genl Hosp 91; **Fac Appt:** Assoc Prof OrS, Univ Fla Coll Med

Scully, Sean P MD [OrS] - **Spec Exp:** Bone Cancer; Sarcoma; Musculoskeletal Tumors; **Hospital:** Cedars Med Ctr - Miami; **Address:** Cedars Medical Ctr, East Bldg, 1400 NW 12th Ave Fl 4, Miami, FL 33136; **Phone:** 305-325-4475; **Board Cert:** Orthopaedic Surgery 95; **Med School:** Univ Rochester 80; **Resid:** Orthopaedic Surgery, Duke Univ Med Ctr 85; **Fellow:** Orthopedic Oncology, Mass General Hosp 87; Research, NIH 88; **Fac Appt:** Clin Prof OrS, Univ Miami Sch Med

Walling, Arthur MD [OrS] - **Spec Exp:** Bone & Muscle Tumors; Foot & Ankle Surgery; **Hospital:** H Lee Moffitt Cancer Ctr & Research Inst; **Address:** 13020 N Telecom Pkwy, Temple Terrace, FL 33637; **Phone:** 813-978-9700; **Board Cert:** Orthopaedic Surgery 82; **Med School:** Creighton Univ 76; **Resid:** Orthopaedic Surgery, Univ South Florida Affil Hosps 80; **Fellow:** Surgical Oncology, Univ Florida 81; **Fac Appt:** Assoc Clin Prof OrS, Univ S Fla Coll Med

Ward, William G MD [OrS] - **Spec Exp:** Bone Tumors; Soft Tissue Tumors; Reconstructive Surgery; **Hospital:** Wake Forest Univ Baptist Med Ctr (page 117); **Address:** Wake Forest Univ Baptist Med Ctr, Dept Ortho, Med Ctr Blvd, Winston Salem, NC 27157-1070; **Phone:** 336-716-4013; **Board Cert:** Orthopaedic Surgery 04; **Med School:** Duke Univ 75; **Resid:** Surgery, Duke Univ Med Ctr 85; Orthopaedic Surgery, Duke Univ Med Ctr 89; **Fellow:** Sports Medicine, Cleveland Clinic 90; Orthopedic Oncology, UCLA Med Ctr 91; **Fac Appt:** Prof OrS, Wake Forest Univ

Midwest

Biermann, J Sybil MD [OrS] - **Spec Exp:** Sarcoma; Bone Cancer; Multiple Myeloma; **Hospital:** Univ Michigan Hlth Sys; **Address:** Univ Michigan Cancer Ctr, 1500 E Medical Ctr Drive, 7304 CCGC, Ann Arbor, MI 48109; **Phone:** 734-936-9594; **Board Cert:** Orthopaedic Surgery 04; **Med School:** Stanford Univ 87; **Resid:** Orthopaedic Surgery, Univ Iowa Hosp 92; **Fellow:** Orthopedic Oncology, Univ Chicago Hosps 93; **Fac Appt:** Assoc Prof OrS, Univ Mich Med Sch

Cheng, Edward MD [OrS] - **Spec Exp:** Bone & Soft Tissue Tumors; **Hospital:** Fairview-Univ Med Ctr - Univ Campus; **Address:** Univ Minnesota Med Ctr, Dept Orthopedic Surg, 2450 Riverside Ave S, rm 200, Minneapolis, MN 55455; **Phone:** 612-273-1177; **Board Cert:** Orthopaedic Surgery 03; **Med School:** Northwestern Univ 83; **Resid:** Surgery, Northwestern Univ 85; Orthopaedic Surgery, Beth Israel Hosp 89; **Fellow:** Surgical Oncology, Mass Genl Hosp 90; **Fac Appt:** Prof OrS, Univ Minn

Clohisy, Dennis MD [OrS] - **Spec Exp:** Bone Cancer; **Hospital:** Fairview-Univ Med Ctr - Univ Campus; **Address:** Oncology Clin @ Masonic Cancer Ctr, 424 Harvard St SE, Minneapolis, MN 55455; **Phone:** 612-273-1177; **Board Cert:** Orthopaedic Surgery 04; **Med School:** Northwestern Univ 83; **Resid:** Orthopaedic Surgery, Univ Minn 90; **Fellow:** Pathology, Wash Univ Med Ctr 87; Musculoskeletal Oncology, Mass Genl Hosp/Harvard 91; **Fac Appt:** Prof OrS, Univ Minn

Joyce, Michael J MD [OrS] - **Spec Exp:** Bone & Musculoskeletal Tumors; Fractures-Non-union & Complex; MusculoskeletalTissue Banking; **Hospital:** Cleveland Clin Fdn (page 92); **Address:** Cleveland Clinic, Dept Orthopaedic Surgery, 9500 Euclid Ave, Desk A41, Cleveland, OH 44195; **Phone:** 216-444-4282; **Board Cert:** Orthopaedic Surgery 85; **Med School:** Univ Louisville Sch Med 76; **Resid:** Surgery, Johns Hopkins Hosp 78; Orthopaedic Surgery, Mass General Hosp 81; **Fellow:** Orthopedic Oncology, Mass General Hosp 82; Trauma, Univ Toronto-Sunnybrook Hosp 83; **Fac Appt:** Assoc Clin Prof OrS, Case West Res Univ

Marks, Kenneth E MD [OrS] - **Spec Exp:** Bone & Musculoskeletal Tumors; Bone Transplant; Joint Replacement; **Hospital:** Cleveland Clin Fdn (page 92); **Address:** Cleveland Clinic, Dept Orthopaedic Surgery, 9500 Euclid Ave, Cleveland, OH 44195-0001; **Phone:** 216-444-2637; **Board Cert:** Orthopaedic Surgery 77; **Med School:** Case West Res Univ 70; **Resid:** Orthopaedic Surgery, Cleveland Clinic 74; Orthopaedic Surgery, Univ Virginia Med Ctr 75; **Fellow:** Orthopaedic Surgery, Oxford Univ 76; **Fac Appt:** Prof OrS, Case West Res Univ

McDonald, Douglas J MD [OrS] - **Spec Exp:** Bone Tumors; Ewing's Sarcoma; Reconstructive Surgery; **Hospital:** Barnes-Jewish Hosp (page 85); **Address:** Center for Advanced Medicine, Orthopaedic Surgery Ctr, 4921 Parkview Pl Fl 6 - Ste A, Box 8605, St Louis, MO 63110; **Phone:** 314-747-2500; **Board Cert:** Orthopaedic Surgery 01; **Med School:** Univ Minn 82; **Resid:** Orthopaedic Surgery, Mayo Clinic 87; **Fellow:** Orthopedic Oncology, Mayo Clinic 88; **Fac Appt:** Prof OrS, Washington Univ, St Louis

Peabody, Terrance MD [OrS] - **Spec Exp:** Soft Tissue Tumors; Bone Tumors; **Hospital:** Univ of Chicago Hosps; **Address:** 5841 S Maryland Ave, MC-3079, Chicago, IL 60637-1463; **Phone:** 773-702-3442; **Board Cert:** Orthopaedic Surgery 04; **Med School:** UC Irvine 85; **Resid:** Orthopaedic Surgery, UC Irvine Med Ctr 90; **Fellow:** Orthopedic Oncology, Univ Chicago 91; **Fac Appt:** Assoc Prof S, Univ Chicago-Pritzker Sch Med

Simon, Michael MD [OrS] - **Spec Exp:** Bone Tumors; Soft Tissue Tumors; Pediatric Orthopaedic Cancers; **Hospital:** Univ of Chicago Hosps; **Address:** 5841 S Maryland Ave, MC 3079, Chicago, IL 60637; **Phone:** 773-702-6144; **Board Cert:** Orthopaedic Surgery 92; **Med School:** Univ Mich Med Sch 67; **Resid:** Surgery, Univ Mich Med Ctr 69; Orthopaedic Surgery, Univ Mich Med Ctr 74; **Fellow:** Orthopedic Oncology, Univ Fla 75; **Fac Appt:** Prof S, Univ Chicago-Pritzker Sch Med

Great Plains and Mountains

Neff, James R MD [OrS] - **Spec Exp:** Musculoskeletal Tumors-Adult & Pediatric; Reconstructive Surgery; Limb Lengthening; **Hospital:** Nebraska Med Ctr; **Address:** UNMC, Dept Orth Surg, 981080 Nebraska Med Ctr, Omaha, NE 68198-1080; **Phone:** 402-559-8000; **Board Cert:** Orthopaedic Surgery 93; **Med School:** Univ Kans 66; **Resid:** Surgery, U Mich Hosp 68; Orthopaedic Surgery, U Mich Hosp 73; **Fellow:** Musculoskeletal Oncology, Fla Univ 74; **Fac Appt:** Prof OrS, Univ Nebr Coll Med

Wilkins, Ross M MD [OrS] - **Spec Exp:** Bone Cancer; **Hospital:** Presby - St Luke's Med Ctr; **Address:** 1601 E 19th Ave, Ste 3300, Denver, CO 80218; **Phone:** 303-837-0072; **Board Cert:** Orthopaedic Surgery 97; **Med School:** Wayne State Univ 78; **Resid:** Orthopaedic Surgery, Univ Colorado Med Ctr 83; **Fellow:** Orthopedic Oncology, Mayo Clinic 84; **Fac Appt:** Assoc Clin Prof OrS, Univ Colorado

West Coast and Pacific

Conrad, Ernest U MD [OrS] - **Spec Exp:** Pediatric Orthopaedic Surgery; Bone Tumors-Adult & Pediatric; Sarcoma; **Hospital:** Chldns Hosp and Regl Med Ctr - Seattle; **Address:** Children's Hospital & Regional Medical Ctr, 4800 Sandpoint Way, MS 6D-1, Seattle, WA 98105; **Phone:** 206-987-5096; **Board Cert:** Orthopaedic Surgery 99; **Med School:** Univ VA Sch Med 79; **Resid:** Orthopaedic Surgery, Hosp for Special Surgery 84; **Fellow:** Orthopedic Oncology, U Fla Coll Med 85; Pediatric Orthopaedic Surgery, Hosp for Sick Chldn 86; **Fac Appt:** Prof OrS, Univ Wash

Eckardt, Jeffrey J MD [OrS] - **Spec Exp:** Bone Tumors; Soft Tissue Tumors; Limb Salvage; **Hospital:** UCLA Med Ctr (page 111); **Address:** UCLA Med Ctr, Dept Ortho Surg/Onc, 1250 16th St, Ste 713, Santa Monica, CA 90404; **Phone:** 310-319-3816; **Board Cert:** Orthopaedic Surgery 81; **Med School:** Cornell Univ-Weill Med Coll 71; **Resid:** Orthopaedic Surgery, UCLA Med Ctr 79; **Fellow:** Orthopedic Oncology, Mayo Clinic 80; **Fac Appt:** Prof OrS, UCLA

Luck Jr, James Vernon MD [OrS] - **Spec Exp:** Hemophilla Related Disease; Hip & Knee Replacement; Musculoskeletal Tumors; **Hospital:** Orthopaedic Hosp; **Address:** 2300 S Flower St, Ste 200, Los Angeles, CA 90007-2660; **Phone:** 213-749-8255; **Board Cert:** Orthopaedic Surgery 00; **Med School:** USC Sch Med 67; **Resid:** Orthopaedic Surgery, Orthopaedic Hosp 73; **Fellow:** Orthopedic Oncology, Orthopaedic Hosp 74; Reconstructive Surgery, Rancho Los Amigos 74

Singer, Daniel I MD [OrS] - **Spec Exp:** Hand Surgery; Bone Cancer; **Hospital:** Queen's Med Ctr - Honolulu; **Address:** Queen's Physicians' Office Blg 1, 1380 Lusitana St, Ste 608, Honolulu, HI 96813-2442; **Phone:** 808-521-8109; **Board Cert:** Orthopaedic Surgery 00; Hand Surgery 00; **Med School:** Boston Univ 79; **Resid:** Surgery, Univ Conn Hlth Ctr 81; Orthopaedic Surgery, Univ Hawaii 84; **Fellow:** Hand Surgery, Thomas Jefferson Univ Med Ctr 85; Microvascular Surgery, St Vincent's Hosp 85; **Fac Appt:** Assoc Prof OrS, Univ Hawaii JA Burns Sch Med

HAND SURGERY

Mid Atlantic

Athanasian, Edward MD [HS] - **Spec Exp:** Bone & Soft Tissue Tumors; Hand & Upper Extremity Fractures; **Hospital:** Hosp For Special Surgery; **Address:** Hospital for Special Surgery, 535 E 70th St, New York, NY 10021; **Phone:** 212-606-1962; **Board Cert:** Orthopaedic Surgery 97; Hand Surgery 99; **Med School:** Columbia P&S 88; **Resid:** Surgery, Beth Israel Hosp 89; Orthopaedic Surgery, Hosp Special Surgery 93; **Fellow:** Hand Surgery, Mayo Clinic 94; Orthopedic Oncology, Meml Sloan Kettering Cancer Ctr 95; **Fac Appt:** Asst Prof OrS, Cornell Univ-Weill Med Coll

West Coast and Pacific

Szabo, Robert M MD [HS] - **Spec Exp:** Peripheral Nerve Surgery; Hand Injuries; Hand & Upper Extremity Tumors; **Hospital:** UC Davis Med Ctr; **Address:** UC Davis, Dept Orthopedics, 4860 Y St, Ste 3800, Sacramento, CA 95817-2307; **Phone:** 916-734-3678; **Board Cert:** Orthopaedic Surgery 98; Hand Surgery 98; **Med School:** SUNY Buffalo 77; **Resid:** Surgery, Mt Sinai Hosp 79; Orthopaedic Surgery, Mt Sinai Hosp 82; **Fellow:** Hand Surgery, UCSD Med Ctr 83; Epidemiology, UC Berkeley 95; **Fac Appt:** Prof OrS, UC Davis

OTOLARYNGOLOGY

*A*n otolaryngologist diagnoses and provides medical and/or surgical therapy prevention of diseases, allergies, neoplasms, deformities, disorders and/or injuries of the ears, nose, sinuses, throat, respiratory and upper alimentary systems, face, jaws and the other head and neck systems. Head and neck oncology, facial plastic and reconstructive surgery and the treatment of disorders of hearing and voice are fundamental areas of expertise.

An otolarayngologist-head and neck surgeon provides comprehensive medical and surgical care for patients with diseases and disorders that affect the ears, nose, throat, the respiratory and upper alimentary systems and related structures of the head and neck.

Certification in the following subspecialty requires additional training and examination.

Training required: *Five years*

PLASTIC SURGERY WITHIN THE HEAD AND NECK:

An otolaryngologist with additional training in plastic and reconstructive procedures within the head, face, neck and associated structures, including cutaneous head and neck oncology and reconstructioin, management of maxillofacial trauma, soft tissue repair and neural surgery.

This field is diverse and involves a wide range of patients, from the newborn to the aged. While both cosmetic and reconstructive surgeries are practiced, there are many additional procedures which interface with them.

LARYNGEAL CANCER
THE CLEVELAND CLINIC

9500 Euclid Avenue • Cleveland, OH 44195
www.clevelandclinic.org/otol
For information or appointments, call 216/444-6691
or 800/223-2273, ext. 45691

THE
CLEVELAND
CLINIC

CLEVELAND CLINIC HEAD AND NECK INSTITUTE: TAKING A NOVEL APPROACH TO VOICE BOX CARCINOMA

Cleveland Clinic experts in Ear Nose and Throat Medicine follow a novel surgical approach in the treatment of early voice box carcinoma that combines endoscopic laser resection and freezing. It is yielding remarkably positive outcomes invoice quality and laryngeal function.

The dual technique was introduced about three years ago by Marshall Strome, M.D., chairman of the Cleveland Clinic Head and Neck Institute, based on his theory that destroying an extra margin of tissue might yield better cancer control rates than laser treatment alone. In early follow-up of patients treated with the combined surgery, however, it was found that the procedure also has a clear advantage in terms of postoperative voice quality.

Overall, patients who underwent the laser/freezing surgery achieved phonatory function and vocal performance that was equal to or better than before surgery and that was even "normal" in many patients. "We have never before seen voices like these in patients treated for laryngeal cancer, and the outcomes are particularly extraordinary considering that some of the patients had fairly large tumors," says Dr. Strome.

Claudio F. Milstein, Ph.D., a speech-language pathologist in the Clinic's Voice Center, analyzed voice and laryngeal function data from 22 patients who underwent the surgery for stage T1-T2 laryngeal squamous cell carcinoma, including several in whom radiation therapy failed. All had moderate to severe impairment preoperatively, but after a mean of 19 months after surgery, most showed significant improvement, with 30% having normal voices and phonatory function. "These findings are remarkable," Dr. Milstein says.

In collaboration with the team at The Taussig Cancer Center, including medical and radiation oncologists and scientists, the staff of the Cleveland Clinic Head and Neck Institute have developed strategies of treatment for inoperable cancers, sometimes reducing the cancer enough to allow surgery. When necessary, innovative chemotherapy and chemo-radiation strategies are used for patients with very advanced cancers.

An internationally recognized leader in head and neck medcine, The Cleveland Clinic is ranked as one of the top hospitals in the nation for otolaryngology by *U.S.News & World Report*.

SPECIAL SERVICE FOR OUT-OF-STATE PATIENTS

The Cleveland Clinic offers a complimentary concierge service exclusively for out-of-state patients and their families. Among other things, Cleveland Clinic Medical Concierge staff assist with coordinating multiple appointments; schedule or confirm air and ground transportation; and assist with hotel and housing reservations.

Call 800/ 223-2273, ext. 55580, or send an e-mail to medicalconcierge@ccf.org.

INSTITUTE FOR HEAD & NECK AND THYROID CANCER

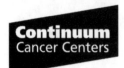

Beth Israel Medical Center
Roosevelt Hospital
St. Luke's Hospital
Long Island College Hospital
New York Eye and Ear Infirmary

Continuum Cancer Centers of New York

Phone (212) 844-8775

THE IDEAL ENVIRONMENT FOR THE CURE OF HEAD AND NECK CANCER

Because of the complexity of their location, cancers of the head and neck present a unique challenge to the patient and the physician. The treatment facility you choose is of paramount importance for the best possible outcome in terms of cure, as well as in maintaining appearance and function, and preserving your quality of life.

Each year, about 38,000 cases of head and neck cancer are diagnosed in America. These cancers affect a number of anatomical sites including the mouth; tongue; tonsils; the larynx or voice box; the nasal cavity and sinuses; the salivary glands; the neck and the thyroid.

WORLD-CLASS PHYSICIANS

The Institute for Head and Neck and Thyroid Cancer—part of Continuum Cancer Centers of New York—encompasses a unique group of clinicians in every discipline relating to these illnesses. Our specialized professionals provide the highest-quality care for patients with benign or malignant tumors in the head and neck region. This multidisciplinary team has unparalleled experience and expertise in managing all head and neck cancers, including the most complex and difficult to treat. They include world-renowned surgeons, radiation oncologists, medical oncologists, radiologists, dental oncologists, pathologists, and skilled nursing care.

Treatment of head and neck tumors can affect quality of life, because the anatomical structures are essential for communication, eating, vision and smell, as well as appearance. Our physicians are leaders in developing and implementing treatments that combine the highest chance for cure with the best possible functional outcome. Preserving the involved organs and their function is often very possible.

TOTAL CARE FOR THE WHOLE PATIENT

Our program is tailored to the full range of patient needs, and to the needs of their families. We provide a full array of patient support services, including speech and swallowing therapists, nutrition counselors, and an onsite cancer library for use by patients and their family members who would like to research their disease in a more detailed manner. In addition, we offer the individualized services of patient navigators who help to ensure that the entire patient and family experience is a positive one.

OPTIMIZING CURE WHILE PRESERVING QUALITY OF LIFE

At the Institute for Head and Neck and Thyroid Cancer, we have developed treatment strategies aimed at a cure, while—at the same time maxmizing preservation of function. Those are important reasons to come to Continuum Cancer Centers of New York. Saving your life is not enough—we also want to preserve your qualty of life.

THE NEW YORK EYE & EAR INFIRMARY

310 East 14th Street • New York, NY 10003
Tel. (212) 979-4000 • Fax. (212) 228-0664
www.nyee.edu
Information and Referral Line: (800) 449-HOPE (4673)

OPHTHALMOLOGY

Ocular Tumor Service: The Infirmary is a major referral center within the Collaborative Ocular Melanoma Study of the National Eye Institute/NIH. New and innovative treatments include radioactive plaques for intraocular tumors and chemotherapy for conjunctival neoplasia. Patients with tumors of the iris, retina, choroid and optic nerve are also treated here.

Oculoplastic, Orbital & Reconstructive Surgery: A leading service in this country and abroad for the treatment of orbital and eyelid cancer, these specialists also commonly see systemic diseases affecting the eye socket, including thyroid disease and lymphoproliferative disorders. A multidisciplinary Ocular Tumor Board meets monthly to discuss the most difficult cases and formulate therapeutic options.

OTOLARYNGOLOGY/ HEAD & NECK SURGERY

Head & Neck Oncology: A team comprised of board-certified surgeons, medical & radiation oncologists, nutritionists and rehabilitation specialists ensure rapid recovery from complex, life saving surgical procedures and return to daily activities.

Thyroid Center: A unique center concentrates on streamlining the diagnosis and treatment of thyroid diseases and cancers with a highly skilled team of surgeons, endocrinologists and radiologists. An area of expertise is cancer resulting from radiation exposure such as Chernobyl.

Facial Plastics and Reconstructive Surgery: Treatment of facial tumors, both benign and cancerous, frequently requires expert reconstruction. Designed to restore the function and appearance of the face, these procedures may be required after appropriate treatment of skin cancers or deep tumors.

Otology–Neuro-otology: These rare cancers can be treated by our highly skilled team of surgeons which includes a neuro-otologist and a neurosurgeon.

Center for the Voice: The Center is cooperatively staffed by a team of specialists able to diagnose cancer of the vocal cords early and rehabilitate the voice after surgical and radiation treatment.

PATHOLOGY & LABORATORY MEDICINE

The laboratory of the Ocular Pathology Service is utilized by ophthalmologists throughout the entire Northeast. The Infirmary is the site of promising studies into diseases and cancers of the eye, ear, nose and throat. Research includes cellular markers of oral cancer risk, non-invasive detection of thyroid cancer, basic cell biology of the growth of ocular melanoma cells, and persistence of biomaterials for repair in plastic and reconstructive surgery.

ABOUT NYEEI

Established in 1820, the Infirmary is the oldest continuously operating specialty hospital in the nation and one of the most experienced in terms of the number of patients it treats and complexity of cases.

Each year the Ophthalmology Department performs more than 16,000 surgeries and sees more than 80,000 visits from outpatients. The Otolaryngology Department performs more than 6,000 surgeries and has some 60,000 outpatient visits. A third clinical department, the Department of Plastic and Reconstructive Surgery, is a natural complement to the Infirmary's other services and annually treats more than 1,000 patients who seek reconstructive surgery as a result of accident, birth defect or cancer, and those who elect cosmetic surgery.

NYEEI is a teaching affiliate of New York Medical College and a member of Continuum Health Partners, Inc.

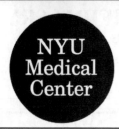

NYU Medical Center

550 First Avenue (at 31st Street)
New York, NY 10016
Physician Referral:
1-888-7-NYU-MED
www.nyumc.org

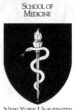

SCHOOL OF MEDICINE

NEW YORK UNIVERSITY

OTOLARYNGOLOGY (EAR, NOSE AND THROAT)

Treating the full spectrum of ear, nose, throat, head and neck disorders, the Department of Otolaryngology at NYU Medical Center provides state-of-the-art patient care and research through the following programs:

COCHLEAR IMPLANTS – the first center in the U.S. to use a multichannel cochlear implant in a profoundly deaf adult, in 1984. Since then we have implanted more than 700 adults and children from the age of 6 months to 85 years.

SINUS AND NASAL DISORDERS – comprehensive diagnosis and minimally invasive treatment of sinus and nasal disorders.

FACIAL PLASTIC SURGERY – plastic and reconstructive surgery for a variety of problems, including nasal obstruction, facial trauma, defects left after removing skin and other facial cancers, facial paralysis and spasm, congenital malformations.

HEAD AND NECK SURGERY – minimally invasive surgery to remove cancers of the head and neck with as little disturbance to everyday function as possible.

SLEEP APNEA – repairing the collapse of soft tissue that leads to snoring and sleep apnea (a dangerous condition in which snorers stop breathing repeatedly during the night, taxing the heart and leaving the snorer unrested).

SKULL BASE SURGERY – minimally invasive treatment of complex skull base tumors.

SWALLOWING DISORDERS – the only center of its kind in New York City, providing comprehensive diagnosis, treatment and therapy for swallowing disorders.

VOICE CENTER – state-of-the-art biofeedback and therapy to rectify problems in speech.

ADVANCED OTOLOGIC MEDICINE & SURGERY – treating patients with disorders of the ear and conditions that affect hearing, balance and facial nerve function.

The cochlear implant program at NYU Medical Center is one of the nation's finest. Since it set the standard in 1984 by implanting a profoundly deaf adult, the Division has been the site of numerous studies and research trials that will continue to improve the technologies available.

Adults and children travel from all over the world to get their cochlear implant at NYU Medical Center. Currently, NYU Medical Center is the only center performing bilateral implants under a special protocol designed to investigate the best method of programming devices, so that patients receive maximum benefits.

PHYSICIAN REFERRAL
1-888-7-NYU-MED
(1-888-769-8633)
www.nyumc.org

OTOLARYNGOLOGY

New England

Catalano, Peter J MD **[Oto]** - **Spec Exp:** Skull Base Tumors & Surgery; Head & Neck Cancer & Surgery; Sinus Surgery-Endoscopic; **Hospital:** Lahey Clin; **Address:** Lahey Clinic - ENT Dept, 5 Central Clinic, 41 Mall Rd, Burlington, MA 01805; **Phone:** 781-744-8451; **Board Cert:** Otolaryngology 90; **Med School:** Mount Sinai Sch Med 85; **Resid:** Surgery, Cedars-Sinai Med Ctr 87; Otolaryngology, Mount Sinai Med Ctr 90; **Fac Appt:** Assoc Prof Oto, Harvard Med Sch

Sasaki, Clarence T MD **[Oto]** - **Spec Exp:** Head & Neck Cancer; Voice/Swallowing Disorders; Sinus Disorders; **Hospital:** Yale - New Haven Hosp; **Address:** Yale Sch Med, Dept Otolaryngology, 333 Cedar St, Box 208041, New Haven, CT 06520-8041; **Phone:** 203-785-2592; **Board Cert:** Otolaryngology 73; **Med School:** Yale Univ 66; **Resid:** Surgery, Dartmouth-Mary Hitchcock Hosp 68; Otolaryngology, Yale-New Haven Hosp 73; **Fellow:** Head and Neck Surgery, Univ of Milan; Skull Base Surgery, Univ Zurich; **Fac Appt:** Prof Oto, Yale Univ

Shapshay, Stanley M MD **[Oto]** - **Spec Exp:** Laryngeal Cancer; Laryngeal Cancer; Vocal Cord Disorders; **Hospital:** Boston Med Ctr; **Address:** 720 Harrison Ave, Ste 601, Boston, MA 02118; **Phone:** 617-638-8124; **Board Cert:** Otolaryngology 75; **Med School:** Med Coll VA 68; **Resid:** Surgery, New England Med Ctr 71; Otolaryngology, Boston Med Ctr 75; **Fellow:** Surgery, Serafimer Hosp/Karolinska Med Sch 72; **Fac Appt:** Prof Oto, Boston Univ

Mid Atlantic

Abramson, Allan MD **[Oto]** - **Spec Exp:** Throat Tumors; Laryngeal Cancer; Head & Neck Surgery; **Hospital:** Long Island Jewish Med Ctr; **Address:** LIJ Med Ctr, Dept Otolaryngology, 270-05 76th Ave, Ste 1120, New Hyde Park, NY 11040; **Phone:** 516-470-7555; **Board Cert:** Otolaryngology 72; **Med School:** SUNY Downstate 67; **Resid:** Surgery, LI Jewish-Hillside Med Ctr 69; Otolaryngology, Mount Sinai Med Ctr 72; **Fac Appt:** Prof Oto, Albert Einstein Coll Med

Arriaga, Moises Alberto MD **[Oto]** - **Spec Exp:** Hearing Loss; Acoustic Nerve Tumors; Balance Disorders; **Hospital:** Allegheny General Hosp; **Address:** 420 E North Ave, Ste 402, Pittsburgh, PA 15212; **Phone:** 412-359-6690; **Board Cert:** Otolaryngology 90; **Med School:** Brown Univ 85; **Resid:** Otolaryngology, Univ Pittsburgh Med Ctr 90; **Fellow:** Neurotology, House Ear Clin 91; **Fac Appt:** Assoc Clin Prof Oto, Univ Pittsburgh

Carrau, Ricardo L. MD **[Oto]** - **Spec Exp:** Skull Base Tumors & Surgery; Nasal & Sinus Cancer; Swallowing Disorders; **Hospital:** UPMC Presby, Pittsburgh (page 114); **Address:** Eye & Ear Institute, 200 Lothrop St, Ste 500, Pittsburg, PA 15213; **Phone:** 412-647-2100; **Board Cert:** Otolaryngology 87; **Med School:** Univ Puerto Rico 81; **Resid:** Surgery, University Hosp 84; Head and Neck Surgery, University Hosp 87; **Fellow:** Head and Neck Oncology, Univ Pittsburgh 90; **Fac Appt:** Assoc Prof Oto, Univ Pittsburgh

Chalian, Ara A MD **[Oto]** - **Spec Exp:** Head & Neck Cancer; Head & Neck Reconstruction; Thyroid Cancer; **Hospital:** Hosp Univ Penn - UPHS (page 115); **Address:** Hospital U Penn, Dept Otolaryngology, 5 Silverstein, 3400 Spruce St, Philadelphia, PA 19104; **Phone:** 215-349-5559; **Board Cert:** Otolaryngology 94; **Med School:** Indiana Univ 88; **Resid:** Surgery, Indiana Univ Hosp 90; Otolaryngology, Indiana Univ Hosp 93; **Fellow:** Molecular Biology, Hosp U Penn 94; Head and Neck Surgery, Hosp U Penn 95; **Fac Appt:** Assoc Prof Oto, Univ Pennsylvania

Cho, Hyun MD [Oto] - **Spec Exp:** Head & Neck Cancer; Laryngeal Disorders; **Hospital:** St Vincent Cath Med Ctrs - Manhattan (page 108); **Address:** St Vincent Catholic Medical Ctr, Spellman 5, 170 W 12th St, New York, NY 10011; **Phone:** 212-888-3784; **Board Cert:** Otolaryngology 82; **Med School:** South Korea 64; **Resid:** Surgery, Beth Israel Med Ctr 72; Otolaryngology, Columbia Presby Med Ctr 82; **Fellow:** Head and Neck Surgery, Beth Israel Med Ctr 74; **Fac Appt:** Assoc Prof Oto, Albert Einstein Coll Med

Close, Lanny G MD [Oto] - **Spec Exp:** Skull Base Surgery; Head & Neck Cancer; Sinus Disorders/Surgery; **Hospital:** NY-Presby Hosp - Columbia Presby Med Ctr (page 103); **Address:** 16 E 60th St, Ste 470, New York, NY 10022; **Phone:** 212-326-8475; **Board Cert:** Otolaryngology 77; **Med School:** Baylor Coll Med 72; **Resid:** Surgery, Johns Hopkins Hosp 74; Otolaryngology, Baylor Affil Hosps 77; **Fellow:** Head and Neck Surgery, MD Anderson Cancer Ctr 79; **Fac Appt:** Prof Oto, Columbia P&S

Cohen, Noel L MD [Oto] - **Spec Exp:** Cochlear Implants; Acoustic Nerve Tumors; Hearing Loss; **Hospital:** NYU Med Ctr (page 104); **Address:** Dept Otolaryngology, 530 1st Ave, Ste 3C, New York, NY 10016; **Phone:** 212-263-7373; **Board Cert:** Otolaryngology 63; **Med School:** Netherlands 57; **Resid:** Otolaryngology, NYU Med Ctr 62; **Fac Appt:** Prof Oto, NYU Sch Med

Costantino, Peter D MD [Oto] - **Spec Exp:** Skull Base Tumors & Craniofacial Surgery; Head & Neck Cancer; Reconstructive Surgery-Face & Skull; **Hospital:** St Luke's - Roosevelt Hosp Ctr - Roosevelt Div (page 93); **Address:** 425 W 59th St Fl 10, New York, NY 10019-1104; **Phone:** 212-262-4444; **Board Cert:** Otolaryngology 90; Facial Plastic & Reconstructive Surgery 00; **Med School:** Northwestern Univ 84; **Resid:** Surgery, Northwestern Meml Hosp 86; Otolaryngology, Northwestern Meml Hosp 89; **Fellow:** Head and Neck Surgery, Northwestern Meml Hosp 90; Skull Base Surgery, Univ Pittsburgh 91; **Fac Appt:** Prof Oto, Columbia P&S

Cummings, Charles MD [Oto] - **Spec Exp:** Head & Neck Surgery; Laryngeal Disorders; **Hospital:** Johns Hopkins Hosp - Baltimore (page 97); **Address:** Johns Hopkins Outpt Ctr, Dept Otolaryngology, 601 N Caroline St Fl 6, Baltimore, MD 21287; **Phone:** 410-955-7400; **Board Cert:** Otolaryngology 68; **Med School:** Univ VA Sch Med 61; **Resid:** Surgery, Univ Va Hosp 65; Otolaryngology, Mass Genl Hosp 68; **Fac Appt:** Prof Oto, Johns Hopkins Univ

Davidson, Bruce J MD [Oto] - **Spec Exp:** Head & Neck Cancer; Thyroid Disorders; **Hospital:** Georgetown Univ Hosp; **Address:** Georgetown Univ Med Ctr, Dept Oto, 3800 Reservoir Rd NW, 1 Gorman, Washington, DC 20007; **Phone:** 202-444-8186; **Board Cert:** Otolaryngology 93; **Med School:** W VA Univ 87; **Resid:** Otolaryngology, Georgetown Univ Med Ctr 92; **Fellow:** Otolaryngology, Memorial Sloan-Kettering Cancer Ctr 94; **Fac Appt:** Asst Prof Oto, Georgetown Univ

Grandis, Jennifer MD [Oto] - **Spec Exp:** Head & Neck Cancer; **Hospital:** UPMC Presby, Pittsburgh (page 114); **Address:** Univ Pittsburgh Med Ctr EELB, 200 Lothrop St, Ste 500, Pittsburgh, PA 15213; **Phone:** 412-647-5280; **Board Cert:** Otolaryngology 94; **Med School:** Univ Pittsburgh 87; **Resid:** Otolaryngology, Univ Pittsburgh Med Ctr 93; **Fellow:** Univ Pittsburgh Med Ctr 92; **Fac Appt:** Prof Oto, Univ Pittsburgh

Har-El, Gady MD [Oto] - **Spec Exp:** Head & Neck Cancer; Sinus & Skull Base Surgery; Thyroid & Parathyroid Cancer & Surgery; **Hospital:** Long Island Coll Hosp (page 93); **Address:** 110 E 59th St, New York, NY 10022; **Phone:** 212-223-1333; **Board Cert:** Otolaryngology 92; **Med School:** Israel 82; **Resid:** Otolaryngology, SUNY Downstate Med Ctr 91; **Fac Appt:** Prof Oto, SUNY Hlth Sci Ctr

Hicks Jr, Wesley L MD/DDS **[Oto]** - **Spec Exp:** Head & Neck Cancer; Reconstructive Surgery; **Hospital:** Roswell Park Cancer Inst (page 107); **Address:** Roswell Park Cancer Inst, Dept Head & Neck Surg, Elm & Carlton Sts, Buffalo, NY 14263; **Phone:** 716-845-3158; **Board Cert:** Otolaryngology 93; **Med School:** SUNY Buffalo 84; **Resid:** Otolaryngology, Manhattan Eye Ear & Throat Hosp; Otolaryngology, New York Hosp/Meml Sloan Kettering Cancer Ctr; **Fellow:** Head and Neck Surgery, Stanford Univ Med Ctr; **Fac Appt:** Assoc Prof Oto, SUNY Buffalo

Hirsch, Barry MD **[Oto]** - **Spec Exp:** Hearing Loss; Ear Infections/Tumors; Skull Base Tumors; **Hospital:** UPMC Presby, Pittsburgh (page 114); **Address:** 200 Lothrop St, Ste 500, Ear Nose & Throat Inst, Dept Otolaryngology, Pittsburgh, PA 15213; **Phone:** 412-647-2100; **Board Cert:** Otolaryngology 82; **Med School:** Univ Pennsylvania 77; **Resid:** Otolaryngology, Univ Pittsburgh Med Ctr 82; **Fellow:** Neurotology, Univ Pittsburgh 85; Neurotology, Univ Zurich; **Fac Appt:** Prof Oto, Univ Pittsburgh

Holliday, Michael J MD **[Oto]** - **Spec Exp:** Head & Neck Cancer; Skull Base Surgery; Neuro-Otology; **Hospital:** Johns Hopkins Hosp - Baltimore (page 97); **Address:** Johns Hopkins Outpatient Ctr, 601 N Caroline St Fl 6, Baltimore, MD 21287; **Phone:** 410-955-3492; **Board Cert:** Otolaryngology 76; **Med School:** Marquette Sch Med 69; **Resid:** Otolaryngology, Johns Hopkins Hosp 76; **Fellow:** Neurotology, Univ Zurich; **Fac Appt:** Assoc Prof Oto, Johns Hopkins Univ

Johnson, Jonas T MD **[Oto]** - **Spec Exp:** Head & Neck Surgery; Head & Neck Cancer; Snoring/Sleep Apnea; **Hospital:** UPMC Presby, Pittsburgh (page 114); **Address:** Univ Physicians UPMC, ENT, Eye & Ear Inst, 200 Lothrop St, Ste 300, Pittsburgh, PA 15213; **Phone:** 412-647-2100; **Board Cert:** Otolaryngology 77; **Med School:** SUNY Upstate Med Univ 72; **Resid:** Surgery, Med Coll Virginia Hosps 74; Otolaryngology, SUNY-Univ Hosp 77; **Fac Appt:** Prof Oto, Univ Pittsburgh

Keane, William M MD **[Oto]** - **Spec Exp:** Head & Neck Cancer & Surgery; Thyroid Cancer; Sinus Disorders/Surgery; **Hospital:** Thomas Jefferson Univ Hosp (page 110); **Address:** 925 Chestnut St Fl 6, Philadelphia, PA 19107; **Phone:** 215-955-6760; **Board Cert:** Otolaryngology 78; **Med School:** Harvard Med Sch 70; **Resid:** Surgery, Strong Meml Hosp 72; Otolaryngology, Univ Penn Hosp 77; **Fac Appt:** Prof Oto, Thomas Jefferson Univ

Kennedy, David W MD **[Oto]** - **Spec Exp:** Sinus Disorders/Surgery; Skull Base Minimally Invasive Surgery; Head & Neck Cancer; **Hospital:** Hosp Univ Penn - UPHS (page 115); **Address:** Hosp Univ Penn, Dept Oto/Head & Neck Surg, 3400 Spruce St, Ravdin Bldg, Fl 5, Philadelphia, PA 19104; **Phone:** 215-662-2777; **Board Cert:** Otolaryngology 78; **Med School:** Ireland 72; **Resid:** Surgery, Johns Hopkins Hosp 74; Otolaryngology, Johns Hopkins Hosp 78; **Fac Appt:** Prof Oto, Univ Pennsylvania

Koch, Wayne Martin MD **[Oto]** - **Spec Exp:** Head & Neck Cancer; Sinus Cancer; **Hospital:** Johns Hopkins Hosp - Baltimore (page 97); **Address:** Johns Hopkins Hosp, Dept Otolaryngology, 601 N Caroline St Fl 6, Baltimore, MD 21287; **Phone:** 410-955-4906; **Board Cert:** Otolaryngology 87; **Med School:** Univ Pittsburgh 82; **Resid:** Otolaryngology, Tufts-Boston Univ Hosps 87; **Fellow:** Surgical Oncology, Johns Hopkins Hosp 89; **Fac Appt:** Assoc Prof Oto, Johns Hopkins Univ

Kraus, Dennis MD **[Oto]** - **Spec Exp:** Head & Neck Cancer; Skull Base Tumors & Surgery; Sinus Cancer; **Hospital:** Meml Sloan Kettering Cancer Ctr (page 100); **Address:** 1275 York Ave, Box 285, Memorial Sloan Kettering Cancer Ctr, New York, NY 10021-6007; **Phone:** 212-639-5621; **Board Cert:** Otolaryngology 90; **Med School:** Univ Rochester 85; **Resid:** Surgery, Cleveland Clinic Hosp 87; Otolaryngology, Cleveland Clinic Hosp 90; **Fellow:** Head and Neck Surgery, Meml Sloan Kettering Cancer Ctr 91; **Fac Appt:** Assoc Prof Oto, Cornell Univ-Weill Med Coll

Krespi, Yosef MD [Oto] - **Spec Exp:** Nasal & Sinus Surgery; Sleep Disorders/Apnea/Snoring; Head & Neck Cancer & Surgery; **Hospital:** St Luke's - Roosevelt Hosp Ctr - Roosevelt Div (page 93); **Address:** 425 W 59th St Fl 10, New York, NY 10019-1128; **Phone:** 212-262-4444; **Board Cert:** Otolaryngology 81; **Med School:** Israel 73; **Resid:** Surgery, Mount Sinai Hosp 76; Otolaryngology, Mount Sinai Hosp 80; **Fellow:** Surgery, Northwestern Meml Hosp 81; **Fac Appt:** Clin Prof Oto, Columbia P&S

Lawson, William MD [Oto] - **Spec Exp:** Sinus Disorders/Surgery; Cosmetic Surgery-Face; Head & Neck Cancer; **Hospital:** Mount Sinai Med Ctr (page 101); **Address:** 5 E 98th St, Fl 8, New York, NY 10029-6501; **Phone:** 212-241-9410; **Board Cert:** Otolaryngology 74; **Med School:** NYU Sch Med 65; **Resid:** Surgery, Bronx VA Hosp 67; Otolaryngology, Mount Sinai Hosp 73; **Fellow:** Otolaryngology, Mount Sinai Hosp 70; **Fac Appt:** Prof Oto, Mount Sinai Sch Med

Linstrom, Christopher MD [Oto] - **Spec Exp:** Cochlear Implants; Acoustic Nerve Tumors; Encephalocele & Cholesteatoma; **Hospital:** New York Eye & Ear Infirm (page 102); **Address:** NY Eye & Ear Infirmary, Dept Otolaryngology, 310 E 14th St Fl 6, New York, NY 10003-4201; **Phone:** 212-979-4200; **Board Cert:** Otolaryngology 87; **Med School:** Canada 82; **Resid:** Surgery, Geo Wash Med Ctr 84; Otolaryngology, New York Hosp 87; **Fellow:** Otology & Neurotology, Michigan Ear Inst 89; **Fac Appt:** Assoc Prof Oto, NY Med Coll

Myers, Eugene MD [Oto] - **Spec Exp:** Head & Neck Surgery; Head & Neck Cancer; Paragangliomas; **Hospital:** UPMC Presby, Pittsburgh (page 114); **Address:** UPMC Hlth Sys, Dept Otolaryngology, 200 Lothrop St Bldg EE1 Fl 3 - Ste 300, Pittsburgh, PA 15213-2546; **Phone:** 412-647-2100; **Board Cert:** Otolaryngology 66; **Med School:** Temple Univ 60; **Resid:** Surgery, VA Hosp 62; Otolaryngology, Mass EE Infirm 65; **Fellow:** Otolaryngology, Harvard Med School 65; Head and Neck Surgery, St Vincent's Hosp 68; **Fac Appt:** Prof Oto, Univ Pittsburgh

O'Malley Jr, Bert W MD [Oto] - **Spec Exp:** Head & Neck Cancer; Sinus Tumors; Skull Base Tumors; **Hospital:** Hosp Univ Penn - UPHS (page 115); **Address:** Hosp Univ Penn, Dept Oto-HNS, 3400 Spruce St, 5 Ravdin, Philadelphia, PA 19104; **Phone:** 215-615-4325; **Board Cert:** Otolaryngology 95; **Med School:** Univ Tex SW, Dallas ; **Resid:** Surgery, UTSW Med Ctr/Parkland Meml Hosp; Otolaryngology, Baylor Coll Med; **Fellow:** Head and Neck Oncology, Univ Pittsburgh; Skull Base Surgery, Univ Pittsburgh; **Fac Appt:** Prof Oto, Univ Pennsylvania

Papel, Ira David MD [Oto] - **Spec Exp:** Rhinoplasty - Cosmetic & Functional; Cosmetic Surgery-Face; Facial Reconstruction & Skin Cancer; **Hospital:** Johns Hopkins Hosp - Baltimore (page 97); **Address:** 1838 Greene Tree Rd, Baltimore, MD 21208; **Phone:** 410-486-3400; **Board Cert:** Otolaryngology 86; Facial Plastic & Reconstructive Surgery 91; **Med School:** Boston Univ 81; **Resid:** Otolaryngology, Johns Hopkins Hosp 86; **Fellow:** Facial Plastic Surgery, UCSF Med Ctr 87; **Fac Appt:** Assoc Prof Oto, Johns Hopkins Univ

Persky, Mark S MD [Oto] - **Spec Exp:** Head & Neck Cancer; Skull Base Tumors; Thyroid Cancer & Surgery; **Hospital:** Beth Israel Med Ctr - Petrie Division (page 93); **Address:** 10 Union Square East, Ste 4J, New York, NY 10003-3314; **Phone:** 212-844-8648; **Board Cert:** Otolaryngology 76; **Med School:** SUNY Upstate Med Univ 72; **Resid:** Otolaryngology, Bellevue Hosp 76; **Fellow:** Head and Neck Surgery, Beth Israel Med Ctr 77; **Fac Appt:** Clin Prof Oto, Albert Einstein Coll Med

Rassekh, Christopher MD [Oto] - **Spec Exp:** Laryngeal Cancer-Organ Preservation; Skull Base Tumors; Salivary Gland Tumors & Surgery; **Hospital:** WV Univ Hosp - Ruby Memorial; **Address:** West Virginia Univ Dept Otolaryngology, PO Box 9200, Morgantown, WV 26506; **Phone:** 304-293-3233; **Board Cert:** Otolaryngology 93; **Med School:** Univ Iowa Coll Med 86; **Resid:** Otolaryngology, U Iowa Med Ctr 92; **Fellow:** Head and Neck Surgery, U Pittsburgh Med Ctr 93; **Fac Appt:** Assoc Prof Oto, W VA Univ

Schantz, Stimson P MD [Oto] - **Spec Exp:** Head & Neck Surgery; Cancer Surgery; **Hospital:** New York Eye & Ear Infirm (page 102); **Address:** 310 E 14th St Fl 6N, New York, NY 10003; **Phone:** 212-979-4535; **Board Cert:** Surgery 94; **Med School:** Univ Cincinnati 75; **Resid:** Surgery, Georgetown Univ Med Ctr 82; Otolaryngology, Univ Illinois Eye & Ear Infirm 80; **Fellow:** Surgical Oncology, MD Anderson Cancer Ctr 84; **Fac Appt:** Prof Oto, NY Med Coll

Shindo, Maisie L MD [Oto] - **Spec Exp:** Head & Neck Cancer & Surgery; Thyroid Cancer; Laryngeal Cancer; **Hospital:** Stony Brook Univ Hosp; **Address:** Stony Brook University Hospital, HSC (T19-090), Stony Brook, NY 11794-8191; **Phone:** 631-444-8242; **Board Cert:** Otolaryngology 89; **Med School:** Univ Saskatchewan 84; **Resid:** Otolaryngology, Los Angeles Co USC Med Ctr 89; **Fellow:** Head and Neck Surgery, Northwestern Univ 91; **Fac Appt:** Assoc Prof Oto, SUNY Stony Brook

Snyderman, Carl H MD [Oto] - **Spec Exp:** Skull Base Tumors & Surgery; Sinus Tumors; Head & Neck Cancer; **Hospital:** UPMC Presby, Pittsburgh (page 114); **Address:** Eye & Ear Institute - Dept of Otolaryngology, 200 Lothrop St, Ste 500, Pittsburgh, PA 15213; **Phone:** 412-647-2100; **Board Cert:** Otolaryngology 87; **Med School:** Univ Chicago-Pritzker Sch Med 82; **Resid:** Otolaryngology, Eye-Ear Hosp/Univ Pittsburgh 87; **Fellow:** Skull Base Surgery, Eye-Ear Hosp/Univ Pittsburgh 88; **Fac Appt:** Assoc Prof Oto, Univ Pittsburgh

Urken, Mark MD [Oto] - **Spec Exp:** Microvascular Reconstruction; Head & Neck Cancer; Thyroid & Parathyroid Surgery; **Hospital:** Beth Israel Med Ctr - Petrie Division (page 93); **Address:** 10 Union Square E, Ste 5B, New York, NY 10003; **Phone:** 212-844-8775; **Board Cert:** Otolaryngology 86; **Med School:** Univ VA Sch Med 81; **Resid:** Otolaryngology, Mount Sinai Hosp 86; **Fellow:** Microvascular Surgery, Mercy Hosp 87; **Fac Appt:** Prof Oto, Mount Sinai Sch Med

Wazen, Jack J MD [Oto] - **Spec Exp:** Skull Base Surgery; Meniere's Disease; Acoustic Nerve Tumors; **Hospital:** NY-Presby Hosp - Columbia Presby Med Ctr (page 103); **Address:** 364 E 69th St, New York, NY 10021-1802; **Phone:** 212-249-3232; **Board Cert:** Otolaryngology 83; **Med School:** Lebanon 78; **Resid:** Surgery, St Lukes Hosp 80; Otolaryngology, Columbia Presby Hosp 83; **Fellow:** Neurotology, Ear Rsch Fdn 84; **Fac Appt:** Assoc Clin Prof Oto, Columbia P&S

Weinstein, Gregory MD [Oto] - **Spec Exp:** Head & Neck Cancer; Laryngeal Cancer-Organ Preservation; **Hospital:** Hosp Univ Penn - UPHS (page 115); **Address:** Hosp Univ Penn, Dept Otolaryngology, 3400 Spruce St, Ravdin 5, Philadelphia, PA 19104; **Phone:** 215-349-5390; **Board Cert:** Otolaryngology 90; **Med School:** NY Med Coll 85; **Resid:** Otolaryngology, Univ Iowa Hosp 90; **Fellow:** Head and Neck Oncology, UC Davis Med Ctr 91; **Fac Appt:** Assoc Prof Oto, Univ Pennsylvania

Woo, Peak MD [Oto] - **Spec Exp:** Voice Disorders; Laryngeal Disorders; Laryngeal Cancer; **Hospital:** Mount Sinai Med Ctr (page 101); **Address:** 5 E 98th St Fl 1, Box 1653, New York, NY 10029-6501; **Phone:** 212-241-9425; **Board Cert:** Otolaryngology 83; **Med School:** Boston Univ 78; **Resid:** Otolaryngology, Boston Univ 83; **Fac Appt:** Prof Oto, Mount Sinai Sch Med

Southeast

Bumpous, Jeffrey MD [Oto] - **Spec Exp:** Head & Neck Cancer; Head & Neck Reconstruction; Thyroid & Parathyroid Cancer & Surgery; **Hospital:** Univ of Louisville Hosp; **Address:** 601 S Floyd St, Ste 604, Louisville, KY 40202-1845; **Phone:** 502-583-8303; **Board Cert:** Otolaryngology 94; **Med School:** Univ Louisville Sch Med 89; **Resid:** Otolaryngology, Univ Louisville Hosp 93; **Fellow:** Head and Neck Surgery, Univ Pittsburgh 94; **Fac Appt:** Asst Prof Oto, Univ Louisville Sch Med

Burkey, Brian MD **[Oto]** - **Spec Exp:** Parotid Gland Tumors; Head & Neck Cancer; Microvascular Reconstruction; **Hospital:** Vanderbilt Univ Med Ctr (page 116); **Address:** Vanderbilt Univ, Dept Otolaryngology, S-2100 MCN, Nashville, TN 37232-2559; **Phone:** 615-322-7267; **Board Cert:** Otolaryngology 92; **Med School:** Univ VA Sch Med 86; **Resid:** Otolaryngology, Univ Mich Med Ctr 91; **Fellow:** Microsurgery, Ohio State Univ; **Fac Appt:** Assoc Prof Oto, Vanderbilt Univ

Cassisi, Nicholas J MD **[Oto]** - **Spec Exp:** Head & Neck Cancer; Voice Disorders; **Hospital:** Shands Hlthcre at Univ of FL (page 109); **Address:** Shands Healthcare at Univ FL, 1600 SW Archer Rd, Box 100264, Gainesville, FL 32610; **Phone:** 352-265-8989; **Board Cert:** Otolaryngology 71; **Med School:** Univ Miami Sch Med 65; **Resid:** Surgery, Jackson Memorial Hosp 67; Otolaryngology, Barnes Hosp - Washington U 71; **Fac Appt:** Prof Oto, Univ Fla Coll Med

Couch, Marion E MD **[Oto]** - **Spec Exp:** Head & Neck Cancer; Thyroid Cancer; **Hospital:** Univ NC Hosps (page 112); **Address:** Univ North Carolina Sch Med - Dept Otolaryngology, CB 7070, Chapel Hill, NC 27599-7070; **Phone:** 919-966-3342; **Board Cert:** Otolaryngology 97; **Med School:** Rush Med Coll 90; **Resid:** Surgery, Johns Hopkins Hosp 91; Otolaryngology, Johns Hopkins Hosp 95; **Fac Appt:** Asst Prof Oto, Univ NC Sch Med

Goodwin, W Jarrard MD **[Oto]** - **Spec Exp:** Head & Neck Cancer; **Hospital:** Univ of Miami Hosp & Clins/Sylvester Comp Canc Ctr; **Address:** Dept Otolaryngology, 1475 NW 12th Ave, Ste 4037, Miami, FL 33136-1015; **Phone:** 305-243-4387; **Board Cert:** Otolaryngology 78; **Med School:** Albany Med Coll 72; **Resid:** Surgery, Univ Miami/Jackson Hosp Meml Hosp 73; Otolaryngology, Univ Miami/Jackson Hosp 77; **Fellow:** Head & Neck Surgical Oncology, MD Anderson Hosp 80; **Fac Appt:** Prof Oto, Univ Miami Sch Med

Lanza, Donald MD **[Oto]** - **Spec Exp:** Skull Base Tumors; Sinus Disorders/Surgery; Rhinitis; **Hospital:** St Anthony's Hosp - St Petersburg; **Address:** 900 Carillon Pkwy, Ste 200, St. Petersburg, FL 33716; **Phone:** 727-573-0074; **Board Cert:** Otolaryngology 90; **Med School:** SUNY Hlth Sci Ctr 85; **Resid:** Surgery, Albany Med Ctr 87; Otolaryngology, Albany Med Ctr 90; **Fellow:** Johns Hopkins Univ 91; Univ Penn

Levine, Paul A MD **[Oto]** - **Spec Exp:** Head & Neck Cancer; Head & Neck Reconstruction; Skull Base Tumors; **Hospital:** Univ Virginia Med Ctr; **Address:** UVA Hlth Systems, Dept Otolaryngology, PO Box 800713, Charlottesville, VA 22908; **Phone:** 434-924-5593; **Board Cert:** Otolaryngology 78; **Med School:** Albany Med Coll 73; **Resid:** Otolaryngology, Yale-New Haven Hosp 77; **Fellow:** Head and Neck Surgery, Stanford Med Ctr 78; **Fac Appt:** Prof Oto, Univ VA Sch Med

Mattox, Douglas MD **[Oto]** - **Spec Exp:** Neuro-Otology; Ear Tumors; **Hospital:** Emory Univ Hosp; **Address:** Emory University Hospital, Dept Otolaryngology, 1365-A Clifton Rd NE, Atlanta, GA 30322; **Phone:** 404-778-3381; **Board Cert:** Otolaryngology 77; **Med School:** Yale Univ 73; **Resid:** Otolaryngology, Stanford Univ Hosp 77; **Fac Appt:** Prof Oto, Emory Univ

McCaffrey, Thomas MD **[Oto]** - **Spec Exp:** Head & Neck Cancer; Thyroid Cancer; Tracheal & Subglottic Stenosis; **Hospital:** H Lee Moffitt Cancer Ctr & Research Inst; **Address:** H Lee Moffitt Cancer Ctr-Dept Otolaryngology-HNS, 12902 Magnolia Drive, Tampa, FL 33612; **Phone:** 813-972-8463; **Board Cert:** Otolaryngology 80; **Med School:** Loyola Univ-Stritch Sch Med 74; **Resid:** Surgery, Mayo Grad Sch Med 76; Otolaryngology, Mayo Grad Med 80; **Fac Appt:** Prof Oto, Univ S Fla Coll Med

McGuirt, W Fredrick MD **[Oto]** - **Spec Exp:** Head & Neck Cancer; Laryngeal Disorders; Salivary Gland Tumors & Surgery; **Hospital:** Wake Forest Univ Baptist Med Ctr (page 117); **Address:** Wake Forest Baptist Med Ctr-Dept Otolaryngology, Medical Center Blvd, Winston Salem, NC 27157; **Phone:** 336-716-4161; **Board Cert:** Otolaryngology 76; **Med School:** Wake Forest Univ 68; **Resid:** Otolaryngology, NC Bapt Hosp 70; Surgery, Iowa Hosp 76; **Fac Appt:** Prof Oto, Wake Forest Univ

Netterville, James MD [Oto] - **Spec Exp:** Head & Neck Surgery; Head & Neck Cancer; Vocal Cord Surgery; **Hospital:** Vanderbilt Univ Med Ctr (page 116); **Address:** Vanderbilt Univ Med Ctr, Dept Otolaryngology, 1301 22nd Ave S, Ste 2900 TVC, Nashville, TN 37232-5555; **Phone:** 615-343-8840; **Board Cert:** Otolaryngology 85; **Med School:** Univ Tenn Coll Med, Memphis 80; **Resid:** Surgery, Methodist Hosp 82; Otolaryngology, Univ Tenn 85; **Fellow:** Surgical Oncology, Univ Iowa 86; **Fac Appt:** Assoc Prof Oto, Vanderbilt Univ

Peters, Glenn E MD [Oto] - **Spec Exp:** Head & Neck Cancer; Skull Base Surgery; Thyroid & Parathyroid Cancer & Surgery; **Hospital:** Univ of Ala Hosp at Birmingham; **Address:** UAB Med Ctr, Div of Head & Neck Surgery, 1530 3rd Ave S, BDB 563 Ave S, Birmingham, AL 35294-0012; **Phone:** 205-934-9766; **Board Cert:** Otolaryngology 85; **Med School:** Louisiana State Univ 80; **Resid:** Surgery, Bapt Med Ctr 82; Otolaryngology, Univ Alabama Hosp 84; **Fellow:** Head & Neck Surgical Oncology, Johns Hopkins Hosp 87; **Fac Appt:** Prof S, Univ Ala

Pitman, Karen MD [Oto] - **Spec Exp:** Head & Neck Cancer & Surgery; Swallowing Disorders; Thyroid & Parathyroid Cancer & Surgery; **Hospital:** Univ Hosps & Clins - Jackson; **Address:** Univ Mississippi Med Ctr, 2500 N State St, Jackson, MS 39216; **Phone:** 601-984-5160; **Board Cert:** Otolaryngology 95; **Med School:** Uniformed Srvs Univ, Bethesda 87; **Resid:** Otolaryngology, Naval Med Ctr 94; **Fellow:** Head and Neck Oncology, Univ Pittsburgh 96; **Fac Appt:** Assoc Prof Oto, Univ Miss

Stringer, Scott Pearson MD [Oto] - **Spec Exp:** Head & Neck Cancer; Nasal & Sinus Disorders; Thyroid & Parathyroid Cancer & Surgery; **Hospital:** Univ Hosps & Clins - Jackson; **Address:** Univ Mississippi Med Ctr, Dept Otolaryngology, 2500 N State St, Jackson, MS 39216-4505; **Phone:** 601-984-5160; **Board Cert:** Otolaryngology 87; **Med School:** Univ Tex SW, Dallas 82; **Resid:** Surgery, Univ Tex SW Med Ctr 84; Otolaryngology, Univ Tex SW Med Ctr 87; **Fac Appt:** Prof Oto, Univ Miss

Valentino, Joseph MD [Oto] - **Spec Exp:** Head & Neck Cancer; **Hospital:** Univ Kentucky Med Ctr; **Address:** 740 S Limestone St, rm B-317, Lexington, KY 40536-0284; **Phone:** 859-257-5405; **Board Cert:** Otolaryngology 93; **Med School:** UMDNJ-RW Johnson Med Sch 87; **Resid:** Otolaryngology, Univ Minn 92; **Fellow:** Otolaryngology, Univ Iowa Coll Med 93; **Fac Appt:** Assoc Prof Oto, Univ KY Coll Med

Weissler, Mark Christian MD [Oto] - **Spec Exp:** Head & Neck Cancer; Laryngotracheal Stenosis; Voice Disorders; **Hospital:** Univ NC Hosps (page 112); **Address:** G0412 Neurosciences Hosp UNC CB#7070, Chapel Hill, NC 27599-7070; **Phone:** 919-843-3796; **Board Cert:** Otolaryngology 85; **Med School:** Boston Univ 80; **Resid:** Surgery, Mass Genl Hosp 82; Otolaryngology, Mass Eye & Ear Infirm 85; **Fellow:** Head and Neck Oncology, Univ Cincinnati 86; **Fac Appt:** Prof Oto, Univ NC Sch Med

Yarbrough, Wendell G MD [Oto] - **Spec Exp:** Head & Neck Cancer; **Hospital:** Vanderbilt Univ Med Ctr (page 116); **Address:** Vaderbilt School of Medicine - Dept Oto, MC 52100, 1301 22nd Ave S, Ste 2900, Nashville, TN 37232; **Phone:** 615-348-8840; **Board Cert:** Otolaryngology 95; **Med School:** Univ NC Sch Med 89; **Resid:** Otolaryngology, UNC Sch Med Hosps 94; **Fellow:** Surgical Oncology, UNC Sch Med Hosps 96; **Fac Appt:** Assoc Prof Oto, Vanderbilt Univ

Midwest

Arts, H Alexander MD [Oto] - **Spec Exp:** Skull Base Tumors & Surgery; Head & Neck Cancer & Surgery; Otology & Neuro-Otology; **Hospital:** Univ Michigan Hlth Sys; **Address:** Univ Michigan Health Systems, Dept Otolaryngology, 1904 Taubman Ctr, 1500 E Medical Center Drive, Ann Arbor, MI 48109; **Phone:** 734-936-8006; **Board Cert:** Otolaryngology 92; **Med School:** Baylor Coll Med 83; **Resid:** Surgery, Univ Washington Med Ctr 85; Otolaryngology, Univ Washington Med Ctr 90; **Fellow:** Neurotology, Univ Virginia 91; **Fac Appt:** Assoc Prof Oto, Univ Mich Med Sch

Bojrab, Dennis I MD [Oto] - **Spec Exp:** Otology & Neuro-Otology; Facial Nerve Disorders; Skull Base Tumors; **Hospital:** Providence Hosp - Southfield; **Address:** Michigan Ear Institute, 30055 Northwestern Hwy, Ste 101, Farmington Hills, MI 48334; **Phone:** 248-865-4444; **Board Cert:** Otolaryngology 85; **Med School:** Indiana Univ 79; **Resid:** Surgery, Butterworth Hosp 81; Otolaryngology, Univ Indiana Sch Med 84; **Fellow:** Skull Base Surgery, Vanderbilt Univ Med Ctr 85; **Fac Appt:** Prof Oto, Wayne State Univ

Bradford, Carol MD [Oto] - **Spec Exp:** Head & Neck Cancer; Melanoma-Head & Neck; Skin Cancer - Head & Neck; **Hospital:** Univ Michigan Hlth Sys; **Address:** A A Taubman Health Care Ctr, 1500 E Medical Center Drive, rm 1904-TC, Ann Arbor, MI 48109-0312; **Phone:** 734-936-8050; **Board Cert:** Otolaryngology 93; **Med School:** Univ Mich Med Sch 86; **Resid:** Otolaryngology, Univ Michigan Med Ctr 92; **Fac Appt:** Prof Oto, Univ Mich Med Sch

Campbell, Bruce H MD [Oto] - **Spec Exp:** Head & Neck Surgery; Head & Neck Cancer; **Hospital:** Froedtert Meml Lutheran Hosp; **Address:** Med Coll Wisc-Dept Oto, 9200 W Wisconsin Ave, Milwaukee, WI 53226; **Phone:** 414-805-5583; **Board Cert:** Otolaryngology 86; **Med School:** Rush Med Coll 80; **Resid:** Otolaryngology, Med Coll Wisc 85; **Fellow:** Head and Neck Surgery, MD Anderson Canc Ctr 87; **Fac Appt:** Prof Oto, Med Coll Wisc

Funk, Gerry Franklin MD [Oto] - **Spec Exp:** Head & Neck Cancer; Head & Neck Reconstruction; Head & Neck Trauma; **Hospital:** Univ Iowa Hosp & Clinics; **Address:** UIHC, Dept Otolaryngology, 200 Hawkins Dr, Iowa City, IA 52242-1009; **Phone:** 319-356-2169; **Board Cert:** Otolaryngology 92; **Med School:** Univ Chicago-Pritzker Sch Med 86; **Resid:** Surgery, LAC-USC Med Ctr 87; Otolaryngology, LAC-USC Med Ctr 91; **Fellow:** Head and Neck Surgery, Univ Iowa Hosp 92; **Fac Appt:** Prof Oto, Univ Iowa Coll Med

Gluckman, Jack L MD [Oto] - **Spec Exp:** Head & Neck Cancer; Head & Neck Surgery; **Hospital:** Univ Hosp - Cincinnati; **Address:** Univ of Cin Med Ctr/Dept Otolaryngology-Head & Neck Surgery, 231 Albert B. Sabin Way Bldg MSB Fl 6th - rm 6505, Box 670528, Cincinnati, OH 45267-0528; **Phone:** 513-558-4152; **Board Cert:** Otolaryngology 90; **Med School:** South Africa 67; **Resid:** Surgery, St James Hosp 71; Otolaryngology, Groote Schuur Hosp 74; **Fellow:** Otolaryngology, Univ Cincinnati Med Ctr 79; **Fac Appt:** Prof Oto, Univ Cincinnati

Haughey, Bruce MD [Oto] - **Spec Exp:** Reconstructive Surgery-Face; Head & Neck Cancer; **Hospital:** Barnes-Jewish Hosp (page 85); **Address:** Barnes Jewish Hosp South, 660 S Euclid Ave, Box 8115, St Louis, MO 63110; **Phone:** 314-362-7509; **Board Cert:** Otolaryngology 84; **Med School:** New Zealand 76; **Resid:** Surgery, Univ Auckland 80; Otolaryngology, Univ Iowa Med Ctr 84; **Fac Appt:** Assoc Prof Oto, Washington Univ, St Louis

Hoffman, Henry T MD [Oto] - **Spec Exp:** Head & Neck Cancer; Head & Neck Surgery; Voice Disorders; **Hospital:** Univ Iowa Hosp & Clinics; **Address:** Univ Iowa Hosp & Clins-Dept Oto, 200 Hawkins Drive, Iowa City, IA 52242; **Phone:** 319-356-2166; **Board Cert:** Otolaryngology 85; **Med School:** UCSD 80; **Resid:** Otolaryngology, Univ Iowa Hosp & Clinics 85; **Fellow:** Head and Neck Oncology, Univ Michigan Hosp 89; **Fac Appt:** Clin Prof Oto, Univ Iowa Coll Med

Kern, Robert MD [Oto] - **Spec Exp:** Head & Neck Cancer; Sinus Disorders/Surgery; Rhinoplasty; **Hospital:** Northwestern Meml Hosp; **Address:** 675 N St Clair St, Ste 15-200, Chicago, IL 60611; **Phone:** 312-695-8182; **Board Cert:** Otolaryngology 90; **Med School:** Jefferson Med Coll 85; **Resid:** Otolaryngology, Wayne State Affil Hosp 90; **Fellow:** Research, Natl Inst Hlth 91; **Fac Appt:** Assoc Prof Oto, Northwestern Univ

Lavertu, Pierre MD [Oto] - **Spec Exp:** Thyroid Cancer; Head & Neck Cancer; Skull Base Tumors; **Hospital:** Univ Hosps of Cleveland; **Address:** Univ Hosps, Dept Oto-Head & Neck Surg, 11100 Euclid Ave, MS 5045, Cleveland, OH 44106-5045; **Phone:** 216-844-4773; **Board Cert:** Otolaryngology 81; **Med School:** Univ Montreal 76; **Resid:** Otolaryngology, Univ Montreal 81; Head and Neck Surgery, Univ Montreal 82; **Fellow:** Head and Neck Surgery, Cleveland Clinic Fdn 83; **Fac Appt:** Prof Oto, Case West Res Univ

Leonetti, John P MD [Oto] - **Spec Exp:** Skull Base Tumors & Surgery; Acoustic Nerve Tumors; Neuro-Otology; **Hospital:** Loyola Univ Med Ctr (page 98); **Address:** Loyola University Medical Ctr, Dept Otolaryngology, 2160 S First Ave Bldg 105 - Ste 1870, Maywood, IL 60153; **Phone:** 708-216-4804; **Board Cert:** Otolaryngology 87; **Med School:** Loyola Univ-Stritch Sch Med 82; **Resid:** Otolaryngology, Loyola Univ Med Ctr 87; Research, House Ear Inst; **Fellow:** Neurotology, Barnes Hosp 88; **Fac Appt:** Prof Oto, Loyola Univ-Stritch Sch Med

Marentette, Lawrence MD [Oto] - **Spec Exp:** Skull Base Tumors & Surgery; Head & Neck Cancer & Surgery; Facial Plastic & Reconstructive Surgery; **Hospital:** Univ Michigan Hlth Sys; **Address:** Univ Michigan Health Systems, Dept Otolaryngology, 1904 Taubman Ctr, 1500 E Medical Center Drive, Ann Arbor, MI 48109; **Phone:** 313-936-7633; **Board Cert:** Otolaryngology 81; Facial Plastic & Reconstructive Surgery 87; **Med School:** Wayne State Univ 76; **Resid:** Otolaryngology, Wayne State Univ 80; **Fellow:** Maxillofacial Surgery, Univ of Zurich 85; **Fac Appt:** Assoc Prof NS, Univ Mich Med Sch

Miyamoto, Richard T MD [Oto] - **Spec Exp:** Neuro-Otology; Acoustic Nerve Tumors; Middle Ear Disorders; **Hospital:** Indiana Univ Hosp (page 90); **Address:** 702 Barnhill Drive, Ste 0860, Indianapolis, IN 46202-5128; **Phone:** 317-274-3556; **Board Cert:** Otolaryngology 75; **Med School:** Univ Mich Med Sch 70; **Resid:** Surgery, Butterworth Hosp 72; Rhinoplasty, Indiana Univ Hosps 75; **Fellow:** Otolaryngology, Otologic Med Grp 78; **Fac Appt:** Prof Oto, Indiana Univ

Olsen, Kerry D MD [Oto] - **Spec Exp:** Head & Neck Cancer & Surgery; Esthesioneuroblastoma; Salivary Gland Tumors & Surgery; **Hospital:** Mayo Med Ctr & Clin - Rochester; **Address:** Mayo Clinic, Dept Otolaryngology, 200 1st St SW, Rochester, MN 55905-0001; **Phone:** 507-284-2544; **Board Cert:** Otolaryngology 81; **Med School:** Mayo Med Sch 76; **Resid:** Otolaryngology, Mayo Clinic 81; **Fac Appt:** Prof Oto, Mayo Med Sch

Pelzer, Harold J MD/DDS [Oto] - **Spec Exp:** Head & Neck Cancer; Swallowing Disorders; **Hospital:** Northwestern Meml Hosp; **Address:** 675 N St Clair, Ste 15-200, Chicago, IL 60611; **Phone:** 312-695-8182; **Board Cert:** Otolaryngology 85; **Med School:** Northwestern Univ 79; **Resid:** Surgery, Northwestern Meml Hosp 83; **Fellow:** Head and Neck Surgery, Northwestern Meml Hosp 85; **Fac Appt:** Asst Prof Oto, Northwestern Univ

Pensak, Myles MD [Oto] - **Spec Exp:** Skull Base Tumors; Facial Paralysis; Vertigo; **Hospital:** Univ Hosp - Cincinnati; **Address:** Univ Cincinnati, Dept Oto/HNS, PO Box 670528, Cincinnati, OH 45267-0528; **Phone:** 513-475-8400; **Board Cert:** Otolaryngology 04; **Med School:** NY Med Coll 78; **Resid:** Surgery, Upstate Med Ctr 80; Otolaryngology, Yale Univ 83; **Fellow:** Otology & Neurotology, EAR Foundation 84; **Fac Appt:** Prof Oto, Univ Cincinnati

Petruzzelli, Guy MD/PhD [Oto] - **Spec Exp:** Head & Neck Cancer & Surgery; Skull Base Tumors; Thyroid Tumors; **Hospital:** Loyola Univ Med Ctr (page 98); **Address:** Loyola Univ Med Ctr, 2160 S 1st Ave, Bldg 105 - rm 1870, Maywood, IL 60153-3304; **Phone:** 708-216-9183; **Board Cert:** Otolaryngology 93; **Med School:** Rush Med Coll 87; **Resid:** Otolaryngology, Univ Pittsburgh Med Ctr 92; **Fellow:** Head and Neck Oncology, Univ Pittsburgh Med Ctr 93; Skull Base Surgery, Univ Pittsburgh Ctr Cranial Base Surg; **Fac Appt:** Prof Oto, Loyola Univ-Stritch Sch Med

Schuller, David MD [Oto] - **Spec Exp:** Head & Neck Cancer; Head & Neck Surgery; **Hospital:** Arthur G James Cancer Hosp & Research Inst (page 105); **Address:** 300 W 10th Ave, rm 518, Columbus, OH 43210; **Phone:** 614-293-8074; **Board Cert:** Otolaryngology 75; **Med School:** Ohio State Univ 70; **Resid:** Otolaryngology, Ohio State Univ Affil Hosps 75; Surgery, Univ Hosps 73; **Fellow:** Head and Neck Surgery, Pack Med Fdn 73; Head and Neck Oncology, Univ Iowa 76; **Fac Appt:** Prof Oto, Ohio State Univ

Siegel, Gordon J MD [Oto] - **Spec Exp:** Head & Neck Cancer; Nasal & Sinus Disorders; Cosmetic Surgery-Face; **Hospital:** Northwestern Meml Hosp; **Address:** 3 E Huron St Fl 1, Chicago, IL 60611-2705; **Phone:** 312-988-7777; **Board Cert:** Otolaryngology 84; **Med School:** Univ Hlth Sci/Chicago Med Sch 78; **Resid:** Otolaryngology, Northwestern Univ 82; **Fac Appt:** Asst Clin Prof Oto, Northwestern Univ

Strome, Marshall MD [Oto] - **Spec Exp:** Sleep Disorders/Apnea; Voice Disorders; Head & Neck Cancer; **Hospital:** Cleveland Clin Fdn (page 92); **Address:** Cleveland Clinic Fdn, 9500 Euclid Ave, Ste A71, Cleveland, OH 44195; **Phone:** 216-444-6686; **Board Cert:** Otolaryngology 70; **Med School:** Univ Mich Med Sch 64; **Resid:** Surgery, Harper Hosp 66; Otolaryngology, Univ Michigan Hosp 70; **Fac Appt:** Prof Oto, Cleveland Cl Coll Med/Case West Res

Teknos, Theodoros N MD [Oto] - **Spec Exp:** Head & Neck Cancer; Thyroid Cancer; Facial Plastic & Reconstructive Surgery; **Hospital:** Univ Michigan Hlth Sys; **Address:** Univ Mich Med Ctr-Dept Otolaryngology-TC 1904, 1500 E Med Ctr Drive, Ann Arbor, MI 48109; **Phone:** 734-936-3172; **Board Cert:** Otolaryngology 97; **Med School:** Harvard Med Sch 91; **Resid:** Otolaryngology, Mass Eye & Ear Hosp 96; **Fellow:** Head and Neck Surgery, Vanderbilt Med Ctr 97; **Fac Appt:** Assoc Prof Oto, Univ Mich Med Sch

Telian, Steven Allen MD [Oto] - **Spec Exp:** Cochlear Implants; Ear Disorders/Surgery; Acoustic Nerve Tumors; **Hospital:** Univ Michigan Hlth Sys; **Address:** Univ Mich Med Ctr, Dept Oto-HNS, 1500 E Med Ctr Dr, Taubman Ctr, rm 1904, Ann Arbor, MI 48109-0312; **Phone:** 734-936-8006; **Board Cert:** Otolaryngology 85; **Med School:** Univ Pennsylvania 80; **Resid:** Otolaryngology, Univ Penn 85; **Fellow:** Neurotology, Univ Mich Med Ctr 86; **Fac Appt:** Prof Oto, Univ Mich Med Sch

Wackym, Phillip MD [Oto] - **Spec Exp:** Cochlear Implants; Acoustic Nerve Tumors; Head & Neck Surgery; **Hospital:** Froedtert Meml Lutheran Hosp; **Address:** 9200 W Wisconsin Ave, Milwaukee, WI 53226; **Phone:** 414-805-3666; **Board Cert:** Otolaryngology 92; **Med School:** Vanderbilt Univ 85; **Resid:** Neurological Surgery, UCLA Med Ctr 87; Head and Neck Surgery, UCLA Med Ctr 91; **Fellow:** Otology & Neurotology, Univ Iowa 92; Neurological Science, UCLA Med Ctr 95; **Fac Appt:** Prof Oto, Med Coll Wisc

Wiet, Richard J MD [Oto] - **Spec Exp:** Acoustic Nerve Tumors; Hearing Loss; Cholesteatoma; **Hospital:** Hinsdale Hosp; **Address:** 950 York Rd, Ste 102, Hinsdale, IL 60521-8608; **Phone:** 630-789-3110; **Board Cert:** Otolaryngology 76; Neurotology 04; **Med School:** Loyola Univ-Stritch Sch Med 71; **Resid:** Otolaryngology, Cincinnati Med Ctr 76; **Fellow:** Neurotology, Univ Zurich/Ear Fdn 79; **Fac Appt:** Clin Prof Oto, Northwestern Univ

Wilson, Keith M MD [Oto] - **Spec Exp:** Head & Neck Cancer & Surgery; Voice Disorders; **Hospital:** Univ Hosp - Cincinnati; **Address:** University of Cincinnati Medical Ctr, 222 Piedmont , Ste 5200, Cincinnati, OH 45219; **Phone:** 513-475-8351; **Board Cert:** Otolaryngology 92; **Med School:** Cornell Univ-Weill Med Coll 86; **Resid:** Otolaryngology, St Louis Univ Med Ctr 91; **Fellow:** Head & Neck Surgical Oncology, Ohio State Med Ctr 92; **Fac Appt:** Assoc Prof Oto, Univ Cincinnati

Wolf, Gregory T MD [Oto] - **Spec Exp:** Head & Neck Cancer; Laryngeal Cancer; **Hospital:** Univ Michigan Hlth Sys; **Address:** Univ Mich Med Ctr, Dept Oto-HNS, 1500 E Med Ctr, Taubman Ctr, rm 1904, Ann Arbor, MI 48109-0312; **Phone:** 734-936-8029; **Board Cert:** Otolaryngology 78; **Med School:** Univ Mich Med Sch 73; **Resid:** Surgery, Georgetown Univ Hosp 75; Otolaryngology, SUNY Upstate Med Ctr 78; **Fac Appt:** Prof Oto, Univ Mich Med Sch

Great Plains and Mountains

Bentz, Brandon G MD [Oto] - **Spec Exp:** Head & Neck Surgery & Cancer; Sarcoma-Head & Neck; Skull Base Tumors; **Hospital:** Univ Utah Hosps and Clins; **Address:** University of Utah Hospitals, Div Otolaryngology, 50 N Medical Drive, rm 3C120, Salt Lake City, UT 84132; **Phone:** 801-581-7515; **Board Cert:** Otolaryngology 01; **Med School:** Northwestern Univ 93; **Resid:** Otolaryngology, Northwestern Univ Med Ctr 97; **Fellow:** Head & Neck Surgical Oncology, Meml Sloan Kettering Cancer Ctr 99; **Fac Appt:** Asst Prof Oto, Univ Utah

Chowdhury, Khalid MD [Oto] - **Spec Exp:** Skull Base Tumors & Surgery; Craniofacial Surgery; **Hospital:** Presby - St Luke's Med Ctr; **Address:** Center for Craniofacial Surgery, 1601 E 19th Ave, Ste 3000, Denver, CO 80218; **Phone:** 305-839-5155; **Board Cert:** Otolaryngology 90; **Med School:** Univ Saskatchewan 82; **Resid:** Surgery, Univ Saskatchewan Hosp 85; Otolaryngology, McGill Univ Hosps 89; **Fellow:** Craniofacial Surgery, Univ Bern Hosp 90; **Fac Appt:** Assoc Prof Oto, Univ Colorado

Jenkins, Herman A. MD [Oto] - **Spec Exp:** Ear Disorders/Surgery; Neuro-Otology; Acoustic Nerve Tumors; **Hospital:** Univ Colorado Hosp; **Address:** Univ Colorado Hlth & Sci Ctr, Dept Otolaryngology, 1635 N Urusla Ave Bldg AOP Fl 6, MC F737, Aurora, CO 80045; **Phone:** 720-848-2820; **Board Cert:** Otolaryngology 77; Neurotology 04; **Med School:** Vanderbilt Univ 70; **Resid:** Surgery, UCLA 72; Otolaryngology, UCLA 77; **Fellow:** Neurotology, Univ Hosp 80; **Fac Appt:** Prof Oto, Univ Colorado

Lydiatt, Daniel D MD [Oto] - **Spec Exp:** Head & Neck Cancer; **Hospital:** Nebraska Med Ctr; **Address:** 981225 Nebraska Medical Ctr, Omaha, NE 68198-1225; **Phone:** 402-559-5268; **Board Cert:** Otolaryngology 92; **Med School:** Univ Nebr Coll Med 83; **Resid:** Otolaryngology, Univ Nebraska Med Ctr 90; **Fellow:** Head and Neck Surgery, MD Anderson Med Ctr 91; **Fac Appt:** Assoc Prof Oto, Univ Nebr Coll Med

Lydiatt, William M MD [Oto] - **Spec Exp:** Head & Neck Cancer; Thyroid Cancer; **Hospital:** Nebraska Med Ctr; **Address:** 981225 Nebraska Medical Ctr, Omaha, NE 68198-1225; **Phone:** 402-559-5268; **Board Cert:** Otolaryngology 94; **Med School:** Univ Nebr Coll Med 88; **Resid:** Otolaryngology, Univ Nebraska Med Ctr 93; **Fellow:** Head and Neck Surgery, Meml Sloan Kettering Cancer Ctr 95; **Fac Appt:** Assoc Prof Oto, Univ Nebr Coll Med

Southwest

Clayman, Gary Lee MD/DMD [Oto] - **Spec Exp:** Thyroid Cancer & Surgery; Salivary Gland Tumors & Surgery; Head & Neck Cancer; **Hospital:** UT MD Anderson Cancer Ctr, The (page 115); **Address:** Univ TX/MD Anderson Cancer Center, 1515 Holcombe Blvd, Box 441, Houston, TX 77030-4009; **Phone:** 713-792-8837; **Board Cert:** Otolaryngology 92; **Med School:** NE Ohio Univ 86; **Resid:** Surgery, Hennepin Co Med Ctr 87; Otolaryngology, Univ Minn 91; **Fellow:** Head and Neck Surgery, MD Anderson Cancer Ctr 93; **Fac Appt:** Prof Oto, Univ Tex, Houston

Coker, Newton J MD [Oto] - **Spec Exp:** Acoustic Nerve Tumors; Cochlear Implants; Bell's Palsy; **Hospital:** Methodist Hosp - Houston; **Address:** Baylor Coll Medicine, One Baylor Plaza, MS NA-102, Houston, TX 77030; **Phone:** 713-798-3200; **Board Cert:** Otolaryngology 81; **Med School:** Med Coll GA 76; **Resid:** Surgery, Med Coll Georgia 78; Otolaryngology, Med Coll Georgia 81; **Fellow:** Otology & Neurotology, University Hosp; **Fac Appt:** Prof Oto, Baylor Coll Med

Daspit, C Phillip MD [Oto] - **Spec Exp:** Hearing Loss & Balance Disorders; Skull Base Tumors & Surgery; Cochlear Implants; **Hospital:** St Joseph's Hosp & Med Ctr - Phoenix; **Address:** 222 W Thomas Rd, Ste 114, Phoenix, AZ 85013; **Phone:** 602-279-5444; **Board Cert:** Otolaryngology 77; **Med School:** Louisiana State Univ 68; **Resid:** Surgery, UCSF Med Ctr 73; Otolaryngology, Ft Miley VA Hosp 77; **Fellow:** Otology & Neurotology, House Ear Inst 78; Skull Base Surgery, House Ear Inst 78; **Fac Appt:** Clin Prof S, Univ Ariz Coll Med

Donovan, Donald Thomas MD [Oto] - **Spec Exp:** Head & Neck Cancer; Voice Disorders; Thyroid Disorders; **Hospital:** Methodist Hosp - Houston; **Address:** 6550 Fannin St, Ste 1727, Houston, TX 77030; **Phone:** 713-798-3380; **Board Cert:** Otolaryngology 81; **Med School:** Baylor Coll Med 76; **Resid:** Surgery, Baylor Affil Hosps 78; Otolaryngology, Baylor Affil Hosps 81; **Fellow:** Head and Neck Surgery, Columbia-Presby Med Ctr 82; **Fac Appt:** Assoc Prof Oto, Baylor Coll Med

Hanna, Ehab Y MD [Oto] - **Spec Exp:** Skull Base Tumors & Surgery; Head & Neck Cancer & Surgery; **Hospital:** UT MD Anderson Cancer Ctr, The (page 115); **Address:** Univ Tex MD Anderson Cancer Ctr, 1515 Holcolmbe Blvd, Unit 441, Houston, TX 77030; **Phone:** 713-745-1815; **Board Cert:** Otolaryngology 94; **Med School:** Egypt 82; **Resid:** Otolaryngology, Cleveland Clinic 89; Otolaryngology, Cleveland Clinic 93; **Fellow:** Otolaryngology, Univ Pittsburgh Med Ctr 94; **Fac Appt:** Asst Prof Oto, Univ Tex, Houston

Medina, Jesus MD [Oto] - **Spec Exp:** Head & Neck Cancer; **Hospital:** OU Med Ctr; **Address:** Univ OK Hlth Sci Ctr, Dept Oto-WP 1360, PO Box 26901, Oklahoma City, OK 73190; **Phone:** 405-271-8047; **Board Cert:** Otolaryngology 80; **Med School:** Peru 74; **Resid:** Surgery, Wayne St Univ Affil Hosp 77; Otolaryngology, Wayne St Univ Affil Hosp 80; **Fellow:** Head and Neck Surgery, Univ Tex Sys Cancer Ctrs 81; **Fac Appt:** Prof Oto, Univ Okla Coll Med

Myers, Jeffrey N MD/PhD [Oto] - **Spec Exp:** Head & Neck Cancer; Melanoma-Head & Neck; Tongue Cancer; **Hospital:** UT MD Anderson Cancer Ctr, The (page 115); **Address:** Univ Texas MD Anderson Cancer Ctr, 1515 Holcombe Blvd, Box 441, Houston, TX 77030; **Phone:** 713-745-2667; **Board Cert:** Otolaryngology 97; **Med School:** Univ Pennsylvania 91; **Resid:** Otolaryngology, Univ Pittsburgh Med Ctr 96; **Fellow:** Head & Neck Surgical Oncology, MD Anderson Cancer Ctr 97; **Fac Appt:** Assoc Prof Oto, Univ Tex, Houston

Nuss, Daniel W MD [Oto] - **Spec Exp:** Head & Neck Cancer; Skull Base Tumors & Surgery; **Hospital:** Meml Med Ctr - Baptist Campus; **Address:** LSU Health Sci Ctr, Dept Otolaryngology, 533 Bolivar St Fl 5, New Orleans, LA 70112; **Phone:** 504-412-1578; **Board Cert:** Otolaryngology 87; **Med School:** Louisiana State Univ 81; **Resid:** Surgery, Charity Hosp 83; Otolaryngology, LSU Med Ctr 87; **Fellow:** Surgical Oncology, MD Anderson Hosp-Univ Tex; Head and Neck Surgery, Ctr Cranial Base Surg-Univ Pittsbur 91; **Fac Appt:** Prof Oto, Louisiana State Univ

Otto, Randal A MD [Oto] - **Spec Exp:** Head & Neck Cancer; Thyroid & Parathyroid Cancer & Surgery; Sinus Disorders/Surgery; **Hospital:** UTSA - Univ Hosp; **Address:** 7703 Floyd Curl Drive, MS 777, San Antonio, TX 78229-3901; **Phone:** 210-567-5655; **Board Cert:** Otolaryngology 87; **Med School:** Univ MO-Columbia Sch Med 81; **Resid:** Pathology, Queens Med Ctr 82; Otolaryngology, Univ Missouri 87; **Fac Appt:** Prof Oto, Univ Tex, San Antonio

Suen, James Y MD [Oto] - **Spec Exp:** Head & Neck Cancer; Vascular Lesions-Head & Neck; Laryngeal Cancer & Disorders; **Hospital:** UAMS Med Ctr; **Address:** Univ Hosp Arkansas Med Scis, 4301 W Markham St, Slot 543, Little Rock, AR 72205; **Phone:** 501-686-8224; **Board Cert:** Otolaryngology 73; **Med School:** Univ Ark 66; **Resid:** Surgery, Univ Arkansas Med Ctr 70; Otolaryngology, Univ Arkansas Med Ctr 73; **Fellow:** Head and Neck Surgery, MD Anderson Cancer Ctr-Tumor Inst 74; **Fac Appt:** Prof Oto, Univ Ark

Weber, Randal S MD [Oto] - **Spec Exp:** Thyroid Cancer; Thyroid & Parathyroid Cancer & Surgery; Skull Base Tumors; **Hospital:** UT MD Anderson Cancer Ctr, The (page 115); **Address:** 1515 Holcombe Blvd, Unit 441, Houston, TX 77030-4009; **Phone:** 713-745-0497; **Board Cert:** Otolaryngology 85; **Med School:** Univ Tenn Coll Med, Memphis 76; **Resid:** Surgery, Baylor Coll Med 82; Otolaryngology, Baylor Coll Med 85; **Fellow:** Head and Neck Surgery, MD Anderson Cancer Ctr 86; **Fac Appt:** Prof Oto, Univ Tex, Houston

Weber, Samuel C MD [Oto] - **Spec Exp:** Thyroid Cancer; **Hospital:** St Luke's Episcopal Hosp - Houston; **Address:** 6624 Fannin St, Ste 1480, Houston, TX 77030-2385; **Phone:** 713-795-5343; **Board Cert:** Otolaryngology 73; **Med School:** Univ Tenn Coll Med, Memphis 65; **Resid:** Surgery, Baylor Coll Med 70; Otolaryngology, Baylor Coll Med 72; **Fac Appt:** Assoc Clin Prof Oto, Baylor Coll Med

West Coast and Pacific

Berke, Gerald S MD [Oto] - **Spec Exp:** Head & Neck Surgery; Head & Neck Cancer; Voice Disorders; **Hospital:** UCLA Med Ctr (page 111); **Address:** 200 UCLA Med Plaza, Ste 550, Los Angeles, CA 90095; **Phone:** 310-825-5179; **Board Cert:** Otolaryngology 84; **Med School:** USC Sch Med 78; **Resid:** Otolaryngology, LAC-USC Med Ctr 79; **Fellow:** Head and Neck Surgery, UCLA Med Ctr 84

Brackmann, Derald E MD [Oto] - **Spec Exp:** Ear Disorders/Surgery; Facial Nerve Disorders; Acoustic Nerve Tumors; **Hospital:** St Vincent's Med Ctr - Los Angeles; **Address:** House Ear Clinic, 2100 W 3rd St, Fl 1st, Los Angeles, CA 90057-1902; **Phone:** 213-483-9930 x8244; **Board Cert:** Otolaryngology 71; **Med School:** Univ IL Coll Med 62; **Resid:** Otolaryngology, LAC/USC Med Ctr 70; **Fellow:** Otology & Neurotology, House Ear Clinic 71; **Fac Appt:** Clin Prof Oto, USC Sch Med

Cohen, James I MD [Oto] - **Spec Exp:** Head & Neck Cancer; Thyroid Surgery; Parathyroid Surgery; **Hospital:** OR Hlth & Sci Univ; **Address:** Oregon Hlth Scis U-PV-01, 3181 SW Sam Jackson Park Rd, Portland, OR 97239; **Phone:** 503-494-5355; **Board Cert:** Otolaryngology 84; **Med School:** Canada 78; **Resid:** Surgery, Univ Minn Med Ctr 80; Otolaryngology, Univ Minn Med Ctr 84; **Fellow:** Head & Neck Surgical Oncology, MD Anderson Hosp 85; **Fac Appt:** Prof Oto, Oregon Hlth Sci Univ

Courey, Mark S MD [Oto] - **Spec Exp:** Laryngeal Disorders; Swallowing Disorders; Laryngeal Cancer; **Hospital:** UCSF - Mt Zion Med Ctr; **Address:** UCSF Voice & Swallowing Ctr, 2330 Post St Fl 5, San Francisco, CA 94115; **Phone:** 415-885-7700; **Board Cert:** Otolaryngology 93; **Med School:** SUNY Buffalo 87; **Resid:** Otolaryngology, SUNY-Buffalo Med Ctr 92; **Fellow:** Laryngology, Vanderbilt Univ 93; **Fac Appt:** Prof Oto, UCSF

De la Cruz, Antonio MD [Oto] - **Spec Exp:** Otosclerosis/Stapedectomy; Acoustic Nerve Tumors; Otology; **Hospital:** St Vincent's Med Ctr - Los Angeles; **Address:** 2100 W 3rd St Fl 1, Los Angeles, CA 90057; **Phone:** 213-483-9930; **Board Cert:** Otolaryngology 73; **Med School:** Costa Rica 67; **Resid:** Surgery, Univ Miami Med Ctr 70; Otolaryngology, Univ Miami Med Ctr 73; **Fellow:** Otology & Neurotology, House Ear Clinic; **Fac Appt:** Clin Prof Oto, USC Sch Med

Donald, Paul MD [Oto] - **Spec Exp:** Skull Base Tumors & Surgery; Head & Neck Cancer; **Hospital:** UC Davis Med Ctr; **Address:** 2521 Stockton Blvd, rm 7200, Sacramento, CA 95817; **Phone:** 916-734-2832; **Board Cert:** Otolaryngology 73; **Med School:** Univ British Columbia Fac Med 64; **Resid:** Surgery, St Paul's Hosp 69; Otolaryngology, Univ Iowa Hosp 73; **Fac Appt:** Prof Oto, UC Davis

Eisele, David W. MD [Oto] - **Spec Exp:** Salivary Gland Tumors & Surgery; Head & Neck Cancer; Thyroid Cancer; **Hospital:** UCSF - Mt Zion Med Ctr; **Address:** UCSF, Dept Otolaryngology, 400 Parnassus Ave, Ste A 730, San Francisco, CA 94143-0342; **Phone:** 415-502-0498; **Board Cert:** Otolaryngology 88; **Med School:** Cornell Univ-Weill Med Coll 82; **Resid:** Surgery, Univ WashMed Ctr 84; Otolaryngology, Univ Wash Med Ctr 88; **Fac Appt:** Prof Oto, UCSF

Fee Jr, Willard E MD [Oto] - **Spec Exp:** Head & Neck Cancer; Parotid Gland Tumors; Thyroid Cancer; **Hospital:** Stanford Univ Med Ctr; **Address:** Cancer Ctr Head & Neck Surg/Clinic B, H75 Lake Wilber Dr, Stanford, CA 94305; **Phone:** 650-723-5416; **Board Cert:** Otolaryngology 74; **Med School:** Univ Colorado 69; **Resid:** Surgery, Wadsworth VA Hosp 71; Otolaryngology, UCLA Med Ctr 74; **Fac Appt:** Prof Oto, Stanford Univ

Futran, Neal D MD/DMD [Oto] - **Spec Exp:** Head & Neck Surgery; Head & Neck Cancer Reconstruction; **Hospital:** Univ Wash Med Ctr; **Address:** U Wash Med Ctr, Oto Office, 1959 NE Pacific St, Box 356515, Seattle, WA 98195-6515; **Phone:** 206-543-3060; **Board Cert:** Otolaryngology 93; **Med School:** Univ Pennsylvania 87; **Resid:** Surgery, Kings Co-SUNY Downstate 85; Otolaryngology, U Rochester Med Ctr 92; **Fellow:** Microvascular Surgery, Mt Sinai Hosp 93; **Fac Appt:** Prof Oto, Univ Wash

Geller, Kenneth Allen MD [Oto] - **Spec Exp:** Airway Disorders; Sinus Surgery-Pediatric; Head & Neck Cancer-Pediatric; **Hospital:** Chldns Hosp - Los Angeles; **Address:** Chldns Hosp, Dept Oto, 4650 Sunset Blvd, MS 58, Los Angeles, CA 90027; **Phone:** 323-669-2145; **Board Cert:** Otolaryngology 78; **Med School:** USC Sch Med 72; **Resid:** Surgery, Wadsworth VA Hosp 75; Otolaryngology, UCLA Hlth Scis Ctr 78; **Fellow:** Pediatric Otolaryngology, Chldns Hosp 79; **Fac Appt:** Assoc Clin Prof Oto, USC Sch Med

Jackler, Robert K MD [Oto] - **Spec Exp:** Neuro-Otology; Skull Base Surgery; Ear Tumors; **Hospital:** Stanford Univ Med Ctr; **Address:** Stanford Univ Med Ctr, Dept Oto-Head & Neck Surg, 801 Welch Rd, Stanford, CA 94305-5739; **Phone:** 650-725-6500; **Board Cert:** Otolaryngology 84; **Med School:** Boston Univ 79; **Resid:** Otolaryngology, UCSF Mee Ctr 84; **Fellow:** Otolaryngology, Oto Med Grp; **Fac Appt:** Prof Oto, Stanford Univ

Kaplan, Michael J MD [Oto] - **Spec Exp:** Head & Neck Surgery; Skull Base Surgery; Head & Neck Cancer; **Hospital:** Stanford Univ Med Ctr; **Address:** Stanford Cancer Center Otolaryngology-Head/Neck Surgery, 801 Welch Rd, Stanford, CA 94305-5739; **Phone:** 650-723-5416; **Board Cert:** Otolaryngology 82; **Med School:** Harvard Med Sch 77; **Resid:** Surgery, Beth Israel-Chldns Hosps 79; Otolaryngology, Mass EE Infirm 82; **Fellow:** Head and Neck Surgery, Univ of VA 84; **Fac Appt:** Prof Oto, Stanford Univ

McMenomey, Sean O MD [Oto] - **Spec Exp:** Otology & Neuro-Otology; Skull Base Tumors & Surgery; Head & Neck Surgery; **Hospital:** OR Hlth & Sci Univ; **Address:** Oregon Health Sci Ctr, Dept Otolaryngology, 3181 SW Sam Jackson Park Rd, Ste PV-01, Portland, OR 97201; **Phone:** 503-494-8135; **Board Cert:** Otolaryngology 93; **Med School:** St Louis Univ 87; **Resid:** Otolaryngology, Oregon Health Sci Ctr 92; **Fellow:** Otology & Neurotology, Baptist Hosp 93; **Fac Appt:** Assoc Prof Oto, Oregon Hlth Sci Univ

Rice, Dale MD [Oto] - **Spec Exp:** Head & Neck Cancer; Sinus Disorders/Surgery; **Hospital:** USC Univ Hosp - R K Eamer Med Plz; **Address:** USC Keck Sch Med, 1200 N State St, Box 795, Los Angeles, CA 90033-1029; **Phone:** 323-442-5790; **Board Cert:** Otolaryngology 76; **Med School:** Univ Mich Med Sch 68; **Resid:** Otolaryngology, Univ Mich Med Ctr 76; Surgery, Univ Mich Med Ctr 70; **Fac Appt:** Prof Oto, USC Sch Med

Singer, Mark I MD [Oto] - **Spec Exp:** Head & Neck Surgery; Head & Neck Cancer; Melanoma; **Hospital:** UCSF - Mt Zion Med Ctr; **Address:** 2380 Sutter St Fl 2, Box 1703, San Francisco, CA 94143-1703; **Phone:** 415-885-7528; **Board Cert:** Otolaryngology 76; **Med School:** Columbia P&S 70; **Resid:** Surgery, Northwestern Meml Hosp 73; Otolaryngology, Northwestern Meml Hosp 76; **Fellow:** Oncology, Northwestern Meml Hosp 76; **Fac Appt:** Prof Oto, UCSF

Sinha, Uttam Kumar MD [Oto] - **Spec Exp:** Head & Neck Cancer; Voice Disorders; **Hospital:** USC Univ Hosp - R K Eamer Med Plz; **Address:** 1200 N State St, Box 795, Los Angeles, CA 90033; **Phone:** 323-226-7315; **Board Cert:** Otolaryngology 98; **Med School:** India 85; **Resid:** Otolaryngology, LAC-USC Med Ctr 95; **Fellow:** Mount Sinai Med Sch 88; LAC-USC Med Ctr 90; **Fac Appt:** Asst Prof Oto, USC Sch Med

Wax, Mark K MD [Oto] - **Spec Exp:** Facial Nerve Disorders; Skull Base Tumors & Surgery; Facial Plastic & Reconstructive Surgery; **Hospital:** OR Hlth & Sci Univ; **Address:** Oregon Hlth Scis Univ-Dept Otolaryngology, 3181 SW Sam Jackson Park Rd, Ste PV-01, Portland, OR 97201; **Phone:** 503-494-5355; **Board Cert:** Otolaryngology 85; Facial Plastic & Reconstructive Surgery 87; **Med School:** Univ Toronto 80; **Resid:** Otolaryngology, Univ Toronto 85; Surgery, Cedars-Sinai Med Ctr 83; **Fellow:** Head and Neck Surgery, St Michaels Hosp 91; **Fac Appt:** Prof Oto, Oregon Hlth Sci Univ

Weisman, Robert A MD [Oto] - **Spec Exp:** Head & Neck Cancer & Reconstruction; Clinical Trials; Thyroid & Parathyroid Cancer & Surgery; **Hospital:** UCSD Med Ctr; **Address:** UCSD Medical Ctr, 200 W Arbor Drive, Ste 149, MC 8891, San Diego, CA 92103-8891; **Phone:** 619-543-2708; **Board Cert:** Otolaryngology 78; **Med School:** Washington Univ, St Louis 73; **Resid:** Head and Neck Surgery, UCLA Med Ctr 78; **Fac Appt:** Prof S, UCSD

Weymuller, Ernest MD [Oto] - **Spec Exp:** Head & Neck Cancer; Sinus Disorders/Surgery; **Hospital:** Univ Wash Med Ctr; **Address:** 1959 NE Pacific St, Box 356161, Seattle, WA 98195-6161; **Phone:** 206-598-4022; **Board Cert:** Otolaryngology 73; **Med School:** Harvard Med Sch 66; **Resid:** Surgery, Vanderbilt Univ Hosp 68; Otolaryngology, Mass Eye and Ear Infirm 73; **Fac Appt:** Prof Oto, Univ Wash

Yueh, Bevan MD [Oto] - **Spec Exp:** Head & Neck Cancer; Hearing Loss; **Hospital:** Univ Wash Med Ctr; **Address:** Surgery Section, VA Puget Sound, 1660 S Columbian Way, MS 112 OTO, Seattle, WA 98108; **Phone:** 206-764-2424; **Board Cert:** Otolaryngology 95; **Med School:** Stanford Univ 89; **Resid:** Otolaryngology, Johns Hopkins Hosp 94; **Fellow:** Otolaryngology, Johns Hopkins Hosp 95; **Fac Appt:** Assoc Prof Oto, Univ Wash

PAIN MEDICINE

a subspecialty of ANESTHESIOLOGY, NEUROLOGY, PHYSICAL MEDICINE & REHABILITATION or PSYCHIATRY

*S*ome physicians who have their primary board certification in anesthesiology, neurology, physical medicine and rehabilitation, or psychiatry have completed additional training and passed an examination in the subspecialty called pain management. These doctors provide a high level of care, either as a primary physcian or consultant, for patients experiencing problems with acute, chronic and/or cancer pain in both hospital and ambulatory settings.

For more information about the main specialties of these physicians, see Anesthesiology, Neurology, Physical Medicine and Rehabilitation or Psychiatry.

Training Required: *Number of years required for primary specialty plus additional training and examination.*

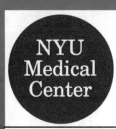

550 First Avenue (at 31st Street)
New York, NY 10016
Physician Referral:
1-888-7-NYU-MED
www.nyumc.org

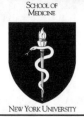

SCHOOL OF MEDICINE

NEW YORK UNIVERSITY

PAIN MANAGEMENT

NYU Medical Center's Pain Management Center, a division of the Department of Anesthesiology, offers state-of-the-art care under the umbrella of the New York University School of Medicine. We offer comprehensive and holistic treatments for pain, including acute, chronic, and cancer pain. Patients receive compassionate and individualized care using the most advanced diagnostic procedures and interventions.

The Pain Management Center fosters a truly multi-disciplinary approach to care, with experienced and dedicated pain specialists trained in anesthesiology, psychology, nursing, neurology, and rehabilitation medicine. We also offer patients an integrative medicine approach that focuses on the mind-body relationship.

The following are examples of treatment methods available through the Pain Management Center:

SPINAL CORD STIMULATION - an electronic implant that blocks pain signals

EPIDURAL BLOCKS - an infusion of medication to the spine that provides relief that can last for weeks while other interventions are applied

NERVE BLOCKS - carries medication to the site of pain in the nerves

IMPLANTABLE PUMPS - provide continuous, targeted relief for intractable pain

BIOFEEDBACK - provides visual and auditory feedback to patients, enabling them to change specific physiological parameters such as muscle tension, heart rate, and temperature.

COGNITIVE-BEHAVIORAL THERAPY - teaches patients to use techniques such as relaxation training, cognitive restructuring, and hypnosis to facilitate better coping skills.

RADIO FREQUENCY LESIONING - provides prolonged relief for chronic pain by targeting specific nerves

The Pain Management Center is also at the frontier of research, testing new drugs designed to reach pain receptors without the side effects of many narcotics. The Center also has a state-of-the-art fluoroscopy suite that enables the pain physician to observe treatments as they are administered, ensuring greater precision and superior outcomes.

Specialists at the NCI-designated NYU Cancer Institute seek to enhance and coordinate the extensive resources of NYU Medical Center to optimize research, treatment, and the ultimate control of cancer.

Our new NYU Clinical Cancer Center is located at 160 East 34th Street. This state-of-the-art 13-level, 85,000-square-foot building serves as "home base" for patients, by providing the latest cancer prevention, screening, diagnostic treatment, genetic counseling, and support services in one central location. The NYU Clinical Cancer Center stands to dramatically improve the lives of people with cancer. As part of NYU Medical Center, patients can access a variety of other non-cancer services throughout the institution.

PHYSICIAN REFERRAL
1-888-7-NYU-MED
(1-888-769-8633)
www.nyumc.org
www.nyuci.org

PAIN MEDICINE

New England

Acquadro, Martin A MD/DMD **[PM]** - **Spec Exp:** Pain-Neuropathic; Headache; Pain-Cancer; **Hospital:** Mass Genl Hosp; **Address:** Mass Genl Hosp, Pain Clinic - ACC324, 15 Parkman St, Boston, MA 02114; **Phone:** 617-726-8810; **Board Cert:** Anesthesiology 89; Internal Medicine 01; Pain Medicine 98; **Med School:** Boston Univ 83; **Resid:** Internal Medicine, Carney Hosp 85; Anesthesiology, Mass Genl Hosp 88; **Fellow:** Pain Medicine, Mass Genl Hosp 88; **Fac Appt:** Asst Clin Prof Anes, Harvard Med Sch

Mid Atlantic

Foley, Kathleen M MD **[PM]** - **Spec Exp:** Palliative Care; Pain-Cancer; **Hospital:** Meml Sloan Kettering Cancer Ctr (page 100); **Address:** Memorial Sloan Kettering Cancer Ctr, Pain & Palliative Care Svc, 1275 York Ave, Box 52, New York, NY 10021-6007; **Phone:** 212-639-7050; **Board Cert:** Neurology 77; **Med School:** Cornell Univ-Weill Med Coll 69; **Resid:** Neurology, New York Hosp 74; **Fellow:** Clinical Genetics, New York Hosp 71; **Fac Appt:** Prof N, Cornell Univ-Weill Med Coll

Jain, Subhash MD **[PM]** - **Spec Exp:** Pain-Cancer; Pain-Pelvic; Reflex Sympathetic Dystrophy (RSD); **Hospital:** NY-Presby Hosp - NY Weill Cornell Med Ctr (page 103); **Address:** 360 S 72nd St, Ste C, New York, NY 10021; **Phone:** 212-439-6100; **Board Cert:** Anesthesiology 94; Pain Medicine 98; **Med School:** India 68; **Resid:** Surgery, St Vincent Med Ctr 77; Anesthesiology, New York Hosp 79; **Fellow:** Pain Medicine, New York Hosp/Meml Sloan Kettering Cancer Ctr 80

Kreitzer, Joel MD **[PM]** - **Spec Exp:** Pain-Back; Pain-Cancer; Pain-Neuropathic; **Hospital:** Mount Sinai Med Ctr (page 101); **Address:** Upper East Side Pain Medicine, PC, 1540 York Ave, New York, NY 10028; **Phone:** 212-288-2180; **Board Cert:** Anesthesiology 90; Pain Medicine 03; **Med School:** Albert Einstein Coll Med 85; **Resid:** Anesthesiology, Mount Sinai Hosp 89; **Fellow:** Pain Medicine, Mount Sinai Hosp 89; **Fac Appt:** Assoc Clin Prof Anes, Mount Sinai Sch Med

Lema, Mark J MD/PhD **[PM]** - **Spec Exp:** Pain-Cancer; Pain-Acute & Perioperative; Pain-Neuropathic; **Hospital:** Roswell Park Cancer Inst (page 107); **Address:** Roswell Park Cancer Inst, Dept Anesthesia & Pain Medicine, Carlton & Elm Sts, Buffalo, NY 14263-0001; **Phone:** 716-845-3240; **Board Cert:** Anesthesiology 87; Pain Medicine 94; **Med School:** SUNY Downstate 82; **Resid:** Anesthesiology, Brigham & Women's Hosp 84; **Fellow:** Physiology, SUNY Buffalo Genl Hosp 78; **Fac Appt:** Prof Anes, SUNY Buffalo

Portenoy, Russell MD **[PM]** - **Spec Exp:** Pain-Cancer; Palliative Care; **Hospital:** Beth Israel Med Ctr - Petrie Division (page 93); **Address:** Beth Israel Med Ctr, Dept Pain Med & Palliative Care, First Ave at 16th St, New York, NY 10003; **Phone:** 212-844-1505; **Board Cert:** Neurology 85; **Med School:** Univ MD Sch Med 80; **Resid:** Neurology, Albert Einstein 84; **Fellow:** Pain Medicine, Meml Sloan-Kettering 85; **Fac Appt:** Prof N, Albert Einstein Coll Med

Weinberger, Michael L MD **[PM]** - **Spec Exp:** Pain-Cancer; Pain-Back & Neck; **Hospital:** NY-Presby Hosp - Columbia Presby Med Ctr (page 103); **Address:** 622 W 168th St, TH5, rm 500, New York, NY 10032-3720; **Phone:** 212-305-7114; **Board Cert:** Internal Medicine 86; Anesthesiology 90; Pain Medicine 03; **Med School:** Columbia P&S 83; **Resid:** Internal Medicine, St Vincent's Hosp 86; Anesthesiology, Columbia-Presby Med Ctr 89; **Fellow:** Pain Medicine, Meml Sloan Kettering Cancer Ctr; **Fac Appt:** Assoc Prof Anes, Colombia

Southeast

Payne, Richard MD [PM] - Spec Exp: Palliative Care; Neurology & Pain Management; **Hospital:** Duke Univ Med Ctr (page 94); **Address:** Duke Inst on Care at the End of Life, 2 Chapel Drive, Box 90968, Durham, NC 27708; **Phone:** 919-660-3553; **Board Cert:** Neurology 84; **Med School:** Harvard Med Sch 77; **Resid:** Internal Medicine, Peter Bent Brigham Hosp 79; Neurology, New York Hosp 82; **Fellow:** Neurological Oncology, Meml Sloan Kettering Cancer Ctr 84

Midwest

Benedetti, Costantino MD [PM] - Spec Exp: Pain-Cancer; Palliative Care; **Hospital:** Ohio St Univ Med Ctr (page 105); **Address:** Ohio State Univ Med Ctr, 300 W 10th Ave, Ste 519, Columbus, OH 43210; **Phone:** 614-293-6040; **Med School:** Italy 72; **Resid:** Anesthesiology, Univ Colorado Hosp; Anesthesiology, Univ Wash Med Ctr; **Fellow:** Pain Medicine, Univ Wash Med Ctr 78; **Fac Appt:** Clin Prof Anes, Ohio State Univ

Swarm, Robert A MD [PM] - Spec Exp: Pain-Acute; Pain-Chronic; Pain-Cancer; **Hospital:** Barnes-Jewish Hosp (page 85); **Address:** Ctr for Advanced Med-Pain Mngmt Ctr, 4921 Parkview Pl, Ste 10A, MS 90-35-706, St Louis, MO 63110; **Phone:** 314-362-8820; **Board Cert:** Anesthesiology 90; Pain Medicine 04; **Med School:** Washington Univ, St Louis 83; **Resid:** Surgery, Barnes Hosp 86; Anesthesiology, Barnes Hosp 89; **Fellow:** Pain Medicine, Univ Sydney; **Fac Appt:** Assoc Prof Anes, Washington Univ, St Louis

Great Plains and Mountains

Weinstein, Sharon MD [PM] - Spec Exp: Pain-Cancer; **Hospital:** Univ Utah Hosps and Clins; **Address:** Huntsman Cancer Inst, Univ Utah, 2000 E Circle of Hope, rm 2151, Salt Lake City, UT 84112; **Phone:** 801-585-0262; **Board Cert:** Neurology 93; Pain Medicine 00; **Med School:** Albert Einstein Coll Med 86; **Resid:** Neurology, Albert Einstein Coll Med 90; **Fellow:** Pain Medicine, Meml Sloan Kettering Cancer Ctr; **Fac Appt:** Assoc Prof Anes, Univ Utah

Southwest

Patt, Richard B MD [PM] - Spec Exp: Pain-Cancer; Palliative Care; Pain-Chronic; **Hospital:** St Luke's Episcopal Hosp - Houston; **Address:** The Pratt Center for Cancer Pain & Wellness, 1920 Woodbury Blvd, Houston, TX 77030; **Phone:** 713-799-2777; **Board Cert:** Anesthesiology 87; Pain Medicine 94; **Med School:** Amer Univ Caribbean, Plymouth 82; **Resid:** Anesthesiology, Montefiore-Weiler Enstein Div 85; **Fellow:** Pain Medicine, Montefiore/Weiler Einstein Div 86

West Coast and Pacific

Du Pen, Stuart L MD [PM] - Spec Exp: Pain-Cancer; Pain-Chronic; **Hospital:** Overlake Hosp Med Ctr; **Address:** 1135 116th Ave NE, Ste 130, Bellevue, WA 98004; **Phone:** 425-990-0400; **Board Cert:** Anesthesiology 72; Pain Medicine 93; **Med School:** St Louis Univ 67; **Resid:** Anesthesiology, Virginia Mason Med Ctr 71; **Fac Appt:** Assoc Clin Prof Anes, Univ Wash

Fishman, Scott M MD [PM] - Spec Exp: Pain-Cancer; Pain-Chronic; Psychiatry in Pain Management; **Hospital:** UC Davis Med Ctr; **Address:** UC Davis Med Ctr, Dept Pain Management, 4860 Y St, Ste 3730, Sacramento, CA 95817; **Phone:** 916-734-7246; **Board Cert:** Internal Medicine 94; Psychiatry 98; **Med School:** Univ Mass Sch Med 90; **Resid:** Internal Medicine, Greenwich Hosp 93; Psychiatry, Mass Genl Hosp 96; **Fellow:** Pain Medicine, Mass Genl Hosp 95; **Fac Appt:** Assoc Prof Anes, UC Davis

Fitzgibbon, Dermot R MD **[PM]** - **Spec Exp:** Pain-Perioperative; Pain-Cancer; **Hospital:** Univ Wash Med Ctr; **Address:** Univ Wash Med Ctr, Dept Anesthesiology, 1959 NE Pacific St, Box 356540, Seattle, WA 98195; **Phone:** 206-598-4260; **Board Cert:** Anesthesiology 96; Pain Medicine 98; **Med School:** Ireland 83; **Resid:** Anesthesiology, St Vincent's Hosp 92; Anesthesiology, Univ Washington Med Ctr 95; **Fellow:** Pain Medicine, Univ Wash-Pain Mngmt Clinic; **Fac Appt:** Assoc Prof Anes, Univ Wash

Ready, L Brian MD **[PM]** - **Spec Exp:** Pain-Cancer; **Hospital:** Tacoma Genl Hosp; **Address:** 316 Martin Luther King Jr Way, Ste 103, Tacoma, WA 98415; **Phone:** 253-403-1375; **Med School:** Canada 67; **Resid:** Anesthesiology, Univ Washington Med Ctr 75

Rosner, Howard L MD **[PM]** - **Spec Exp:** Spinal Interventional Pain; Pain-Cancer; Pain-Back; **Hospital:** Cedars-Sinai Med Ctr (page 88); **Address:** 444 S San Vincente Blvd, Ste 1101, Los Angeles, CA 90048; **Phone:** 310-423-9612; **Board Cert:** Anesthesiology 89; Pain Medicine 93; **Med School:** Univ Miami Sch Med 80; **Resid:** Anesthesiology, Mass Genl Hosp 83; **Fellow:** Pain Medicine, Columbia-Presby Med Ctr

PATHOLOGY

A *pathologist deals with the causes and nature of disease and contributes to diagnosis, prognosis and treatment through knowledge gained by the laboratory application of the biologic, chemical and physical sciences.*

A pathologist uses information gathered from the microscopic examination of tissue specimens, cells and body fluids, and from clinical laboratory tests on body fluids and secretions for the diagnosis, exclusion and monitoring of the disease.

Training required: *Five to seven years*

Certification in the following subspecialty requires additional training and examination.

DERMATOPATHOLOGY:

A dermatopathologist has the expertise to diagnose and monitor diseases of the skin including infectious, immunologic, degenerative and neoplastic diseases. This entails the examination and interpretation of specially prepared tissue sections, cellular scrapings and smears of skin lesions by means of routine and special (electron and fluorescent) microscopes.

PHYSICIAN LISTINGS

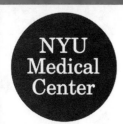

NYU
Medical
Center

550 First Avenue (at 31st Street)
New York, NY 10016
Physician Referral:
1-888-7-NYU-MED
www.nyumc.org

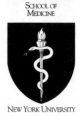

SCHOOL OF
MEDICINE

NEW YORK UNIVERSITY

PATHOLOGY:
Your Consultants in Diagnosis

You've finally found a general practitioner you trust, you're grateful to your dermatologist for botoxing those wrinkles (and spotting that melanoma), and you cherish your relationship with your pediatrician. But chances are, you've never even thought about the pathologists who make the diagnoses on all your family's test results and biopsies.

We're involved in every stage of patient care, from diagnosis and staging to telling your surgeon whether the abnormal tissue they see is malignant or inflammatory helping them select treatments. We are the cornerstone of your cancer diagnosis and treatment team.

CYTOPATHOLOGY: We are national leaders in minimally invasive procedures such as fine needle aspiration (FNA) biopsy, a quick, relatively painless way to obtain cells from a variety of lumps, such as those in the breast, lymph nodes, salivary glands, and thyroid gland. We conduct the biopsies ourselves and review the results with you and your physician. You can have your test, diagnosis, and treatment plan the same day. Our clinic is one of the largest in the city, seeing over 50,000 cytology specimens a year and 5000 fine needle aspirates.

MOLECULAR PATHOLOGY: Molecular testing is an integral part of cancer diagnosis. We can study chromosomal abnormalities to better understand the patient's precise type of cancer and what treatments are likely to work best. We also support our cancer researchers at NYU by providing a tumor bank of tissue samples so that future generations will benefit from the cutting-edge research being conducted at NYU.

SURGICAL PATHOLOGY: Our nationally renowned specialists in gastrointestinal, gynecologic, breast, pediatric, neurologic, urologic, and hematologic malignancies guide surgeons and oncologists in their treatment decisions. With about 43,000 surgical specimens examined each year, we see many malignancies that don't fit the usual mold, so we are able to spot tumor types that are frequently misdiagnosed

PATHOLOGY

New England

Bell, Debra A MD [Path] - **Spec Exp:** Gynecologic Pathology; Ovarian Cancer; **Hospital:** Mass Genl Hosp; **Address:** Pathology Assocs, 55 Fruit St, WRN 105, Boston, MA 02114; **Phone:** 617-726-3977; **Board Cert:** Anatomic Pathology 80; Cytopathology 89; **Med School:** Albany Med Coll 76; **Resid:** Pathology, NYU Med Ctr 81; **Fellow:** Cytopathology, Meml Sloan Kettering Cancer Ctr 82; **Fac Appt:** Assoc Prof Path, Harvard Med Sch

Bhan, Atul Kumar MD [Path] - **Spec Exp:** Immunopathology; Liver Disease; Liver Cancer; **Hospital:** Mass Genl Hosp; **Address:** Mass Genl Hosp, Dept Path, 55 Fruit St, Warren 501, Boston, MA 02114-2620; **Phone:** 617-726-2588; **Board Cert:** Anatomic Pathology 76; Immunopathology 85; **Med School:** India 65; **Resid:** Pathology, Boston Univ Hosp 71; Pathology, Chldns Univ Hosp 74; **Fac Appt:** Prof Path, Harvard Med Sch

Connolly, James Leo MD [Path] - **Spec Exp:** Breast Pathology; Breast Cancer; **Hospital:** Beth Israel Deaconess Med Ctr - Boston; **Address:** BIDMC, Dept Path, 330 Brookline Ave, rm ES 112, Boston, MA 02215-5400; **Phone:** 617-667-4344; **Board Cert:** Anatomic Pathology 80; **Med School:** Vanderbilt Univ 74; **Resid:** Anatomic Pathology, Beth Israel Hosp 78; **Fac Appt:** Prof Path, Harvard Med Sch

DeLellis, Ronald A MD [Path] - **Spec Exp:** Thyroid Cancer; Endocrine Tumors; **Hospital:** Rhode Island Hosp; **Address:** Rhode Island Hospital, Dept Pathology, 593 Eddy St, Providence, RI 02903; **Phone:** 401-444-5154; **Board Cert:** Anatomic Pathology 97; **Med School:** Tufts Univ 66; **Resid:** Anatomic Pathology, Mass Genl Hosp 67; Pathology, Natl Inst Hlth 71; **Fac Appt:** Prof Path, Brown Univ

Fletcher, Christopher MD [Path] - **Spec Exp:** Soft Tissue Tumors; Sarcoma; Surgical Pathology; **Hospital:** Brigham & Women's Hosp (page 87); **Address:** Brigham & Women's Hospital, Dept Pathology, 75 Francis St, Boston, MA 02115-6110; **Phone:** 617-732-8558; **Med School:** England 81; **Resid:** Pathology, St Thomas Hosp 85; **Fellow:** Pathology, St Thomas Hosp; **Fac Appt:** Prof Path, Harvard Med Sch

Harris, Nancy L MD [Path] - **Spec Exp:** Lymphoma; Hematopathology; **Hospital:** Mass Genl Hosp; **Address:** Mass Genl Hosp, Dept Path, 55 Fruit St, Warren 219, Boston, MA 02114; **Phone:** 617-726-5155; **Board Cert:** Anatomic Pathology 78; Clinical Pathology 78; **Med School:** Stanford Univ 70; **Resid:** Pathology, Beth Israel Hosp 78; **Fellow:** Immunopathology, Mass Genl Hosp 80; **Fac Appt:** Prof Path, Harvard Med Sch

Mark, Eugene J MD [Path] - **Spec Exp:** Lung Cancer; Cardiac Pathology; Forensic Pathology; **Hospital:** Mass Genl Hosp; **Address:** Mass Genl Hosp, Dept Path, 55 Fruit St, Warren 246, Boston, MA 02114; **Phone:** 617-726-8891; **Board Cert:** Anatomic Pathology 73; Dermatopathology 75; **Med School:** Harvard Med Sch 67; **Resid:** Pathology, Mass Genl Hosp 72; Pathology, Mass Genl Hosp 79; **Fellow:** Pathology, Dantonsspital 66; **Fac Appt:** Assoc Prof Path, Harvard Med Sch

Odze, Robert D MD [Path] - **Spec Exp:** Gastrointestinal Pathology and Cancer; Liver Pathology; Inflammatory Bowel Disease; **Hospital:** Brigham & Women's Hosp (page 87); **Address:** Brigham & Women's Hospital, Dept Pathology, 75 Francis St, Boston, MA 02115; **Phone:** 617-732-7549; **Board Cert:** Anatomic Pathology 90; **Med School:** McGill Univ 84; **Resid:** Surgery, McGill Univ 87; Pathology, McGill Univ 90; **Fellow:** Gastrointestinal Pathology, New England Deaconess Med Ctr 91; **Fac Appt:** Assoc Prof Path, Harvard Med Sch

Schnitt, Stuart J MD [Path] - **Spec Exp:** Breast Pathology; Breast Cancer; **Hospital:** Beth Israel Deaconess Med Ctr - Boston; **Address:** Beth Israel Deaconess Med Ctr, Dept Pathology, 330 Brookline Ave, Boston, MA 02215-5400; **Phone:** 617-667-4344; **Board Cert:** Anatomic & Clinical Pathology 83; **Med School:** Albany Med Coll 79; **Resid:** Anatomic Pathology, Beth Israel Deaconess Med Ctr; **Fellow:** Surgical Pathology, Beth Israel Deaconess Med Ctr; **Fac Appt:** Assoc Prof Path, Harvard Med Sch

Young, Robert H MD [Path] - **Spec Exp:** Ovarian Cancer; Breast Cancer; **Hospital:** Mass Genl Hosp; **Address:** Mass Genl Hosp, Dept Path, 55 Fruit St Bldg Warren - rm 215, Boston, MA 02114; **Phone:** 617-726-8892; **Board Cert:** Anatomic Pathology 80; **Med School:** Ireland 74; **Resid:** Pathology, Mass Genl Hosp 79; Pathology, Dublin Univ 77; **Fac Appt:** Prof Path, Harvard Med Sch

Mid Atlantic

Burger, Peter MD [Path] - **Spec Exp:** Brain Tumors; Neuropathology; **Hospital:** Johns Hopkins Hosp - Baltimore (page 97); **Address:** 600 N Wolfe St, Pathology 710, Baltimore, MD 21287; **Phone:** 410-955-8378; **Board Cert:** Anatomic Pathology 76; Neuropathology 76; **Med School:** Northwestern Univ 66; **Resid:** Anatomic Pathology, Duke Univ Med Ctr 73; **Fellow:** Neuropathology, Duke Univ Med Ctr 73

Dorfman, Howard D MD [Path] - **Spec Exp:** Bone Tumor Pathology; Soft Tissue Tumors; Joint Pathology; **Hospital:** Montefiore Med Ctr; **Address:** Orthopaedic Pathology Div, 111 E 210th St, Bronx, NY 10467-2401; **Phone:** 718-920-5622; **Board Cert:** Anatomic Pathology 58; **Med School:** SUNY Downstate 51; **Resid:** Pathology, Mt Sinai Hosp 53; Surgical Pathology, Columbia-Presby Med Ctr 58; **Fellow:** Pathology, Mt Sinai Med Ctr 54; **Fac Appt:** Prof Path, Albert Einstein Coll Med

Epstein, Jonathan MD [Path] - **Spec Exp:** Bladder Cancer; Urologic Cancer & Pathology; Prostate Cancer; **Hospital:** Johns Hopkins Hosp - Baltimore (page 97); **Address:** 401 N Broadway, Weinberg 2242, Baltimore, MD 21231; **Phone:** 410-955-5043; **Board Cert:** Anatomic Pathology 86; **Med School:** Boston Univ 81; **Resid:** Pathology, Johns Hopkins Hosp 85; **Fellow:** Pathology, Meml Sloan Kettering Cancer Ctr 84; **Fac Appt:** Prof Path, Johns Hopkins Univ

Frizzera, Glauco MD [Path] - **Spec Exp:** Hematopathology; Lymph Node Pathology; Lymphoma; **Hospital:** NY-Presby Hosp - NY Weill Cornell Med Ctr (page 103); **Address:** 525 E 68th St, Starr - 737A, New York, NY 10021-4870; **Phone:** 212-746-6401; **Board Cert:** Anatomic Pathology 97; **Med School:** Italy 64; **Resid:** Pathology, Univ Bologna 69; **Fellow:** Hematology, Univ Chicago 74; **Fac Appt:** Prof Path, Cornell Univ-Weill Med Coll

Gupta, Prabodh K MD [Path] - **Spec Exp:** Lung Pathology; Cervical Pathology; **Hospital:** Hosp Univ Penn - UPHS (page 113); **Address:** Hosp Univ Penn - Cytopathology, 3400 Spruce St, 6 Founders, Philadelphia, PA 19104; **Phone:** 215-662-3238; **Board Cert:** Anatomic Pathology 75; Cytopathology 89; **Med School:** India 65; **Resid:** Pathology, All India Inst Med Scis 67; **Fellow:** Pathology, Mass Genl Hosp 68; **Fac Appt:** Prof Path, Univ Pennsylvania

Hoda, Syed A F MD [Path] - **Spec Exp:** Breast Cancer; **Hospital:** NY-Presby Hosp - NY Weill Cornell Med Ctr (page 103); **Address:** 525 E 68th St, 1028 Starr, New York, NY 10021; **Phone:** 212-746-2700; **Board Cert:** Anatomic & Clinical Pathology 01; Cytopathology 91; **Med School:** Pakistan 84; **Resid:** Anatomic & Clinical Pathology, Tulane Univ Affil Hosps 90; **Fellow:** Cytopathology, Meml Sloan Kettering Cancer Ctr 91; Pathology, Meml Sloan Kettering Cancer Ctr 92; **Fac Appt:** Assoc Clin Prof Path, Cornell Univ-Weill Med Coll

Hruban, Ralph H MD [Path] - **Spec Exp:** Gastrointestinal Pathology; Pancreatic Cancer; **Hospital:** Johns Hopkins Hosp - Baltimore (page 97); **Address:** Johns Hopkins Hosp, Dept Pathology, 401 N Broadway Bldg Weinberg - rm 2242, Baltimore, MD 21231; **Phone:** 410-955-9132; **Board Cert:** Anatomic Pathology 90; **Med School:** Johns Hopkins Univ 85; **Resid:** Pathology, Johns Hopkins Hosp 90; **Fellow:** Meml Sloan Kettering Cancer Ctr 89; **Fac Appt:** Prof Path, Johns Hopkins Univ

Huvos, Andrew G MD [Path] - **Spec Exp:** Bone Tumors; Head & Neck Tumors; **Hospital:** Meml Sloan Kettering Cancer Ctr (page 100); **Address:** Meml Sloan Kettering Cancer Ctr, Dept Pathology, 1275 York Ave, New York, NY 10021-6007; **Phone:** 212-639-5905; **Board Cert:** Anatomic Pathology 98; **Med School:** Germany 63; **Resid:** Pathology, Meml Cancer Hosp 69; **Fellow:** Surgical Pathology, Columbia Presby Hosp 67; **Fac Appt:** Prof Path, Cornell Univ-Weill Med Coll

Jaffe, Elaine S MD [Path] - **Spec Exp:** Lymphoma; Hematopathology; **Hospital:** Natl Inst of Hlth - Clin Ctr; **Address:** Natl Cancer Inst. NIH-Lab Pathology, 10 Center Drive Bldg 10 - rm 2N202 MSC 1500, Bethesda, MD 20892; **Phone:** 301-496-0183; **Board Cert:** Anatomic Pathology 74; **Med School:** Univ Pennsylvania 69; **Resid:** Pathology, Clinical Ctr/NIH 72; Pathology; **Fellow:** Hematopathology, Natl Cancer Inst 74; **Fac Appt:** Clin Prof Path, Geo Wash Univ

Katzenstein, Anna-Luise A MD [Path] - **Spec Exp:** Lung Cancer; Pulmonary Pathology; Vasculitis; **Hospital:** Univ. Hosp.- SUNY Upstate; **Address:** SUNY Upstate Medical Univ, 766 Irving Ave, Weiskotten, rm 2106, Syracuse, NY 13210; **Phone:** 315-464-7125; **Board Cert:** Anatomic Pathology 76; **Med School:** Johns Hopkins Univ 71; **Resid:** Pathology, Univ Hospital 75; **Fellow:** Surgical Pathology, Barnes Hosp-Wash Univ 76; **Fac Appt:** Prof Path, SUNY Upstate Med Univ

Knowles, Daniel MD [Path] - **Spec Exp:** Lymph Node Pathology; Bone Marrow Pathology; Lymphoma; **Hospital:** NY-Presby Hosp - NY Weill Cornell Med Ctr (page 103); **Address:** Cornell-Weill Medical College, Dept Pathology, 1300 York Ave, rm C302, New York, NY 10021; **Phone:** 212-746-6464; **Board Cert:** Anatomic Pathology 78; Immunopathology 84; **Med School:** Univ Chicago-Pritzker Sch Med 73; **Resid:** Anatomic Pathology, Columbia-Presby Med Ctr 78; **Fellow:** Immunopathology, Rockefeller Univ 77; **Fac Appt:** Prof Path, Cornell Univ-Weill Med Coll

Kurman, Robert J MD [Path] - **Spec Exp:** Gynecologic Pathology; Ovarian Cancer; Uterine Cancer; **Hospital:** Johns Hopkins Hosp - Baltimore (page 97); **Address:** Johns Hopkins Hosp, Dept Pathology, 401 N Broadway, Weinberg-2242, Baltimore, MD 21231; **Phone:** 410-955-0471; **Board Cert:** Anatomic Pathology 72; Obstetrics & Gynecology 80; **Med School:** SUNY Upstate Med Univ 68; **Resid:** Pathology, Peter Bent Brigham Hosp/Mass Genl Hosp 77; Obstetrics & Gynecology, LAC Hosp/USC 78; **Fellow:** Obstetrics & Gynecology, Harvard Univ 73; **Fac Appt:** Prof Path, Johns Hopkins Univ

Li Volsi, Virginia A MD [Path] - **Spec Exp:** Endocrine Cancer; Thyroid Cancer; Gynecologic Cancer; **Hospital:** Hosp Univ Penn - UPHS (page 113); **Address:** Hosp Univ Penn - Pathology, 3400 Spruce St, Philadelphia, PA 19104; **Phone:** 215-662-6544; **Board Cert:** Anatomic Pathology 74; **Med School:** Columbia P&S 69; **Resid:** Anatomic Pathology, Presbyterian Hosp 74; **Fac Appt:** Prof Path, Univ Pennsylvania

McCormick, Steven MD [Path] - **Spec Exp:** Ophthalmic Pathology/Cancer; Head & Neck Pathology; **Hospital:** New York Eye & Ear Infirm (page 102); **Address:** 310 E 14th St, New York, NY 10003; **Phone:** 212-979-4156; **Board Cert:** Anatomic Pathology 88; **Med School:** W VA Univ 84; **Resid:** Anatomic Pathology, W Va Univ Hosp 88; **Fellow:** Ophthalmic Pathology, W Va Univ Hosp 88; **Fac Appt:** Assoc Prof Path, NY Med Coll

Melamed, Jonathan MD [Path] - **Spec Exp:** Prostate Cancer; Tumor Banking; **Hospital:** NYU Med Ctr (page 104); **Address:** NYU Medical Ctr, Dept Pathology, 160 First Ave, New York, NY 10016; **Phone:** 212-263-8927; **Board Cert:** Anatomic & Clinical Pathology 92; **Med School:** South Africa 85; **Resid:** Pathology, Lenox Hill Hosp 91; **Fellow:** Pathology, Meml Sloan Kettering Cancer Ctr 92; Urologic Pathology, Meml Sloan Kettering Cancer Ctr 93; **Fac Appt:** Assoc Prof Path, NYU Sch Med

Mies, Carolyn MD [Path] - **Spec Exp:** Breast Cancer; **Hospital:** Hosp Univ Penn - UPHS (page 113); **Address:** Hosp Univ Penn - Surgical Pathology, 3400 Spruce St, Founders 6, Philadelphia, PA 19104; **Phone:** 215-662-6503; **Board Cert:** Anatomic Pathology 80; **Med School:** Rush Med Coll 80; **Resid:** Pathology, Tufts-New England Med Ctr 82; Pathology, New England Deaconess Hosp 84; **Fellow:** Surgical Pathology, Meml Sloan Kettering Cancer Ctr 86; **Fac Appt:** Assoc Prof Path, Univ Pennsylvania

Montgomery, Elizabeth A MD [Path] - **Spec Exp:** Barrett's Esophagus; Esophageal Cancer; Gastrointestinal Pathology; **Hospital:** Johns Hopkins Hosp - Baltimore (page 97); **Address:** Johns Hopkins Univ, Dept Pathology, 720 Rutland Ave, Ross 632, Baltimore, MD 21205; **Phone:** 410-955-3511; **Board Cert:** Anatomic Pathology 88; Cytopathology 94; **Med School:** Geo Wash Univ 84; **Resid:** Pathology, Walter Reed AMC 88; **Fac Appt:** Assoc Prof Path, Johns Hopkins Univ

Orenstein, Jan M MD/PhD [Path] - **Spec Exp:** Prostate Cancer; Tumor Banking; **Hospital:** G Washington Univ Hosp; **Address:** Geo Wash Univ Med Ctr-Path, Ross 502, 2300 Eye St NW, Washington, DC 20037; **Phone:** 202-994-2943; **Board Cert:** Anatomic Pathology 77; **Med School:** SUNY Downstate 71; **Resid:** Pathology, Presby Hosp 73; **Fellow:** Pathology, Natl Cancer Inst-NIH 77; **Fac Appt:** Prof Path, Geo Wash Univ

Patchefsky, Arthur S MD [Path] - **Spec Exp:** Breast Cancer; Pulmonary Pathology; **Hospital:** Fox Chase Cancer Ctr (page 95); **Address:** Fox Chase Cancer Center, 7701 Burholme Ave, rm C4333, Philadelphia, PA 19111; **Phone:** 215-728-5390; **Board Cert:** Anatomic Pathology 69; **Med School:** Hahnemann Univ 63; **Resid:** Pathology, John Hopkins Hosp 66; Pathology, Hosp U Penn 67; **Fellow:** Pathology, Meml Sloan Kettering Cancer Ctr 68; **Fac Appt:** Prof Path, Thomas Jefferson Univ

Rosen, Paul P MD [Path] - **Spec Exp:** Breast Pathology; Breast Cancer; **Hospital:** NY-Presby Hosp - NY Weill Cornell Med Ctr (page 103); **Address:** New York Presbyterian, Dept Pathology, 525 E 68th St, Starr 103, New York, NY 10021-4870; **Phone:** 212-746-6482; **Board Cert:** Anatomic Pathology 98; **Med School:** Columbia P&S 64; **Resid:** Pathology, Presby Hosp 66; Pathology, VA Hosp 68; **Fellow:** Pathology, Meml Hosp Cancer Ctr 70; **Fac Appt:** Prof Path, Cornell Univ-Weill Med Coll

Ross, Jeffrey S MD [Path] - **Spec Exp:** Urologic Cancer & Disease; Prostate Cancer & Disease; Breast Cancer; **Hospital:** Albany Med Ctr; **Address:** Albany Med Coll, Dept Path, New Scotland Ave, MC 81, Albany, NY 12208; **Phone:** 518-262-5471; **Board Cert:** Anatomic & Clinical Pathology 74; **Med School:** SUNY Buffalo 70; **Resid:** Pathology, Mass Genl Hosp 74; **Fellow:** Pathology, Harvard Med Sch 74; **Fac Appt:** Prof Path, Albany Med Coll

Sanchez, Miguel A MD [Path] - **Spec Exp:** Breast Cancer; Thyroid Cancer; **Hospital:** Englewood Hosp & Med Ctr; **Address:** Englewood Hosp & Med Ctr, Dept Pathology, 350 Engle St, Englewood, NJ 07631-1898; **Phone:** 201-894-3423; **Board Cert:** Anatomic Pathology 75; Clinical Pathology 79; Cytopathology 91; **Med School:** Spain 69; **Resid:** Pathology, Englewood Hosp 72; Pathology, Temple Univ 73; **Fellow:** Pathology, Meml Sloan Kettering Cancer Ctr 74; **Fac Appt:** Assoc Prof Path, Mount Sinai Sch Med

Schiller, Alan L MD **[Path]** - **Spec Exp:** Bone & Joint Pathology; Soft Tissue Pathology; Bone Tumors; **Hospital:** Mount Sinai Med Ctr (page 101); **Address:** Mt Sinai Sch Med, Dept Pathology, 1 Gustave Levy Pl, Box 1194, New York, NY 10029-6500; **Phone:** 212-241-8014; **Board Cert:** Anatomic Pathology 73; **Med School:** Univ Hlth Sci/Chicago Med Sch 67; **Resid:** Pathology, Mass Genl Hosp 72; **Fac Appt:** Prof Path, Mount Sinai Sch Med

Silverberg, Steven G MD **[Path]** - **Spec Exp:** Gynecologic Cancer & Pathology; Breast Cancer & Pathology; Urologic Pathology; **Hospital:** Univ of MD Med Sys; **Address:** University of Maryland Medical Ctr, Dept Pathology, 22 S Greene St, Baltimore, MD 21201; **Phone:** 410-328-5072; **Board Cert:** Anatomic Pathology 69; **Med School:** Johns Hopkins Univ 62; **Resid:** Pathology, Yale-New Haven Hosp 65; **Fellow:** Surgical Pathology, Meml Sloan Kettering Cancer Ctr 66; **Fac Appt:** Prof Path, Univ MD Sch Med

Silverman, Jan F MD **[Path]** - **Spec Exp:** Breast Cancer; Lung Cancer; Gastrointestinal Pathology; **Hospital:** Allegheny General Hosp; **Address:** Allegheny Gen Hosp-Dept Lab Medicine, 320 E North Ave, Pittsburgh, PA 15212; **Phone:** 412-359-6886; **Board Cert:** Anatomic & Clinical Pathology 75; Cytopathology 89; **Med School:** Med Coll VA ; **Resid:** Pathology, Medical College of VA 75; **Fellow:** Surgical Pathology, Medical College of VA 75; **Fac Appt:** Prof Path, Drexel Univ Coll Med

Swerdlow, Steven H MD **[Path]** - **Spec Exp:** Lymphoma; Hematopathology; Transplant Pathology; **Hospital:** UPMC Presby, Pittsburgh (page 114); **Address:** UPMC-Presby Hosp, Div Hematopathology, 200 Lothrop St, rm C606, Pittsburgh, PA 15213-2582; **Phone:** 412-647-5191; **Board Cert:** Anatomic Pathology 79; Clinical Pathology 79; **Med School:** Harvard Med Sch 75; **Resid:** Pathology, Beth Israel Hosp 79; **Fellow:** Hematopathology, Vanderbilt Univ 81; Hematopathology, St Bartholmew's Hosp 83; **Fac Appt:** Prof Path, Univ Pittsburgh

Tomaszewski, John E MD **[Path]** - **Spec Exp:** Breast Cancer; Head & Neck Cancer; Ovarian, Uterine Cancer; **Hospital:** Hosp Univ Penn - UPHS (page 113); **Address:** Hosp Univ Penn, Dept Pathology & Lab Med, 3400 Spruce St, 6 Founders Bldg, Ste 6056, Philadelphia, PA 19104; **Phone:** 215-662-6852; **Board Cert:** Anatomic Pathology 82; Immunopathology 83; **Med School:** Univ Pennsylvania 77; **Resid:** Pathology, Hosp Univ Penn 82; **Fellow:** Surgical Pathology, Hosp Univ Penn 83; **Fac Appt:** Prof Path, Univ Pennsylvania

Travis, William MD **[Path]** - **Spec Exp:** Pulmonary Pathology; Lung Cancer; Interstitial Lung Disease; **Hospital:** Meml Sloan Kettering Cancer Ctr (page 100); **Address:** Meml Sloan-Kettering Cancer Ctr, Dept Pathology, 1275 York Ave, New York, NY 10021; **Phone:** 212-639-5905; **Board Cert:** Anatomic & Clinical Pathology 85; **Med School:** Univ Fla Coll Med 81; **Resid:** Anatomic Pathology, New England Deaconess Hosp 83; Clinical Pathology, Mayo Clinic 85; **Fellow:** Surgical Pathology, Mayo Clinic 86

Yousem, Samuel A. MD **[Path]** - **Spec Exp:** Pulmonary Pathology; Transplant-Lung (Pathology); Lung Cancer & Disease; **Hospital:** UPMC Presby, Pittsburgh (page 114); **Address:** Dept Pathology, A-610, 200 Lothrop St, Pittsburgh, PA 15213; **Phone:** 412-647-6193; **Board Cert:** Anatomic Pathology 85; Cytopathology 97; **Med School:** Univ MD Sch Med 81; **Resid:** Pathology, Stanford Univ Med Ctr 83; **Fellow:** Surgical Pathology, Stanford Univ Med Ctr 84; **Fac Appt:** Prof Path, Univ Pittsburgh

Southeast

Amin, Mahul MD **[Path]** - **Spec Exp:** Genitourinary Pathology; Bladder Pathology; **Hospital:** Emory Univ Hosp; **Address:** Emory Univ Hosp, 1364 Clifton Rd NE, Ste G-167, Atlanta, GA 30322; **Phone:** 404-712-0190; **Board Cert:** Anatomic & Clinical Pathology 96; **Med School:** India 83; **Resid:** Pathology, Henry Ford Hosp 92; **Fellow:** Surgical Pathology, MD Anderson Cancer Ctr 93; **Fac Appt:** Prof Path, Emory Univ

Banks, Peter MD [Path] - **Spec Exp:** Hematopathology; Lymphoma; **Hospital:** Carolinas Med Ctr; **Address:** Dept Pathology, 1000 Blythe Blvd, 4th Fl Lab, Charlotte, NC 28203; **Phone:** 704-355-2251; **Board Cert:** Anatomic Pathology 97; **Med School:** Harvard Med Sch 71; **Resid:** Pathology, National Cancer Inst 74; Pathology, Duke Univ Med Ctr 75; **Fellow:** Surgical Pathology, Univ Minn Med Ctr 76; **Fac Appt:** Prof Path, Univ NC Sch Med

Behm, Frederick G MD [Path] - **Hospital:** St Jude Children's Research Hosp; **Address:** St Jude Children's Research Hosp, 332 N Lauderdale St, Memphis, TN 38105; **Phone:** 901-495-3300; **Board Cert:** Anatomic & Clinical Pathology 80; Hematology 83; **Med School:** Med Coll Wisc 74; **Resid:** Pathology, Medical Coll of Va 79; **Fac Appt:** Assoc Prof Path, Univ Tenn Coll Med, Memphis

Bostwick, David MD [Path] - **Spec Exp:** Urologic Pathology; Prostate Cancer; Bladder Cancer; **Address:** 4355 Innflake Drive, Glen Allen, VA 23060; **Phone:** 804-967-9225; **Board Cert:** Anatomic Pathology 85; **Med School:** Univ MD Sch Med 79; **Resid:** Pathology, Stanford Univ 81; **Fellow:** Surgical Pathology, Stanford Univ 84; **Fac Appt:** Clin Prof Path, Univ VA Sch Med

Braylan, Raul MD [Path] - **Spec Exp:** Hematopathology; Leukemia; Lymphoma; **Hospital:** Shands Hlthcre at Univ of FL (page 109); **Address:** University of Florida, Dept Hematopathology, Box 100275, Gainesville, FL 32610; **Phone:** 352-392-3477; **Board Cert:** Anatomic Pathology 72; **Med School:** Argentina 60; **Resid:** Anatomic Pathology, Mt Sinai Hosp 65; Anatomic Pathology, Einstein Affil Hosps 67; **Fellow:** Anatomic Pathology, Meml Sloan Kettering Cancer Hosp 68; Hematopathology, Univ Chicago Hosps 73; **Fac Appt:** Prof Path, Univ Fla Coll Med

Crawford, James M MD/PhD [Path] - **Spec Exp:** Liver Pathology; Gastrointestinal Pathology; Gastrointestinal Cancer; **Hospital:** Shands Hlthcre at Univ of FL (page 109); **Address:** Univ Florida, Dept Pathology, 1600 SW Archer Rd, rm M649, Box 100275, Gainesville, FL 32610; **Phone:** 352-392-3741; **Board Cert:** Anatomic Pathology 87; **Med School:** Duke Univ 82; **Resid:** Pathology, Brigham & Women's Hosp 84; **Fellow:** Gastrointestinal Pathology, Brigham & Women's Hosp 87; **Fac Appt:** Prof Path, Univ Fla Coll Med

Lage, Janice MD [Path] - **Spec Exp:** Obstetric Pathology; Gynecologic Pathology; Breast Pathology; **Hospital:** MUSC Med Ctr; **Address:** MUSC Med Ctr, Dept Path, 165 Ashley Ave, Ste 309, Box 250908, Charleston, SC 29425; **Phone:** 843-792-3121; **Board Cert:** Anatomic Pathology 01; **Med School:** Washington Univ, St Louis 80; **Resid:** Pathology, Barnes Hosp/Wash Univ 82; Obstetrics & Gynecology, Barnes Hosp/Wash Univ 83; **Fellow:** Surgical Pathology, Barnes Hosp/Wash Univ 84; **Fac Appt:** Prof Path, Med Univ SC

Masood, Shahla MD [Path] - **Spec Exp:** Breast Cancer; Breast Pathology; **Hospital:** Shands Jacksonville (page 109); **Address:** Shands Jacksonville, Dept Pathology, 655 W 8th St, Jacksonville, FL 32209-6511; **Phone:** 904-244-4387; **Board Cert:** Anatomic Pathology 98; Cytopathology 90; **Med School:** Iran 73; **Resid:** Anatomic Pathology, University Hospital 77; **Fac Appt:** Assoc Prof Path, Univ Fla Coll Med

McCurley, Thomas L MD [Path] - **Spec Exp:** Hematopathology; Lymphoma; **Hospital:** Vanderbilt Univ Med Ctr (page 116); **Address:** Vanderbilt Univ Hosp, Dept Pathology, 21st & Garland Ave, Nashville, TN 37232; **Phone:** 615-343-9167; **Board Cert:** Anatomic & Clinical Pathology 81; Immunopathology 86; Hematology 99; **Med School:** Vanderbilt Univ 74; **Resid:** Internal Medicine, UCSF Med Ctr 76; Pathology, Vanderbilt Univ Med Ctr 81; **Fellow:** Hematopathology, Vanderbilt Univ Med Ctr 84; **Fac Appt:** Assoc Prof Path, Vanderbilt Univ

Mills, Stacey E MD [Path] - **Spec Exp:** Breast Pathology; ENT Cancer; Surgical Pathology; **Hospital:** Univ Virginia Med Ctr; **Address:** Univ VA Hlth System, Dept Pathology, PO Box 800214, OMS Fl 3 - rm 3874, Charlottesville, VA 22908-0214; **Phone:** 434-982-4406; **Board Cert:** Anatomic Pathology 99; **Med School:** Univ VA Sch Med 77; **Resid:** Pathology, Univ Virginia Med Ctr 80; **Fellow:** Pathology, Univ Virginia 81; **Fac Appt:** Prof Path, Univ VA Sch Med

Murphy, William M MD [Path] - **Spec Exp:** Bladder Cancer; Prostate Cancer; Kidney Cancer (Adult); **Hospital:** Shands Hlthcre at Univ of FL (page 109); **Address:** Shands at Univ Florida - Dept Pathology, 1600 SW Archer Rd, rm 3109, Gainesville, FL 32610; **Phone:** 352-265-0432; **Board Cert:** Anatomic Pathology 99; **Med School:** Harvard Med Sch 67; **Resid:** Pathology, Case Western Reserve Univ 71; **Fellow:** Immunology, Cleveland Clinic 72; **Fac Appt:** Prof Path, Univ Fla Coll Med

Nicosia, Santo MD [Path] - **Spec Exp:** Ovarian Cancer; **Hospital:** H Lee Moffitt Cancer Ctr & Research Inst; **Address:** 12901 Bruce B Downs Blvd, MDC Box 11, Tampa, FL 33612-4742; **Phone:** 813-974-3133; **Board Cert:** Anatomic Pathology 78; Cytopathology 90; **Med School:** Italy 67; **Resid:** Anatomic Pathology, Michael Reese Hosp 72; Obstetrics & Gynecology, Catholic Univ Hosps; **Fellow:** Hosp Univ Penn 73; **Fac Appt:** Prof Path, Univ S Fla Coll Med

Page, David L MD [Path] - **Spec Exp:** Breast Cancer; Skin Cancer; **Hospital:** Vanderbilt Univ Med Ctr (page 116); **Address:** Vanderbilt Univ, MCN, 1161 21st Ave S, rm C 3309, Nashville, TN 37232-2561; **Phone:** 615-322-3759; **Board Cert:** Anatomic Pathology 72; Dermatopathology 74; **Med School:** Johns Hopkins Univ 66; **Resid:** Pathology, Mass Genl Hosp 69; Pathology, Johns Hopkins Hosp 72; **Fac Appt:** Prof Path, Vanderbilt Univ

Sewell, C Whitaker MD [Path] - **Spec Exp:** Breast Pathology; Surgical Pathology; **Hospital:** Emory Univ Hosp; **Address:** Emory Univ Hosp, Dept Pathology, 1364 Clifton Rd NE, rm H187, Atlanta, GA 30322; **Phone:** 404-712-7003; **Board Cert:** Anatomic Pathology 74; Clinical Pathology 74; **Med School:** Emory Univ 69; **Resid:** Pathology, Emory Univ Hosp 74; **Fac Appt:** Prof Path, Emory Univ

Weiss, Sharon MD [Path] - **Spec Exp:** Soft Tissue Pathology; Surgical Pathology; Sarcoma; **Hospital:** Emory Univ Hosp; **Address:** Emory Univ Hosp, Dept Path, 1364 Clifton Rd NE, Fl H180, Atlanta, GA 30322; **Phone:** 404-712-0708; **Board Cert:** Anatomic Pathology 74; **Med School:** Johns Hopkins Univ 71; **Resid:** Pathology, Johns Hopkins Hosp 75; **Fac Appt:** Prof Path, Emory Univ

Midwest

Balla, Andre K MD/PhD [Path] - **Spec Exp:** Prostate Cancer; Gynecologic Pathology; Tumor Banking; **Hospital:** Univ of IL Med Ctr at Chicago; **Address:** Univ IL at Chicago, Dept Path, 1819 W Polk St, rm 446, MC 847, Chicago, IL 60612; **Phone:** 312-996-3879; **Board Cert:** Anatomic & Clinical Pathology 88; **Med School:** Brazil 72; **Resid:** Pathology, Hahnemann Univ Hosp 88; **Fellow:** Clinical Immunology, Scripps Clin Rsch Fdn 81; **Fac Appt:** Prof Path, Univ IL Coll Med

Cho, Kathleen R MD [Path] - **Spec Exp:** Gynecologic Pathology; Ovarian Cancer; Cervical Cancer; **Hospital:** Univ Michigan Hlth Sys; **Address:** Univ Michigan -Life Sciences Bldg, 210 Washtenaw Ave, rm 5401, Ann Arbor, MI 48109-2216; **Phone:** 734-764-1549; **Board Cert:** Anatomic Pathology 90; **Med School:** Vanderbilt Univ 84; **Resid:** Pathology, Johns Hopkins Hosp 88; **Fellow:** Gynecologic Pathology, Johns Hopkins Hosp 90; **Fac Appt:** Prof Path, Univ Mich Med Sch

Cohen, Michael B MD [Path] - **Spec Exp:** Prostate Cancer; Urologic Pathology; **Hospital:** Univ Iowa Hosp & Clinics; **Address:** Univ Iowa - Dept Pathology, 200 Hawkins Drive, rm C670GH, Iowa City, IA 52242; **Phone:** 319-384-9609; **Board Cert:** Anatomic Pathology 98; Cytopathology 96; **Med School:** Albany Med Coll 82; **Resid:** Pathology, UCSF Hosps-Clinics 87; **Fellow:** Cytopathology, UCSF Hosps-Clinics 87; **Fac Appt:** Prof Path, Univ Iowa Coll Med

Goldblum, John R MD [Path] - **Spec Exp:** Soft Tissue Pathology-Sarcoma; Esophageal Cancer; Gastrointestinal Stromal Tumors; **Hospital:** Cleveland Clin Fdn (page 92); **Address:** Cleveland Clinic, Chairman, Dept. Anatomic Pathology L25, 9500 Euclid Ave, Cleveland, OH 44195; **Phone:** 216-444-8238; **Board Cert:** Anatomic Pathology 93; **Med School:** Univ Mich Med Sch 89; **Resid:** Anatomic Pathology, Univ Michigan Hosps 93; **Fac Appt:** Prof Path, Cleveland Cl Coll Med/Case West Res

Greenson, Joel K MD [Path] - **Spec Exp:** Liver Cancer & Disease; Gastrointestinal Tumors & Disorders; **Hospital:** Univ Michigan Hlth Sys; **Address:** University of Michigan Hospitals, Dept Pathology, 1500 E Medical Center Drive, rm 2G332, Ann arbor, MI 48109-0054; **Phone:** 734-936-6776; **Board Cert:** Anatomic & Clinical Pathology 88; **Med School:** Univ Mich Med Sch 84; **Resid:** Pathology, Cedars-Sinai Med Ctr 88; **Fellow:** Gastrointestinal Pathology, Johns Hopkins Hosp 90; **Fac Appt:** Assoc Prof Path, Univ Mich Med Sch

Kurtin, Paul J MD [Path] - **Spec Exp:** Lumph Node Pathology; Bone Marrow Pathology; Lymphoma; **Hospital:** Mayo Med Ctr & Clin - Rochester; **Address:** Mayo Clinic, Hilton Bldg, 200 First St, rm 1156, Rochester, MN 55905; **Phone:** 507-284-4939; **Board Cert:** Anatomic & Clinical Pathology 83; Hematology 88; **Med School:** Med Coll Wisc 79; **Resid:** Anatomic Pathology, Brigham & Women's Hosp 83; **Fellow:** Hematopathology, Brigham & Women's Hosp 84; **Fac Appt:** Prof Path, Mayo Med Sch

Myers, Jeffrey L MD [Path] - **Spec Exp:** Lung Cancer; Lung Pathology; **Hospital:** Mayo Med Ctr & Clin - Rochester; **Address:** Mayo Clinic, Dept Pathology, 200 First St, Rochester, MN 55905; **Phone:** 507-284-2656; **Board Cert:** Anatomic Pathology 86; **Med School:** Washington Univ, St Louis 81; **Resid:** Anatomic Pathology, Barnes Jewish Hosp 84; **Fellow:** Surgical Pathology, U Alabama Med Ctr 85; **Fac Appt:** Prof Path, Mayo Med Sch

Nascimento, Anthony MD [Path] - **Spec Exp:** Bone & Soft Tissue Pathology; Head & Neck Pathology; **Hospital:** Mayo Med Ctr & Clin - Rochester; **Address:** Mayo Clinic - Dept Pathology, 200 First St SW, Rochester, MN 55905; **Phone:** 507-284-1187; **Board Cert:** Anatomic Pathology 79; **Med School:** Brazil ; **Resid:** Pathology, Univ Mississippi Med Ctr; **Fellow:** Anatomic Pathology, Meml Sloan-Kettering Cancer Ctr; Surgical Pathology, Mayo Clinic

Perlman, Elizabeth J MD [Path] - **Spec Exp:** Wilms' Tumor; Pediatric Tumors; **Hospital:** Children's Mem Hosp; **Address:** Children's Memorial Hosp, 2300 Children's Plaza, Box 17, Chicago, IL 60614; **Phone:** 773-880-4306; **Board Cert:** Anatomic Pathology 90; Pediatric Pathology 91; **Med School:** Johns Hopkins Univ 84; **Resid:** Pathology, Johns Hopkins Hosp 88; **Fellow:** Pediatric Pathology, Johns Hopkins Hosp 90; **Fac Appt:** Prof Path, Northwestern Univ

Scheithauer, Bernd MD [Path] - **Spec Exp:** Brain Tumors; Pituitary Cancer & Disorders; Neuro-Pathology; **Hospital:** Mayo Med Ctr & Clin - Rochester; **Address:** Mayo Clinic, Dept Pathology, 200 First St SW, Rochester, MN 55905; **Phone:** 507-284-8350; **Board Cert:** Anatomic Pathology 79; Neuropathology 79; **Med School:** Loma Linda Univ 73; **Resid:** Anatomic Pathology, Stanford Med Ctr 76; Neuropathology, Stanford Med Ctr 78; **Fac Appt:** Prof Path, Mayo Med Sch

Suster, Saul M MD [Path] - **Spec Exp:** Lung Cancer; Mediastinal Cancer; Surgical Pathology; **Hospital:** Ohio St Univ Med Ctr (page 105); **Address:** Ohio State University Med Ctr, E-411 Doan Hall, Dept Pathology, 410 W 10th Ave, Columbus, OH 43210; **Phone:** 614-293-7625; **Board Cert:** Anatomic & Clinical Pathology 88; **Med School:** Ecuador 76; **Resid:** Anatomic Pathology, Tel Aviv Univ Med Ctr 84; Anatomic & Clinical Pathology, Mt Sinai Med Ctr 88; **Fellow:** Surgical Pathology, Yale-New Haven Hosp 90; **Fac Appt:** Prof Path, Ohio State Univ

Ulbright, Thomas M MD [Path] - **Spec Exp:** Testicular Cancer; Gynecologic Pathology; **Hospital:** Indiana Univ Hosp (page 90); **Address:** Indiana University Hospital, Dept Pathology, 550 N University Blvd, rm 3465, Indianapolis, IN 46202; **Phone:** 317-274-3486; **Board Cert:** Anatomic Pathology 80; **Med School:** Washington Univ, St Louis 75; **Resid:** Pathology, Barnes Jewish Hosp 78; Surgical Pathology, Barnes Jewish Hosp 79; **Fellow:** Gynecologic Pathology, St Johns Mercy Med Ctr 80; **Fac Appt:** Prof Path, Indiana Univ

Unni, K Krishnan MD [Path] - **Spec Exp:** Bone Tumors; Lung Cancer; **Hospital:** Mayo Med Ctr & Clin - Rochester; **Address:** Mayo Medical Lab, Dept Pathology, 200 First St SW, Rochester, MN 55905-0001; **Phone:** 507-284-1193; **Board Cert:** Anatomic Pathology 69; **Med School:** India 62; **Resid:** Pathology, Mayo Grad Sch 70; **Fellow:** Pathology, Mayo Clinic 74; **Fac Appt:** Prof Path, Mayo Med Sch

Great Plains and Mountains

Pour, Parviz M MD [Path] - **Spec Exp:** Pancreatic Cancer; Prostate Cancer; Nutrition & Cancer; **Hospital:** Nebraska Med Ctr; **Address:** University of Nebraska Medical Ctr, 600 S 42nd St, Omaha, NE 68198-6805; **Phone:** 402-559-4495; **Board Cert:** Anatomic Pathology 79; **Med School:** Germany 63; **Resid:** Pathology, Hannover University Med Ctr 70; Anatomic Pathology, Nebraska Med Ctr 74; **Fac Appt:** Prof Path, Univ Nebr Coll Med

Weisenburger, Dennis MD [Path] - **Spec Exp:** Hematopathology; Lymphoma; **Hospital:** Nebraska Med Ctr; **Address:** Univ Nebr Med Ctr, Dept Path, 983135 Nebraska Medical Center, Omaha, NE 68198-3135; **Phone:** 402-559-7688; **Board Cert:** Anatomic & Clinical Pathology 79; **Med School:** Univ Minn 74; **Resid:** Anatomic Pathology, Univ Iowa Hosps 78; **Fellow:** Hematology, City of Hope Natl Med Ctr 80; **Fac Appt:** Prof Path, Univ Nebr Coll Med

Southwest

Allred, D Craig MD [Path] - **Spec Exp:** Breast Cancer; Breast Pathology; **Hospital:** Methodist Hosp - Houston; **Address:** Baylor Coll Med - Breast Center, One Baylor Plaza, BCM 600, Houston, TX 77030; **Phone:** 713-798-1626; **Board Cert:** Anatomic Pathology 84; **Med School:** Univ Utah 79; **Resid:** Anatomic Pathology, Univ Conn Hlth Ctr 83; **Fellow:** Immunopathology, Univ Conn Hlth Ctr 82; **Fac Appt:** Prof Path, Baylor Coll Med

Bruner, Janet M MD [Path] - **Spec Exp:** Brain Tumors; Neuro-Pathology; **Hospital:** UT MD Anderson Cancer Ctr, The (page 115); **Address:** MD Anderson Cancer Ctr, 1515 Holcombe Ave, Unit 85, Houston, TX 77030; **Phone:** 713-792-6127; **Board Cert:** Anatomic Pathology 97; Neuropathology 84; **Med School:** Med Coll OH 79; **Resid:** Anatomic & Clinical Pathology, Med Coll Ohio Hosp 82; **Fellow:** Neurological Pathology, Baylor Coll Med 84; **Fac Appt:** Prof Path, Univ Tex, Houston

Cagle, Philip MD [Path] - **Spec Exp:** Pulmonary Pathology; Lung Cancer & Disease; Mesothelioma; **Hospital:** Methodist Hosp - Houston; **Address:** Methodist Hospital, Dept Pathology, 6565 Fannin St, Houston, TX 77030; **Phone:** 713-441-6478; **Board Cert:** Anatomic & Clinical Pathology 85; **Med School:** Univ Tenn Coll Med, Memphis 81; **Fac Appt:** Prof Path, Baylor Coll Med

Colby, Thomas V MD [Path] - **Spec Exp:** Pulmonary Pathology; Surgical Pathology; Lung Cancer; **Hospital:** Mayo Clin Hosp - Scottsdale; **Address:** Mayo Clinic, Dept Path, 13400 E Shea Blvd, Scottsdale, AZ 85259; **Phone:** 480-301-8021; **Board Cert:** Anatomic Pathology 78; **Med School:** Univ Mich Med Sch 74; **Resid:** Anatomic Pathology, Stanford Univ Hosp 78; **Fellow:** Surgical Pathology, Stanford Univ Hosp; **Fac Appt:** Prof Path, Mayo Med Sch

Foucar, M Kathryn MD **[Path]** - **Spec Exp:** Leukemia; Lymph Node Pathology; Bone Marrow Pathology; **Hospital:** Univ NM Hlth & Sci Ctr; **Address:** TriCore Reference Laboratories, 1001 Woodward Pl NE, Albuquerque, NM 87102; **Phone:** 505-938-8457; **Board Cert:** Anatomic & Clinical Pathology 78; **Med School:** Ohio State Univ 74; **Resid:** Anatomic Pathology, Univ NM Health & Sci Ctr 76; Anatomic Pathology, Univ Minn Med Ctr 78; **Fellow:** Surgical Pathology, Univ Minn Med Ctr 79; **Fac Appt:** Prof Path, Univ New Mexico

Grogan, Thomas M MD **[Path]** - **Spec Exp:** Immunopathology; Lymphoma; **Hospital:** Univ Med Ctr - Tucson; **Address:** Univ Med Ctr, Dept Path, 1501 N Campbell Ave, rm 5212, Tucson, AZ 85724; **Phone:** 520-626-7477; **Board Cert:** Anatomic Pathology 76; **Med School:** Geo Wash Univ 71; **Resid:** Pathology, Letterman Army Med Ctr 76; **Fellow:** Immunopathology, Stanford Univ Sch Med 79; **Fac Appt:** Prof Path, Univ Ariz Coll Med

Hamilton, Stanley R MD **[Path]** - **Spec Exp:** Surgical Pathology; Gastrointestinal Pathology; Liver Pathology; **Hospital:** UT MD Anderson Cancer Ctr, The (page 115); **Address:** Univ Texas MD Anderson Cancer Ctr, 1515 Holcombe Blvd, Unit 85, Houston, TX 77030-4009; **Phone:** 713-792-2040; **Board Cert:** Anatomic & Clinical Pathology 78; **Med School:** Indiana Univ 73; **Resid:** Pathology, Johns Hopkins Hosp 78; **Fellow:** St Marks Hosp 79; **Fac Appt:** Prof Path, Univ Tex, Houston

Kinney, Marsha C MD **[Path]** - **Spec Exp:** Hematopathology; Lymphoma; Leukemia; **Hospital:** UTSA - Univ Hosp; **Address:** Univ Tex Hlth & Sci Ctr, Dept Path, 7703 Floyd Curl Drive, , MC 7750, San Antonio, TX 78229-3900; **Phone:** 210-567-4098; **Board Cert:** Anatomic & Clinical Pathology 85; Hematology 98; **Med School:** Univ Tex SW, Dallas 81; **Resid:** Pathology, Vanderbilt Univ Med Ctr 85; **Fellow:** Hematopathology, Vanderbilt Univ Med Ctr 88; **Fac Appt:** Prof Path, Univ Tex, San Antonio

Leslie, Kevin O MD **[Path]** - **Spec Exp:** Pulmonary Pathology; Lung Cancer; Surgical Pathology; **Hospital:** Mayo Clin Hosp - Scottsdale; **Address:** Mayo Clinic, Scottsdale, Dept Lab Med & Path, 13400 E Shea Blvd, Scottsdale, AZ 85259; **Phone:** 480-301-8021; **Board Cert:** Anatomic & Clinical Pathology 82; **Med School:** Albert Einstein Coll Med 76; **Resid:** Anatomic & Clinical Pathology, Unic Colorado Health Sci Ctr 82; **Fellow:** Surgical Pathology, Stanford Univ Med Ctr 83; **Fac Appt:** Prof Path, Mayo Med Sch

Logrono, Roberto MD **[Path]** - **Spec Exp:** Pancreatic Pathology; Lymph Node Pathology; Gastrointestinal Submucosal Masses; **Hospital:** UT Med Br Hosp at Galveston; **Address:** Univ Texas Med Br, Dept Path, 301 University Blvd, rm 9.300 John Sealy Annex, Galveston, TX 77555-0548; **Phone:** 409-772-8438; **Board Cert:** Anatomic & Clinical Pathology 91; Cytopathology 95; **Med School:** Dominican Republic 82; **Resid:** Anatomic Pathology, St Barnabas Med Ctr 91; **Fellow:** Cytopathology, Univ Wisc Med Ctr 95; **Fac Appt:** Assoc Prof Path, Univ Tex Med Br, Galveston

Moran, Cesar A MD **[Path]** - **Spec Exp:** Lung Cancer; Mediastinal Cancer; Mesothelioma; **Hospital:** UT MD Anderson Cancer Ctr, The (page 115); **Address:** MD Anderson Cancer Ctr, Dept Pathology, 1515 Holcombe Blvd, rm G1-3738, Houston, TX 77030; **Phone:** 713-792-8134; **Board Cert:** Anatomic Pathology 92; **Med School:** Guatemala 81; **Resid:** Anatomic & Clinical Pathology, Mt Sinai Med Ctr 88; **Fellow:** Surgical Pathology, Yale- New Haven Med Ctr 89; **Fac Appt:** Prof Path, Univ Tex, Houston

Prieto, Victor G MD/PhD **[Path]** - **Spec Exp:** Dermatopathology; Melanoma; Skin Cancer; **Hospital:** UT MD Anderson Cancer Ctr, The (page 115); **Address:** MD Anderson Cancer Ctr, Dept Pathology, 1515 Holcombe Blvd, Box 85, Houston, TX 77030; **Phone:** 713-792-0918; **Board Cert:** Anatomic Pathology 95; Dermatopathology 97; **Med School:** Spain 86; **Resid:** Pathology, NY Hosp-Cornell Med Ctr 93; **Fellow:** Pathology, Meml Sloan Kettering Cancer Ctr 95; Dermatopathology, NY Hosp-Cornell Med Ctr 96; **Fac Appt:** Assoc Prof Path, Univ Tex, Houston

Silva, Elvio G MD [Path] - **Spec Exp:** Gynecologic Pathology; Gynecologic Cancer; **Hospital:** UT MD Anderson Cancer Ctr, The (page 115); **Address:** MD Anderson Cancer Ctr, Dept Pathology, 1515 Holcombe Blvd, Box 85, Houston, TX 77030; **Phone:** 713-792-3154; **Board Cert:** Anatomic Pathology 97; **Med School:** Argentina 69; **Resid:** Pathology, National Univ Med Ctr 75; Anatomic Pathology, Univ Toronto 78; **Fellow:** Surgical Pathology, MD Anderson Cancer Ctr 79; **Fac Appt:** Prof Path, Univ Tex, Houston

Thor, Ann D MD [Path] - **Spec Exp:** Breast Cancer; Gynecologic Cancer; **Hospital:** OU Med Ctr; **Address:** Univ Oklahoma Hlth Sci Ctr, BMSB 451, 940 Stanton L Young Blvd, Oklahoma City, OK 73104; **Phone:** 405-271-2422; **Board Cert:** Anatomic Pathology 87; Cytopathology 89; **Med School:** Vanderbilt Univ 81; **Resid:** Pathology, Vanderbilt Univ 83; **Fellow:** Immunopathology, Natl Cancer Inst 86; Gynecologic Pathology, Mass Genl Hosp 90; **Fac Appt:** Prof Path, Univ Okla Coll Med

Wheeler, Thomas M MD [Path] - **Spec Exp:** Thyroid Disorders; Thyroid Cancer; **Hospital:** Ben Taub General Hosp; **Address:** Baylor Coll Med, Dept Pathology, One Baylor Plaza, rm T203, Houston, TX 77030; **Phone:** 713-798-4664; **Board Cert:** Anatomic & Clinical Pathology 99; Cytopathology 90; **Med School:** Baylor Coll Med 77; **Resid:** Pathology, Baylor Coll Med 81; **Fac Appt:** Prof Path, Baylor Coll Med

West Coast and Pacific

Arber, Daniel A MD [Path] - **Spec Exp:** Bone Marrow Pathology; Lymph Node Pathology; Spleen Pathology; **Hospital:** Stanford Univ Med Ctr; **Address:** Clinic Laboratories, Stanford University Medical Ctr, 300 Pasteur Drive, rm H1507, MC 5627, Stanford, CA 94305; **Phone:** 650-725-5604; **Board Cert:** Anatomic Pathology 91; Hematology 93; **Med School:** Univ Tex, San Antonio 86; **Resid:** Anatomic & Clinical Pathology, Scott & White Meml Hosp 95; **Fellow:** Hematopathology, City of Hope Natl Med Ctr 93; **Fac Appt:** Prof Path, Stanford Univ

Bollen, Andrew W MD [Path] - **Spec Exp:** Neuro-Pathology; Brain Tumors; Brain Infections; **Hospital:** UCSF Med Ctr; **Address:** Dept Pathology/Neuropathology, 513 Parnassus Ave, rm HSW408, San Francisco, CA 94143-0511; **Phone:** 415-476-5236; **Board Cert:** Clinical Pathology 93; Anatomic Pathology 92; Neuropathology 92; **Med School:** UCSD 85; **Resid:** Anatomic Pathology, UCSF Med Ctr 91; **Fellow:** Neuropathology, UCSF Med Ctr 89; **Fac Appt:** Prof Path, UCSF

Chandrasoma, Parakrama T MD [Path] - **Spec Exp:** Gastrointestinal Pathology; Gastrointestinal Cancer; Neuro-Pathology; **Hospital:** LAC & USC Med Ctr; **Address:** LAC-USC Med Ctr, Dept Path, 1200 N State St, rm 16-905, Los Angeles, CA 90033; **Phone:** 323-226-4600; **Board Cert:** Anatomic Pathology 82; **Med School:** Sri Lanka 71; **Resid:** Anatomic Pathology, Univ Sri Lanka 78; Anatomic Pathology, LAC-USC Med Ctr 82; **Fac Appt:** Prof Path, USC Sch Med

Cochran, Alistair J MD [Path] - **Spec Exp:** Melanoma-Sentinel Node; Dermatopathology; **Hospital:** UCLA Med Ctr (page 111); **Address:** UCLA Med Ctr, Dept Path & Med, 10833 Le Conte Ave, rm 13-145CHS, Box 951713, Los Angeles, CA 90095-1713; **Phone:** 310-825-2743; **Med School:** Scotland 66; **Resid:** Dermatopathology, Western Infirmary 68; **Fellow:** Immunology, Karolinska Inst 70; **Fac Appt:** Prof Path, UCLA

Cote, Richard J MD [Path] - **Spec Exp:** Sentinel Node Pathology; Bladder Cancer; Breast Cancer; **Hospital:** USC Norris Canc Comp Ctr; **Address:** 1441 Eastlake Ave, rm 2424, Los Angeles, CA 90033; **Phone:** 323-865-3270; **Board Cert:** Anatomic Pathology 87; **Med School:** Univ Chicago-Pritzker Sch Med 80; **Resid:** Pathology, New York Hosp-Cornell 87; **Fellow:** Pathology, Meml Sloan-Kettering Cancer Ctr 90; **Fac Appt:** Prof Path, USC Sch Med

Dail, David H MD [Path] - **Spec Exp:** Lung Cancer & Disease; Pulmonary Pathology; **Hospital:** Virginia Mason Med Ctr; **Address:** Virginia Mason Medical Ctr, Dept Pathology, C6-PTH, 1100 9th Ave, Box 900, Seattle, WA 98101; **Phone:** 206-223-6861; **Board Cert:** Anatomic Pathology 78; **Med School:** Med Coll Wisc 68; **Resid:** Pathology, UCSD Med Ctr 75; **Fac Appt:** Clin Prof Path, Univ Wash

Dubeau, Louis MD [Path] - **Spec Exp:** Ovarian Cancer; Breast Cancer; **Hospital:** USC Norris Canc Comp Ctr; **Address:** USC Norris Cancer Ctr, Dept Pathology, 1441 Eastlake Ave, rm 7320, Los Angeles, CA 90033-1048; **Phone:** 323-865-0720; **Board Cert:** Anatomic Pathology 84; **Med School:** McGill Univ 79; **Resid:** Anatomic Pathology, McGill Univ Med Ctr 84; **Fac Appt:** Assoc Prof Path, USC Sch Med

Hammar, Samuel P MD [Path] - **Spec Exp:** Lung Cancer & Disease; Pulmonary Pathology; **Hospital:** Harrison Meml Hosp; **Address:** Diagnostic Specialties Laboratory, 700 Lebo Blvd, Bremerton, WA 98310; **Phone:** 360-479-7707; **Board Cert:** Anatomic & Clinical Pathology 75; **Med School:** Univ Wash 70

Hendrickson, Michael MD [Path] - **Spec Exp:** Gynecologic Cancer; Gynecologic Pathology; **Hospital:** Stanford Univ Med Ctr; **Address:** Stanford Univ Med Ctr, Surg Path Lab, 300 Pasteur Drive, rm H2110, Stanford, CA 94305; **Phone:** 650-498-6460; **Board Cert:** Anatomic Pathology 75; **Med School:** Stanford Univ 71; **Resid:** Anatomic Pathology, Stanford Univ Med Sch 74; **Fac Appt:** Prof Path, Stanford Univ

Koss, Michael N MD [Path] - **Spec Exp:** Pulmonary Pathology; Lung Cancer; Mediastinal Cancer; **Hospital:** USC Norris Canc Comp Ctr; **Address:** Hoffman Medical Research Bldg, rm 209, 2011 Zonal Ave, Los Angeles, CA 90033; **Phone:** 323-226-6507; **Board Cert:** Anatomic Pathology 79; **Med School:** Stanford Univ 70; **Resid:** Pathology, Columbia Presby Med Ctr 74; **Fellow:** Renal Pathology, Columbia Presby Med Ctr 75; Pulmonary Pathology, Armed Forces Inst of Pathology 78; **Fac Appt:** Prof Path, USC Sch Med

Le Boit, Philip E MD [Path] - **Spec Exp:** Cutaneous Lymphoma; Skin Cancer; Dermatopathology; **Hospital:** UCSF Med Ctr; **Address:** UCSF - Dermatopathology Section, 1701 Divisadero St, Ste 350, San Francisco, CA 94115; **Phone:** 415-353-7546; **Board Cert:** Anatomic Pathology 83; Clinical Pathology 86; Dermatopathology 83; **Med School:** Albany Med Coll 79; **Resid:** Anatomic Pathology, UCSF Med Ctr 81; Clinical Pathology, Mt Sinai Hosp 82; **Fellow:** Dermatopathology, New York Hosp-Cornell Med Ctr; **Fac Appt:** Prof Path, UCSF

Ljung, Britt-Marie E MD [Path] - **Spec Exp:** Breast Cancer; **Hospital:** UCSF - Mt Zion Med Ctr; **Address:** UCSF - Dept Pathology, Box 1785, San Francisco, CA 94143; **Phone:** 415-885-7301; **Board Cert:** Anatomic Pathology 85; Cytopathology 89; **Med School:** Sweden 75; **Resid:** Pathology, Karolinska Hosp 79; Anatomic Pathology, UCLA Med Ctr 83; **Fac Appt:** Prof Path, UCSF

Nathwani, Bharat N MD [Path] - **Spec Exp:** Hematopathology; Leukemia; Lymphoma; **Hospital:** LAC & USC Med Ctr; **Address:** LAC & USC Med Ctr, Dept Pathology, 1200 N State St, rm 2422, Los Angeles, CA 90033-4526; **Phone:** 323-226-7064; **Board Cert:** Anatomic Pathology 77; **Med School:** India 69; **Resid:** Pathology, JJ Group-Grant Med Ctr 72; Pathology, Rush-Presby-St Luke's Med Ctr; **Fellow:** Hematopathology, City Hope Natl Med Ctr; **Fac Appt:** Prof Path, USC Sch Med

Rubin, Brian P MD [Path] - **Spec Exp:** Bone & Soft Tissue Tumors; Sarcoma; **Hospital:** Univ Wash Med Ctr; **Address:** Univ Wash Med Ctr, Hosp Path, 1959 NE Pacific St, rm BB-220, Seattle, WA 98195; **Phone:** 206-598-5024; **Board Cert:** Anatomic Pathology 99; **Med School:** Cornell Univ-Weill Med Coll 95; **Resid:** Pathology, Brigham & Women's Hosp 00; **Fac Appt:** Asst Prof Path, Univ Wash

Rutgers, Joanne MD [Path] - **Spec Exp:** Gynecologic & Cancer Pathology; Cytopathology; Gastrointestinal Pathology; **Hospital:** Long Beach Meml Med Ctr; **Address:** 2801 Atlantic Ave, Long Beach, CA 90806; **Phone:** 562-933-0717; **Board Cert:** Clinical Pathology 92; Anatomic Pathology 85; Pathology 97; Cytopathology 97; **Med School:** UCSD 81; **Resid:** Pathology, Montefiore Med Ctr 83; Pathology, NYU 85; **Fellow:** Gynecologic Pathology, Mass Genl Hosp 89; **Fac Appt:** Assoc Clin Prof Path, UCLA

Sibley, Richard K MD [Path] - **Spec Exp:** Kidney Cancer & Pathology; Breast Cancer & Pathology; Liver Cancer & Pathology; **Hospital:** Stanford Univ Med Ctr; **Address:** Stanford University Medical Ctr, Dept Pathology, 300 Pasteur Drive, rm H2110, MC 5243, Stanford, CA 94305; **Phone:** 650-723-7211; **Board Cert:** Anatomic Pathology 75; **Med School:** Univ Tex SW, Dallas 71; **Resid:** Anatomic Pathology, Univ Chicago Hosps 74; **Fellow:** Stanford Univ Med Ctr 75; **Fac Appt:** Prof Path, Stanford Univ

Triche, Timothy J MD/PhD [Path] - **Spec Exp:** Pediatric Pathology; Sarcoma; **Hospital:** Chldns Hosp - Los Angeles; **Address:** Chldns Hosp of Los Angeles, Dept Path, 4650 Sunset Blvd, MS 43, Los Angeles, CA 90027; **Phone:** 323-669-4516; **Board Cert:** Anatomic Pathology 75; **Med School:** Tulane Univ 71; **Resid:** Anatomic Pathology, Barnes Hosp-Wash Univ 73; Surgical Pathology, Barnes Hosp 74; **Fellow:** Pathology, Natl Cancer Inst 75; **Fac Appt:** Prof Path, USC Sch Med

True, Lawrence D MD [Path] - **Spec Exp:** Urologic Pathology; Prostate Cancer; Bladder Cancer; **Hospital:** Univ Wash Med Ctr; **Address:** Univ Wash Med Ctr, Dept Anatomic Path, 1959 NE Pacific St, rm BB220, Box 356100, Seattle, WA 98195-6100; **Phone:** 206-598-4027; **Board Cert:** Anatomic Pathology 81; **Med School:** Tulane Univ 71; **Resid:** Pathology, Univ Colo Hlth Sci Ctr 80; **Fac Appt:** Prof Path, Univ Wash

Warnke, Roger A MD [Path] - **Spec Exp:** Lymphoma; Hematopathology; **Hospital:** Stanford Univ Med Ctr; **Address:** Stanford Univ, Dept Pathology, 300 Pasteur, Ste L235, Stanford, CA 94305; **Phone:** 650-725-5167; **Board Cert:** Anatomic Pathology 75; **Med School:** Washington Univ, St Louis 71; **Resid:** Pathology, Stanford Univ Med Ctr 73; **Fellow:** Surgical Pathology, Stanford Univ Med Ctr 75; Immunology, Stanford Univ Med Ctr 76; **Fac Appt:** Prof Path, Stanford Univ

Weiss, Lawrence M MD [Path] - **Spec Exp:** Lymphoma; Hematopathology; Adrenal Pathology; **Hospital:** City of Hope Natl Med Ctr & Beckman Rsch (page 89); **Address:** City of Hope Natl Med Ctr, Div Pathology, 1500 E Duarte Rd, Duarte, CA 91010-0269; **Phone:** 626-359-8111 x62456; **Board Cert:** Anatomic Pathology 85; **Med School:** Univ MD Sch Med 81; **Resid:** Pathology, Brigham & Women's Hosp 83; **Fellow:** Pathology, Stanford Univ Hosp 84

PEDIATRICS

A *pediatrician is concerned with the physical, emotional and social health of children from birth to young adulthood. Care encompasses a broad spectrum of health services ranging from preventive healthcare to the diagnosis and treatment of acute and chronic diseases.*

A pediatrician deals with biological, social and environmental influences on the developing child, and with the impact of disease and dysfunction on development.

Training required: *Three years*

PEDIATRIC HEMATOLOGY/ONCOLOGY

A pediatrician trained in the combination of pediatrics, hematology and oncology to recognize and manage pediatric blood disorders and cancerous diseases.

PEDIATRIC ALLERGY AND IMMUNOLOGY

An allergist-immunologist is trained in evaluation, physical and laboratory diagnosis and management of disorders

PHYSICIAN LISTINGS:

PEDIATRIC HEMATOLOGY/ONCOLOGY

PEDIATRIC ALLERGY & IMMUNOLOGY

involving the immune system. Selected examples of such conditions include asthma, anaphylaxis, rhinitis, eczema and adverse reactions to drugs, foods and insect stings as well as immune deficiency diseases (both acquired and congenital), defects in host defense and problems related to autoimmune disease, organ transplantation or malignancies of the immune system. As our understanding of the immune system develops, the scope of this specialty is widening.

Training programs are available at some medical centers to provide individuals with expertise in both allergy/immunology and pediatric pulmonology. Such individuals are candidates for dual certification.

Training required: Prior certification in pediatrics plus two years in allergy/immunology.

PHYSICIAN LISTINGS

PEDIATRIC ENDOCRINOLOGY

Mid Atlantic	400
Southeast	400
Midwest	400
Southwest	400

PEDIATRIC OTOLARYNGOLOGY

New England	401
Mid Atlantic	401
West Coast & Pacific	401

PEDIATRIC ENDOCRINOLOGY

A pediatrician who provides expert care to infants, children and adolescents who have diseases that result from an abnormality in the endocrine glands (glands which secrete hormones) These diseases include diabetes mellitus, growth failure, unusual size for age, early or late pubertal development, birth defects, the genital region and disorders of the thyroid, the adrenal and pituitary glands.

PEDIATRIC OTOLARYNGOLOGY

A pediatric otolaryngologist has special expertise in the management of infants and children with disorders that include congenital and acquired conditions involving the aerodigestive tract, nose and paranasal sinuses, the ear and other areas of the head and neck. The pediatric otolaryngologist has special skills in the diagnosis, treatment and management of childhood disorders of voice, speech, language and hearing.

PEDIATRIC SURGERY

A surgeon with expertise in the management of surgical conditions in premature and newborn infants, children and adolescents.

PHYSICIAN LISTINGS

PEDIATRIC SURGERY

PEDIATRICS

377

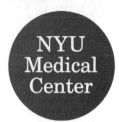

NYU
Medical
Center

550 First Avenue (at 31st Street)
New York, NY 10016
Physician Referral:
1-888-7-NYU-MED
www.nyumc.org

PEDIATRIC HEMATOLOGY PROGRAM

For decades, children with chronic blood diseases have come to NYU Medical Center's Pediatric Hematology Program for comprehensive medical care, including a full range of psychosocial support services to meet every need. Members of the program's expert staff are guided by a patient- and family-centered approach to care, with all the advantages of a leading academic medical center at their fingertips.

The Program addresses the needs of patients with red blood cell disorders, including a variety of anemias and thalassemias – problems of hemoglobin metabolism – as well as vascular problems and malformations, coagulation disorders, and numerous other hemostatic abnormalities.

Patients requiring hospitalization are treated on the pediatric floor of Tisch Hospital, where they benefit from its advanced diagnostic and therapeutic expertise and the support of all pediatric subspecialties. Families are actively encouraged to become knowledgeable about their children's disease and its management. Our multidisciplinary team works closely with the patient's primary care physician to coordinate both medical and psychosocial care.

PSYCHOSOCIAL SERVICES

To help children and families cope with their disease and to prevent later psychological trauma, our behavioral health professionals are committed to a holistic approach to patient care. Among the services we provide are art therapy, relaxation training, play therapy, psychiatric evaluation, neuropsychological assessment, individual and group counseling, and patient education.

THE PEDIATRIC SPECIAL HEMATOLOGY LABORATORY

As a service to clinicians, the Pediatric Special Hematology Laboratory provides comprehensive hemostasis and red cell testing. Tests have been adapted so that small quantities of blood can be drawn from pediatric patients. The Laboratory's repertoire of test procedures is routinely upgraded to incorporate the latest developments in the field. It strives to provide fast, precise test information that leads to effective treatments while maintaining rigorous quality control standards.

Children with cancer or chronic blood diseases receive comprehensive outpatient care at the Steven D. Hassenfeld Center for Children with Cancer and Blood Disorders – a pediatric day hospital at NYU that provides fully coordinated care at a state-of-the-art facility. The medical team works hand in hand with a behavioral science team consisting of a full-time psychologist, social worker, and child life specialist. Most therapies and procedures are performed on an ambulatory basis. In addition to examining rooms and doctors' offices, the Center comprises the day hospital, an on-site laboratory, and a playroom.

PHYSICIAN REFERRAL
1-888-7-NYU-MED
(1-888-769-8633)
www.nyumc.org

PEDIATRIC HEMATOLOGY-ONCOLOGY

New England

Albritton, Karen H MD **[PHO]** - **Spec Exp:** Sarcoma; Adolescent/Young Adult Cancers; **Hospital:** Dana-Farber Cancer Inst (page 87); **Address:** Dand Farber Cancer Inst, 44 Binney St, JFG08, Boston, MA 02115; **Phone:** 617-532-5122; **Board Cert:** Internal Medicine 96; Pediatrics 96; Medical Oncology 01; Pediatric Hematology-Oncology 02; **Med School:** Univ Tex, San Antonio 92; **Resid:** Internal Medicine & Pediatrics, Univ NC Hosps 96; **Fellow:** Hematology and Oncology, Univ NC Hosps 00

Altman, Arnold MD **[PHO]** - **Spec Exp:** Leukemia; **Hospital:** CT Chldns Med Ctr; **Address:** Connecticut Children's Med Ctr-Dept Hem-Onc, 282 Washington St, Ste 2J, Hartford, CT 06106; **Phone:** 860-545-9630; **Board Cert:** Pediatrics 71; Pediatric Hematology-Oncology 74; **Med School:** Johns Hopkins Univ 65; **Resid:** Pediatrics, Chldns Hosp Med Ctr 70; **Fellow:** Pediatric Hematology-Oncology, Chldns Hosp Med Ctr 72; **Fac Appt:** Prof Ped, Univ Conn

Diller, Lisa R MD **[PHO]** - **Spec Exp:** Brain Tumors; Neuroblasatoma; Cancer Survivors-Late Effects of Therapy; **Hospital:** Dana-Farber Cancer Inst (page 87); **Address:** Dana-Farber Cancer Inst, 44 Binney St, Dana 362, Boston, MA 02115; **Phone:** 617-632-5642; **Board Cert:** Pediatric Hematology-Oncology 00; **Med School:** UCSD 85; **Resid:** Pediatrics, Chldns Hosp 88; **Fellow:** Pediatric Hematology-Oncology, Chldns Hosp-Dana Farber Cancer Inst 91; **Fac Appt:** Assoc Prof Ped, Harvard Med Sch

Grier, Holcombe E MD **[PHO]** - **Spec Exp:** Bone Cancer; Ewing's Sarcoma; Rhabdomyosarcoma; **Hospital:** Dana-Farber Cancer Inst (page 87); **Address:** Dana Farber Cancer Inst, 44 Binney St, G350, Boston, MA 02115; **Phone:** 617-632-3971; **Board Cert:** Pediatrics 83; Internal Medicine 80; Pediatric Hematology-Oncology 98; **Med School:** Univ Pennsylvania 76; **Resid:** Pediatrics, NC Meml Hosp 80; Internal Medicine, NC Meml Hosp 80; **Fellow:** Pediatric Oncology, Dana Farber Children's Hosp 84; **Fac Appt:** Assoc Prof Ped, Harvard Med Sch

Homans, Alan C MD **[PHO]** - **Spec Exp:** Leukemia; **Hospital:** FAHC - Med Ctr Campus; **Address:** Children's Specialty Ctr, 111 Colchester Ave,Modular B, Rm 113, Burlington, VT 05401; **Phone:** 802-847-2850; **Board Cert:** Pediatrics 85; Pediatric Hematology-Oncology 87; **Med School:** Ohio State Univ 79; **Resid:** Pediatrics, Med Ctr Hosp 81; Pediatrics, Univ Massachusetts Med Ctr 81; **Fellow:** Pediatric Hematology-Oncology, Rhode Island Hosp 85; **Fac Appt:** Prof Ped, Univ VT Coll Med

Israel, Mark A MD **[PHO]** - **Spec Exp:** Neuro-Oncology; Brain Tumors; Neuroblastoma; **Hospital:** Dartmouth - Hitchcock Med Ctr; **Address:** Norris Cotton Cancer Ctr, One Medical Center Drive, Lebanon, NH 03756; **Phone:** 603-653-3611; **Board Cert:** Pediatrics 82; **Med School:** Albert Einstein Coll Med 73; **Resid:** Pediatrics, Chldns Hosp Med Ctr 75; **Fellow:** Pediatric Hematology-Oncology, Natl Cancer Inst 81; **Fac Appt:** Prof Ped, Dartmouth Med Sch

Kieran, Mark MD/PhD **[PHO]** - **Spec Exp:** Brain Tumors; **Hospital:** Children's Hospital - Boston; **Address:** Dana Farber Cancer Inst, 44 Binney St, Shields Warren Ste 331, Boston, MA 02115; **Phone:** 617-632-4271; **Board Cert:** Pediatrics 00; Pediatric Hematology-Oncology 96; **Med School:** Canada 86; **Resid:** Pediatrics, Montreal Chldns Hosp 92; **Fellow:** Pediatric Hematology-Oncology, Chldns Hosp 95; **Fac Appt:** Asst Prof Ped, Harvard Med Sch

Kretschmar, Cynthia S MD [PHO] - **Spec Exp:** Brain Tumors; Neuroblastoma; Drug Discovery & Development; **Hospital:** Tufts-New England Med Ctr; **Address:** Floating Hosp, Div Pediatric Hem/Onc, 750 Washington St, NEMC 14, Boston, MA 02111; **Phone:** 617-636-5535; **Board Cert:** Pediatrics 84; Pediatric Hematology-Oncology 87; **Med School:** Yale Univ 78; **Resid:** Pediatrics, Yale-New Haven Hosp 81; **Fellow:** Pediatric Hematology-Oncology, Dana Farber Cancer Inst 84; **Fac Appt:** Prof Ped, Tufts Univ

Weinstein, Howard J MD [PHO] - **Spec Exp:** Bone Marrow Transplant; Leukemia; Lymphoma; **Hospital:** Mass Genl Hosp; **Address:** 55 Fruit St, Yawkey 8B-8893, Boston, MA 02114-2622; **Phone:** 617-724-3315; **Board Cert:** Pediatrics 77; **Med School:** Univ MD Sch Med 72; **Resid:** Pediatrics, Mass Genl Hosp 74; **Fellow:** Pediatric Hematology-Oncology, Dana Farber Cancer Inst/Chldns Hosp 77; **Fac Appt:** Prof Ped, Harvard Med Sch

Wolfe, Lawrence C MD [PHO] - **Spec Exp:** Leukemia; Neuro-Oncology; Cancer Survivors-Late Effects of Therapy; **Hospital:** Tufts-New England Med Ctr; **Address:** Floating Hosp, Div Pediatric Hem/Onc, 750 Washington St, NEMC 14, Boston, MA 02111; **Phone:** 617-636-5535; **Board Cert:** Pediatrics 81; Pediatric Hematology-Oncology 87; **Med School:** Harvard Med Sch 76; **Resid:** Pediatrics, Chldns Hosp 78; **Fellow:** Pediatric Hematology-Oncology, Chldns Hosp 91; **Fac Appt:** Assoc Prof Ped, Tulane Univ

Mid Atlantic

Arceci, Robert John MD/PhD [PHO] - **Spec Exp:** Leukemia; Histiocytosis; Bone Marrow Transplant; **Hospital:** Johns Hopkins Hosp - Baltimore (page 97); **Address:** Sidney Kimmel Comp Cancer Ctr, Bunting-Blaustein Cancer Rsch Bldg, 1650 Orleans St, CRB 2M51, Baltimore, MD 21231; **Phone:** 410-502-7519; **Board Cert:** Pediatrics 87; Pediatric Hematology-Oncology 98; **Med School:** Univ Rochester 81; **Resid:** Pediatrics, Chldns Hosp 83; **Fellow:** Pediatric Hematology-Oncology, Chldns Hosp/Dana Farber Cancer Ctr 86; **Fac Appt:** Prof Ped, Johns Hopkins Univ

Brecher, Martin L MD [PHO] - **Spec Exp:** Brain Tumors; Lymphoma; Hodgkin's Disease; **Hospital:** Roswell Park Cancer Inst (page 107); **Address:** Roswell Park Cancer Inst, Dept Pediatrics, Elm & Carlton Sts, Buffalo, NY 14263; **Phone:** 716-845-2333; **Board Cert:** Pediatrics 77; Pediatric Hematology-Oncology 78; **Med School:** SUNY Buffalo 72; **Resid:** Pediatrics, Buffalo Chldns Hosp 75; **Fellow:** Hematology and Oncology, Buffalo Chldns Hosp/Roswell Park Cancer Inst 77; **Fac Appt:** Prof Ped, SUNY Buffalo

Brodeur, Garrett MD [PHO] - **Spec Exp:** Neuroblastoma; **Hospital:** Chldns Hosp of Philadelphia, The; **Address:** Children's Hosp of Philadelphia, 3615 Civic Center Blvd, Ste 902ARC, Philadelphia, PA 19104-4318; **Phone:** 215-590-3025; **Board Cert:** Pediatrics 80; Pediatric Hematology-Oncology 80; **Med School:** Washington Univ, St Louis 75; **Resid:** Pediatrics, St Louis Childrens Hosp 77; **Fellow:** Pediatric Hematology-Oncology, St Jude Childrens Rsch Hosp 79; **Fac Appt:** Prof Ped, Univ Pennsylvania

Bussel, James MD [PHO] - **Spec Exp:** Platelet Disorders; Autoimmunity/Immune Deficiency; Bleeding/Coagulation Disorders; **Hospital:** NY-Presby Hosp - NY Weill Cornell Med Ctr (page 103); **Address:** 525 E 68th St, Ste P-695, New York, NY 10021-4870; **Phone:** 212-746-3474; **Board Cert:** Pediatrics 79; Pediatric Hematology-Oncology 81; **Med School:** Columbia P&S 75; **Resid:** Pediatrics, Chldns Hosp 78; **Fellow:** Pediatric Hematology-Oncology, NY Hosp 81; **Fac Appt:** Prof Ped, Cornell Univ-Weill Med Coll

Cairo, Mitchell S MD **[PHO]** - **Spec Exp:** Bone Marrow Transplant; Leukemia; Lymphoma; **Hospital:** NY-Presby Hosp - Columbia Presby Med Ctr (page 103); **Address:** Babies & Chldns Hosp, Columbia Presby Med Ctr, 161 Fort Washington Ave Fl 7 - rm 754, New York, NY 10032; **Phone:** 212-305-8316; **Board Cert:** Pediatrics 80; Pediatric Hematology-Oncology 82; **Med School:** UCSF 76; **Resid:** Pediatrics, UCLA Med Ctr 78; **Fellow:** Pediatric Hematology-Oncology, Indiana Univ Med Ctr 81; **Fac Appt:** Prof Ped, Columbia P&S

Carroll, William L MD **[PHO]** - **Spec Exp:** Pediatric Cancers; Leukemia; **Hospital:** NYU Med Ctr (page 104); **Address:** NYU Med Ctr, Div Ped Hem/Onc, 317 E 34th St Fl 8, Box 1208, New York, NY 10016; **Phone:** 212-263-8414; **Board Cert:** Pediatrics 84; Pediatric Hematology-Oncology 87; **Med School:** UC Irvine 78; **Resid:** Pediatrics, Chldns Hosp Med Ctr 81; **Fellow:** Pediatric Hematology-Oncology, Stanford Univ 84; Pediatric Hematology-Oncology, Stanford Univ 87; **Fac Appt:** Prof Ped, NYU Sch Med

Chen, Allen R MD/PhD **[PHO]** - **Spec Exp:** Bone Marrow Transplant-Pediatric; Hodgkin's Disease Immunotherapy; Graft vs Host Disease; **Hospital:** Johns Hopkins Hosp - Baltimore (page 97); **Address:** Johns Hopkins Hosp, Div Peds Oncology, 600 N Wolfe St, CMSC 800, Baltimore, MD 21287; **Phone:** 410-955-7385; **Board Cert:** Pediatrics 02; **Med School:** Duke Univ 86; **Resid:** Pediatrics, Chldns Hosp Med Ctr 89; **Fellow:** Hematology and Oncology, Fred Hutchinson Cancer Ctr 93; Pediatric Hematology-Oncology, Fred Hutchinson Cancer Ctr 94; **Fac Appt:** Asst Prof Ped, Johns Hopkins Univ

Civin, Curt Ingraham MD **[PHO]** - **Spec Exp:** Pediatric Cancers; Leukemia; Bone Marrow Transplant; **Hospital:** Johns Hopkins Hosp - Baltimore (page 97); **Address:** 1650 Orleans St, Ste 2M44, Baltimore, MD 21231-1000; **Phone:** 410-955-8816; **Board Cert:** Pediatrics 79; Pediatric Hematology-Oncology 80; **Med School:** Harvard Med Sch 74; **Resid:** Pediatrics, Chldns Hosp 76; **Fellow:** Pediatric Hematology-Oncology, Natl Cancer Inst 79; **Fac Appt:** Prof Ped, Johns Hopkins Univ

Drachtman, Richard MD **[PHO]** - **Spec Exp:** Pediatric Cancers; Sickle Cell Disease; **Hospital:** Robert Wood Johnson Univ Hosp - New Brunswick (page 106); **Address:** Cancer Inst of New Jersey, 195 Little Albany St, New Brunswick, NJ 08903-1928; **Phone:** 732-235-5437; **Board Cert:** Pediatrics 00; Pediatric Hematology-Oncology 00; **Med School:** Univ Hlth Sci/Chicago Med Sch 84; **Resid:** Pediatrics, N Shore Univ Hosp 88; **Fellow:** Pediatric Hematology-Oncology, Mount Sinai 91; **Fac Appt:** Assoc Prof Ped, UMDNJ-RW Johnson Med Sch

Dunkel, Ira J MD **[PHO]** - **Spec Exp:** Retinoblastoma; Brain & Spinal Cord Tumors; Brain Cancer; **Hospital:** Meml Sloan Kettering Cancer Ctr (page 100); **Address:** Memorial Sloan Kettering Cancer Ctr, Dept Pediatrics, 1275 York Ave, rm H-1102, New York, NY 10021; **Phone:** 212-639-2153; **Board Cert:** Pediatric Hematology-Oncology 00; Pediatrics 89; **Med School:** Duke Univ 85; **Resid:** Pediatrics, Duke University 88; **Fellow:** Pediatric Hematology-Oncology, Memorial-Sloan Kettering 92

Frantz, Christopher N MD **[PHO]** - **Spec Exp:** Solid Tumors; Neuroblastoma; **Hospital:** Alfred I duPont Hosp for Children; **Address:** Alfred I duPont Hosp for Chldn, 1600 Rockland Rd, Box 269, Wilmington, DE 19899; **Phone:** 302-651-5500; **Board Cert:** Pediatrics 77; Pediatric Hematology-Oncology 98; **Med School:** Albert Einstein Coll Med 71; **Resid:** Pediatrics, Chldns Hosp 76; **Fellow:** Pediatric Hematology-Oncology, Chldns Hosp/Dana Farber Cancer Inst 79

Garvin, James MD/PhD **[PHO]** - **Spec Exp:** Bone Marrow Transplant; Brain Tumors; Pediatric Cancers; **Hospital:** NY-Presby Hosp - Columbia Presby Med Ctr (page 103); **Address:** 161 Fort Washington Ave, rm 718, New York, NY 10032; **Phone:** 212-305-9770; **Board Cert:** Pediatrics 82; Pediatric Hematology-Oncology 84; **Med School:** Jefferson Med Coll 76; **Resid:** Pediatrics, Chldns Hosp 78; Pediatrics, Middlesex Hosp 79; **Fellow:** Pediatric Hematology-Oncology, Dana Farber Cancer Inst/Childrens Hosp 82; **Fac Appt:** Clin Prof Ped, Columbia P&S

Green, Daniel M MD [PHO] - **Spec Exp:** Wilms' Tumor; Fertility in Cancer Survivors; Cancer Survivors-Late Effects of Therapy; **Hospital:** Roswell Park Cancer Inst (page 107); **Address:** Roswell Park Cancer Inst, Dept Pediatrics, Elm & Carlton Sts, Buffalo, NY 14263; **Phone:** 716-845-2334; **Board Cert:** Pediatrics 86; Pediatric Hematology-Oncology 97; **Med School:** St Louis Univ 73; **Resid:** Pediatrics, Boston City Hosp 75; **Fellow:** Pediatric Hematology-Oncology, Chldn's Hosp Med Ctr 78; **Fac Appt:** Prof Ped, SUNY Buffalo

Grupp, Stephan A MD [PHO] - **Spec Exp:** Stem Cell Transplant; Neuroblastoma; Bone Marrow Transplant; **Hospital:** Chldns Hosp of Philadelphia, The; **Address:** Childrens Hosp - Oncology, 3615 Civic Ctr Blvd, Abramson 902, Philadelphia, PA 19104; **Phone:** 215-590-2821; **Board Cert:** Pediatric Hematology-Oncology 02; **Med School:** Univ Cincinnati 87; **Resid:** Pediatrics, Chldns Hosp 90; **Fellow:** Pediatric Hematology-Oncology, Dana Farber Cancer Inst/Chldns Hosp 92; **Fac Appt:** Asst Prof Ped, Univ Pennsylvania

Halpern, Steven MD [PHO] - **Spec Exp:** Leukemia; Brain Tumors; Hemophilia; **Hospital:** Hackensack Univ Med Ctr (page 96); **Address:** 30 Prospect Ave Fl 1-WFAN, Hackensack, NJ 07601; **Phone:** 201-996-5437; **Board Cert:** Pediatrics 81; Pediatric Hematology-Oncology 82; **Med School:** Univ Hlth Sci/Chicago Med Sch 76; **Resid:** Pediatrics, St Christopher's Hosp for Children 79; **Fellow:** Pediatric Hematology-Oncology, Childrens Hospital 82; **Fac Appt:** Asst Prof Ped, UMDNJ-NJ Med Sch, Newark

Harris, Michael B MD [PHO] - **Spec Exp:** Leukemia & Lymphoma; Bone Tumors; Sarcoma-Soft Tissue; **Hospital:** Hackensack Univ Med Ctr (page 96); **Address:** Tomorrows Chldns Inst - JM Sanzari Chldns Hosp, 30 Prospect Ave Bldg Imus Fl 1 - Ste TCI - rm PC116, Hackensack, NJ 07601; **Phone:** 201-996-5437; **Board Cert:** Pediatrics 74; Pediatric Hematology-Oncology 74; **Med School:** Albert Einstein Coll Med 69; **Resid:** Pediatrics, Chldns Hosp 71; **Fellow:** Pediatric Hematology-Oncology, Chldns Hosp 74; **Fac Appt:** Prof Ped, UMDNJ-NJ Med Sch, Newark

Helman, Lee Jay MD [PHO] - **Spec Exp:** Solid Tumors; **Hospital:** Natl Inst of Hlth - Clin Ctr; **Address:** National Cancer Inst, NIH, 10 Center Drive Bldg 10 - rm 13N 240, Bethesda, MD 20892-1928; **Phone:** 301-496-4257; **Board Cert:** Internal Medicine 83; Medical Oncology 85; **Med School:** Univ MD Sch Med 80; **Resid:** Internal Medicine, Barnes Hosp 83; **Fellow:** Oncology, Natl Inst Hlth 86

Hinkle, Andrea S MD [PHO] - **Spec Exp:** Cancer Survivors-Late Effects of Therapy; **Hospital:** Univ of Rochester Strong Meml Hosp; **Address:** Golisano Childrens Hosp at Strong, 601 Elmwood Ave, Box 777, Rochester, NY 14642; **Phone:** 585-275-2981; **Board Cert:** Pediatrics 99; Pediatric Hematology-Oncology 00; **Med School:** Brown Univ 87; **Resid:** Pediatrics, Boston City Hosp 91; **Fellow:** Pediatric Hematology-Oncology, Chldns Natl Med Ctr 94; **Fac Appt:** Asst Prof Ped, Univ Rochester

Jakacki, Regina MD [PHO] - **Spec Exp:** Neuro-Oncology; **Hospital:** Chldns Hosp of Pittsburgh - UPMC (page 114); **Address:** Children's Hospital Pittsburgh, 3705 Fifth Ave Fl 4B - Ste 385, Pittsburgh, PA 15213; **Phone:** 412-692-5055; **Board Cert:** Pediatric Hematology-Oncology 00; **Med School:** Univ Pennsylvania 85; **Resid:** Pediatrics, Children's Hosp 88; **Fellow:** Pediatric Hematology-Oncology, Childrens Hosp 91; **Fac Appt:** Assoc Prof Ped, Univ Pittsburgh

Kamen, Barton A MD/PhD [PHO] - **Spec Exp:** Drug Development; **Hospital:** Robert Wood Johnson Univ Hosp - New Brunswick (page 106); **Address:** Cancer Inst of New Jersey, 195 Little Albany St, rm 3507, New Brunswick, NJ 08903; **Phone:** 732-235-8131; **Board Cert:** Pediatrics 81; Pediatric Hematology-Oncology 87; **Med School:** Case West Res Univ 76; **Resid:** Pediatrics, Yale-New Haven Hosp 78; **Fellow:** Pediatric Hematology-Oncology, Yale-New Haven Hosp 80; **Fac Appt:** Prof Ped, UMDNJ-RW Johnson Med Sch

Keller Jr, Frank G MD [PHO] - **Hospital:** WV Univ Hosp - Ruby Memorial; **Address:** West Virginia Univ HSC, Dept Pediatric Hem/Onc, One Medical Center Drive, Box 9214, Morgantown, WV 26506; **Phone:** 304-293-1217; **Board Cert:** Pediatric Hematology-Oncology 02; **Med School:** Univ NC Sch Med 86; **Resid:** Pediatrics, Vanderbilt Univ Med Ctr 90; **Fellow:** Pediatric Hematology-Oncology, Duke Univ Med Ctr 93

Korones, David MD [PHO] - **Spec Exp:** Brain Tumors; Palliative Care; Pediatric Oncology; **Hospital:** Univ of Rochester Strong Meml Hosp; **Address:** Golisano Childrens Hosp at Strong, 601 Elmwood Ave, Box 777, Rochester, NY 14642-8777; **Phone:** 585-275-2981; **Board Cert:** Pediatrics 87; Pediatric Hematology-Oncology 98; **Med School:** Vanderbilt Univ 83; **Resid:** Pediatrics, Strong Meml Hosp 86; **Fellow:** Pediatrics, Yale Univ 88; Pediatric Hematology-Oncology, Strong Meml Hosp 91; **Fac Appt:** Assoc Prof Ped, Univ Rochester

Kushner, Brian H MD [PHO] - **Spec Exp:** Neuroblastoma; Bone Marrow Transplant; Immunotherapy; **Hospital:** Meml Sloan Kettering Cancer Ctr (page 100); **Address:** 1275 York Ave, rm H1113, New York, NY 10021-6007; **Phone:** 212-639-6793; **Board Cert:** Pediatrics 83; Pediatric Hematology-Oncology 87; **Med School:** Johns Hopkins Univ 76; **Resid:** Pediatrics, Columbia-Presbyn Med Ctr 78; Pediatrics, NY Hosp 79; **Fellow:** Pediatric Hematology-Oncology, Boston Chldns Hosp 80; Pediatric Hematology-Oncology, Meml Sloan Kettering Cancer Ctr 86; **Fac Appt:** Prof Ped, Cornell Univ-Weill Med Coll

Lange, Beverly MD [PHO] - **Spec Exp:** Leukemia; Central Nervous System Tumors; **Hospital:** Chldns Hosp of Philadelphia, The; **Address:** Chldns Hosp Philadelphia, 34th & Civic Ctr Blvd, Philadelphia, PA 19104; **Phone:** 215-590-2249; **Board Cert:** Pediatrics 76; Pediatric Hematology-Oncology 97; **Med School:** Temple Univ 71; **Resid:** Pediatrics, Philadelphia Genl Hosp 73; **Fellow:** Pediatric Oncology, Chldns Hosp; **Fac Appt:** Prof Ped, Univ Pennsylvania

Lanzkowsky, Philip MD [PHO] - **Spec Exp:** Anemia; Leukemia; **Hospital:** Schneider Chldn's Hosp; **Address:** 269-01 76th Ave, Ste CH102, New Hyde Park, NY 11040-1434; **Phone:** 718-470-3201; **Board Cert:** Pediatrics 66; Pediatric Hematology-Oncology 74; **Med School:** South Africa 54; **Resid:** Pediatrics, Red Cross War Meml Chldns Hosp 60; Pediatrics, St Mary's Hosp 61; **Fellow:** Pediatric Hematology-Oncology, Duke Univ Med Ctr 62; Pediatric Hematology-Oncology, Univ UT Hosp 63; **Fac Appt:** Prof Ped, Albert Einstein Coll Med

Lipton, Jeffrey M MD/PhD [PHO] - **Spec Exp:** Bone Marrow Failure Disorders; Stem Cell Transplant; **Hospital:** Schneider Chldn's Hosp; **Address:** Div Hem-Onc & Stem Cell Transplant, 269-01 76th Ave, rm 255, MC-07670, New Hyde Park, NY 11040-1433; **Phone:** 718-470-3460; **Board Cert:** Pediatrics 81; **Med School:** St Louis Univ 75; **Resid:** Pediatrics, Boston Chldns Hosp 77; **Fellow:** Pediatric Hematology-Oncology, Boston Chldns Hosp/Dana Farber Cancer Inst 79; **Fac Appt:** Prof Ped, Albert Einstein Coll Med

Maris, John M MD [PHO] - **Spec Exp:** Neuroblastoma; Clinical Trials; **Hospital:** Chldns Hosp of Philadelphia, The; **Address:** Childrens Hosp - Oncology ARC 902A, 3615 Civic Center Blvd, Philadelphia, PA 19104-4318; **Phone:** 215-590-2821; **Board Cert:** Pediatric Hematology-Oncology 04; **Med School:** Univ Pennsylvania 89; **Resid:** Pediatrics, Chldns Hosp 92; **Fellow:** Pediatric Hematology-Oncology, Chldns Hosp 96

Meek, Rita MD [PHO] - **Hospital:** Alfred I duPont Hosp for Children; **Address:** Dupont Hosp for Children, Div Hem-Onc, 1600 Rockland Rd, PO Box 269, Wilmington, DE 19899; **Phone:** 302-651-5500; **Board Cert:** Pediatrics 79; Pediatric Hematology-Oncology 80; **Med School:** Geo Wash Univ 74; **Resid:** Pediatrics, Childns Hosp Natl Med Ctr 77; **Fellow:** Pediatric Hematology-Oncology, Chldns Hosp Natl Med Ctr 79; **Fac Appt:** Assoc Clin Prof Ped, Jefferson Med Coll

Meyers, Paul MD [PHO] - **Spec Exp:** Pediatric Cancers; Bone Tumors; Sarcoma; **Hospital:** Meml Sloan Kettering Cancer Ctr (page 100); **Address:** 1275 York Ave, Box 471, New York, NY 10021-6007; **Phone:** 212-639-5952; **Board Cert:** Pediatrics 78; Pediatric Hematology-Oncology 78; **Med School:** Mount Sinai Sch Med 73; **Resid:** Pediatrics, Mt Sinai Hosp 76; **Fellow:** Pediatric Hematology-Oncology, NY Hosp-Cornell 79; **Fac Appt:** Assoc Prof Ped, Cornell Univ-Weill Med Coll

O'Reilly, Richard MD [PHO] - **Spec Exp:** Bone Marrow Transplant; **Hospital:** Meml Sloan Kettering Cancer Ctr (page 100); **Address:** 1275 York Ave, rm H1409, New York, NY 10021; **Phone:** 212-639-5957; **Board Cert:** Pediatrics 74; **Med School:** Univ Rochester 68; **Resid:** Pediatrics, Chldrns Hosp 72; **Fellow:** Infectious Disease, Chldrns Hosp 73; **Fac Appt:** Prof Ped, Cornell Univ-Weill Med Coll

Parker, Robert MD [PHO] - **Spec Exp:** Pediatric Cancer; Bleeding/Coagulation Disorders; Platelet Disorders; **Hospital:** Stony Brook Univ Hosp; **Address:** Stony Brook Univ Hosp, Dept Peds, HSC T-11, Rm 029, Stony Brook, NY 11794-8111; **Phone:** 631-444-7720; **Board Cert:** Pediatrics 83; Pediatric Hematology-Oncology 84; **Med School:** Brown Univ 76; **Resid:** Internal Medicine, Roger Williams Med Ctr 77; Pediatrics, Rhode Island Hosp 79; **Fellow:** Pediatric Hematology-Oncology, Natl Cancer Inst 81; Hematology, Natl Cancer Inst 84; **Fac Appt:** Assoc Prof Ped, SUNY Stony Brook

Rausen, Aaron MD [PHO] - **Spec Exp:** Leukemia & Lymphoma; Bone Tumors & Soft Tissue Sarcomas; Retinoblastoma; **Hospital:** NYU Med Ctr (page 104); **Address:** NYU Medical Ctr, 317 E 34th St Fl 8, New York, NY 10016-4974; **Phone:** 212-263-7144; **Board Cert:** Pediatrics 60; Pediatric Hematology-Oncology 74; **Med School:** SUNY Downstate 54; **Resid:** Pediatrics, Bellevue Hosp 56; Pediatrics, Mount Sinai 59; **Fellow:** Hematology, Chldns Hosp 61; **Fac Appt:** Prof Ped, NYU Sch Med

Reaman, Gregory MD [PHO] - **Spec Exp:** Leukemia; Lymphoma; Cancer Survivors-Late Effects of Therapy; **Hospital:** Chldns Natl Med Ctr; **Address:** 111 Michigan Ave NW, Washington, DC 20010-2916; **Phone:** 202-884-2147; **Board Cert:** Pediatrics 78; Pediatric Hematology-Oncology 78; **Med School:** Loyola Univ-Stritch Sch Med 73; **Resid:** Hematology, Montreal Chldns Hosp 75; Pediatrics, Montreal Chldns Hosp 76; **Fellow:** Pediatric Oncology, Natl Cancer Inst 79; **Fac Appt:** Prof Ped, Geo Wash Univ

Rheingold, Susan R MD [PHO] - **Spec Exp:** Leukemia; Clinical Trials; Complementary Medicine; **Hospital:** Chldns Hosp of Philadelphia, The; **Address:** Chldns Hosp Phila - Div Oncology, 34th & Civic Ctr Blvd, Philadelphia, PA 19104; **Phone:** 215-590-3025; **Board Cert:** Pediatrics 03; Pediatric Hematology-Oncology 00; **Med School:** Univ Pennsylvania 92; **Resid:** Pediatrics, Johns Hopkins Hosp 95; **Fellow:** Pediatric Hematology-Oncology, Chldns Hosp 99; **Fac Appt:** Asst Prof Ped, Univ Pennsylvania

Ritchey, Arthur MD [PHO] - **Spec Exp:** Leukemia; Bleeding/Coagulation Disorders; **Hospital:** Chldns Hosp of Pittsburgh - UPMC (page 114); **Address:** Chldns Hosp, Div Hem Onc, 3705 Fifth Ave, Desoto Wing 4B, Ste 385, Pittsburgh, PA 15213; **Phone:** 412-692-5055; **Board Cert:** Pediatrics 77; Pediatric Hematology-Oncology 00; **Med School:** Univ Cincinnati 72; **Resid:** Pediatrics, Johns Hopkins Hosp 75; **Fellow:** Pediatric Hematology-Oncology, Yale-New Haven Hosp 80; **Fac Appt:** Prof Ped, Univ Pittsburgh

Schwartz, Cindy Lee MD [PHO] - **Spec Exp:** Hodgkin's Disease; Bone Cancer; Cancer Survivors-Late Effects of Therapy; **Hospital:** Johns Hopkins Hosp - Baltimore (page 97); **Address:** 600 N Wolfe St, CMSC-800, Baltimore, MD 21287; **Phone:** 410-955-2457; **Board Cert:** Pediatrics 85; Pediatric Hematology-Oncology 02; **Med School:** Brown Univ 79; **Resid:** Pediatrics, Johns Hopkins Hosp 82; **Fellow:** Pediatric Hematology-Oncology, Johns Hopkins Hosp 85; **Fac Appt:** Assoc Prof Ped, Johns Hopkins Univ

Steinherz, Peter G MD **[PHO]** - **Spec Exp:** Leukemia & Lymphoma; Pediatric Cancers; Wilms' Tumor; **Hospital:** Meml Sloan Kettering Cancer Ctr (page 100); **Address:** Memorial Sloan Kettering Cancer Ctr, 1275 York Ave, Box 411, New York, NY 10021; **Phone:** 212-639-7951; **Board Cert:** Pediatrics 73; Pediatric Hematology-Oncology 78; **Med School:** Albert Einstein Coll Med 68; **Resid:** Pediatrics, NY Cornell Med Ctr 71; **Fellow:** Pediatric Hematology-Oncology, NY Cornell Med Ctr 75; **Fac Appt:** Prof Ped, Cornell Univ-Weill Med Coll

Weiner, Michael MD **[PHO]** - **Spec Exp:** Hodgkin's Disease; Lymphoma; Leukemia; **Hospital:** NY-Presby Hosp - Columbia Presby Med Ctr (page 103); **Address:** 161 Fort Washington Ave, Irving Pavilion-FL 7, New York, NY 10032-3710; **Phone:** 212-305-9770; **Board Cert:** Pediatrics 80; Pediatric Hematology-Oncology 80; **Med School:** SUNY Hlth Sci Ctr 72; **Resid:** Pediatrics, Montefiore Med Ctr 74; **Fellow:** Pediatric Hematology-Oncology, NYU Med Ctr 76; Pediatric Hematology-Oncology, Johns Hopkins Hosp 77; **Fac Appt:** Prof Ped, Columbia P&S

Wexler, Leonard MD **[PHO]** - **Spec Exp:** Rhabdomyosarcoma; Bone Cancer; **Hospital:** Meml Sloan Kettering Cancer Ctr (page 100); **Address:** 1275 York Ave, Box 210, New York, NY 10021; **Phone:** 212-639-7990; **Board Cert:** Pediatrics 00; Pediatric Hematology-Oncology 00; **Med School:** Boston Univ 85; **Resid:** Pediatrics, Montefiore Med Ctr 88; **Fellow:** Pediatric Hematology-Oncology, National Cancer Inst 91; **Fac Appt:** Assoc Prof Ped, Columbia P&S

Southeast

Barbosa, Jerry L MD **[PHO]** - **Spec Exp:** Pediatric Cancers; **Hospital:** All Children's Hosp; **Address:** All Children's Hosp, Div Ped Hem/Onc, 880 6th St S, Ste 140, St Petersburg, FL 33701; **Phone:** 727-892-4175; **Board Cert:** Pediatrics 76; Pediatric Hematology-Oncology 78; **Med School:** Spain 69; **Resid:** Pediatrics, Rhode Island Hosp 74; **Fellow:** Pediatric Hematology-Oncology, Med Coll VA 76; **Fac Appt:** Assoc Clin Prof Ped, Univ S Fla Coll Med

Barredo, Julio C MD **[PHO]** - **Spec Exp:** Cancer Survivors-Late Effects of Therapy; Clinical Trials; **Hospital:** MUSC Med Ctr; **Address:** Med Univ South Carolina Med Ctr, 135 Rutledge Ave, PO Box 250558, Charleston, SC 29425; **Phone:** 843-792-2957; **Board Cert:** Pediatrics 00; Pediatric Hematology-Oncology 00; **Med School:** Peru 82; **Resid:** Pediatrics, Kings Co Hosp 87; **Fellow:** Pediatric Hematology-Oncology, Chldns Hosp/USC; **Fac Appt:** Prof Ped, Med Univ SC

Bertolone, Salvatore MD **[PHO]** - **Spec Exp:** Bone Marrow Transplant; Kasabach-Merritt Syndrome (KMS); Sickle Cell Disease; **Hospital:** Kosair Chldn's Hosp; **Address:** Kosair Childrens Hosp-Ped Hem/Onc, 571 S Floyd, rm 445, Louisville, KY 40202-3820; **Phone:** 502-852-8450; **Board Cert:** Pediatrics 75; Pediatric Hematology-Oncology 76; **Med School:** Univ Louisville Sch Med 70; **Resid:** Pediatrics, Univ Louisville 72; **Fellow:** Pediatric Hematology-Oncology, Univ Colorado 74; **Fac Appt:** Prof Ped, Univ Louisville Sch Med

Breitfeld, Philip P MD **[PHO]** - **Spec Exp:** Sarcoma; Clinical Trials; **Hospital:** Duke Univ Med Ctr (page 94); **Address:** Duke Univ Med Ctr, Box 2916, Durham, NC 27710; **Phone:** 919-684-3401; **Board Cert:** Pediatrics 84; Pediatric Hematology-Oncology 98; **Med School:** Univ Rochester 79; **Resid:** Pediatrics, Univ Rochester Med Ctr 82; **Fellow:** Pediatric Hematology-Oncology, Chldns Hosp 85; **Fac Appt:** Assoc Prof Ped, Duke Univ

Castleberry Jr, Robert P MD **[PHO]** - **Spec Exp:** Neuroblastoma; Leukemia; **Hospital:** Children's Hospital - Birmingham; **Address:** Univ of Ala Hosp at Birmingham-Dept Ped, 1600 7th Ave S, Ste ACC 512, Birmingham, AL 35233; **Phone:** 205-939-9285; **Board Cert:** Pediatrics 77; Pediatric Hematology-Oncology 98; **Med School:** Med Coll GA 71; **Resid:** Pediatrics, Chldns Hosp-Univ Ala 73; **Fellow:** Pediatric Hematology-Oncology, Univ of Ala Hosp 75; **Fac Appt:** Prof Ped, Univ Ala

Falletta, John MD **[PHO]** - **Hospital:** Duke Univ Med Ctr (page 94); **Address:** Duke Univ, N Pavillion, Ste 9000, 2400 Pratt St, Box 2991, Durham, NC 27705; **Phone:** 919-668-5111; **Board Cert:** Pediatrics 72; Pediatric Hematology-Oncology 74; **Med School:** Univ Kans 66; **Resid:** Pediatrics, Texas Childrens Hosp 71; **Fellow:** Pediatric Hematology-Oncology, Baylor 73; **Fac Appt:** Prof Ped, Duke Univ

Frangoul, Haydar MD **[PHO]** - **Spec Exp:** Stem Cell Transplant; **Hospital:** Vanderbilt Univ Med Ctr (page 116); **Address:** Vanderbilt Chldrns Hosp-Dept Ped Hem Onc, 2220 Pierce Ave, rm 397 PRB, Nashville, TN 37232-6310; **Phone:** 615-936-1762; **Board Cert:** Pediatrics 01; Pediatric Hematology-Oncology 00; **Med School:** Amer Univ Beirut 90; **Resid:** Pediatrics, Duke Univ Med Ctr 93; **Fellow:** Pediatric Hematology-Oncology, Duke Univ Med Ctr 94; **Fac Appt:** Asst Prof Ped, Vanderbilt Univ

Friedman, Henry S MD **[PHO]** - **Spec Exp:** Neuro-Oncology, Adult & Pediatric; Brain Tumors; **Hospital:** Duke Univ Med Ctr (page 94); **Address:** Brain Tumor Ctr at Duke University, Rm 047 Baker House, DUMC, Box 3624, Durham, NC 27710; **Phone:** 919-684-5301; **Board Cert:** Pediatrics 82; Pediatric Hematology-Oncology 82; **Med School:** SUNY Upstate Med Univ 77; **Resid:** Pediatrics, SUNY Upstate Med Ctr 80; **Fellow:** Pediatric Hematology-Oncology, Duke Univ Med Ctr 83; **Fac Appt:** Prof Ped, Duke Univ

Gold, Stuart H MD **[PHO]** - **Spec Exp:** Leukemia; Brain Tumors; Cancer Survivors-Late Effects of Therapy; **Hospital:** Univ NC Hosps (page 112); **Address:** Univ North Carolina - Dept Pediatrics, Div Hem/Onc, Gravely Clinical Bldg, CB 7220, Chapel Hill, NC 27599-7220; **Phone:** 919-966-1178; **Board Cert:** Pediatrics 86; Pediatric Hematology-Oncology 87; **Med School:** Vanderbilt Univ 81; **Resid:** Pediatrics, Univ Colorado Hlth Sci Ctr 84; **Fellow:** Pediatric Hematology-Oncology, Univ Colorado Hlth Sci Ctr 89; **Fac Appt:** Prof Ped, Univ NC Sch Med

Graham-Pole, John R MD **[PHO]** - **Spec Exp:** Bone Marrow Transplant; Palliative Care; Arts in the Healing Process; **Hospital:** Shands Hlthcre at Univ of FL (page 109); **Address:** Shands Hosp, Dept Ped Hem-Onc, 1600 SW Archer Rd, rm M401, Gainesville, FL 32610-0296; **Phone:** 352-392-5633; **Board Cert:** Pediatrics 83; Pediatric Hematology-Oncology 87; **Med School:** England 66; **Resid:** Pediatrics, Hosp Sick Chldn; Pediatrics, Royal Hosp Sick Chldn; **Fellow:** Pediatric Hematology-Oncology, Royal Hosp Sick Chldn; **Fac Appt:** Prof Ped, Univ Fla Coll Med

Horwitz, Edwin MD **[PHO]** - **Spec Exp:** Stem Cell Transplant; **Hospital:** St Jude Children's Research Hosp; **Address:** St Jude Children's Research Hosp-Dept Hem Onc, 332 N Lauderdale, MS 321, Memphis, TN 38105; **Phone:** 901-495-3695; **Board Cert:** Pediatric Hematology-Oncology 98; **Med School:** Indiana Univ 88; **Resid:** Pediatrics, Chldns Hosp/ Washington Univ 91; **Fellow:** Pediatric Hematology-Oncology, Chldns Hosp/ Washington Univ 94

Hudson, Melissa MD **[PHO]** - **Spec Exp:** Cancer Survivors-Late Effects of Therapy; Hodgkin's Disease; **Hospital:** St Jude Children's Research Hosp; **Address:** St Jude Children's Research Hosp, 322 N Lauderdale St, MS 735, Memphis, TN 38105; **Phone:** 901-495-3384; **Board Cert:** Pediatrics 88; Pediatric Hematology-Oncology 98; **Med School:** Univ Tex SW, Dallas 83; **Resid:** Pediatrics, Univ Texas Affil Hosps 86; **Fellow:** Pediatric Hematology-Oncology, MD Anderson Cancer Ctr 89

Kreissman, Susan G MD **[PHO]** - **Spec Exp:** Neuroblastoma; Clinical Trials; **Hospital:** Duke Univ Med Ctr (page 94); **Address:** Duke Univ Med Ctr, Box 2916, Durham, NC 27710; **Phone:** 919-684-3401; **Board Cert:** Pediatrics 98; Pediatric Hematology-Oncology 04; **Med School:** Mount Sinai Sch Med 85; **Resid:** Pediatrics, Chldns Hosp 88; **Fellow:** Pediatric Hematology-Oncology, Chldns Hosp/Dana Farber Cancer Inst 91; **Fac Appt:** Assoc Prof Ped, Duke Univ

Kurtzberg, Joanne MD [PHO] - **Spec Exp:** Stem Cell Transplant; Bone Marrow Transplant; **Hospital:** Duke Univ Med Ctr (page 94); **Address:** Duke Univ Med Ctr, Box 3350, 2400 Pratt St, Ste 1400, Durham, NC 27785; **Phone:** 919-668-1100; **Board Cert:** Pediatrics 82; Pediatric Hematology-Oncology 82; **Med School:** NY Med Coll 76; **Resid:** Pediatrics, Dartmouth Med Ctr 77; Pediatrics, Upstate Med Ctr 79; **Fellow:** Pediatric Hematology-Oncology, Upstate Med Ctr 80; Pediatric Hematology-Oncology, Duke Med Ctr 83; **Fac Appt:** Prof Ped, Duke Univ

Lauer, Stephen MD [PHO] - **Spec Exp:** Leukemia; Germ Cell Tumors; **Hospital:** Emory Univ Hosp; **Address:** 2015 Upper Gate Rd, Atlanta, GA 30322; **Phone:** 404-727-1380; **Board Cert:** Pediatrics 75; Pediatric Hematology-Oncology 78; **Med School:** Med Coll Wisc 70; **Resid:** Pediatrics, Milwaukee Chldns Hosp 73; **Fellow:** Pediatric Hematology-Oncology, Milwaukee Chldns Hosp 77; **Fac Appt:** Prof Ped, Emory Univ

Moscow, Jeffrey A MD [PHO] - **Spec Exp:** Pediatric Cancers; **Hospital:** Univ Kentucky Med Ctr; **Address:** Univ Kentucky - Kentucky Clinic, 740 S Limestone, rm J457, Lexington, KY 40536; **Phone:** 859-257-4554; **Board Cert:** Pediatrics 88; Pediatric Hematology-Oncology 00; **Med School:** Dartmouth Med Sch 82; **Resid:** Pediatrics, UTSW Med Sch; **Fellow:** Pediatric Hematology-Oncology, Natl Cancer Inst

Pui, Ching Hon MD [PHO] - **Spec Exp:** Leukemia; Lymphoma; **Hospital:** St Jude Children's Research Hosp; **Address:** St Jude Chldns Rsch Hosp, 332 N Lauderdale St, Memphis, TN 38105; **Phone:** 901-495-3335; **Board Cert:** Pediatrics 80; Pediatric Hematology-Oncology 82; **Med School:** Taiwan 76; **Resid:** Pediatrics, St Jude Chldns Rsch Hosp 79; **Fellow:** Hematology and Oncology, St Jude Chldns Rsch Hosp 81; **Fac Appt:** Prof Ped, Univ Tenn Coll Med, Memphis

Rosoff, Phillip M MD [PHO] - **Spec Exp:** Cancer Survivors-Late Effects of Therapy; Down Syndrome; Leukemia; **Hospital:** Duke Univ Med Ctr (page 94); **Address:** Duke Univ Med Ctr, Box 2916, Durham, NC 27710-0001; **Phone:** 919-684-3401; **Board Cert:** Pediatrics 84; Pediatric Hematology-Oncology 02; **Med School:** Case West Res Univ 78; **Resid:** Pediatrics, Chldns Hosp 80; **Fellow:** Pediatric Hematology-Oncology, Chldns Hosp/Dana Farber Cancer Inst 84; **Fac Appt:** Assoc Prof Ped, Duke Univ

Sandler, Eric MD [PHO] - **Spec Exp:** Bone Marrow Transplant; Leukemia; Clinical Trials; **Hospital:** Wolfson Chldns Hosp; **Address:** 807 Childrens Way, Jacksonville, FL 32207-8426; **Phone:** 904-390-3793; **Board Cert:** Pediatrics 00; Pediatric Hematology-Oncology 00; **Med School:** Univ VT Coll Med 85; **Resid:** Pediatrics, UCSF Med Ctr 88; **Fellow:** Pediatric Hematology-Oncology, Univ Fla Med Sch 91; **Fac Appt:** Assoc Prof Ped, Mayo Med Sch

Sandlund Jr, John T MD [PHO] - **Spec Exp:** Lymphoma, Non-Hodgkin's; Leukemia & Lymphoma; Ataxia-Telangiectasia (A-T); **Hospital:** St Jude Children's Research Hosp; **Address:** St Jude Children's Research Hosp, 332 N Lauderdale St, MS 260, Memphis, TN 38105; **Phone:** 901-495-3300; **Board Cert:** Pediatrics 86; Pediatric Hematology-Oncology 87; **Med School:** Ohio State Univ 80; **Resid:** Pediatrics, Columbus Chldns Hosp 83; **Fellow:** Hematology, National Cancer Inst 86; Research, National Cancer Inst 87

Tebbi, Cameron MD [PHO] - **Spec Exp:** Adolescent/Young Adult Cancers; Hemophilia; **Hospital:** St Joseph's Hosp - Tampa; **Address:** 3001 W Martin Luther King Jr Blvd, Tampa, FL 33607; **Phone:** 813-870-4243; **Board Cert:** Pediatrics 74; Pediatric Hematology-Oncology 80; **Med School:** Iran 68; **Resid:** Pediatrics, Cincinnati Chldns Hosp 72; Pediatric Hematology-Oncology, MD Anderson Cancer Inst 72; **Fellow:** Pediatric Hematology-Oncology, St Louis Chldns Hosp 73; Medical Oncology, Ontario Cancer Inst 74

Toledano, Stuart R MD **[PHO]** - **Spec Exp:** Leukemia; Solid Tumors; **Hospital:** Jackson Meml Hosp; **Address:** Univ Miami, Dept Peds-Div Ped Hem/Onc, (R-131) P.O. Box 016960, Miami, FL 33101; **Phone:** 305-585-5635; **Board Cert:** Pediatrics 86; Pediatric Hematology-Oncology 86; **Med School:** SUNY Buffalo 72; **Resid:** Pediatrics, Montefiore Med Ctr 75; **Fellow:** Pediatric Hematology-Oncology, Montefiore Med Ctr 75; **Fac Appt:** Prof Ped, Univ Miami Sch Med

Wang, Winfred C MD **[PHO]** - **Spec Exp:** Sickle Cell Disease; Bone Marrow Failure Disorders; Anemia-Aplastic; **Hospital:** St Jude Children's Research Hosp; **Address:** St Jude Chldn Rsch Hosp, 332 N Lauderdale St, rm R6010, Memphis, TN 38105-2729; **Phone:** 901-495-5700; **Board Cert:** Pediatrics 72; Pediatric Hematology-Oncology 74; **Med School:** Univ Chicago-Pritzker Sch Med 67; **Resid:** Pediatrics, Montefiore Med Ctr 69; Pediatrics, Kauikeolani Chldn's Hosp 70; **Fellow:** Pediatric Hematology-Oncology, Univ California 75; **Fac Appt:** Prof Ped, Univ Tenn Coll Med, Memphis

Whitlock, James A MD **[PHO]** - **Spec Exp:** Leukemia; **Hospital:** Vanderbilt Univ Med Ctr (page 116); **Address:** Vanderbilt Univ Med Ctr-Pediatrics, 2220 Pierce Ave, Nashville, TN 37232; **Phone:** 615-936-1762; **Board Cert:** Pediatrics 89; Pediatric Hematology-Oncology 00; **Med School:** Vanderbilt Univ 84; **Resid:** Pediatrics, Vanderbilt Univ Med Ctr 87; **Fellow:** Pediatric Hematology-Oncology, Vanderbilt Univ Med Ctr 90; **Fac Appt:** Assoc Prof Ped, Vanderbilt Univ

Woods, William G MD **[PHO]** - **Spec Exp:** Leukemia; Neuroblastoma; **Hospital:** Chldns Hlthcare Atlanta - Egleston; **Address:** AFLAC Cancer Ctr, 2015 Uppergate Drive, rm 404, Atlanta, GA 30322; **Phone:** 404-785-6170; **Board Cert:** Pediatrics 76; Pediatric Hematology-Oncology 78; **Med School:** Univ Pennsylvania 72; **Resid:** Pediatrics, Minnesota Hosp 75; **Fellow:** Hematology, Minnesota Hosp 77; **Fac Appt:** Prof Ped, Emory Univ

Midwest

Arndt, Carola A MD **[PHO]** - **Spec Exp:** Sarcoma; Brain Tumors; Stem Cell Transplant; **Hospital:** Mayo Med Ctr & Clin - Rochester; **Address:** Mayo Clinic - Dept Pediatrics, 200 1st St SW, Rochester, MN 55905; **Phone:** 507-284-2695; **Board Cert:** Pediatrics 82; Pediatric Hematology-Oncology 87; **Med School:** Boston Univ 78; **Resid:** Pediatrics, Naval Reg Med Ctr 81; **Fellow:** Pediatric Hematology-Oncology, Natl Inst Hlth 84

Camitta, Bruce MD **[PHO]** - **Spec Exp:** Anemia-Aplastic; Leukemia; Bone Marrow Transplant; **Hospital:** Chldns Hosp - Wisconsin; **Address:** Medical College of Wisconsin, 8701 Watertown Plank Rd, Milwaukee, WI 53226; **Phone:** 414-456-4170; **Board Cert:** Pediatrics 71; Pediatric Hematology-Oncology 76; **Med School:** Johns Hopkins Univ 66; **Resid:** Pediatrics, Children's Hosp 68; Pediatrics, Johns Hopkins Hosp 69; **Fellow:** Pediatric Hematology-Oncology, Children's Hosp 73; **Fac Appt:** Prof Ped, Med Coll Wisc

Castle, Valerie MD **[PHO]** - **Spec Exp:** Neuroblastoma; Bleeding/Coagulation Disorders; Cancer Survivors-Late Effects of Therapy; **Hospital:** Univ Michigan Hlth Sys; **Address:** Univ Mich Comp Cancer Ctr & Geriatric Ctr, 1500 E Med Ctr Drive, Ann Arbor, MI 48109-0938; **Phone:** 734-936-9814; **Board Cert:** Pediatrics 00; Pediatric Hematology-Oncology 98; **Med School:** McMaster Univ 83; **Resid:** Pediatrics, McMaster Univ Med Ctr 86; **Fellow:** Pediatric Hematology-Oncology, Univ Mich Hosps 89; **Fac Appt:** Prof Ped, Univ Mich Med Sch

Cohn, Susan L MD **[PHO]** - **Spec Exp:** Neuroblastoma; **Hospital:** Children's Mem Hosp; **Address:** 2300 Childrens Plz, Box 30, Children's Memorial Hospital, Chicago, IL 60614; **Phone:** 773-880-4562; **Board Cert:** Pediatrics 85; Pediatric Hematology-Oncology 87; **Med School:** Univ IL Coll Med 80; **Resid:** Pediatrics, Michael Reese Hosp 84; **Fellow:** Hematology and Oncology, Children's Memorial Hosp 85; **Fac Appt:** Prof Ped, Northwestern Univ

Davies, Stella M MD/PhD [PHO] - **Spec Exp:** Leukemia; Bone Marrow Transplant; Stem Cell Transplant; **Hospital:** Cincinnati Chldns Hosp Med Ctr; **Address:** Cincinnati Chldns Hosp Med Ctr, 3333 Burnet Ave, MLC 7015, Cincinnati, OH 45229-3039; **Phone:** 513-636-2469; **Med School:** England 81; **Resid:** Pediatrics, Univ Newcastle-Upon-Tyne 85; **Fellow:** Pediatric Hematology-Oncology, Univ Minn 93; **Fac Appt:** Prof Ped, Univ Cincinnati

Fallon, Robert J MD/PhD [PHO] - **Spec Exp:** Lymphoma; Hodgkin's Disease; Stem Cell Transplant; **Hospital:** Riley Chldns Hosp (page 90); **Address:** Riley Childrens Hospital, 702 Barnhill Drive, rm 4340, Indianapolis, IN 46202; **Phone:** 317-274-8784; **Board Cert:** Internal Medicine 83; Medical Oncology 85; **Med School:** NYU Sch Med 80; **Resid:** Internal Medicine, Brigham & Womens Hosp 83; **Fellow:** Hematology and Oncology, Brigham & Womens Hosp/Dana Farber Cancer Inst 85; **Fac Appt:** Prof Ped, Indiana Univ

Ferrara, James MD [PHO] - **Spec Exp:** Bone Marrow Transplant; Graft vs Host Disease; Inflammatory Cytokines; **Hospital:** Univ Michigan Hlth Sys; **Address:** Univ Michigan Comprehensive Cancer Ctr, 1500 E Medical Center Drive, Ste 6308, Ann Arbor, MI 48109-0942; **Phone:** 734-615-1340; **Board Cert:** Pediatrics 04; **Med School:** Georgetown Univ 80; **Resid:** Pediatrics, Children's Hosp 82; **Fellow:** Pediatric Hematology-Oncology, Children's Hosp 85; **Fac Appt:** Prof Ped, Univ Mich Med Sch

Friebert, Sarah E MD [PHO] - **Spec Exp:** Palliative Care; **Hospital:** Children's Hosp & Med Ctr-Akron; **Address:** Children's Hospital Medical Ctr of Akron, One Perkins Sq, Akron, OH 44308; **Phone:** 330-543-8730; **Board Cert:** Pediatrics 04; Pediatric Hematology-Oncology 00; **Med School:** Case West Res Univ 93; **Resid:** Pediatrics, Chldns Hosp 96; **Fellow:** Pediatric Hematology-Oncology, Rainbow Babies-Chldns Hosp 99

Goldman, Stewart MD [PHO] - **Spec Exp:** Neuro-Oncology; Brain Tumors; **Hospital:** Children's Mem Hosp; **Address:** Childrens Meml Hosp, Div Hem/Onc, 2300 Childrens Plaza, Box 30, Chicago, IL 60614; **Phone:** 773-880-4562; **Board Cert:** Pediatrics 97; Pediatric Hematology-Oncology 04; **Med School:** Loyola Univ-Stritch Sch Med 85; **Resid:** Pediatrics, Univ Chicago Hosps 88; **Fellow:** Pediatric Hematology-Oncology, Univ Chicago 91

Hayani, Ammar MD [PHO] - **Spec Exp:** Leukemia; Sarcoma; Bone Marrow Failure Disorders; **Hospital:** Adv Christ Med Ctr; **Address:** Hope Children's Hospital, 4440 W 95th St, Ste 4091, Oak Lawn, IL 60453-2600; **Phone:** 708-346-4094; **Board Cert:** Pediatrics 89; Pediatric Hematology-Oncology 98; **Med School:** Syria 82; **Resid:** Pediatrics, Louisiana State Univ 87; **Fellow:** Pediatric Hematology-Oncology, Baylor Coll Med 91

Hayashi, Robert J MD [PHO] - **Spec Exp:** Bone Marrow Transplant; Cancer Survivors-Late Effects of Therapy; Leukemia; **Hospital:** St Louis Chldns Hosp; **Address:** St Louis Children's Hosp, Div Ped Hem/Oncology, One Children's Pl Fl 9S, St Louis, MO 63110; **Phone:** 314-454-6018; **Board Cert:** Pediatrics 00; Pediatric Hematology-Oncology 00; **Med School:** Washington Univ, St Louis 86; **Resid:** Pediatrics, St Louis Children's Hosp 89; **Fellow:** Pediatric Hematology-Oncology, Johns Hopkins Hosp 92; **Fac Appt:** Asst Prof Ped, Washington Univ, St Louis

Hetherington, Maxine MD [PHO] - **Spec Exp:** Brain Tumors; **Hospital:** Chldns Mercy Hosps & Clinics; **Address:** Childrens Mercy Hosptial, 2401 Gillham Rd, Kansas City, MO 64108; **Phone:** 816-234-3265; **Board Cert:** Pediatrics 83; Pediatric Hematology-Oncology 87; **Med School:** Univ Tenn Coll Med, Memphis 78; **Resid:** Pediatrics, Childrens Med Ctr 81; **Fellow:** Pediatric Hematology-Oncology, Univ Texas Hlth Sci Ctr 87; **Fac Appt:** Assoc Prof Ped, Univ MO-Kansas City

Hilden, Joanne M MD [PHO] - **Spec Exp:** Pediatric & Infant Rare Cancers; Central Nervous System Tumors; Palliative Care; **Hospital:** Cleveland Clin Fdn (page 92); **Address:** Cleveland Clin Fdn, Dept Ped Hem/Onc, 9500 Euclid Ave, MS S20, Cleveland, OH 44195; **Phone:** 216-444-8407; **Board Cert:** Pediatrics 99; Pediatric Hematology-Oncology 02; **Med School:** Univ Minn 88; **Resid:** Pediatrics, Univ Minn 91; **Fellow:** Pediatric Hematology-Oncology, Univ Minn 94

Himelstein, Bruce MD [PHO] - **Spec Exp:** Palliative Care; **Hospital:** Chldns Hosp - Wisconsin; **Address:** Chldns Hosp of Wisconsin, 9000 W Wisconsin Ave, Milwaukee, WI 53226; **Phone:** 414-266-2775; **Board Cert:** Pediatrics 90; Pediatric Hematology-Oncology 02; **Med School:** NYU Sch Med 87; **Resid:** Pediatric Surgery, Albert Einstein Coll Med 90; **Fellow:** Pediatric Hematology-Oncology, Chldns Hosp 93; **Fac Appt:** Assoc Prof Ped, Med Coll Wisc

Hutchinson, Raymond MD [PHO] - **Spec Exp:** Bone Marrow Transplant; Leukemia; Hodgkin's Disease; **Hospital:** Univ Michigan Hlth Sys; **Address:** Cancer Ctr/Geriatrics Ctr, 1500 E Medical Center Drive, rm B1-207, Box 0914, Ann Arbor, MI 48109-0914; **Phone:** 734-936-8456; **Board Cert:** Pediatrics 79; Pediatric Hematology-Oncology 80; **Med School:** Harvard Med Sch 73; **Resid:** Pediatrics, New England Med Ctr 75; **Fellow:** Pediatric Hematology-Oncology, Childrens Hosp 78; **Fac Appt:** Prof Ped, Univ Mich Med Sch

Luchtman-Jones, Lori MD [PHO] - **Spec Exp:** Leukemia; Bleeding/Coagulation Disorders; Brain Tumors; **Hospital:** St Louis Chldns Hosp; **Address:** Pediatric Hematology-Oncology, 9 South, 1 Childrens Place, Box 8116, Saint Louis, MO 63110; **Phone:** 314-454-6018; **Board Cert:** Pediatrics 99; Pediatric Hematology-Oncology 04; **Med School:** UCSD 87; **Resid:** Pediatrics, UCSD School Med 90; **Fellow:** Pediatric Hematology-Oncology, Washington Univ 95; **Fac Appt:** Asst Prof Ped, Washington Univ, St Louis

Manera, Ricarchito MD [PHO] - **Spec Exp:** Leukemia; Brain Tumors; Lymphoma; **Hospital:** Loyola Univ Med Ctr (page 98); **Address:** Loyola University Med Ctr, 2160 S First Ave, Maywood, IL 60611; **Phone:** 708-327-9136; **Board Cert:** Pediatrics 03; Pediatric Hematology-Oncology 04; **Med School:** Philippines 84; **Resid:** Pediatrics, Bronx-Lebanon Hosp Ctr 95; **Fellow:** Pediatric Hematology-Oncology, MD Anderson Cancer Ctr 94; Pediatric Hematology-Oncology, Columbia-Presbyterian Med Ctr 96; **Fac Appt:** Asst Prof Ped, Loyola Univ-Stritch Sch Med

Morgan, Elaine MD [PHO] - **Spec Exp:** Leukemia; Palliative Care; **Hospital:** Children's Mem Hosp; **Address:** Children's Meml Hosp, Div Hem/Onc, 2300 Children's Plaza, Box 30, Chicago, IL 60614; **Phone:** 773-880-4562; **Board Cert:** Pediatrics 76; Pediatric Hematology-Oncology 78; **Med School:** Univ Pennsylvania 71; **Resid:** Pediatrics, Chldns Hosp 74; **Fellow:** Pediatric Hematology-Oncology, Chldns Hosp Med Ctr 75; Chldns Meml Med Ctr 76; **Fac Appt:** Assoc Prof Ped, Northwestern Univ

Nachman, James MD [PHO] - **Spec Exp:** Leukemia & Lymphoma; Bone Tumors; Hodgkin's Disease; **Hospital:** Univ of Chicago Hosps; **Address:** Univ Chicago Hosps, 5841 S Maryland Ave, MC 4060, Chicago, IL 60637; **Phone:** 773-702-6808; **Board Cert:** Pediatrics 79; Pediatric Hematology-Oncology 80; **Med School:** Johns Hopkins Univ 74; **Resid:** Pediatrics, Chldns Meml Hosp 77; Pediatrics, Fell-Wylers Chldns Hosp 80; **Fellow:** Pediatric Hematology-Oncology, Chldns Meml Hosp 79; **Fac Appt:** Prof Ped, Univ Chicago-Pritzker Sch Med

Neglia, Joseph MD [PHO] - **Spec Exp:** Cancer Survivors-Late Effects of Therapy; **Hospital:** Fairview-Univ Med Ctr - Univ Campus; **Address:** Univ Minnesota-Div Ped Hem/Oncology, 420 Delaware St SE, MMC 484, Minneapolis, MN 55455; **Phone:** 612-626-2778; **Board Cert:** Pediatrics 86; Pediatric Hematology-Oncology 87; **Med School:** Loma Linda Univ 81; **Resid:** Pediatrics, Baylor Coll Med 84; **Fellow:** Pediatric Hematology-Oncology, Univ Minn Hosp 87; **Fac Appt:** Prof Ped, Univ Minn

O'Leary, Maura C MD [PHO] - **Spec Exp:** Cancer Survivors-Late Effects of Therapy; Clinical Trials; **Hospital:** Chldns Hosp and Clinics - Minneapolis; **Address:** Children's Health Care Hem/Oncology Clinic, 2525 Chicago Ave S, Ste 4150, Minneapolis, MN 55404; **Phone:** 612-813-5940; **Board Cert:** Pediatrics 80; Pediatric Hematology-Oncology 80; **Med School:** Georgetown Univ 73; **Resid:** Pediatrics, NY Presby Hosp-Cornell 77; **Fellow:** Pediatric Hematology-Oncology, Fairview-Univ Med Ctr 80

Puccetti, Diane MD [PHO] - **Spec Exp:** Brain Tumors; Neuro-Oncology; Cancer Survivors-Late Effects of Therapy; **Hospital:** Univ WI Hosp & Clins; **Address:** 600 Highland Ave, rm K4-440, Madison, WI 53792; **Phone:** 608-263-6420; **Board Cert:** Pediatrics 89; Pediatric Hematology-Oncology 90; **Med School:** Med Coll OH 85; **Resid:** Pediatrics, UC-Irvine Med Ctr 86; Pediatrics, Med Coll Ohio 88; **Fellow:** Pediatric Hematology-Oncology, Riley Hosp Chldn 91; **Fac Appt:** Asst Clin Prof Ped, Univ Wisc

Salvi, Sharad MD [PHO] - **Spec Exp:** Leukemia; Bleeding/Coagulation Disorders; **Hospital:** Adv Christ Med Ctr; **Address:** Hope Chldns Hosp, 4440 W 95th St, rm 4091, Oak Lawn, IL 60453; **Phone:** 708-346-4094; **Board Cert:** Pediatrics 82; Pediatric Hematology-Oncology 82; **Med School:** India 74; **Resid:** Pediatrics, Lincoln Meml Hosp 79; **Fellow:** Pediatric Hematology-Oncology, Chldns Hosp/Roswell Park Meml Cancer Inst 81

Sondel, Paul M MD [PHO] - **Spec Exp:** Immunotherapy; Stem Cell Transplant; **Hospital:** Univ WI Hosp & Clins; **Address:** Univ Wisc Clinics, 600 Highland Ave, K4/448 Clin Sci Ctr, Madison, WI 53792-0001; **Phone:** 608-263-6200; **Board Cert:** Pediatrics 81; **Med School:** Harvard Med Sch 77; **Resid:** Pediatrics, Univ Minn Hosp 78; Pediatrics, Univ Wisc Hosp 80; **Fellow:** Research, Sidney Farber Cancer Inst/Harvard 77; **Fac Appt:** Prof Ped, Univ Wisc

Tannous, Raymond MD [PHO] - **Spec Exp:** Wilms' Tumor; Leukemia & Lymphoma; Pain-Cancer; **Hospital:** Univ Iowa Hosp & Clinics; **Address:** Univ Iowa Hosps & Clinics-Dept Peds, 2528 JCP, Iowa City, IA 52242; **Phone:** 319-356-1905; **Board Cert:** Pediatrics 76; Pediatric Hematology-Oncology 78; **Med School:** France 72; **Resid:** Pediatrics, St Jude Chldns Rsch Hosp 76; **Fellow:** Pediatric Hematology-Oncology, St Jude Chldns Rsch Hosp 77; **Fac Appt:** Assoc Prof Ped, Univ Iowa Coll Med

Valentino, Leonard A MD [PHO] - **Spec Exp:** Bleeding/Coagulation Disorders; Thrombotic Disorders; **Hospital:** Rush Univ Med Ctr; **Address:** Presby-St Luke's Profl Bldg, Ste 718, 1725 W Harrison St, Chicago, IL 60612-3828; **Phone:** 312-942-5983; **Board Cert:** Pediatrics 00; Pediatric Hematology-Oncology 98; **Med School:** Creighton Univ 84; **Resid:** Pediatrics, Univ Illinios Med Ctr 87; **Fellow:** Pediatric Hematology-Oncology, UCLA Med Ctr 90; **Fac Appt:** Assoc Prof Ped, Rush Med Coll

Vik, Terry A MD [PHO] - **Spec Exp:** Neuroblastoma; Clinical Trials; Cancer Survivors-Late Effects of Therapy; **Hospital:** Riley Chldns Hosp (page 90); **Address:** Riley Hosp Children, 702 Barnhill Dr, Riley 4340, Indianapolis, IN 46202; **Phone:** 317-274-2143; **Board Cert:** Pediatrics 87; Pediatric Hematology-Oncology 04; **Med School:** Johns Hopkins Univ 83; **Resid:** Pediatrics, UCLA Med Ctr 86; **Fellow:** Pediatric Hematology-Oncology, Chldns Hosp 89; **Fac Appt:** Assoc Prof Ped, Indiana Univ

Great Plains and Mountains

Abromowitch, Minnie MD [PHO] - **Hospital:** Children's Hosp - Omaha; **Address:** Children's Memorial Hospital-Dept Ped Hem Onc, 8200 Dodge St, Omaha, NE 68198; **Phone:** 402-955-3950; **Board Cert:** Pediatrics 80; Pediatric Hematology-Oncology 82; **Med School:** Canada 72; **Resid:** Pediatrics, Hospital for Sick Children 76; **Fellow:** Pediatric Hematology-Oncology, Univ Manitoba 78; Pediatric Hematology-Oncology, St Jude Chldns Research Hosp 80; **Fac Appt:** Assoc Prof Ped, Univ Nebr Coll Med

Bruggers, Carol S MD [PHO] - **Spec Exp:** Leukemia; Clinical Trials; **Hospital:** Primary Children's Med Ctr; **Address:** Primary Children's Medical Ctr, 100 N Medical Drive, Ste 1400, Salt Lake City, UT 84113; **Phone:** 801-588-2680; **Board Cert:** Pediatrics 00; Pediatric Hematology-Oncology 00; **Med School:** Mich State Univ 84; **Resid:** Pediatrics, Univ Colorado Health Sci Ctr 87; **Fellow:** Pediatric Hematology-Oncology, Duke Univ Med Ctr 91; **Fac Appt:** Assoc Prof Med, Univ Utah

Coccia, Peter MD [PHO] - **Spec Exp:** Bone Marrow Transplant; Leukemia & Lymphoma; Solid Tumors; **Hospital:** Nebraska Med Ctr; **Address:** Univ Nebr Med Ctr, Dept Peds, 982168 Nebraska Med Ctr, Omaha, NE 68198-2168; **Phone:** 402-559-7257; **Board Cert:** Clinical Pathology 72; Hematology 75; Pediatrics 76; Pediatric Hematology-Oncology 76; **Med School:** SUNY Upstate Med Univ 68; **Resid:** Pathology, Upstate Med Ctr 70; Pediatrics, Univ Minn 73; **Fellow:** Pediatric Hematology-Oncology, Univ Minn 74; **Fac Appt:** Prof Ped, Univ Nebr Coll Med

Johnston, J Martin MD [PHO] - **Spec Exp:** Leukemia; Lymphoma; Hemophilia; **Hospital:** St. Luke's Reg Med Ctr - Boise; **Address:** 100 E Idaho St, Boise, ID 83712; **Phone:** 208-381-2782; **Board Cert:** Pediatric Hematology-Oncology 02; **Med School:** Duke Univ 84; **Resid:** Pediatrics, Univ Utah 88; **Fellow:** Pediatric Hematology-Oncology, Wash Univ 91

Manco-Johnson, Marilyn MD [PHO] - **Spec Exp:** Hemophilia; Thrombotic Disorders; **Hospital:** Chldn's Hosp - Denver, The; **Address:** Univ Colorado Hlth Sci Ctr, Hemophilia Ctr, Box 6507, MS F416, Aurora, CO 80045-0507; **Phone:** 303-724-0365; **Board Cert:** Pediatrics 79; Pediatric Hematology-Oncology 80; **Med School:** Jefferson Med Coll 74; **Resid:** Pediatrics, Univ Colorado Affil Hosps 77; **Fellow:** Pediatric Hematology-Oncology, Chldn's Hosp/Colorado Med Ctr 81; **Fac Appt:** Prof Ped, Univ Colorado

Odom, Lorrie F MD [PHO] - **Spec Exp:** Leukemia; Solid Tumors; Cancer Survivors-Late Effects of Therapy; **Hospital:** Presby - St Luke's Med Ctr; **Address:** Childhood Hem/Onc Assocs, 1601 S 19th Ave, Ste 5100, Denver, CO 80218; **Phone:** 303-832-2462; **Board Cert:** Pediatrics 74; Pediatric Hematology-Oncology 76; **Med School:** Univ Colorado 69; **Resid:** Pediatrics, Childrens Hosp 72; **Fellow:** Pediatric Hematology-Oncology, Dana-Farber Cancer Inst 74; Pediatric Hematology-Oncology, Univ Colorado Med Ctr 75; **Fac Appt:** Prof Ped, Univ Colorado

Southwest

Abella, Esteban MD [PHO] - **Spec Exp:** Leukemia; Anemia-Aplastic, Leukemia; Neuroblastoma; **Hospital:** Banner Desert Med Ctr; **Address:** 1450 S Dobson, Ste A-108, Mesa, AZ 85202; **Phone:** 480-833-1123; **Board Cert:** Pediatrics 98; Pediatric Hematology-Oncology 02; **Med School:** Dominican Republic 85; **Resid:** Pediatrics, Chldns Hosp of MI 88; **Fellow:** Pediatric Hematology-Oncology, Chldns Hosp of MI 91; **Fac Appt:** Prof Ped, Wayne State Univ

Berg, Stacey MD [PHO] - **Hospital:** Texas Chldns Hosp - Houston; **Address:** Texas Chldns Cancer Ctr, Ped Hem-Onc, 6621 Fannin St, MC 3-3320, Houston, TX 77030; **Phone:** 832-824-4588; **Board Cert:** Pediatrics 00; Pediatric Hematology-Oncology 00; **Med School:** Univ Pittsburgh 85; **Resid:** Pediatrics, Chldns Hosp 88; **Fellow:** Pediatric Hematology-Oncology, Natl Inst Hlth 91

Blaney, Susan MD [PHO] - **Spec Exp:** Brain Tumors; Neuro-Oncology; **Hospital:** Texas Chldns Hosp - Houston; **Address:** 6621 Fannin St #CC 1410.0.0, Houston, TX 77030; **Phone:** 832-822-1482; **Board Cert:** Pediatrics 98; Pediatric Hematology-Oncology 98; **Med School:** Med Coll OH 84; **Resid:** Pediatrics, Letterman AMC 87; **Fellow:** Pediatric Oncology, Walter Reed AMC 90; **Fac Appt:** Assoc Prof Ped, Baylor Coll Med

Bleyer, W Archie MD [PHO] - **Spec Exp:** Adolescent/Young Adult Cancers; Brain & Spinal Cord Tumors; Clinical Trials; **Hospital:** UT MD Anderson Cancer Ctr, The (page 115); **Address:** Univ Texas/MD Anderson Cancer Ctr, 1515 Holcombe Blvd, MC 241, Houston, TX 77030-4009; **Phone:** 713-792-8516; **Board Cert:** Pediatrics 86; Pediatric Hematology-Oncology 86; **Med School:** Univ Rochester 69; **Resid:** Pediatrics, Univ Washington Med Ctr 71; Pediatric Hematology-Oncology, Natl Cancer Inst 74; **Fellow:** Pediatric Hematology-Oncology, Univ Washington 75; Radiation Oncology, Univ Washington 86; **Fac Appt:** Prof Ped, Univ Tex, Houston

Corey, Seth MD [PHO] - **Spec Exp:** Multiple Myeloma; Leukemia; **Hospital:** UT MD Anderson Cancer Ctr, The (page 115); **Address:** MD Anderson Cancer Ctr, 1515 Holcombe Blvd, Houston, TX 77030; **Phone:** 713-792-6615; **Board Cert:** Pediatrics 86; Pediatric Hematology-Oncology 87; **Med School:** Tulane Univ 82; **Resid:** Pediatrics, St Louis Chldns Hosp 85; **Fellow:** Hematology and Oncology, Tufts Med Sch 92; Hematology and Oncology, Boston Chldns-Dana Farber Ctr 89; **Fac Appt:** Assoc Prof Ped, Univ Tex, Houston

Dreyer, ZoAnn E MD [PHO] - **Spec Exp:** Cancer Survivors-Late Effects of Therapy; Leukemia in Infants; **Hospital:** Texas Chldns Hosp - Houston; **Address:** Texas Childrens Hosp, Clinical Care Ctr, 6701 Fannin Fl 14, MC CC1410, Houston, TX 77030; **Phone:** 832-822-4242; **Board Cert:** Pediatrics 88; Pediatric Hematology-Oncology 98; **Med School:** UC Davis 82; **Resid:** Pediatrics, Baylor Affil Hosps 85; **Fellow:** Pediatric Hematology-Oncology, Baylor Coll Med 88; **Fac Appt:** Assoc Prof Ped, Baylor Coll Med

Goldman, Stanton C MD [PHO] - **Spec Exp:** Leukemia; Lymphoma; Stem Cell Transplant; **Hospital:** Med City Dallas Hosp; **Address:** 7777 Forest Ln, Ste D-400, Dallas, TX 75230; **Phone:** 972-566-6647; **Board Cert:** Pediatrics 01; Pediatric Hematology-Oncology 04; **Med School:** Boston Univ 90; **Resid:** Pediatrics, Chldns Natl Med Ctr; **Fellow:** Pediatric Hematology-Oncology, Johns Hopkins Hosp

Graham, Michael L MD [PHO] - **Spec Exp:** Bone Marrow Transplant; Leukemia; Stem Cell Transplant; **Hospital:** Univ Med Ctr - Tucson; **Address:** Univ Arizona Hlth Science Ctr, 1501 N Campbell Ave, rm 4341, Box 245073, Tucson, AZ 85724-5073; **Phone:** 520-626-6527; **Board Cert:** Pediatrics 80; Pediatric Hematology-Oncology 84; **Med School:** Brown Univ 75; **Resid:** Pediatrics, Johns Hopkins Hosp 78; Pediatric Hematology-Oncology, Johns Hopkins Hosp 80; **Fellow:** Medical Oncology, Yale-New Haven Hosp 82; **Fac Appt:** Assoc Prof PHO, Univ Ariz Coll Med

Kane, Javier R MD [PHO] - **Spec Exp:** Palliative Care; **Hospital:** Santa Rosa Children's Hosp; **Address:** Santa Rosa Chldns Hosp, 333 N Santa Rosa, San Antonio, TX 78207; **Phone:** 210-704-2187; **Board Cert:** Pediatrics 00; **Med School:** Mexico 86; **Resid:** Pediatrics, Austin Med Ed Prog; **Fellow:** Pediatric Hematology-Oncology, Univ Tennessee; **Fac Appt:** Assoc Prof Ped, Univ Tex, San Antonio

Murphy, Sharon B MD [PHO] - **Spec Exp:** Lymphoma, Non-Hodgkin's; Leukemia; **Hospital:** UTSA - Univ Hosp; **Address:** UTHSCSA - Children's Cancer Research Inst, 8403 Floyd Curl Drive, MS 7784, San Antonio, TX 78229-3900; **Phone:** 210-562-9000; **Board Cert:** Pediatrics 90; Pediatric Hematology-Oncology 90; **Med School:** Harvard Med Sch 69; **Resid:** Pediatrics, Univ Colorado Med Ctr 71; **Fellow:** Pediatric Hematology-Oncology, Chldns Hosp 73; **Fac Appt:** Prof Ped, Univ Tex, San Antonio

Raney Jr, R Beverly MD [PHO] - **Spec Exp:** Rhabdomyosarcoma; Sarcoma-Soft Tissue; **Hospital:** UT MD Anderson Cancer Ctr, The (page 115); **Address:** MD Anderson Cancer Ctr, 1515 Holcombe Blvd, Unit 87, Houston, TX 77030; **Phone:** 713-792-6624; **Board Cert:** Pediatrics 71; Pediatric Hematology-Oncology 74; **Med School:** Univ Pennsylvania 65; **Resid:** Pediatrics, NC Meml Hosp 68; **Fellow:** Pediatric Hematology-Oncology, Duke Med Ctr 73; Pediatric Hematology-Oncology, Chldns Hosp 74; **Fac Appt:** Prof Ped, Univ Tex, Houston

Scher, Charles D MD [PHO] - **Spec Exp:** Sickle Cell Anemia; Leukemia; **Hospital:** Tulane Univ Med Ctr Hosp & Clin; **Address:** Tulane University Hospital, Dept Pediatrics, 1430 Tulane Ave, Box SL-37, New Orleans, LA 70112; **Phone:** 504-588-5412; **Board Cert:** Pediatrics 72; **Med School:** Univ Pennsylvania 65; **Resid:** Pediatrics, Bronx Muni Hosp Ctr 67; Pediatrics, Chldns Hosp Med Ctr 72; **Fellow:** Pediatric Hematology-Oncology, Chldns Hosp Med Ctr 74; **Fac Appt:** Prof Ped, Tulane Univ

Tomlinson, Gail E MD [PHO] - **Spec Exp:** Cancer Survivors-Late Effects of Therapy; Cancer Genetics; Liver & Kidney Cancer; **Hospital:** Chldns Med Ctr of Dallas; **Address:** UT Southwestern Med Ctr, 5323 Harry Hines Blvd, Dallas, TX 75390-8593; **Phone:** 214-648-4907; **Board Cert:** Pediatrics 01; Pediatric Hematology-Oncology 02; **Med School:** Geo Wash Univ 84; **Resid:** Pediatrics, Chldns Hosp Natl Med Ctr 87; **Fellow:** Pediatric Hematology-Oncology, MD Anderson Cancer Ctr 89; Pediatric Hematology-Oncology, Univ Texas SW Med Ctr 92; **Fac Appt:** Assoc Prof Ped, Univ Tex SW, Dallas

Wall, Donna A MD [PHO] - **Spec Exp:** Bone Marrow & Stem Cell Transplant; Immune Deficiency/SCIDS; **Hospital:** Methodist Hosp - Houston; **Address:** Texas Transplant Inst, 8201 Ewing Halsell, Ste 280, San Antonio, TX 78229; **Phone:** 210-575-7138; **Board Cert:** Pediatrics 86; Pediatric Hematology-Oncology 87; **Med School:** Canada 81; **Resid:** Pediatrics, NY Presby Hosp-Columbia Univ; Pediatrics, New England Med Ctr; **Fellow:** Pediatric Hematology-Oncology, Dana Farber Cancer Inst

Warrier, Rajasekharan MD [PHO] - **Spec Exp:** Leukemia; Sickle Cell Disease; Clinical Trials; **Hospital:** Children's Hospital - New Orleans; **Address:** Childrens Hosp - New Orleans Dept Ped Hem/Onc, 200 Henry Clay Ave, Ste 4109, New Orleans, LA 70118-5720; **Phone:** 504-896-9740; **Board Cert:** Pediatrics 77; Pediatric Hematology-Oncology 80; **Med School:** India 73; **Resid:** Pediatrics, Henry Ford Hosp 77; **Fellow:** Pediatric Hematology-Oncology, Wayne State Univ 79; **Fac Appt:** Prof Ped, Louisiana State Univ

Winick, Naomi J MD [PHO] - **Spec Exp:** Leukemia; **Hospital:** Chldns Med Ctr of Dallas; **Address:** Univ Texas Health Science Ctr-Peds, 5323 Harry Hines Blvd, Dallas, TX 75390-9063; **Phone:** 214-456-2382; **Board Cert:** Pediatrics 84; Pediatric Hematology-Oncology 87; **Med School:** Northwestern Univ 78; **Resid:** Pediatrics, Babies Hosp-Columbia Presbyterian Med Ctr 81; **Fellow:** Pediatric Hematology-Oncology, Sloan-Kettering Cancer Ctr 83; **Fac Appt:** Prof Ped, Univ Tex SW, Dallas

Yeager, Andrew M MD [PHO] - **Spec Exp:** Stem Cell Transplant; **Hospital:** Univ Med Ctr - Tucson; **Address:** Arizona Cancer Ctr, 1515 N Campbell Ave, Ste 2956, Tuscon, AZ 85724; **Phone:** 520-626-0662; **Board Cert:** Pediatrics 79; Pediatric Hematology-Oncology 80; **Med School:** Johns Hopkins Univ 75; **Resid:** Pediatrics, Johns Hopkins Hosp 78; **Fellow:** Pediatric Hematology-Oncology, Johns Hopkins Hosp 80; **Fac Appt:** Prof Ped, Univ Ariz Coll Med

West Coast and Pacific

Andrews, Robert G MD [PHO] - **Spec Exp:** Bone Marrow Transplant; Leukemia; Lymphoma; **Hospital:** Chldns Hosp and Regl Med Ctr - Seattle; **Address:** Fred Hutchinson Cancer Researcg Ctr, D2-373, 1100 Fairview Ave N, Seattle, WA 98109-1024; **Phone:** 206-288-1024; **Board Cert:** Pediatrics 84; Pediatric Hematology-Oncology 84; **Med School:** Univ Minn 76; **Resid:** Internal Medicine, New England Med Ctr 79; **Fellow:** Pediatric Hematology-Oncology, Children's Hosp Med Ctr 83; **Fac Appt:** Clin Prof Ped, Univ Wash

Ducore, Jonathan M MD [PHO] - **Spec Exp:** Brain Tumors; Bone & Soft Tissue Tumors; Bleeding/Coagulation Disorders; **Hospital:** UC Davis Med Ctr; **Address:** UC Davis Med Ctr, Dept Pediatrics, 2516 Stockton Blvd, Sacramento, CA 95817; **Phone:** 916-734-2781; **Board Cert:** Pediatrics 78; Pediatric Hematology-Oncology 78; **Med School:** Duke Univ 73; **Resid:** Pediatrics, Chldns Med Ctr 75; **Fellow:** Pediatric Hematology-Oncology, Univ Colorado Med Ctr 77; Cancer Research, Natl Cancer Inst 80; **Fac Appt:** Assoc Prof Ped, UC Davis

Feig, Stephen A MD **[PHO]** - **Spec Exp:** Leukemia; Bone Marrow Transplant; Anemia; **Hospital:** UCLA Med Ctr (page 111); **Address:** Mattel Chldns Hosp @ UCLA, Dept Pediatric Hem/Onc, 10833 Le Conte Ave, rm A2-410 MDCC, Los Angeles, CA 90095; **Phone:** 310-825-6708; **Board Cert:** Pediatrics 68; Pediatric Hematology-Oncology 74; **Med School:** Columbia P&S 63; **Resid:** Pediatrics, Mt Sinai Hosp 66; **Fellow:** Pediatric Hematology-Oncology, Chldns Hosp 72; **Fac Appt:** Prof Ped, UCLA

Finklestein, Jerry Z MD **[PHO]** - **Spec Exp:** Ovarian Cancer; Cervical Cancer; **Hospital:** Long Beach Meml Med Ctr; **Address:** 2653 Elm Ave, Ste 200, Long Beach, CA 90806-1600; **Phone:** 562-492-1062; **Board Cert:** Pediatrics 80; Pediatric Hematology-Oncology 74; **Med School:** McGill Univ 63; **Resid:** Pediatrics, Montreal Chldns Hosp 66; **Fellow:** Hematology and Oncology, LA Chldns Hosp 68; **Fac Appt:** Clin Prof Ped, UCLA

Finlay, Jonathan MD **[PHO]** - **Spec Exp:** Brain Tumors; **Hospital:** Chldns Hosp - Los Angeles; **Address:** Chldrns Hosp - LA Ped Hem-Onc, 4650 Sunset Blvd, MS 54, Los Angeles, CA 90027; **Phone:** 323-906-8147; **Board Cert:** Pediatrics 84; Pediatric Hematology-Oncology 87; **Med School:** England 73; **Resid:** Pediatrics, Univ Birmingham 75; Pediatrics, Christie Hosp 76; **Fellow:** Pediatric Allergy & Immunology, Univ Wisconsin Hosp 78; Pediatric Hematology-Oncology, Univ Wisconsin Hosp 80; **Fac Appt:** Prof Ped, NYU Sch Med

Friedman, Debra L MD **[PHO]** - **Spec Exp:** Cancer Survivors-Late Effects of Therapy; Hodgkin's Disease; Retinoblastoma; **Hospital:** Chldns Hosp and Regl Med Ctr - Seattle; **Address:** Childrens Hosp & Regl Med Ctr, Div Hem/Onc, 4800 Sand Point Way NE, MS 6D1, Seattle, WA 98105; **Phone:** 206-987-2106; **Board Cert:** Pediatric Hematology-Oncology 98; **Med School:** UMDNJ-RW Johnson Med Sch 91; **Resid:** Pediatrics, Chldns Hosp 94; **Fellow:** Pediatric Hematology-Oncology, Chldns Hosp 97; **Fac Appt:** Asst Prof Ped, Univ Wash

Geyer, J Russell MD **[PHO]** - **Spec Exp:** Brain Tumors; **Hospital:** Chldns Hosp and Regl Med Ctr - Seattle; **Address:** Chldns Hosp & Reg Med Ctr - Div Hem/Onc, 4800 Sands Point Way NE, MS 6D1, Seattle, WA 98105; **Phone:** 206-987-2106; **Board Cert:** Pediatrics 83; Pediatric Hematology-Oncology 87; **Med School:** Wayne State Univ 77; **Resid:** Pediatrics, Chldns Hosp Michigan 80; **Fellow:** Pediatric Hematology-Oncology, Univ Michigan Med Ctr 81; **Fac Appt:** Prof Ped, Univ Wash

Glader, Bertil MD **[PHO]** - **Spec Exp:** Genetic Blood Disorders; **Hospital:** Stanford Univ Med Ctr; **Address:** 1000 Welch Rd, Ste 300, Palo Alto, CA 94305; **Phone:** 650-497-8953; **Board Cert:** Pediatrics 82; Pediatric Hematology-Oncology 82; Hematology 83; **Med School:** Northwestern Univ 68; **Resid:** Pediatrics, Chldns Hosp Med Ctr 73; **Fellow:** Hematology, Chldns Hosp Med Ctr 75; **Fac Appt:** Prof Ped, Stanford Univ

Godder, Kamar MD/PhD **[PHO]** - **Spec Exp:** Stem Cell Transplant; Leukemia; Palliative Care; **Hospital:** Doernbecher Chldns Hosp/OHSU; **Address:** OHSU Div of Ped Hematology, 3181 SW Sam Jackson Park Rd, MC CDRCP, Portland, OR 97239; **Phone:** 503-494-0829; **Board Cert:** Pediatrics 89; Pediatric Hematology-Oncology 98; **Med School:** Israel 80; **Resid:** Pediatrics, Hadassah-Mt Scopus 84; **Fellow:** Pediatric Hematology-Oncology, Meml Sloan Kettering 88; **Fac Appt:** Prof PHO, Oregon Hlth Sci Univ

Hawkins, Douglas MD **[PHO]** - **Spec Exp:** Bone Tumors; Ewing's & Rhadomyosarcoma; Leukemia; **Hospital:** Chldns Hosp and Regl Med Ctr - Seattle; **Address:** Children's Hospital & Regional Medical Center-Dept Hem-Onc, 4800 Sand Point Way, MS B6553, Seattle, WA 98105; **Phone:** 206-987-2106; **Board Cert:** Pediatrics 01; Pediatric Hematology-Oncology 04; **Med School:** Harvard Med Sch 90; **Resid:** Pediatrics, Univ Washington Med Ctr 93; **Fellow:** Pediatric Hematology-Oncology, Fred Hutchinson Cancer Research Ctr 96

Horn, Biljana N MD [PHO] - **Spec Exp:** Bone Marrow Transplant; Brain Tumors; **Hospital:** UCSF Med Ctr; **Address:** UCSF Med Ctr, Peds BMT Program, 505 Parnassus Ave, rm M-659, San Francisco, CA 94143; **Phone:** 415-476-2188; **Board Cert:** Pediatrics 05; Pediatric Hematology-Oncology 04; **Med School:** Yugoslavia 83; **Resid:** Pediatrics, Rainbow Babies & Chldns Hosp 91; **Fellow:** Pediatric Hematology-Oncology, Natl Cancer Inst 94; Pediatric Neuro-Oncology, UCSF 98; **Fac Appt:** Asst Prof Ped, UCSF

Kadota, Richard P MD [PHO] - **Spec Exp:** Bone Marrow Transplant; Brain Tumors; Clinical Trials; **Hospital:** Children's Hosp and Hlth Ctr - San Diego; **Address:** Children's Hospital, San Diego, 3020 Children's Way, MC 5035, San Diego, CA 92123; **Phone:** 858-576-5811; **Board Cert:** Pediatrics 84; Pediatric Hematology-Oncology 84; **Med School:** Northwestern Univ 79; **Resid:** Pediatrics, Mayo Clinic 83; **Fellow:** Pediatric Hematology-Oncology, Mayo Clinic 85; **Fac Appt:** Clin Prof Ped, UCSD

Kapoor, Neena MD [PHO] - **Spec Exp:** Bone Marrow Transplant; **Hospital:** Chldns Hosp - Los Angeles; **Address:** Childrens Hosp at Los Angeles-Rsch Immunology/BMT, 4650 Sunset Blvd, MS 62, Los Angeles, CA 90027; **Phone:** 323-669-2546; **Board Cert:** Pediatrics 78; Pediatric Hematology-Oncology 96; **Med School:** India 72; **Resid:** Pediatrics, Rhode Island Hosp 76; **Fellow:** Pediatric Hematology-Oncology, Meml Sloan-Kettering Cancer Ctr 78; **Fac Appt:** Prof Ped, USC Sch Med

Kung, Faith MD [PHO] - **Spec Exp:** Leukemia; Lymphoma; **Hospital:** UCSD Med Ctr; **Address:** UCSD Med Ctr, Div Ped Hem/Oncology, 200 W Arbor Drive, San Diego, CA 92103; **Phone:** 619-543-6845; **Board Cert:** Pediatrics 62; Pediatric Hematology-Oncology 74; **Med School:** Univ VA Sch Med 57; **Resid:** Pediatrics, NC Meml Hosp 60; **Fellow:** Pediatric Hematology-Oncology, Chldns Hosp/Babies Hosp 62; **Fac Appt:** Prof Ped, UCSD

Link, Michael P MD [PHO] - **Spec Exp:** Stem Cell Transplant; **Hospital:** Stanford Univ Med Ctr; **Address:** 1000 Welch Rd, Ste 300, Palo Alto, CA 94304; **Phone:** 650-723-5535; **Board Cert:** Pediatrics 79; Pediatric Hematology-Oncology 80; **Med School:** Stanford Univ 74; **Resid:** Pediatrics, Chldns Hosp Med Ctr 76; **Fellow:** Hematology and Oncology, Dana Farber Cancer Inst 79; **Fac Appt:** Prof Ped, Stanford Univ

Marina, Neyssa MD [PHO] - **Spec Exp:** Sarcoma; Cancer Survivors-Late Effects of Therapy; Germ Cell Tumors; **Hospital:** Lucile Packard Chldns Hosp/Stanford Univ Med Ctr; **Address:** Pediatric Hematology & Oncology, 725 Walsh Rd-Clinic E, Palo Alto, CA 94304; **Phone:** 650-497-8953; **Board Cert:** Pediatrics 87; Pediatric Gastroenterology 98; **Med School:** Puerto Rico 83; **Resid:** Pediatrics, Univ Pediatric Hosp 86; **Fellow:** Pediatric Hematology-Oncology, St Jude Children's Hosp 89; **Fac Appt:** Prof Ped, Stanford Univ

Matthay, Katherine K MD [PHO] - **Spec Exp:** Neuroblastoma; Bone Marrow & Stem Cell Transplant; **Hospital:** UCSF Med Ctr; **Address:** UCSF, Dept Ped Onc, 505 Parnassus Ave, Box 0106, San Francisco, CA 94143; **Phone:** 415-476-0603; **Board Cert:** Pediatrics 79; Pediatric Hematology-Oncology 80; **Med School:** Univ Pennsylvania 73; **Resid:** Pediatrics, Univ Colorado 76; **Fellow:** Pediatric Hematology-Oncology, UCSF 79; **Fac Appt:** Prof Ped, UCSF

Nicholson, Henry MD [PHO] - **Spec Exp:** Brain Tumors; Cancer Survivors-Late Effects of Therapy; **Hospital:** Doernbecher Chldns Hosp/OHSU; **Address:** OR Hlth Scis Univ, 3181 SW Sam Jackson Park Rd, MC CDRC-P, Portland, OR 97239; **Phone:** 503-494-1543; **Board Cert:** Pediatrics 99; Pediatric Hematology-Oncology 99; **Med School:** Med Coll GA 85; **Resid:** Pediatrics, Chldns National Med Ctr 88; **Fellow:** Pediatric Hematology-Oncology, Chldns National Med Ctr 91

Pendergrass, Thomas W MD [PHO] - **Spec Exp:** Sarcoma; Leukemia & Lymphoma; Retinoblastoma; **Hospital:** Chldns Hosp and Regl Med Ctr - Seattle; **Address:** Children's Hospital Regional Medical Ctr, 4800 Sandpoint Way NE, Box 5371, Seattle, WA 98105; **Phone:** 206-987-2106; **Board Cert:** Pediatrics 78; **Med School:** Univ Tenn Coll Med, Memphis 71; **Resid:** Pediatrics, Children's Memorial Hosp 73; **Fellow:** Pediatric Hematology-Oncology, Children's Hosp Med Ctr 77; **Fac Appt:** Prof Ped, Univ Wash

Russo, Carolyn MD [PHO] - **Spec Exp:** Brain Tumors; Cancer Survivors-Late Effects of Therapy; Palliative Care; **Hospital:** Kaiser Permanente Santa Clara Med Ctr; **Address:** Kaiser Permanente Santa Clara Med Ctr-Dept Ped Hem Onc, 900 Kiely Blvd, Basement, Santa Clara, CA 95051; **Phone:** 408-236-5028; **Board Cert:** Pediatrics 88; Pediatric Hematology-Oncology 98; **Med School:** UCLA 84; **Resid:** Pediatrics, Harbor-UCLA Med Ctr 87; **Fellow:** Pediatric Hematology-Oncology, Stanford Med Ctr 90

Siegel, Stuart E MD [PHO] - **Spec Exp:** Leukemias & Solid Tumors; Infections in Pediatric Cancer; Psychosocial Aspects of Pediatric Cancer; **Hospital:** Chldns Hosp - Los Angeles; **Address:** Children's Hospital, 4650 Sunset Blvd, MS 54, Los Angeles, CA 90027-6062; **Phone:** 323-669-2205; **Board Cert:** Pediatrics 73; Pediatric Hematology-Oncology 76; **Med School:** Boston Univ 67; **Resid:** Pediatrics, Univ Minnesota Hosps 69; **Fellow:** Pediatric Hematology-Oncology, Natl Cancer Inst 72; **Fac Appt:** Prof Ped, USC Sch Med

Wilkinson, Robert W MD [PHO] - **Hospital:** Kapiolani Med Ctr for Women & Chldn; **Address:** Kapiolani Med Ctr for Women & Children, 1319 Punahou St, Ste 1050, Honolulu, HI 96826; **Phone:** 808-942-8144; **Board Cert:** Pediatrics 86; Pediatric Hematology-Oncology 86; **Med School:** Tulane Univ 67; **Resid:** Pediatrics, Los Angeles Co-USC Med Ctr 71; **Fellow:** Pediatric Hematology-Oncology, Los Angeles Co-USC Med Ctr 72; **Fac Appt:** Assoc Prof Ped, Univ Hawaii JA Burns Sch Med

PEDIATRIC ALLERGY & IMMUNOLOGY
Mid Atlantic

Kamani, Naynesh R MD [PA&I] - **Spec Exp:** Stem Cell Transplant; Immunotherapy for Cancer; Bone Marrow Transplant; **Hospital:** Chldns Natl Med Ctr; **Address:** Chldns Natl Med Ctr, Div Hematology, 111 Michigan Ave NW, Washington, DC 20010; **Phone:** 202-884-5000; **Board Cert:** Pediatrics 83; Pediatric Allergy & Immunology 83; Diagnostic Lab Immunology 86; **Med School:** Ethiopia 75; **Resid:** Pediatrics, Downstate Med Ctr-Kings Co Hosp 81; **Fellow:** Pediatric Allergy & Immunology, Children's Hosp 83; **Fac Appt:** Prof Ped, Geo Wash Univ

PEDIATRIC ENDOCRINOLOGY
Mid Atlantic

Sklar, Charles A MD [PEn] - **Spec Exp:** Cancer Survivors-Late Effects of Therapy; Growth Disorders in Childhood Cancer; Pituitary Disorders; **Hospital:** Meml Sloan Kettering Cancer Ctr (page 100); **Address:** 1275 York Ave, Box 151, New York, NY 10021; **Phone:** 212-639-8138; **Board Cert:** Pediatrics 79; Pediatric Endocrinology 80; **Med School:** USC Sch Med 74; **Resid:** Pediatrics, Childrens Hosp 76; **Fellow:** Pediatric Endocrinology, UCSF Med Ctr 79; **Fac Appt:** Assoc Prof Ped, Cornell Univ-Weill Med Coll

Southeast

Meacham, Lillian R MD [PEn] - **Spec Exp:** Growth Disorders in Childhood Cancer; Cancer Survivors-Late Effects of Therapy; **Hospital:** Emory Univ Hosp; **Address:** Emory Childrens Ctr, 2040 Ridgewood Drive NE, Altanta, GA 30322; **Phone:** 404-727-5753; **Board Cert:** Pediatrics 99; Pediatric Endocrinology 99; **Med School:** Emory Univ 84; **Resid:** Pediatrics, Emory Univ Hosp 87; **Fellow:** Pediatric Endocrinology, Emory Univ 90; **Fac Appt:** Assoc Prof Ped, Emory Univ

Midwest

Zimmerman, Donald MD [PEn] - **Spec Exp:** Growth/Development Disorders; Thyroid Cancer; Thyroid Disorders; **Hospital:** Children's Mem Hosp; **Address:** 2300 Children's Pl, Box 54, Chicago, IL 60614; **Phone:** 773-880-4440; **Board Cert:** Internal Medicine 77; Endocrinology 79; Pediatrics 83; Pediatric Endocrinology 83; **Med School:** Univ IL Coll Med 74; **Resid:** Internal Medicine, Johns Hopkins Hosp 77; Pediatrics, Mayo Grad Sch Med 81; **Fellow:** Endocrinology, Diabetes & Metabolism, Mayo Grad Sch Med 80; **Fac Appt:** Prof Ped, Northwestern Univ

Southwest

Waguespack, Steven G MD [PEn] - **Spec Exp:** Thyroid Cancer; Cancer Survivors-Late Effects of Therapy; **Hospital:** UT MD Anderson Cancer Ctr, The (page 115); **Address:** MD Anderson Cancer Ctr, Div Endocrinology, 1515 Holcombe Blvd, Unit 435, Houston, TX 77030; **Phone:** 713-792-2841; **Board Cert:** Internal Medicine 98; Pediatrics 99; Endocrinology, Diabetes & Metabolism 02; Pediatric Endocrinology 03; **Med School:** Univ Tex, Houston 94; **Resid:** Internal Medicine & Pediatrics, Indiana Univ Hosp 98; **Fellow:** Endocrinology, Indiana Univ 02; **Fac Appt:** Asst Prof Ped, Univ Tex, Houston

PEDIATRIC OTOLARYNGOLOGY

New England

McGill, Trevor MD [PO] - **Spec Exp:** Head & Neck Tumors; Cholesteatoma/Hemangiomas; Lymphatic Malformations; **Hospital:** Children's Hospital - Boston; **Address:** Dept of Otolaryngology, 300 Longwood Ave, Fegan 9, Boston, MA 02115; **Phone:** 617-355-6460; **Board Cert:** Otolaryngology 88; **Med School:** Ireland 67; **Resid:** Otolaryngology, Royal Natl Throat Nose&Ear Hosp 74; **Fellow:** Otolaryngology, Mass Eye&Ear Infirmary 76; **Fac Appt:** Prof Oto, Harvard Med Sch

Mid Atlantic

Potsic, William P MD [PO] - **Spec Exp:** Ear Disorders/Surgery; Ear Tumors; Hearing Disorders; **Hospital:** Chldns Hosp of Philadelphia, The; **Address:** Childrens Hosp of Philadelphia, 34 St & Civic Center Blvd, Wood Bldg, Fl 1, Philadelphia, PA 19104; **Phone:** 215-590-3440; **Board Cert:** Otolaryngology 74; **Med School:** Emory Univ 69; **Resid:** Otolaryngology, Univ Chicago Hosps 74; **Fac Appt:** Prof Oto, Univ Pennsylvania

West Coast and Pacific

Crockett, Dennis M MD [PO] - **Spec Exp:** Head & Neck Cancer; Airway Reconstruction; **Hospital:** Chldns Hosp - Los Angeles; **Address:** USC Health Consultation Ctr #2, 1520 San Pablo St, Ste 4600, Los Angeles, CA 90033; **Phone:** 323-442-5790; **Board Cert:** Otolaryngology 85; **Med School:** USC Sch Med 79; **Resid:** Otolaryngology, LAC-USC Med Ctr 84; **Fellow:** Pediatrics, Boston Chldns Hosp 85; **Fac Appt:** Assoc Prof Oto, USC Sch Med

PEDIATRIC SURGERY

Mid Atlantic

Colombani, Paul M MD **[PS]** - **Spec Exp:** Thoracic Surgery; Transplant-Kidney & Liver; Cancer Surgery; **Hospital:** Johns Hopkins Hosp - Baltimore (page 97); **Address:** 600 N Wolfe St, Box CMSC 7-113, Baltimore, MD 21287; **Phone:** 410-955-2717; **Board Cert:** Surgery 03; Pediatric Surgery 03; **Med School:** Univ KY Coll Med 76; **Resid:** Surgery, Geo Wash Univ Hosp 81; **Fellow:** Pediatric Surgery, Johns Hopkins Hosp 83; **Fac Appt:** Prof S, Johns Hopkins Univ

Ginsburg, Howard B MD **[PS]** - **Spec Exp:** Neonatal Surgery; Tumor Surgery; Pediatric Urology; **Hospital:** NYU Med Ctr (page 104); **Address:** 530 1st Ave, Ste 10W, NYU Medical Ctr, Div Pediatric Surgery, New York, NY 10016-6402; **Phone:** 212-263-7391; **Board Cert:** Surgery 78; Pediatric Surgery 01; **Med School:** Univ Cincinnati 72; **Resid:** Surgery, NYU-Bellvue Hosp 77; Pediatric Surgery, Columbia-Presby Med Ctr 79; **Fellow:** Pediatric Surgery, Mass Genl Hosp 80; **Fac Appt:** Assoc Prof S, NYU Sch Med

La Quaglia, Michael MD **[PS]** - **Spec Exp:** Cancer Surgery; Neuroblastoma; Liver Tumors; **Hospital:** Meml Sloan Kettering Cancer Ctr (page 100); **Address:** 1275 York Ave, Ste 1176, New York, NY 10021-6007; **Phone:** 212-639-7002; **Board Cert:** Surgery 94; Pediatric Surgery 97; **Med School:** UMDNJ-NJ Med Sch, Newark 76; **Resid:** Surgery, Mass Genl Hosp 83; **Fellow:** Cardiothoracic Surgery, Broadgreen Ctr; Pediatric Surgery, Chldns Hosp 85; **Fac Appt:** Prof PS, Cornell Univ-Weill Med Coll

Stolar, Charles JH MD **[PS]** - **Spec Exp:** Pediatric Cancers; Neonatal Surgery; Diaphragmatic hernia; **Hospital:** NY-Presby Hosp - Columbia Presby Med Ctr (page 103); **Address:** Morgan Stanley Children's Hospital of NewYork-Presbyterian, 3959 Broadway, Fl 2 - rm 212 North, New York, NY 10032; **Phone:** 212-305-2305; **Board Cert:** Surgery 01; Pediatric Surgery 95; **Med School:** Georgetown Univ 74; **Resid:** Surgery, Univ Illinois Hosp 80; **Fellow:** Pediatric Surgery, Chldns Hosp Natl Med Ctr 82; **Fac Appt:** Prof S, Columbia P&S

Wiener, Eugene MD **[PS]** - **Spec Exp:** Cancer Surgery; **Hospital:** Chldns Hosp of Pittsburgh - UPMC (page 114); **Address:** Chldns Hosp, Dept Ped Surgery, 3705 5th Ave, Fl 4A, DeSoto Wing, rm 480, Pittsburgh, PA 15213; **Phone:** 412-692-7280; **Board Cert:** Surgery 82; Pediatric Surgery 95; **Med School:** Med Coll VA 64; **Resid:** Surgery, Med Coll Va Hosps 71; **Fac Appt:** Prof PS, Univ Pittsburgh

Southeast

Davidoff, Andrew MD **[PS]** - **Spec Exp:** Neuroblastoma; Cancer Surgery; Pediatric Surgery; **Hospital:** St Jude Children's Research Hosp; **Address:** St Jude Chldns Rsch Hosp, Dept Surg, 332 N Lauderdale St, Memphis, TN 38105; **Phone:** 901-495-4060; **Board Cert:** Surgery 95; Pediatric Surgery 98; **Med School:** Univ Pennsylvania 87; **Resid:** Surgery, Duke Med Ctr 94; **Fellow:** Pediatric Surgery, Chldns Hosp 96; **Fac Appt:** Assoc Prof S, Univ Tenn Coll Med, Memphis

Drucker, David E MD **[PS]** - **Spec Exp:** Thoracic Surgery; Cancer Surgery; Gastrointestinal Surgery; **Hospital:** Meml Regl Hosp - Hollywood; **Address:** 1150 N 35th Ave, Ste 555, Hollywood, FL 33021-5431; **Phone:** 954-981-0072; **Board Cert:** Surgery 97; Pediatric Surgery 99; Surgical Critical Care 02; **Med School:** Brown Univ 82; **Resid:** Surgery, Med Coll VA Hosps 88; **Fellow:** Pediatric Surgery, Chldns Hosp 90

Morgan III, Walter M MD [PS] - **Spec Exp:** Germ Cell Tumors; Neuroblastoma; Bone Cancer; **Hospital:** Vanderbilt Univ Med Ctr (page 116); **Address:** Vanderbilt Children's Hosp-Dept Ped Surgery, 2200 Children's Way, Ste 4150, Nashville, TN 37232; **Phone:** 615-936-1050; **Board Cert:** Surgery 89; Pediatric Surgery 01; **Med School:** Vanderbilt Univ 82; **Resid:** Surgery, Johns Hopkins Hosp 88; **Fellow:** Pediatric Surgery, Johns Hopkins Hosp 90; **Fac Appt:** Asst Prof PS, Vanderbilt Univ

Paidas, Charles N MD [PS] - **Spec Exp:** Tumor Surgery; Chest Wall Deformities; **Hospital:** Tampa Genl Hosp; **Address:** 17 Davis Blvd, Ste 100, Tampa, FL 33606; **Phone:** 813-259-8700; **Board Cert:** Surgery 99; Pediatric Surgery 01; Surgical Critical Care 02; **Med School:** NY Med Coll 81; **Resid:** Surgery, NY Med Coll Affil Hosps 87; **Fellow:** Pediatric Surgery, Johns Hopkins Hosp 91; **Fac Appt:** Assoc Prof PS, Univ S Fla Coll Med

Shochat, Stephen J MD [PS] - **Spec Exp:** Cancer Surgery; Chest Wall Deformities; **Hospital:** St Jude Children's Research Hosp; **Address:** St Jude Children's Research Hospital, Dept Surgery, 332 N Lauderdale St, Memphis, TN 38105; **Phone:** 901-495-2911; **Board Cert:** Surgery 69; Thoracic Surgery 75; Pediatric Surgery 95; **Med School:** Med Coll VA 63; **Resid:** Surgery, Barnes Hospital 64; Pediatric Surgery, Boston Children's Hosp 68; **Fellow:** Thoracic Surgery, George Washington U Med Ctr 74; **Fac Appt:** Prof S, Univ Tenn Coll Med, Memphis

Skinner, Michael A MD [PS] - **Spec Exp:** Endocrine Cancers; Thyroid Cancer; **Hospital:** Duke Univ Med Ctr (page 94); **Address:** Duke Univ Med Ctr, Box 3815, Durham, NC 27710; **Phone:** 919-681-5077; **Board Cert:** Surgery 00; Pediatric Surgery 03; **Med School:** Rush Med Coll 84; **Resid:** Surgery, Duke Univ Med Ctr 91; **Fellow:** Pediatric Surgery, Indiana Univ 93; **Fac Appt:** Assoc Prof S, Duke Univ

Weinberger, Malvin MD [PS] - **Spec Exp:** Neonatal Surgery; Trauma; Cancer Surgery; **Hospital:** Miami Children's Hosp; **Address:** 3200 SW 60th Ct, Ste 201, Miami, FL 33155-4070; **Phone:** 305-662-8320; **Board Cert:** Surgery 70; Pediatric Surgery 95; **Med School:** Temple Univ 62; **Resid:** Surgery, Temple Univ Hosp 69; Pediatric Surgery, Chldns Hosp/Ohio St Univ Hosp 71; **Fac Appt:** Assoc Clin Prof S, Univ Miami Sch Med

Midwest

Aiken, John Judson MD [PS] - **Spec Exp:** Tumor Surgery-Pediatric; Chest Wall Deformities; Hernia; **Hospital:** Chldns Hosp - Wisconsin; **Address:** 9000 W Wisconsin Ave, Ste 403, Milwaukee, WI 53226; **Phone:** 414-266-6550; **Board Cert:** Surgery 04; Pediatric Surgery 00; **Med School:** Univ Cincinnati 84; **Resid:** Surgery, Mass Genl Hosp 91; **Fellow:** Pediatric Surgery, Chldns Hosp; **Fac Appt:** Assoc Prof S, Med Coll Wisc

Alexander, Frederick MD [PS] - **Spec Exp:** Transplant-Small Bowel; Solid Tumors; Congenital Gastrointestinal Anomalies; **Hospital:** Cleveland Clin Fdn (page 92); **Address:** Cleveland Clinic, Dept Pediatric Surgery, 9500 Euclid Ave, M14, Cleveland, OH 44195-0001; **Phone:** 216-445-6846; **Board Cert:** Pediatric Surgery 99; **Med School:** Columbia P&S 76; **Resid:** Surgery, Brigham-Womens Hosp 84; **Fellow:** Pediatric Surgery, Chldns Hosp 86; **Fac Appt:** Assoc Prof PS, Ohio State Univ

Grosfeld, Jay L MD [PS] - **Spec Exp:** Cancer Surgery; **Hospital:** Riley Chldns Hosp (page 90); **Address:** 702 Barnhill Drive, Ste 2500, Indianapolis, IN 46202-5200; **Phone:** 317-274-4682; **Board Cert:** Surgery 89; Pediatric Surgery 82; **Med School:** NYU Sch Med 61; **Resid:** Surgery, Bellevue-NYU Hosp 66; Pediatric Surgery, Ohio State Univ 70; **Fellow:** Pediatric Hematology-Oncology, Chldns Hosp 70; **Fac Appt:** Prof S, Indiana Univ

Great Plains and Mountains

Haase, Gerald M MD **[PS]** - **Spec Exp:** Cancer Surgery; **Hospital:** Chldn's Hosp - Denver, The; **Address:** 1056 E 19th Ave, Ste B190, Denver, CO 80218; **Phone:** 303-861-6182; **Board Cert:** Surgery 95; Surgical Critical Care 96; Pediatric Surgery 97; **Med School:** Tufts Univ 72; **Resid:** Surgery, Univ Colo Hlth Sci Ctr 77; Pediatric Surgery, Boston Chldns Hosp 75; **Fellow:** Pediatric Surgery, Columbus Chldns Hosp 79; **Fac Appt:** Clin Prof S, Univ Colorado

Southwest

Jackson, Richard MD **[PS]** - **Spec Exp:** Cancer Surgery; Neonatal Surgery; Robotic Surgery; **Hospital:** Arkansas Chldns Hosp; **Address:** Arkansas Chldns Hosp - Ped Surgery, 800 Marshall St, MS 837, Little Rock, AR 72202; **Phone:** 501-364-1446; **Board Cert:** Surgery 97; Pediatric Surgery 01; Surgical Critical Care 98; **Med School:** W VA Univ 83; **Resid:** Surgery, W Va Univ Hosps 88; Pediatric Surgery, Chldns Hosp 89; **Fellow:** Pediatric Critical Care Medicine, Chldns Hosp-Univ Pittsburgh 90; Pediatric Surgery, Chldns Hosp-Univ Pittsburgh 92; **Fac Appt:** Assoc Prof S, Univ Ark

West Coast and Pacific

Sawin, Robert S MD **[PS]** - **Spec Exp:** Cancer Surgery; Thoracic Surgery; Neonatal Surgery-Gastrointestinal; **Hospital:** Chldns Hosp and Regl Med Ctr - Seattle; **Address:** 4800 Sand Point Way NE, MS G0035, Dept Surg, Box 359300, Seattle, WA 98105; **Phone:** 206-987-2039; **Board Cert:** Surgery 98; Surgical Critical Care 91; Pediatric Surgery 99; **Med School:** Univ Pittsburgh 82; **Resid:** Surgery, Brigham Women's Hosp 87; **Fellow:** Pediatric Surgery, Chldns Hosp 89; **Fac Appt:** Prof S, Univ Wash

Pediatrics
New England

Sallan, Stephen MD **[Ped]** - **Spec Exp:** Pediatric Oncology; Leukemia; **Hospital:** Children's Hospital - Boston; **Address:** Dana Farber Cancer Institute, Dept Ped Oncology, 44 Binney St, Ste 1642, Boston, MA 02115; **Phone:** 617-632-3316; **Board Cert:** Pediatrics 72; **Med School:** Wayne State Univ 67; **Resid:** Pediatrics, Chldns Hosp 69; Pediatrics, Hosp Sick Chldn 70; **Fellow:** Pediatric Oncology, Chldns Hosp Med Ctr 75; **Fac Appt:** Prof Ped, Harvard Med Sch

Schechter, Neil L MD **[Ped]** - **Spec Exp:** Developmental & Behavioral Disorders; Pain Management; Pain-Cancer; **Hospital:** CT Chldns Med Ctr; **Address:** St Francis Hosp, Dept Peds, 114 Woodland St, Hartford, CT 06105; **Phone:** 860-714-4931; **Board Cert:** Pediatrics 79; **Med School:** Mich State Univ 73; **Resid:** Pediatrics, Univ Conn Hlth Ctr 77; **Fellow:** Developmental-Behavioral Pediatrics, Chldns Hosp Med Ctr/Harvard 79; **Fac Appt:** Prof Ped, Univ Conn

Mid Atlantic

Sahler, Olle Jane Z MD **[Ped]** - **Spec Exp:** Behavioral Pediatrics; Complementary Medicine in Cancer; Palliative Care; **Hospital:** Univ of Rochester Strong Meml Hosp; **Address:** Univ Rochester Med Ctr - Dept Pediatrics, 601 Elmwood Ave, Box 777, Rochester, NY 14642-8777; **Phone:** 585-275-3935; **Board Cert:** Pediatrics 79; **Med School:** Univ Rochester 71; **Resid:** Pediatrics, Duke Univ Med Ctr 73; **Fellow:** Behavioral Pediatrics, Rochester Univ 77; **Fac Appt:** Prof Ped, Univ Rochester

Southwest

Levetown, Marcia MD **[Ped]** - **Spec Exp:** Palliative Care; Pain Management; **Hospital:** Methodist Hosp - Houston; **Address:** Methodist Hosp-Director Palliative Care Prog, 6565 Fannin St Bldg Main 796, Houston, TX 77030; **Phone:** 713-441-0427; **Board Cert:** Pediatrics 04; **Med School:** Med Coll VA 86; **Resid:** Pediatrics, Baylor Coll Med 89; **Fellow:** Pediatric Critical Care Medicine, DC Chldns Hosp 91; Pain Medicine, MD Anderson Cancer Ctr 96

Oeffinger, Kevin MD **[Ped]** - **Spec Exp:** Cancer Survivors-Late Effects of Therapy; **Hospital:** Chldns Med Ctr of Dallas; **Address:** Univ Texas SW Med Ctr, 6263 Harry Hines Blvd, Dallas, TX 75390-9067; **Phone:** 214-648-1399; **Board Cert:** Family Medicine 00; **Med School:** Univ Tex, San Antonio 84; **Resid:** Family Medicine, Baylor Coll Med 85; **Fellow:** Family Medicine, Fam Practice Faculty Dev Ctr 99; Natl Cancer Inst 00; **Fac Appt:** Prof FMed, Univ Tex SW, Dallas

PLASTIC SURGERY

A *plastic surgeon deals with the repair, reconstruction or replacement of physical defects of form or function involving the skin, musculoskeletal system, craniomaxillofacial structures, hand, extremities, breast and trunk and external genitalia. He/she uses aesthetic surgical principles not only to improve undesirable qualities of normal structures (commonly called "cosmetic surgery") but in all reconstructive procedures as well.*

A plastic surgeon possesses special knowledge and skill in the design and surgery of grafts, flaps, free tissue transfer and replantation. Competence in the management of complex wounds, the use of implantable materials, and in tumor surgery is required.

Training required: *Five to seven years*

PLASTIC SURGERY WITHIN THE HEAD AND NECK:

A plastic surgeon with additional training in plastic and reconstructive procedures within the head, face, neck and associated structures, including cutaneous head and neck oncology and reconstruction, management of maxillofacial trauma, soft tissue repair and neural surgery.

PHYSICIAN LISTINGS

407

The field is diverse and involved a wide range of patients, from the newborn to the aged. While both cosmetic and reconstructive surgery are practiced, there are many additional procedures which interface with them.

SURGERY OF THE HAND

(See Hand Surgery under Orthopaedic Surgery)

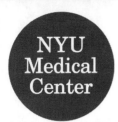

NYU Medical Center

550 First Avenue (at 31st Street)
New York, NY 10016
Physician Referral:
1-888-7-NYU-MED
www.nyumc.org

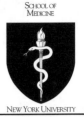

SCHOOL OF MEDICINE

NEW YORK UNIVERSITY

PLASTIC SURGERY

The Institute of Reconstructive Plastic Surgery at NYU Medical Center is the country's largest plastic surgery unit. It has pioneered techniques that have revolutionized reconstructive surgery and transformed the lives of patients, including children and cancer survivors. The Institute is a true multidisciplinary center, where patients and their families are supported by teams of physicians and other healthcare professionals. The residency program is one of the country's most prestigious and attracts applicants from around the world.

Our programs include:

BODY CONTOURING — liposuction and the reduction of excess skin that results following bariatric surgery

BREAST SURGERY — microsurgery is used to reconstruct breasts following mastectomy or other cancer surgery; services also include breast augmentation and reduction

CLEFT LIP AND PALATE — this unit pioneered a technique that uses small orthodontic appliances to achieve dramatic improvements in appearance; speech therapy is a key part of our comprehensive approach to treatment

COSMETIC SURGERY — a wide range of affordable effective treatments, including chin implants, face and eyelid lifts, and skin rejuvenation

CRANIOFACIAL — the unit was the first to use a technique called distraction, which involves stretching and lengthening the bones in children with deficient upper and lower jaws, to improve appearance and vital functions such as breathing and eating

EARS — this clinic offers a range of services that include correcting protruding ears and surgically building new ears for children who are born without them; both appearance and hearing are dealt with by teams of healthcare givers

HEAD AND NECK — brings together all types of plastic surgery, including microsurgery, to improve the lives of cancer patients who have undergone surgery

HEMANGIOMAS AND VASCULAR MALFORMATIONS — these are dramatically improved through the use of surgery, and lasers and catheters that embolize blood vessels; psychologists and geneticists consult with families

NERVE CENTER — treats patients whose nerves have been damaged in accidents or who have Bell's palsy. Also, children with a birth injury of the upper extremities

Specialists at the NCI-designated NYU Cancer Institute seek to enhance and coordinate the extensive resources of NYU Medical Center to optimize research, treatment, and the ultimate control of cancer.

Our new NYU Clinical Cancer Center is located at 160 East 34th Street. This state-of-the-art 13-level, 85,000-square-foot building serves as "home base" for patients, by providing the latest cancer prevention, screening, diagnostic treatment, genetic counseling, and support services in one central location. The NYU Clinical Cancer Center stands to dramatically improve the lives of people with cancer. As part of NYU Medical Center, patients can access a variety of other non-cancer services throughout the institution.

PHYSICIAN REFERRAL
1-888-7-NYU-MED
(1-888-769-8633)
www.nyumc.org
www.nyuci.org

PLASTIC SURGERY

New England

Ariyan, Stephan MD [PIS] - **Spec Exp:** Melanoma; Head & Neck Surgery; Reconstructive Surgery; **Hospital:** Yale - New Haven Hosp; **Address:** 60 Temple St, Ste 7C, New Haven, CT 06510-2716; **Phone:** 203-786-3000; **Board Cert:** Plastic Surgery 78; **Med School:** NY Med Coll 66; **Resid:** Surgery, Yale-New Haven Hosp 75; Plastic Surgery, Yale-New Haven Hosp 76; **Fellow:** Surgical Oncology, Yale-New Haven Hosp 71; **Fac Appt:** Clin Prof S, Yale Univ

Collins, Eva Dale MD [PIS] - **Spec Exp:** Breast Cancer; Breast Reconstruction; **Hospital:** Dartmouth - Hitchcock Med Ctr; **Address:** Darthmouth-Hitchcock Med Ctr, Div Plas Surgery, One Medical Center Drive, Lebanon, NH 03756; **Phone:** 603-653-3907; **Board Cert:** Plastic Surgery 97; **Med School:** Emory Univ 89; **Resid:** Plastic Surgery, Washington Univ Med Ctr 94; **Fellow:** Microsurgery, Washington Univ Med Ctr 95; **Fac Appt:** Assoc Prof S, Dartmouth Med Sch

May Jr, James W MD [PIS] - **Spec Exp:** Cosmetic Surgery; Breast Reconstruction; Hand Surgery; **Hospital:** Mass Genl Hosp; **Address:** Mass Genl Hosp, 15 Parkman St, WACC 453, Boston, MA 02114; **Phone:** 617-726-8220; **Board Cert:** Surgery 75; Plastic Surgery 77; **Med School:** Northwestern Univ 69; **Resid:** Plastic Surgery, Mass Genl Hosp 75; **Fellow:** Hand Surgery, Univ Louisville; **Fac Appt:** Prof S, Harvard Med Sch

Stadelmann, Wayne K MD [PIS] - **Spec Exp:** Melanoma-Head & Neck; Breast Reconstruction; Reconstructive Surgery; **Hospital:** Concord Hospital; **Address:** 248 Pleasant St, Ste 201, Concord, NH 03301; **Phone:** 603-224-5200; **Board Cert:** Plastic Surgery 99; **Med School:** Univ Chicago-Pritzker Sch Med 90; **Resid:** Surgery, Univ Chicago Hosps 94; Plastic Surgery, Univ S Florida/H Lee Moffit Cancer Ctr 97

Stahl, Richard S MD [PIS] - **Spec Exp:** Breast Cosmetic & Reconstructive Surgery; Abdominal Wall Reconstruction; Bronchopleural Fistula Repair; **Hospital:** Yale - New Haven Hosp; **Address:** 5 Durham Rd, Guilford, CT 06437; **Phone:** 203-458-4440; **Board Cert:** Surgery 01; Plastic Surgery 84; **Med School:** Vanderbilt Univ 76; **Resid:** Surgery, Yale New Haven Hosp 81; Plastic Surgery, Emory Univ Med Ctr 83; **Fac Appt:** Clin Prof S, Yale Univ

Mid Atlantic

Bartlett, Scott P MD [PIS] - **Spec Exp:** Craniofacial Surgery/Reconstruction; Pediatric Plastic Surgery; Facial Reconstruction After Skin Cancer; **Hospital:** Hosp Univ Penn - UPHS (page 113); **Address:** Hosp Univ Penn, 3400 Spruce St, Philadelphia, PA 19104-4227; **Phone:** 215-662-4000; **Board Cert:** Plastic Surgery 87; **Med School:** Washington Univ, St Louis 75; **Resid:** Surgery, Mass Genl Hosp 83; Plastic Surgery, Mass Genl Hosp 85; **Fellow:** Craniofacial Surgery, Hosp Univ Penn 86; **Fac Appt:** Assoc Prof PIS, Univ Pennsylvania

Bucky, Louis P MD [PIS] - **Spec Exp:** Cosmetic Surgery; Breast Reconstruction; **Hospital:** Pennsylvania Hosp (page 113); **Address:** 230 W Washington Square, Ste 101, Philadelphia, PA 19106; **Phone:** 215-829-6320; **Board Cert:** Plastic Surgery 97; **Med School:** Harvard Med Sch 86; **Resid:** Surgery, Mass Genl Hosp 92; Plastic Surgery, Mass Genl Hosp 94; **Fellow:** Microsurgery, Meml Sloan Kettering 95; Craniofacial Surgery, Miami Chldns Hosp; **Fac Appt:** Assoc Prof S, Univ Pennsylvania

Cordeiro, Peter G MD [PIS] - **Spec Exp:** Plastic & Reconstructive Surgery; Breast Reconstruction; Facial Reconstructive Surgery; **Hospital:** Meml Sloan Kettering Cancer Ctr (page 100); **Address:** Meml Sloan Kettering Cancer Ctr, 1275 York Ave, rm C1193, New York, NY 10021-6007; **Phone:** 212-639-2521; **Board Cert:** Surgery 98; Plastic Surgery 94; **Med School:** Harvard Med Sch 83; **Resid:** Surgery, New Eng Deaconess Hosp-Harvard 89; Plastic Surgery, NYU Med Ctr 91; **Fellow:** Microsurgery, Meml Sloan-Kettering Cancer Ctr. 92; Craniofacial Surgery, Univ Miami; **Fac Appt:** Assoc Prof S, Cornell Univ-Weill Med Coll

Hoffman, Lloyd MD [PIS] - **Spec Exp:** Cosmetic Surgery-Face; Liposuction; Breast Reconstruction; **Hospital:** NY-Presby Hosp - NY Weill Cornell Med Ctr (page 103); **Address:** 12 E 68th St, New York, NY 10021; **Phone:** 212-861-1640; **Board Cert:** Plastic Surgery 89; Hand Surgery 92; **Med School:** Northwestern Univ 78; **Resid:** Surgery, New York Hosp 83; Plastic Surgery, NYU Med Ctr 86; **Fellow:** Hand Surgery, NYU Med Ctr 87; **Fac Appt:** Assoc Prof PIS, Cornell Univ-Weill Med Coll

Loree, Thom R MD [PIS] - **Spec Exp:** Head & Neck Cancer; Thyroid Cancer; Reconstructive Surgery; **Hospital:** Roswell Park Cancer Inst (page 107); **Address:** Roswell Park Cancer Inst, Div Head & Neck Surgery, Elm & Carlton Sts, Buffalo, NY 14263; **Phone:** 716-845-3158; **Board Cert:** Plastic Surgery 04; Surgery 97; **Med School:** Geo Wash Univ 82; **Resid:** Surgery, St Lukes-Roosevelt Hosp 87; Plastic Surgery, St Lukes-Roosevelt Hosp 89; **Fellow:** Head & Neck Surgical Oncology, Meml Sloan-Kettering Cancer Ctr 90; **Fac Appt:** Assoc Prof S, SUNY Buffalo

Noone, R Barrett MD [PIS] - **Spec Exp:** Breast Reconstruction; Cosmetic Surgery; **Hospital:** Bryn Mawr Hosp; **Address:** 888 Glenbrook Ave, Bryn Mawr, PA 19010-2506; **Phone:** 610-527-4833; **Board Cert:** Surgery 72; Plastic Surgery 74; **Med School:** Univ Pennsylvania 65; **Resid:** Surgery, Hosp Univ Penn 71; Plastic Surgery, Hosp Univ Penn 73; **Fac Appt:** Clin Prof S, Univ Pennsylvania

Slezak, Sheri MD [PIS] - **Spec Exp:** Breast Reconstruction; **Hospital:** Univ of MD Med Sys; **Address:** Univ Maryland, Dept Plastic Surgery, 22 S Greene St, rm S8D12, Baltimore, MD 21201; **Phone:** 410-328-2360; **Board Cert:** Plastic Surgery 91; **Med School:** Harvard Med Sch 80; **Resid:** Surgery, Columbia-Presby Med Ctr 85; Plastic Surgery, Johns Hopkins Hosp 89; **Fac Appt:** Assoc Prof PIS, Univ MD Sch Med

Spear, Scott L MD [PIS] - **Spec Exp:** Breast Reconstruction; Cosmetic Surgery-Face; **Hospital:** Georgetown Univ Hosp; **Address:** Georgetown Univ Hosp, Div Plastic Surg, 3800 Reservoir Rd NW, Washington, DC 20007; **Phone:** 202-444-8612; **Board Cert:** Plastic Surgery 81; **Med School:** Univ Chicago-Pritzker Sch Med 72; **Resid:** Surgery, Beth Israel Hosp 78; Plastic Surgery, Univ Miami Hosps 80; **Fellow:** Plastic Surgery, Hosp St Louis 81; **Fac Appt:** Prof PIS, Georgetown Univ

Sultan, Mark MD [PIS] - **Spec Exp:** Breast Reconstruction; Cosmetic Surgery-Breast; Cosmetic Surgery-Face; **Hospital:** St Luke's - Roosevelt Hosp Ctr - Roosevelt Div (page 93); **Address:** 1100 Park Ave, New York, NY 10128; **Phone:** 212-360-0700; **Board Cert:** Plastic Surgery 92; **Med School:** Columbia P&S 82; **Resid:** Surgery, Columbia-Presby Hosp 87; Plastic Surgery, Columbia-Presby Hosp 90; **Fellow:** Head and Neck Surgery, Emory Univ Hosp 89; **Fac Appt:** Assoc Prof S, Columbia P&S

Whitaker, Linton A MD [PIS] - **Spec Exp:** Cosmetic Surgery-Face; Craniofacial Surgery/Reconstruction; Facial Tumors; **Hospital:** Hosp Univ Penn - UPHS (page 113); **Address:** Hosp Univ Penn -10 Penn Tower, 3400 Spruce St, Philadelphia, PA 19104; **Phone:** 215-662-2048; **Board Cert:** Surgery 70; Plastic Surgery 78; **Med School:** Tulane Univ 62; **Resid:** Surgery, Dartmouth Affl Hosp 69; Plastic Surgery, Hosp Univ Penn 71; **Fac Appt:** Prof PIS, Univ Pennsylvania

Southeast

Caffee, H Hollis MD **[PIS]** - **Spec Exp:** Breast Reconstruction; Microsurgery; Hand Surgery; **Hospital:** Shands Hlthcre at Univ of FL (page 109); **Address:** Univ Florida, Div Plastic Surgery, P.O. Box 100286, Gainesville, FL 32610-0286; **Phone:** 352-265-8402; **Board Cert:** Plastic Surgery 79; Hand Surgery 97; **Med School:** Univ Fla Coll Med 68; **Resid:** Surgery, Harbor Genl Hosp 75; Plastic Surgery, UCLA Med Ctr 77; **Fac Appt:** Prof PIS, Univ Fla Coll Med

Fix, R Jobe MD **[PIS]** - **Spec Exp:** Breast Reconstruction; Hand Surgery; Microsurgery; **Hospital:** Univ of Ala Hosp at Birmingham; **Address:** Univ of Alabama Hosp, Div Plastic Surg, 510 S 20th St, FOT-Ste 1102, Birmingham, AL 35294; **Phone:** 205-934-3358; **Board Cert:** Surgery 97; Hand Surgery 01; Plastic Surgery 91; **Med School:** Univ Nebr Coll Med 82; **Resid:** Surgery, Valley Med Ctr 87; Plastic Surgery, Univ Ala Hosp 89; **Fac Appt:** Prof PIS, Univ Ala

Georgiade, Gregory MD **[PIS]** - **Spec Exp:** Breast Reconstruction; Cleft Palate/Lip; **Hospital:** Duke Univ Med Ctr (page 94); **Address:** Duke Univ Med Ctr, Box 3960, Durham, NC 27710-0001; **Phone:** 919-684-3039; **Board Cert:** Plastic Surgery 81; Surgery 90; **Med School:** Duke Univ 73; **Resid:** Surgery, Duke Univ Med Ctr 78; Plastic Surgery, Duke Univ Med Ctr 80; **Fac Appt:** Prof S, Duke Univ

Hester Jr, T Roderick MD **[PIS]** - **Spec Exp:** Cosmetic Surgery-Face; Breast Reconstruction; **Hospital:** Emory Univ Hosp; **Address:** 3200 Downwood Cir, Ste 640, Atlanta, GA 30327; **Phone:** 404-351-0051; **Board Cert:** Plastic Surgery 80; Surgery 73; **Med School:** Emory Univ 67; **Resid:** Surgery, Emory Affil Hosps 72

Maxwell, G Patrick MD **[PIS]** - **Spec Exp:** Breast Reconstruction; **Hospital:** Baptist Hosp; **Address:** 2021 Church St, Ste 806, Baptist Medical Plaza Two, Nashville, TN 37203; **Phone:** 615-284-8200; **Board Cert:** Plastic Surgery 81; **Med School:** Vanderbilt Univ 72; **Resid:** Surgery, Johns Hopkins Hosp 76; Plastic Surgery, Johns Hopkins Hosp 79; **Fellow:** Microsurgery, Davies Med Ctr; **Fac Appt:** Asst Clin Prof PIS, Vanderbilt Univ

McCraw, John MD **[PIS]** - **Spec Exp:** Breast Reconstruction; **Hospital:** Univ Hosps & Clins - Jackson; **Address:** University of Mississippi Medical Ctr, Div Plastic Surgery, 2500 N State St, Jackson, MS 32916; **Phone:** 601-815-1343; **Board Cert:** Surgery 72; Plastic Surgery 74; **Med School:** Univ MO-Columbia Sch Med 66; **Resid:** Orthopaedic Surgery, Duke U Med Ctr 69; Surgery, Univ Florida Med Ctr 72; **Fellow:** Plastic Surgery, Univ Florida Med Ctr 73; **Fac Appt:** Prof PIS, Univ Miss

Smith Jr, David J MD **[PIS]** - **Spec Exp:** Breast Reconstruction; Burns; **Hospital:** Univ of S FL - Tampa; **Address:** Univ South Florida, Div Plastic Surg, 4 Columbia Drive, rm 650, Tampa, FL 33606; **Phone:** 813-259-0964; **Board Cert:** Plastic Surgery 81; **Med School:** Indiana Univ 73; **Resid:** Plastic Surgery, Ind Univ 80; Surgery, Emory Univ-Grady Hosp 78; **Fellow:** Hand Surgery, Univ Louisville; **Fac Appt:** Prof S, Univ S Fla Coll Med

Vasconez, Luis O MD **[PIS]** - **Spec Exp:** Cosmetic Surgery-Face; Breast Reconstruction; **Hospital:** Univ of Ala Hosp at Birmingham; **Address:** Faculty Office Twr 1102, 510 20th St S, Birmingham, AL 35294-3411; **Phone:** 205-934-3245; **Board Cert:** Surgery 70; Plastic Surgery 71; **Med School:** Washington Univ, St Louis 62; **Resid:** Surgery, Strong Meml Hosp 70; Plastic Surgery, Shands Hosp-Univ FL 69; **Fac Appt:** Prof S, Univ Ala

Midwest

Brandt, Keith MD [PIS] - **Spec Exp:** Breast Reconstruction; Reconstructive Surgery; Microsurgery; **Hospital:** Barnes-Jewish Hosp (page 85); **Address:** 660 S Euclid, Box 8238, St Louis, MO 63110-1010; **Phone:** 314-747-0541; **Board Cert:** Surgery 99; Plastic Surgery 03; Hand Surgery 95; **Med School:** Univ Tex, Houston 83; **Resid:** Surgery, Univ Nebraska Med Ctr 89; Plastic Surgery, Univ Tennessee 91; **Fellow:** Hand Surgery, Wash Univ 92; Microsurgery, Wash Univ 93; **Fac Appt:** Assoc Prof S, Washington Univ, St Louis

Coleman, John J MD [PIS] - **Spec Exp:** Cancer Reconstruction; Breast Reconstruction; Head & Neck Surgery; **Hospital:** Indiana Univ Hosp (page 90); **Address:** 545 Barnhill Dr, Emerson Hall, Ste 232, Indianapolis, IN 46202-5120; **Phone:** 317-274-8106; **Board Cert:** Surgery 98; Plastic Surgery 81; **Med School:** Harvard Med Sch 73; **Resid:** Surgery, Emory Univ Affil Hosp 78; Plastic Surgery, Emory Univ Affil Hosp 79; **Fellow:** Surgical Oncology, Univ Maryland Med Ctr; **Fac Appt:** Prof S, Indiana Univ

Cram, Albert E MD [PIS] - **Spec Exp:** Belt Lipectomy; Breast Augmentation; Breast Reconstruction; **Hospital:** Mercy Med Ctr - Cedar Rapids; **Address:** Univ Iowa Hosps & Clinics, Dept Plastic Surg, 501 12th Ave, Ste 102, Coralville, IA 52241; **Phone:** 319-337-3740; **Board Cert:** Plastic Surgery 89; **Med School:** Univ Nebr Coll Med 69; **Resid:** Surgery, Univ Iowa Hosps 74; Plastic Surgery, Univ Chicago Hosps 87; **Fac Appt:** Prof Emeritus S, Univ Iowa Coll Med

Walton Jr, Robert Lee MD [PIS] - **Spec Exp:** Cosmetic Surgery-Face; Nasal Reconstruction; Breast Reconstruction; **Hospital:** Univ of Chicago Hosps; **Address:** Dept Plas & Reconstruction Surg, 5841 S Maryland Ave, MC 6035, Chicago, IL 60637-1463; **Phone:** 773-702-6302; **Board Cert:** Plastic Surgery 80; Hand Surgery 00; **Med School:** Univ Kans 72; **Resid:** Surgery, Johns Hopkins Hosp 74; Plastic Surgery, Yale-New Haven Hosp 78; **Fellow:** Hand Surgery, Hartford Hosp 78; **Fac Appt:** Prof PIS, Univ Chicago-Pritzker Sch Med

Wilkins, Edwin G MD [PIS] - **Spec Exp:** Breast Reconstruction; Lower Limb Reconstruction; Microsurgery; **Hospital:** Univ Michigan Hlth Sys; **Address:** Univ Mich, Div Plastic Surg, 1500 E Med Ctr Drive, rm 2130 Taubman Ctr, Ann Arbor, MI 48109-0340; **Phone:** 734-998-6022; **Board Cert:** Plastic Surgery 91; **Med School:** Wake Forest Univ 81; **Resid:** Surgery, Charlotte Meml Hosp 86; Plastic Surgery, Vanderbilt Univ Med Ctr 88; **Fellow:** Reconstructive Microsurgery, Univ Louisville Sch Med 89; **Fac Appt:** Assoc Prof PIS, Univ Mich Med Sch

Yetman, Randall John MD [PIS] - **Spec Exp:** Breast Reconstruction; **Hospital:** Cleveland Clin Fdn (page 92); **Address:** 9500 Euclid Ave, Desk A-60, Cleveland, OH 44195; **Phone:** 216-444-6908; **Board Cert:** Plastic Surgery 84; **Med School:** Univ Miami Sch Med 74; **Resid:** Plastic Surgery, NY Hosp-Cornell Med Ctr 79; **Fellow:** Plastic Surgery, Cleveland Clin Fdn

Southwest

Robb, Geoffrey L MD [PIS] - **Spec Exp:** Breast Reconstructiion; Head & Neck Cancer Reconstruction; Facial Reconstructive Surgery; **Hospital:** UT MD Anderson Cancer Ctr, The (page 115); **Address:** 1515 Holcombe Blvd, Unit 443, Houston, TX 77030; **Phone:** 713-794-1247; **Board Cert:** Otolaryngology 79; Plastic Surgery 86; **Med School:** Univ Miami Sch Med 74; **Resid:** Otolaryngology, Naval Reg Med Ctr 79; Plastic Surgery, Univ Pittsburgh 85; **Fellow:** Microvascular Surgery, Univ Pittsburgh; **Fac Appt:** Prof PIS, Univ Tex, Houston

Rohrich, Rod J MD [PIS] - **Spec Exp:** Nasal Surgery; Cosmetic Surgery-Face & Breast; Breast Reconstruction; **Hospital:** Zale Lipshy Univ Hosp - Dallas; **Address:** Univ Tex SW Med Ctr, Plastic/Recon Surg, 5323 Harry Hines Blvd, Dallas, TX 75390-9132; **Phone:** 214-648-3119; **Board Cert:** Plastic Surgery 87; Hand Surgery 90; **Med School:** Baylor Coll Med 79; **Resid:** Plastic Surgery, Univ Mich Hosp 85; Plastic Surgery, Radcliffe Infirm/Oxford; **Fellow:** Hand Surgery, Mass Genl Hosp-Harvard 87; **Fac Appt:** Clin Prof PIS, Univ Tex SW, Dallas

Schusterman, Mark A MD [PIS] - **Spec Exp:** Breast Reconstruction; Cancer Reconstructive Surgery; Cosmetic Surgery-Face & Breast; **Hospital:** St Luke's Episcopal Hosp - Houston; **Address:** 6624 Fannin St, Ste 1420, Houston, TX 77030; **Phone:** 713-794-0368; **Board Cert:** Surgery 86; Plastic Surgery 89; **Med School:** Univ Louisville Sch Med 80; **Resid:** Surgery, Univ Hosp 85; Pediatric Surgery, Univ Pitts Med Ctr 87; **Fellow:** Microsurgery, Univ Pitts Med Ctr 88; **Fac Appt:** Clin Prof PIS, Baylor Coll Med

West Coast and Pacific

Andersen, James S MD [PIS] - **Spec Exp:** Cancer Reconstruction; Breast Reconstruction; Head & Neck Reconstruction; **Hospital:** City of Hope Natl Med Ctr & Beckman Rsch (page 89); **Address:** City of Hope National Cancer Ctr, Div Plastic Surgery, 1500 E Duarte Rd, Duarte, CA 91011; **Phone:** 626-301-8278; **Board Cert:** Plastic Surgery 94; **Med School:** Jefferson Med Coll 83; **Resid:** Surgery, Hosp U Penn 89; Plastic Surgery, Hosp U Penn 91; **Fellow:** Microsurgery, USC Med Ctr 92; **Fac Appt:** Assoc Clin Prof S, USC Sch Med

Isik, F Frank MD [PIS] - **Spec Exp:** Cancer Reconstruction; Breast Reconstruction; **Hospital:** Univ Wash Med Ctr; **Address:** Univ Wash Med Ctr, Div Plastic Surg, 1959 NE Pacific St, Box 356410, Seattle, WA 98108; **Phone:** 206-543-5516; **Board Cert:** Surgery 01; Plastic Surgery 97; **Med School:** Mount Sinai Sch Med 85; **Resid:** Surgery, Boston Univ Hosps 90; Plastic Surgery, Univ Wash 95; **Fellow:** Pathology, NIH / Univ Wash 92; **Fac Appt:** Prof PIS, Univ Wash

Jewell, Mark L MD [PIS] - **Spec Exp:** Lipoplasty-Ultrasonic; Facial Rejuvenation; Breast Reconstruction; **Hospital:** Sacred Heart Med Ctr; **Address:** 630 E 13th Ave, Eugene, OR 97401; **Phone:** 541-683-3234; **Board Cert:** Plastic Surgery 81; **Med School:** Univ Kans 73; **Resid:** Surgery, LAC-Harbor Med Ctr 76; Plastic Surgery, Erlanger Hosp 79; **Fellow:** Burn Surgery, LAC-USC Med Ctr 77; **Fac Appt:** Asst Clin Prof PIS, Oregon Hlth Sci Univ

Mathes, Stephen MD [PIS] - **Spec Exp:** Breast Reconstruction; Reconstructive Surgery; Microsurgery; **Hospital:** UCSF Med Ctr; **Address:** 350 Parnassus Ave, Ste 509, San Francisco, CA 94117; **Phone:** 415-476-9548; **Board Cert:** Surgery 93; Plastic Surgery 79; **Med School:** Louisiana State Univ 68; **Resid:** Surgery, Emory Affil Hosp 75; Plastic Surgery, Emory Affil Hosp 77; **Fac Appt:** Prof PIS, UCSF

Miller, Timothy Alden MD [PIS] - **Spec Exp:** Cosmetic Surgery-Face; Nasal & Eyelid Reconstruction; Skin Cancer; **Hospital:** UCLA Med Ctr (page 111); **Address:** UCLA Med Ctr, Div Plastic Surg, 200 UCLA Med Plaza, Ste 465, Los Angeles, CA 90095-8344; **Phone:** 310-825-5644; **Board Cert:** Surgery 71; Plastic Surgery 73; **Med School:** UCLA 63; **Resid:** Surgery, Johns Hopkins Hosp; Thoracic Surgery, UCLA Med Ctr 69; **Fellow:** Plastic Surgery, Univ Pittsburgh 71; **Fac Appt:** Prof S, UCLA

Sherman, Randolph MD [PIS] - **Spec Exp:** Facial Paralysis; Breast Reconstruction; Limb Surgery/Reconstruction; **Hospital:** USC Univ Hosp - R K Eamer Med Plz; **Address:** 1450 San Pablo St, Ste 2000, Los Angeles, CA 90033-4680; **Phone:** 323-442-6482; **Board Cert:** Surgery 04; Plastic Surgery 86; Hand Surgery 00; **Med School:** Univ MO-Columbia Sch Med 77; **Resid:** Surgery, UCSF Hosps 81; Surgery, State Univ of New York 83; **Fellow:** Plastic Surgery, USC Med Ctr 85; **Fac Appt:** Prof S, USC Sch Med

PSYCHIATRY

A *psychiatrist specializes in the prevention, diagnosis and treatment of mental, addictive and emotional disorders such as schizophrenia and other psychotic disorders, mood disorders, anxiety disorders, substance-related disorders, sexual and gender identity disorders and adjustment disorders. The psychiatrist is able to understand the biologic, psychologic and social components of illness, and therefore is uniquely prepared to treat the whole person. A psychiatrist is qualified to order diagnostic laboratory tests and to prescribe medications, evaluate and treat psychologic and interpersonal problems and to intervene with families who are coping with stress, crises and other problems in living.*

Training required: *Four years*

Certification in one of the following subspecialties requires additional training and examination.

ADDICTION PSYCHIATRY:

A psychiatrist who focuses on the evaluation and treatment of individuals with alcohol, drug, or other substance-related disorders and of individuals with the dual diagnosis of substance-related and other psychiatric disorders.

CHILD AND ADOLESCENT PSYCHIATRY:

A psychiatrist with additional training in the diagnosis and treatment of developmental, behavioral, emotional and mental disorders of childhood and adolescence.

PHYSICIAN LISTINGS

417

GERIATRIC PSYCHIATRY:

A psychiatrist with expertise in the prevention, evaluation, diagnosis and treatment of mental and emotional disorders in the elderly. The geriatric psychiatrist seeks to improve the psychiatric care of the elderly both in health and in disease.

PSYCHIATRY

New England

Greenberg, Donna B MD [Psyc] - **Spec Exp:** Psychiatry in Cancer; **Hospital:** Mass Genl Hosp; **Address:** Mass General Hospital, Warren 605, 55 Fruit St, Boston, MA 02114-2696; **Phone:** 617-726-2984; **Board Cert:** Internal Medicine 78; Psychiatry 90; **Med School:** Univ Rochester 75; **Resid:** Internal Medicine, Boston City Hosp 78; Psychiatry, Mass Genl Hosp 89; **Fellow:** Psychiatry, Mass Genl Hosp 79; **Fac Appt:** Assoc Prof Psyc, Harvard Med Sch

Rauch, Paula K MD [Psyc] - **Spec Exp:** Psychiatry in Childhood Cancer; Children/Families facing Severe Illness; Parent Guidance in Parental Cancer; **Hospital:** Mass Genl Hosp; **Address:** Mass General Hospital, Dept Child Psychiatry, Wang Bldg, Ste 725, Boston, MA 02114; **Phone:** 617-724-5600; **Board Cert:** Psychiatry 90; Child & Adolescent Psychiatry 91; **Med School:** Univ Cincinnati 81; **Resid:** Psychiatry, Mass Genl Hosp 84; **Fac Appt:** Asst Prof Psyc, Harvard Med Sch

Mid Atlantic

Basch, Samuel MD [Psyc] - **Spec Exp:** Psychopharmacology; Psychoanalysis; Psychiatry in Physical Illness/Cancer; **Hospital:** Mount Sinai Med Ctr (page 101); **Address:** 10 E 85th St, Ste 1B, New York, NY 10028-0778; **Phone:** 212-427-0344; **Board Cert:** Psychiatry 70; **Med School:** Hahnemann Univ 61; **Resid:** Psychiatry, Mount Sinai Hosp 65; **Fellow:** Psychoanalysis, Columbia Presby 76; **Fac Appt:** Clin Prof Psyc, Mount Sinai Sch Med

Breitbart, William MD [Psyc] - **Spec Exp:** Psychiatry in Cancer; AIDS/HIV; Pain & Palliative Care; **Hospital:** Meml Sloan Kettering Cancer Ctr (page 100); **Address:** Meml Sloan Kettering, 1242 2nd Ave, New York, NY 10021; **Phone:** 212-639-4770; **Board Cert:** Internal Medicine 82; Psychiatry 86; **Med School:** Albert Einstein Coll Med 78; **Resid:** Internal Medicine, Bronx Muni Hosp Ctr 82; Psychiatry, Bronx Muni Hosp Ctr 84; **Fellow:** Psychiatric Oncology, Meml Sloan Kettering Cancer Ctr 86; **Fac Appt:** Prof Psyc, Cornell Univ-Weill Med Coll

Holland, Jimmie C B MD [Psyc] - **Spec Exp:** Psychiatry in Cancer; Bereavement; **Hospital:** Meml Sloan Kettering Cancer Ctr (page 100); **Address:** Dept Psychiatry & Behavioral Science, 1242 Second Ave, New York, NY 10021-6804; **Phone:** 212-639-3904; **Board Cert:** Psychiatry 66; **Med School:** Baylor Coll Med 52; **Resid:** Psychiatry, Mass Genl Hosp 55; Psychiatry, EJ Meyer Meml Hosp 57; **Fac Appt:** Prof Psyc, Cornell Univ-Weill Med Coll

Klagsbrun, Samuel C MD [Psyc] - **Spec Exp:** Psychiatry in Cancer; Psychiatry in Terminal Illness; **Hospital:** Four Winds Hosp; **Address:** Four Winds Hospital, 800 Cross River Rd, Katonah, NY 10536; **Phone:** 914-763-8151; **Board Cert:** Psychiatry 77; **Med School:** Univ Hlth Sci/Chicago Med Sch 62; **Resid:** Psychiatry, Yale-New Haven Hosp 66; **Fac Appt:** Clin Prof Psyc, Albert Einstein Coll Med

Kunkel, Elisabeth J MD [Psyc] - **Spec Exp:** Psychiatry in Cancer; Psychiatry in Physical Illness; **Hospital:** Thomas Jefferson Univ Hosp (page 110); **Address:** Thomas Jefferson Univ, 1020 Samson St, Thompson Bldg, Ste 1652, Philadelphia, PA 19107; **Phone:** 215-955-6683; **Board Cert:** Psychiatry 89; Geriatric Psychiatry 94; Addiction Psychiatry 98; **Med School:** McGill Univ 83; **Resid:** Psychiatry, NYU Med Ctr 87; **Fellow:** Liason Psychiatry, Meml Sloan Kettering Cancer Ctr 89; **Fac Appt:** Prof Psyc, Jefferson Med Coll

Lederberg, Marguerite MD **[Psyc]** - **Spec Exp:** Psychiatry in Cancer; **Hospital:** Meml Sloan Kettering Cancer Ctr (page 100); **Address:** 1242 2nd Ave, New York, NY 10021; **Phone:** 212-639-3911; **Board Cert:** Pediatrics 70; Psychiatry 80; **Med School:** Yale Univ 61; **Resid:** Pediatrics, Stanford Univ Med Ctr 64; Psychiatry, Stanford Univ Med Ctr 77; **Fellow:** Ambulatory Pediatrics, Stanford Univ Med Ctr 68; **Fac Appt:** Clin Prof Psyc, Cornell Univ-Weill Med Coll

Midwest

Riba, Michelle MD **[Psyc]** - **Spec Exp:** Psychiatry in Cancer; **Hospital:** Univ Michigan Hlth Sys; **Address:** Univ Mich Med Ctr, Dept Psyc, 1500 E Medical Center Drive Bldg MCHC - rm F6236, Ann Arbor, MI 48109-0295; **Phone:** 734-764-6879; **Board Cert:** Psychiatry 91; **Med School:** Univ Conn 85; **Resid:** Psychiatry, Univ Connecticut 89; **Fac Appt:** Assoc Clin Prof Psyc, Univ Mich Med Sch

Southwest

Valentine, Alan D MD **[Psyc]** - **Spec Exp:** Psychiatry in Cancer; Palliative Care; **Hospital:** UT MD Anderson Cancer Ctr, The (page 115); **Address:** Neuro-Oncology Unit 431, MD Anderson Cancer Ctr, PO Box 301402, Houston, TX 77230-1402; **Phone:** 713-792-7546; **Board Cert:** Psychiatry 92; Geriatric Psychiatry 94; **Med School:** Univ Tex, Houston ; **Resid:** Psychiatry, Univ Texas Affil Hosps; **Fac Appt:** Assoc Prof Psyc, Univ Tex, Houston

West Coast and Pacific

Fann, Jesse R MD **[Psyc]** - **Spec Exp:** Psychiatry in Physical Illness; Psychiatry in Neurological Disorders; Psychiatry in Cancer; **Hospital:** Univ Wash Med Ctr; **Address:** University of Washington Medical Ctr, 1959 NE Pacific St, Box 356560, Seattle, WA 98195; **Phone:** 206-543-3925; **Board Cert:** Psychiatry 94; **Med School:** Northwestern Univ 89; **Resid:** Psychiatry, Univ Washington Med Ctr 93; **Fellow:** Liason Psychiatry, Univ Washington Med Ctr 95; **Fac Appt:** Asst Prof Psyc, Univ Wash

Spiegel, David MD **[Psyc]** - **Spec Exp:** Hypnosis; Psychiatry in Cancer; Post Traumatic Stress Disorder; **Hospital:** Stanford Univ Med Ctr; **Address:** Stanford Univ Sch Med, Dept Psyc-Behav Scis, 401 Quarry Rd, rm 2325, Stanford, CA 94305-5718; **Phone:** 650-723-6421; **Board Cert:** Psychiatry 76; **Med School:** Harvard Med Sch 71; **Resid:** Psychiatry, Mass Mental Hlth Ctr 74; Psychiatry, Cambridge Hosp-Harvard Med Sch 74; **Fellow:** Community Psychiatry, Harvard Med Sch 74; **Fac Appt:** Prof Psyc, Stanford Univ

Strouse, Thomas B MD **[Psyc]** - **Spec Exp:** Psychiatry in Cancer; Pain-Cancer; Psychiatry in Physical Illness; **Hospital:** Cedars-Sinai Med Ctr (page 88); **Address:** Cedars-Sinai Outpatient Cancer Ctr, 8700 Beverly Blvd, Ste C2000, Los Angeles, CA 90048-1804; **Phone:** 310-423-0637; **Board Cert:** Psychiatry 93; Pain Medicine 00; **Med School:** Case West Res Univ 87; **Resid:** Psychiatry, UCLA Med Ctr 91; **Fac Appt:** Asst Clin Prof Psyc, UCLA

PULMONARY DISEASE

a subspecialty of INTERNAL MEDICINE

*A*n *internist who treats diseases of the lungs and airways. The pulmonologist diagnosis and treats cancer, pneumonia, pleurisy, asthma, occupational diseases, bronchitis, sleep disorders, emphysema and other complex disorders of the lungs.*

Training required: Three years in internal medicine plus additional training and examination for certification in pulmonary disease.

INTERNAL MEDICINE: An internist is a personal physician who provides long-term, comprehensive care in the office and the hospital, managing both common and complex illness of adolescents, adults and the elderly. Internists are trained in the diagnosis and treatment of cancer, infections and diseases affecting the heart, blood, kidneys, joints and digestive, respiratory and vascular systems. They are also trained in the essentials of primary care internal medicine, which incorporates an understanding of disease prevention, wellness, substance abuse, mental health and effective treatment of common problems of the eyes, ears, skin, nervous system and reproductive organs.

PHYSICIAN LISTINGS

421

PULMONARY DISEASE

New England

Matthay, Richard MD [Pul] - **Spec Exp:** Lung Cancer; Asthma; Lupus/SLE, Scleroderma; **Hospital:** Yale - New Haven Hosp; **Address:** 333 Cedar St, rm 105-LCI, Box 208057, New Haven, CT 06520-3206; **Phone:** 203-785-4198; **Board Cert:** Internal Medicine 73; Pulmonary Disease 76; Critical Care Medicine 97; **Med School:** Tufts Univ 70; **Resid:** Internal Medicine, Univ Colorado Med Ctr 73; **Fellow:** Pulmonary Disease, Univ Colorado Med Ctr 75; **Fac Appt:** Prof Med, Yale Univ

Mid Atlantic

Libby, Daniel MD [Pul] - **Spec Exp:** Asthma; Lung Cancer; Interstitial Lung Disease; **Hospital:** NY-Presby Hosp - NY Weill Cornell Med Ctr (page 103); **Address:** 407 E 70th St, New York, NY 10021-5302; **Phone:** 212-628-6611; **Board Cert:** Internal Medicine 77; Pulmonary Disease 80; **Med School:** Baylor Coll Med 74; **Resid:** Internal Medicine, New York Hosp 77; **Fellow:** Pulmonary Disease, New York Hosp 79; **Fac Appt:** Clin Prof Med, Cornell Univ-Weill Med Coll

Smith, James P MD [Pul] - **Spec Exp:** Emphysema; Lung Cancer; Asthma; **Hospital:** NY-Presby Hosp - NY Weill Cornell Med Ctr (page 103); **Address:** 170 E 77th St, New York, NY 10021-1912; **Phone:** 212-879-2180; **Board Cert:** Internal Medicine 67; Pulmonary Disease 68; **Med School:** Georgetown Univ 60; **Resid:** Internal Medicine, NY Hosp-Cornell Med Ctr 62; Internal Medicine, NY Hosp-Cornell Med Ctr 65; **Fellow:** Pulmonary Disease, NY Hosp-Cornell Med Ctr 66; **Fac Appt:** Clin Prof Med, Cornell Univ-Weill Med Coll

Steinberg, Harry MD [Pul] - **Spec Exp:** Asthma; Emphysema; Lung Cancer; **Hospital:** Long Island Jewish Med Ctr; **Address:** LI Jewish Med Ctr, Dept Med, 270-05 76th Ave, New Hyde Park, NY 11040-1496; **Phone:** 718-470-7230; **Med School:** Temple Univ 66; **Resid:** Internal Medicine, LI Jewish Med Ctr 69; Pulmonary Critical Care Medicine, LI Jewish Med Ctr 70; **Fellow:** Pulmonary Disease, Hosp Univ Penn 74; **Fac Appt:** Clin Prof Med, Albert Einstein Coll Med

Teirstein, Alvin MD [Pul] - **Spec Exp:** Sarcoidosis; Interstitial Lung Disease; Lung Cancer; **Hospital:** Mount Sinai Med Ctr (page 101); **Address:** Mount Sinai Med Ctr, Pulmonary Assoc., 1 Gustave Levy Pl, Box 1232, New York, NY 10029; **Phone:** 212-241-5656; **Board Cert:** Internal Medicine 61; Pulmonary Disease 69; **Med School:** SUNY Downstate 53; **Resid:** Internal Medicine, Mt Sinai Med Ctr 57; **Fellow:** Pulmonary Disease, Mt Sinai Med Ctr 54; Pulmonary Disease, VA Med Ctr 56; **Fac Appt:** Prof Med, Mount Sinai Sch Med

Unger, Michael MD [Pul] - **Spec Exp:** Lung Cancer; Bronchoscopy - Interventional; Cancer Prevention; **Hospital:** Fox Chase Cancer Ctr (page 95); **Address:** Fox Chase Cancer Center, 7701 Burholme Ave, Philadelphia, PA 19111; **Phone:** 215-728-6900; **Board Cert:** Internal Medicine 77; Pulmonary Disease 78; **Med School:** France 71; **Resid:** Internal Medicine, Mt Sinai Med Sers 74; **Fellow:** Pulmonary Disease, Cornell-NY Hosp 76; **Fac Appt:** Clin Prof Med, Thomas Jefferson Univ

White, Dorothy MD [Pul] - **Spec Exp:** Lung Cancer; AIDS/HIV; **Hospital:** Meml Sloan Kettering Cancer Ctr (page 100); **Address:** 1275 York Ave, rm H803, Box 13, New York, NY 10021; **Phone:** 212-639-8022; **Board Cert:** Internal Medicine 80; Pulmonary Disease 84; **Med School:** SUNY Hlth Sci Ctr 77; **Resid:** Internal Medicine, New York Hosp 80; Internal Medicine, Meml Sloan Kettering Inst 81; **Fellow:** Pulmonary Disease, Yale-New Haven Hosp 84; **Fac Appt:** Assoc Prof Med, Cornell Univ-Weill Med Coll

Southeast

Alberts, W Michael MD [Pul] - **Spec Exp:** Lung Cancer; **Hospital:** H Lee Moffitt Cancer Ctr & Research Inst; **Address:** 13000 Bruce B Downs Blvd, Ste 111C, Tampa, FL 33612; **Phone:** 813-972-8436; **Board Cert:** Internal Medicine 80; Critical Care Obstetrics 87; Pulmonary Disease 82; **Med School:** Univ IL Coll Med 77; **Resid:** Internal Medicine, Ohio State Univ Hosp 80; **Fellow:** Internal Medicine, UCSD Med Ctr 83; **Fac Appt:** Prof Med, Univ S Fla Coll Med

Garver Jr, Robert MD [Pul] - **Spec Exp:** Lung Cancer; Lung Disease; **Hospital:** Univ of Ala Hosp at Birmingham; **Address:** 1900 Univ Blvd, Birmingham, AL 35233; **Phone:** 205-934-7556; **Board Cert:** Internal Medicine 84; Pulmonary Disease 86; **Med School:** Johns Hopkins Univ 81; **Resid:** Internal Medicine, Johns Hopkins Hosp 84; **Fellow:** Pulmonary Disease, NHLBI 85; **Fac Appt:** Prof Pul, Univ Ala

Goldman, Allan Larry MD [Pul] - **Spec Exp:** Occupational Lung Disease; Airway Disorders; Lung Cancer; **Hospital:** Tampa Genl Hosp; **Address:** USF Coll Med, Dept Internal Medicine, 12901 Bruce B Downs Blvd, Box MDC19, Tampa, FL 33612-4742; **Phone:** 813-974-2271; **Board Cert:** Internal Medicine 72; Pulmonary Disease 72; **Med School:** Univ Minn 68; **Resid:** Internal Medicine, Brooke Army Hosp 70; **Fellow:** Pulmonary Disease, Walter Reed Army Hosp 72; **Fac Appt:** Prof Med, Univ S Fla Coll Med

Midwest

Jett, James R MD [Pul] - **Spec Exp:** Lung Cancer; Mesothelioma; Thymoma; **Hospital:** Mayo Med Ctr & Clin - Rochester; **Address:** Mayo Clinic, Thoracic Diseases, 200 First St SW, Rochester, MN 55905; **Phone:** 507-284-3764; **Board Cert:** Internal Medicine 76; Pulmonary Disease 78; **Med School:** Univ MO-Columbia Sch Med 73; **Resid:** Internal Medicine, Mayo Clinic 76; **Fellow:** Pulmonary Disease, Mayo Clinic 78; **Fac Appt:** Prof Med, Mayo Med Sch

McLennan, Geoffrey MD [Pul] - **Spec Exp:** Lung Cancer Diagnosis/Bronchoscopy; Emphysema; Chronic Obstructive Lung Disease (COPD); **Hospital:** Univ Iowa Hosp & Clinics; **Address:** Univ Iowa Hosp & Clinics, 200 Hawkins Drive, Ste 4900JPP, Iowa City, IA 52242; **Phone:** 319-353-8201; **Med School:** Australia ; **Resid:** Internal Medicine, Royal Adelaide Medical Sch; **Fellow:** Pulmonary Disease, Queen Elizabeth Hosp; **Fac Appt:** Prof Med, Univ Iowa Coll Med

Silver, Michael MD [Pul] - **Spec Exp:** Chronic Obstructive Lung Disease (COPD); Lung Cancer; Asthma; **Hospital:** Rush Univ Med Ctr; **Address:** 1725 W Harrison St, Prof Bldg 3, rm 054, Chicago, IL 60612; **Phone:** 312-942-6744; **Board Cert:** Internal Medicine 84; Pulmonary Disease 88; Critical Care Medicine 99; **Med School:** Albany Med Coll 81; **Resid:** Internal Medicine, Rush-Presby-St Luke's Med Ctr 85; **Fellow:** Pulmonary Critical Care Medicine, Rush-Presby-St Luke's Med Ctr 87; **Fac Appt:** Assoc Prof Med, Rush Med Coll

West Coast and Pacific

Patterson, James R MD [Pul] - **Spec Exp:** Lung Cancer; Asthma; Chronic Obstructive Lung Disease (COPD); **Hospital:** Providence Portland Med Ctr; **Address:** 507 NE 47th Ave, Ste 103, Portland, OR 97213; **Phone:** 503-215-2300; **Board Cert:** Internal Medicine 72; Pulmonary Disease 01; **Med School:** Columbia P&S 68; **Resid:** Internal Medicine, Columbia-Presby Med Ctr 70; **Fellow:** Pulmonary Disease, Fitzsimons Army Med Ctr 73; **Fac Appt:** Clin Prof Med, Oregon Hlth Sci Univ

RADIOLOGY

A *radiologist utilizes radiologic methodologies to diagnose and treat disease. Physicians practicing in the field of radiology most often specialize in radiology, diagnostic radiology, radiation oncology or radiological physics.*

Training required: *Four years in radiology plus additional training and examination.*

RADIATION ONCOLOGY

A subspecialist in radiation oncology deals with the therapeutic applications of radiant energy and its modifiers and the study and management of disease, especially malignant tumors.

DIAGNOSTIC RADIOLOGY

A radiologist who utilizes X-ray, radionuclides, ultrasound and electromagnetic radiation to diagnose and treat disease.

Training required: *Four years*

INTERVENTIONAL RADIOLOGY

A radiologist who diagnoses and treats diseases by various radiologic imaging modalities. These include fluoroscopy, digital radiography, computed tomography, sonography and magnetic resonance imaging.

NEURORADIOLOGY

A radiologist who diagnoses and treats diseases utilizing imaging procedures as they relate to the brain, spine and spinal cord, head, neck and organs of special sense in adults and children.

Certification in subspecialties such as Pediatric Radiology and Interventional Radiology require additional training and examination.

NUCLEAR MEDICINE

A nuclear medicine specialist employs the properties of radioactive atoms and molecules in the diagnosis and treatment of disease, and in research. Radiation detection and imaging instrument systems are used to detect disease as it changes the function and metabolism of normal cells, tissues and organs. A wide variety of diseases can be found in this way, usually before the structure of the organ involved by the disease can be seen to be abnormal by any other techniques. Early detection of coronary artery disease (including acute heart attack); early cancer detection and evaluation of the effect of tumor treatment; diagnosis of infection and inflammation anywhere in the body; and early detection of blood clot in the lungs, are all possible with *these techniques. Unique forms or radioactive molecules can attack and kill cancer cells (e.g., lymphoma, thyroid cancer) or can relieve the severe pain of cancer that has spread to bone.*

The nuclear medicine specialist has special knowledge in the biologic effects of radiation exposure, the fundamentals of the physical sciences and the principles and operation of radiation detection and imaging instrumentation systems.

Training required: *Three years*

PHYSICIAN LISTINGS

NUCLEAR MEDICINE

RADIATION ONCOLOGY
FOX CHASE CANCER CENTER

333 Cottman Avenue
Philadelphia, Pennsylvania 19111-2497
Phone: 1-888-FOX CHASE • Fax: 215-728-2702 • www.fccc.edu

Fox Chase Cancer Center has one of the most comprehensive radiation oncology facilities in the world. Specially trained board-certified radiation oncologists are skilled in both standard and unique radiation therapies. We are constantly seeking innovative ways to use existing technology and identifying new therapies to help our patients. Major treatment interests include breast cancer, brain cancer, esophageal and other gastrointestinal cancers, gynecologic cancers, head and neck cancers, lung cancers, prostate and other genitourinary cancers and sarcomas.

Fox Chase's radiation oncology program includes intensity-modulated radiation therapy (IMRT) and low-dose-rate and high-dose-rate radiation implants (brachytherapy) as well as conventional external-beam radiation therapy. We offer treatment with radiation alone, as part of a multidisciplinary regimen or through clinical trials to determine the most effective approaches for specific cancers. Researchers in the department carry out studies in radiation biology and physics to enhance the effectiveness of therapy.

Fox Chase uses sophisticated imaging tools during the treatment planning and daily treatment sessions to target the cancer better and spare any healthy surrounding tissue undue exposure to radiation. For example, Fox Chase was the first and remains one of the only centers in North America to use a clinical MRI treatment simulator.

Fox Chase radiation oncologists were also among the first to combine CT scanning and three-dimensional treatment simulation in a process called CT simulation—a convenient, one-stop treatment-planning process for patients. Computers process an extensive CT scan, using a prototype spiral CT scanner, and then accomplish the simulation procedure electronically. Digitally reconstructed radiographs replace the X-rays taken during conventional simulation and improve the radiation oncologists' ability to treat the cancer.

Because of our outstanding reputation as a leader in cancer therapy, we frequently work with the world's foremost makers of medical equipment to test prototypes and develop the best applications. As a result, Fox Chase patients can benefit from the newest approaches in radiation therapy and other technologies long before they are available at other centers in the region or even the nation.

INTENSITY MODULATED RADIATION THERAPY

Fox Chase Cancer Center offers the most precise radiation therapy available for treating women with breast cancer and men with prostate cancer through our region's most comprehensive and experienced program of image-guided intensity-modulated radiation therapy (IMRT). Where appropriate, patients with certain head and neck, gastrointestinal or gynecologic cancers also receive IMRT at Fox Chase.

IMRT—the newest generation of precision-targeted, conformal radiation therapy—permits delivery of powerful radiation doses with extremely high precision while sparing surrounding healthy tissue.

With IMRT throughout their course of radiation therapy, prostate cancer patients at Fox Chase experience fewer side effects related to changes in bladder and rectal function. For women with breast cancer, the precise technology of IMRT minimizes skin irritation and helps avoid possible long-term effects on the lungs and heart.

RADIATION ONCOLOGY

RENOWNED EXPERTS. COMPASSIONATE CARE.

NYU's Department of Radiation Oncology offers a program of thoroughly integrated, multidisciplinary care for adults and children. Individualized treatment is designed using some of the most sophisticated radiation therapy technologies currently available.

ADVANCED TECHNOLOGY

Increased accuracy in targeting tumors and sparing normal tissue with:

* 3-D conformal treatment planning and state-of-the-art CT Simulators
* Three new top-of-the-line linear accelerators used in the delivery of electron and photon beam therapy
* Intensity Modulated Radiation Therapy (IMRT)
* Respiratory Gating

A VARIETY OF TREATMENT OPTIONS

* NYU has piloted the use of a special prone table that spares heart and lung tissue during radiation of the breast
* High Dose Rate Brachytherapy for gynecologic cancer and other malignancies
* Permanent Prostate Seed Implant Program
* Stereotactic radiosurgery with linear accelerators or Gamma Knife

RECENT HIGHLIGHTS

* A brand-new, dedicated outpatient facility
* A unique Center of Excellence Award for Locally Advanced Breast Cancer Research awarded by the U.S. Department of Defense
* Investigator-initiated clinical trials available only at NYU, as well as access to trials via cooperative groups
* Support servies include referrals on-site interdisciplinary programs for patient education, nutrition, counseling, social work services, and access to complementary therapies.

Specialists at the NCI-designated NYU Cancer Institute seek to enhance and coordinate the extensive resources of NYU Medical Center to optimize research, treatment, and the ultimate control of cancer.

Our new NYU Clinical Cancer Center is located at 160 East 34th Street. This state-of-the-art 13-level, 85,000-square-foot building serves as "home base" for patients, by providing the latest cancer prevention, screening, diagnostic treatment, genetic counseling, and support services in one central location. The NYU Clinical Cancer Center stands to dramatically improve the lives of people with cancer. As part of NYU Medical Center, patients can access a variety of other non-cancer services throughout the institution.

PHYSICIAN REFERRAL
1-888-7-NYU-MED
(1-888-769-8633)
www.nyumc.org
www.nyuci.org

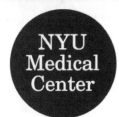

NYU Medical Center

550 First Avenue (at 31st Street)
New York, NY 10016
Physician Referral:
1-888-7-NYU-MED
www.nyumc.org

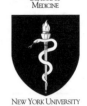

RADIOLOGY:
The Diagnostic Core of Modern Medicine

LEADING EDGE TECHNOLOGY

Focusing on a broad variety of cancers including breast, colon, & lung, NYU Medical Center houses some of the most advanced radiologyequipment in the world, including:

- Multi-detector 64 slice CT
- New multi-Channel MRI technology including two 3-Tesla clinical scanners and 7-Tesla research scanner
- Brand new, high resolution/high sensitivity PET/CT
- Full-field digital mammography as well as standard analog films
- Stereotactic biopsy capability
- Bone densitometry
- Advanced breast MR Imaging
- Digital fluoroscopy
- Advanced digital subtraction angiography with 3D Capabilities
- Minimally invasive techniques including radiofrequency ablationand chemoembilization
- State-of-the-art SPECT gamma cameras
- Radioimmunotherapy for Non-Hodgkin's Lymphoma

ON THE HORIZON

As part of a major academic medical center, our cancer experts collaborate inother aspects of medicine as well. The Department is the 9th largest recipient of NIH research funding in the US and first in New York.

A DRIVER OF CROSS-DISCIPLINARY CLINICAL EXCELLENCE

Radiology plays an increasingly pivotal role in medical, clinical, and translational research. With an explosion of imaging technologies, researchers at NYU are making rapid strides in the understanding of complex diseases.No longer merely a supportive discipline, radiology has been transformed into a dynamic driver of medical knowledge itself. For example, the new imaging technologies allow physicians to observe minute changes in tumor activity during cancer treatment, adjust the dosage accordingly, and monitor the disease process with a depth and precision that would have previously been unimaginable.

PHYSICIAN REFERRAL
1-888-7-NYU-MED
(1-888-769-8633)
www.nyumc.org

RADIATION ONCOLOGY

The Radiation Treatment Center at M. D. Anderson treats more than 4,300 new patients annually and is the most comprehensive technologically advanced facility of its kind in the world. Because our radiation oncologists are highly specialized, they may have seen hundreds or even thousands of patients with the same tumor type. That depth of experience gives them a facile ability to evaluate patients and plan optimal treatment.

Radiation Treatment Center Services include consultation, evaluation, and treatment of all malignant diseases in which radiation therapy plays a role. Approximately 50% of all patients with cancer receive radiation therapy as part of their cancer care. Specialized services include, intensity modulated radiation therapy, three-dimensional conformal treatment planning, image-guided prostate seed implants, stereotactic radiosurgery, total body irradiation, total skin electron treatment and brachytherapy.

Radiation Treatment Center care teams are organized by tumor type, promoting expertise and depth of experience, whether the cancer is common or rare, or whether treatment is straightforward or complex. Each patient's proposed treatment plan is reviewed in a department-wide consultation after being determined in a multidisciplinary conference, giving patients the benefit of many specialists contributing to their care plans. Ongoing reviews during treatment monitor quality and appropriateness of care.

Our full-time faculty are leaders in their fields because of their commitment to translating clinical and basic research to better patient care. They publish their findings in journals edited, read and relied on by other physicians. The radiation oncology department at M. D. Anderson is the only one in Texas given full membership status in the Radiation Therapy Oncology Group, an international organization of scholar-physicians who perform research in radiation oncology. Monitoring of equipment and instrumentation exceeds standards set by federal and state agencies.

The University of Texas M. D. Anderson Cancer Center is one of the world's most productive and highly regarded academic institutions devoted to cancer patient care, research, education and prevention.

Created by the Texas Legislature in 1941, M. D. Anderson was among the nation's first three Comprehensive Cancer Centers designated in 1971. M. D. Anderson has ranked as one of the top two cancer hospitals since *U.S.News & World Report* began its annual survey of "best hospitals" in 1990 and has been recognized number one for cancer care three times in the last four years. M. D. Anderson holds the highest level of accreditation from the Joint Commission on Accreditation of Healthcare Organizations.

Since the first patient was registered in 1944, almost 600,000 patients have come to M. D. Anderson for cancer care in the form of surgery, radiation therapy, chemotherapy, immuno-therapy and supportive therapies. The multi-disciplinary approach to treating cancer was pioneered at M. D. Anderson.

RADIATION ONCOLOGY

New England

Choi, Noah C MD [RadRO] - **Spec Exp:** Lung Cancer; Esophageal Cancer; **Hospital:** Mass Genl Hosp; **Address:** Mass Genl Hosp, Dept Rad Onc, 100 Blossom St, Cox 307, Boston, MA 02114; **Phone:** 617-726-6050; **Board Cert:** Therapeutic Radiology 70; **Med School:** South Korea 63; **Resid:** Radiation Oncology, Princess Margaret Hosp; **Fac Appt:** Assoc Prof Rad, Harvard Med Sch

D'Amico, Anthony V MD/PhD [RadRO] - **Spec Exp:** Prostate Cancer; Brachytherapy; **Hospital:** Brigham & Women's Hosp (page 87); **Address:** Brigham & Women's Hosp, Dept Rad Onc, 75 Francis St, Ste L2, Boston, MA 02115; **Phone:** 617-732-6313; **Board Cert:** Radiation Oncology 99; **Med School:** Univ Pennsylvania 90; **Resid:** Radiation Oncology, Hosp Univ Penn 94; **Fac Appt:** Assoc Prof RadRO, Harvard Med Sch

Haffty, Bruce MD [RadRO] - **Spec Exp:** Breast Cancer; Lung Cancer; Head & Neck Cancer; **Hospital:** Yale - New Haven Hosp; **Address:** Dept Therapeutic Radiology, 20 York St, HRT-133, New Haven, CT 06504; **Phone:** 203-785-2959; **Board Cert:** Radiation Oncology 88; **Med School:** Yale Univ 84; **Resid:** Radiation Oncology, Yale-New Haven Hosp 88; **Fac Appt:** Prof Rad TR, Yale Univ

Harris, Jay R MD [RadRO] - **Spec Exp:** Breast Cancer; **Hospital:** Brigham & Women's Hosp (page 87); **Address:** Dana Farber Cancer Inst, 44 Binney St, rm 1622, Boston, MA 02115; **Phone:** 617-632-2291; **Board Cert:** Therapeutic Radiology 99; **Med School:** Stanford Univ 70; **Resid:** Radiation Oncology, Joint Ctr Rad Ther 76; **Fellow:** Radium Therapy, Harvard Med Sch 77; **Fac Appt:** Prof RadRO, Harvard Med Sch

Hug, Eugen B MD [RadRO] - **Spec Exp:** Brain Tumors; Prostate Cancer; **Hospital:** Dartmouth - Hitchcock Med Ctr; **Address:** Dartmouth-Hitchcock Med Ctr-Dept Rad Oncology, 1 Medical Center Drive, Lebanon, NH 03756; **Phone:** 603-650-6614; **Board Cert:** Radiation Oncology 94; **Med School:** Germany 87; **Resid:** Radiation Therapy, Mass Genl Hosp 92; **Fellow:** Radiation Oncology, Mass Genl Hosp 93; **Fac Appt:** Prof RadRO, Dartmouth Med Sch

Knisely, Jonathan MD [RadRO] - **Spec Exp:** Brain Tumors; Stereotactic Radiosurgery; Gastrointestinal Cancer; **Hospital:** Yale - New Haven Hosp; **Address:** Yale University School Medicine, Dept Therapeutic Radiology, 15 York St Bldg Hunter - Ste HRT 1, New Haven, CT 06520-8040; **Phone:** 203-785-2960; **Board Cert:** Internal Medicine 89; Radiation Oncology 93; **Med School:** Univ Pennsylvania 86; **Resid:** Internal Medicine, Michael Reese Hosp 89; Radiation Oncology, Univ Toronto Med Ctr 91; **Fac Appt:** Assoc Prof Rad TR, Yale Univ

Loeffler, Jay S MD [RadRO] - **Spec Exp:** Spinal Cord Tumors; Stereotactic Radiosurgery; Brain Tumors; **Hospital:** Mass Genl Hosp; **Address:** Mass Gen Hospital, Radiation Oncology, 100 Blossom St, Boston, MA 02114; **Phone:** 617-724-1548; **Board Cert:** Therapeutic Radiology 86; **Med School:** Brown Univ 82; **Resid:** Radiation Oncology, Harvard Joint Ctr for Rad Ther 86; **Fellow:** Cancer Biology, Harvard Sch Pub Hlth 85; **Fac Appt:** Prof RadRO, Harvard Med Sch

Peschel, Richard E MD [RadRO] - **Spec Exp:** Prostate Cancer; **Hospital:** Yale - New Haven Hosp; **Address:** Yale-New Haven Hospital, Dept Therapeutic Radiology, 20 York St, rm HRT 141, New Haven, CT 06510; **Phone:** 203-785-2958; **Board Cert:** Therapeutic Radiology 82; **Med School:** Yale Univ 77; **Resid:** Radiation Therapy, Yale-New Haven Hosp 81; **Fac Appt:** Prof Rad TR, Yale Univ

Recht, Abram MD [RadRO] - **Spec Exp:** Breast Cancer; Gastrointestinal Cancer; Gynecologic Cancer; **Hospital:** Beth Israel Deaconess Med Ctr - Boston; **Address:** Beth Israel Deaconess Med Ctr, 330 Brookline Ave, Boston, MA 02215; **Phone:** 617-667-2345; **Board Cert:** Therapeutic Radiology 84; **Med School:** Johns Hopkins Univ 80; **Resid:** Radiation Oncology, Joint Ctr RadiationTherapy 84; **Fac Appt:** Assoc Prof RadRO, Harvard Med Sch

Roberts, Kenneth MD [RadRO] - **Spec Exp:** Pediatric Cancers; Lymphoma; Hodgkin's Disease; **Hospital:** Yale - New Haven Hosp; **Address:** 15 York St, Hunter Bldg HRT 138, New Haven, CT 06520; **Phone:** 203-785-2957; **Board Cert:** Internal Medicine 87; Medical Oncology 89; Radiation Oncology 95; **Med School:** Duke Univ 84; **Resid:** Internal Medicine, Ohio State Univ Hosps 87; Radiation Oncology, Duke Univ Med Ctr 92; **Fellow:** Hematology and Oncology, Duke Univ Med Ctr 89; **Fac Appt:** Assoc Prof Rad TR, Yale Univ

Shipley, William U MD [RadRO] - **Spec Exp:** Bladder Cancer; Prostate Cancer; **Hospital:** Mass Genl Hosp; **Address:** Mass Genl Hosp, Dept Rad Onc, 100 Blossom St, Cox 347, Boston, MA 02114; **Phone:** 617-726-8146; **Board Cert:** Therapeutic Radiology 75; **Med School:** Harvard Med Sch 66; **Resid:** Surgery, Mass Genl Hosp 71; Radium Therapy, Mass Genl Hosp 73; **Fellow:** Radium Therapy, Royal Marsden Hosp 74; **Fac Appt:** Prof Rad, Harvard Med Sch

Tarbell, Nancy MD [RadRO] - **Spec Exp:** Pediatric Brain Tumors; Proton Beam Therapy; **Hospital:** Mass Genl Hosp; **Address:** Massachusetts Genl Hosp-Bulfinch 360A, 55 Fruit St, Boston, MA 02114; **Phone:** 617-724-1836; **Board Cert:** Therapeutic Radiology 83; **Med School:** SUNY Upstate Med Univ 79; **Resid:** Radiation Therapy, Harvard Med School 83; **Fac Appt:** Prof RadRO, Harvard Med Sch

Underhill, Kelly J MD [RadRO] - **Spec Exp:** Brachytherapy; Breast Cancer; Gynecologic Cancer; **Hospital:** Dartmouth - Hitchcock Med Ctr; **Address:** Norris Cotton Cancer Ctr, One Medical Center Drive, Lebanon, NH 03756; **Phone:** 603-650-6600; **Board Cert:** Radiation Oncology 98; **Med School:** Queens Univ 92; **Resid:** Radiation Oncology, Queens Univ 97; **Fellow:** Brachytherapy, Meml Sloan Kettering Med Ctr 98

Wazer, David E MD [RadRO] - **Spec Exp:** Breast Cancer; Melanoma; **Hospital:** Rhode Island Hosp; **Address:** 593 Eddy St, Providence, RI 02903; **Phone:** 401-444-8311; **Board Cert:** Radiation Oncology 88; **Med School:** NYU Sch Med 82; **Resid:** Radiation Oncology, Tufts New England Med Ctr 88; **Fellow:** Neurological Chemistry, NYU Med Ctr 84; **Fac Appt:** Prof RadRO, Tufts Univ

Wilson, Lynn D MD [RadRO] - **Spec Exp:** Lymphoma, Cutaneous T Cell (CTCL); Lymphoma, Cutaneous B Cell (CBCL); Lung Cancer; **Hospital:** Yale - New Haven Hosp; **Address:** Yale University School Medicine, Dept Therapeutic Radiology, HRT 136, 333 Cedar St, New Haven, CT 06510; **Phone:** 203-737-1202; **Board Cert:** Radiation Oncology 04; **Med School:** Geo Wash Univ 90; **Resid:** Therapeutic Radiology, Yale-New Haven Hosp 94; **Fac Appt:** Assoc Prof Rad TR, Yale Univ

Mid Atlantic

Berg, Christine D MD [RadRO] - **Spec Exp:** Breast Cancer; **Hospital:** Natl Inst of Hlth - Clin Ctr; **Address:** 6130 Executive Blvd, Bethesda, MD 20892-7340; **Phone:** 301-496-8544; **Board Cert:** Internal Medicine 80; Medical Oncology 83; Therapeutic Radiology 99; **Med School:** Northwestern Univ 77; **Resid:** Internal Medicine, Northwestern Meml Hosp 81; Radiation Oncology, Georgetown Univ Hosp 86; **Fellow:** Medical Oncology, Natl Cancer Inst-NIH 84

Berson, Anthony M MD **[RadRO]** - **Spec Exp:** Prostate Cancer; Breast Cancer; Lung Cancer; **Hospital:** St Vincent Cath Med Ctrs - Manhattan (page 108); **Address:** 325 W 15th St, New York, NY 10011-5903; **Phone:** 212-604-6081; **Board Cert:** Radiation Oncology 90; **Med School:** Hahnemann Univ 84; **Resid:** Radiation Oncology, UCSF Med Ctr 89; **Fellow:** Neoplastic Diseases, Lawrence Berkeley Lab 87; **Fac Appt:** Assoc Prof RadRO, NY Med Coll

Coia, Lawrence R MD **[RadRO]** - **Spec Exp:** Esophageal Cancer; Brachytherapy-HDR; Conformal Radiotherapy; **Hospital:** Comm Mem Hosp - Toms River; **Address:** Community Memorial Hospital, Dept Radiation Oncology, 99 Hwy 37 W, Toms River, NJ 08755-6498; **Phone:** 732-557-8148; **Board Cert:** Therapeutic Radiology 82; **Med School:** Temple Univ 76; **Resid:** Radiation Oncology, Thos Jefferson Univ Hosp 81; **Fac Appt:** Assoc Clin Prof Rad, Univ Pennsylvania

Constine III, Louis S MD **[RadRO]** - **Spec Exp:** Pediatric Cancers; Lymphoma; Cancer Survivors-Late Effects of Therapy; **Hospital:** Univ of Rochester Strong Meml Hosp; **Address:** 601 Elmwood Ave, Box 647, Rochester, NY 14642; **Phone:** 585-275-5622; **Board Cert:** Pediatrics 78; Therapeutic Radiology 81; Pediatric Hematology-Oncology 78; **Med School:** Johns Hopkins Univ 73; **Resid:** Pediatrics, Moffitt Hosp-UCSF Med Ctr 75; Pediatrics, Stanford Hosp Med Ctr 76; **Fellow:** Radiation Therapy, Stanford Hosp Med Ctr 81; Pediatric Hematology-Oncology, Univ Wash/Chldns Ortho Hosp 78; **Fac Appt:** Prof RadRO, Univ Rochester

Cooper, Jay MD **[RadRO]** - **Spec Exp:** Head & Neck Cancer; Skin Cancer; Chemo-Radiation Combined Therapy; **Hospital:** Maimonides Med Ctr (page 99); **Address:** Maimonides Cancer Ctr, 6300 8th Ave, Brooklyn, NY 11220; **Phone:** 718-765-2750; **Board Cert:** Therapeutic Radiology 77; **Med School:** NYU Sch Med 73; **Resid:** Radiation Oncology, NYU Med Ctr 77; **Fac Appt:** Prof RadRO, SUNY Downstate

Curran Jr, Walter J MD **[RadRO]** - **Spec Exp:** Lung Cancer; Brain Tumors; Gastrointestinal & Esophageal Cancer; **Hospital:** Thomas Jefferson Univ Hosp (page 110); **Address:** Thomas Jefferson Univ Hosp, Dept Rad Onc, 111 S 11th St, Bodine Ctr, Philadelphia, PA 19107; **Phone:** 215-955-6701; **Board Cert:** Therapeutic Radiology 86; **Med School:** Med Coll GA 82; **Resid:** Radiation Therapy, Hosp Univ Penn 86; **Fac Appt:** Prof RadRO, Jefferson Med Coll

DeWeese, Theodore L MD **[RadRO]** - **Spec Exp:** Urologic Cancer; Prostate Cancer; **Hospital:** Johns Hopkins Hosp - Baltimore (page 97); **Address:** Johns Hopkins Medicine, Dept Rad Oncology, 401 N Broadway, Weinberg Bldg, Ste 1440, Baltimore, MD 21231; **Phone:** 410-955-7068; **Board Cert:** Radiation Oncology 95; **Med School:** Univ Colorado 90; **Resid:** Radiation Oncology, Johns Hopkins Hosp 94; **Fellow:** Urologic Oncology, Johns Hopkins Hosp 95; **Fac Appt:** Prof RadRO, Johns Hopkins Univ

Dritschilo, Anatoly MD **[RadRO]** - **Spec Exp:** Breast Cancer; Prostate Cancer; **Hospital:** Georgetown Univ Hosp; **Address:** Georgetown Univ Hosp, Dept Radiation Medicine, 3800 Reservoir Rd NW, Washington, DC 20007; **Phone:** 202-687-2144; **Board Cert:** Therapeutic Radiology 77; **Med School:** UMDNJ-NJ Med Sch, Newark 73; **Resid:** Radiation Therapy, Harvard Joint Rad Ther Ctr 77

Ennis, Ronald D MD **[RadRO]** - **Spec Exp:** Brachytherapy; Prostate Cancer; Pancreatic Cancer; **Hospital:** St Luke's - Roosevelt Hosp Ctr - Roosevelt Div (page 93); **Address:** St Luke's Roosevelt Hosp-Roosevelt Div, Dept Rad Onc, 1000 10th Ave, Lower Level, New York, NY 10019; **Phone:** 212-523-7165; **Board Cert:** Radiation Oncology 05; **Med School:** Yale Univ 90; **Resid:** Therapeutic Radiology, Yale-New Haven Hosp 94

435

Flickinger, John C MD [RadRO] - **Spec Exp:** Neuro-Oncology; Brain & Spinal Tumors; **Hospital:** UPMC Presby, Pittsburgh (page 114); **Address:** UPMC Cancer Ctr, Radiation Oncology, 22 Lothrop St Fl 3, Pittsburgh, PA 15213; **Phone:** 412-647-3600; **Board Cert:** Therapeutic Radiology 85; **Med School:** Univ Chicago-Pritzker Sch Med 81; **Resid:** Radium Therapy, Mass General Hosp 85; **Fac Appt:** Prof RadRO, Univ Pittsburgh

Formenti, Silvia C MD [RadRO] - **Spec Exp:** Breast Cancer; Prostate Cancer; Chemo-Radiation Combined Therapy; **Hospital:** NYU Med Ctr (page 104); **Address:** NYU Med Ctr, Dept Radiation Oncology, 566 First Ave, New York, NY 10016-6402; **Phone:** 212-263-2601; **Board Cert:** Radiation Oncology 91; **Med School:** Italy 80; **Resid:** Internal Medicine, San Carlo Borromeo Hosp 83; Medical Oncology, Univ of Pavia Med Ctr 85; **Fellow:** Radiation Oncology, USC Med Ctr 90; **Fac Appt:** Asst Prof RadRO, NYU Sch Med

Glassburn, John R MD [RadRO] - **Spec Exp:** Gynecologic Cancer; **Hospital:** Pennsylvania Hosp (page 113); **Address:** Pennsylvania Hospital, Dept Radiation Oncology, 800 Spruce St, Philadelphia, PA 19107; **Phone:** 215-829-3873; **Board Cert:** Therapeutic Radiology 73; **Med School:** Hahnemann Univ 66; **Resid:** Radiology, Hahnemann Hosp 72; **Fac Appt:** Clin Prof Rad, Univ Pennsylvania

Glatstein, Eli MD [RadRO] - **Spec Exp:** Lymphoma; Lung Cancer; Photodynamic Therapy; **Hospital:** Hosp Univ Penn - UPHS (page 113); **Address:** Hosp Univ Penn, Dept Rad Onc, 3400 Spruce St, Donner Bldg Fl 2, Philadelphia, PA 19104; **Phone:** 215-662-3383; **Board Cert:** Therapeutic Radiology 72; **Med School:** Stanford Univ 64; **Resid:** Radium Therapy, Stanford Med Ctr 70; **Fellow:** Radiological Biology, Hammersmith Hosp 72; **Fac Appt:** Prof RadRO, Univ Pennsylvania

Goodman, Robert L MD [RadRO] - **Spec Exp:** Breast Cancer; Lymphoma; **Hospital:** St Barnabas Med Ctr; **Address:** St Barnabas Med Ctr, Dept Rad Onc, 94 Old Short Hills Rd, Livingston, NJ 07039; **Phone:** 973-322-5637; **Board Cert:** Internal Medicine 71; Therapeutic Radiology 74; Medical Oncology 75; **Med School:** Columbia P&S 66; **Resid:** Internal Medicine, Beth Israel Hosp 70; Radium Therapy, Harvard Joint Ctr Rad Therapy 74; **Fellow:** Hematology, Presby Hosp 69

Greenberger, Joel S MD [RadRO] - **Spec Exp:** Lung Cancer; Esophageal Cancer; **Hospital:** UPMC Presby, Pittsburgh (page 114); **Address:** Univ Pittsburgh Cancer Inst, 5150 Centre Ave, Pittsburgh, PA 15232; **Phone:** 412-647-3600; **Board Cert:** Therapeutic Radiology 77; **Med School:** Harvard Med Sch 71; **Resid:** Radium Therapy, Harvard Med Ctr 77; **Fac Appt:** Prof RadRO, Univ Pittsburgh

Harrison, Louis MD [RadRO] - **Spec Exp:** Brachytherapy; Head & Neck Cancer; Radiation Therapy-Intraoperative; **Hospital:** Beth Israel Med Ctr - Petrie Division (page 93); **Address:** Beth Israel Med Ctr, Dept Rad Onc, 10 Union Square East, Ste 4G, New York, NY 10003-3314; **Phone:** 212-844-8087; **Board Cert:** Therapeutic Radiology 86; **Med School:** SUNY Downstate 82; **Resid:** Therapeutic Radiology, Yale-New Haven Hosp 86; **Fac Appt:** Prof RadRO, Albert Einstein Coll Med

Horwitz, Eric MD [RadRO] - **Spec Exp:** Prostate Cancer; Brachytherapy; Head & Neck Cancer; **Hospital:** Fox Chase Cancer Ctr (page 95); **Address:** Fox Chase Cancer Ctr, Dept Radiation Oncology, 333 Cottman Ave, Philadelphia, PA 19111; **Phone:** 215-728-2995; **Board Cert:** Radiation Oncology 99; **Med School:** Albany Med Coll 92; **Resid:** Radiation Oncology, William Beaumont Hosp 97; **Fac Appt:** Assoc Prof RadRO, Temple Univ

Isaacson, Steven MD [RadRO] - **Spec Exp:** Brain Tumors; Neuro-Oncology; Arteriovenous Malformations; **Hospital:** NY-Presby Hosp - Columbia Presby Med Ctr (page 103); **Address:** Columbia Presby Med Ctr, Dept Radiation Oncolgy, 622 W 168th St, BHN-B11, New York, NY 10032; **Phone:** 212-305-2611; **Board Cert:** Radiation Oncology 88; Otolaryngology 78; **Med School:** Jefferson Med Coll 73; **Resid:** Otolaryngology, Hosp Univ Penn 78; Radiation Oncology, SUNY Hlth Sci Ctr 88; **Fac Appt:** Assoc Prof RadRO, Columbia P&S

Konski, Andre MD [RadRO] - **Spec Exp:** Esophageal Cancer; Rectal Cancer; Prostate Cancer; **Hospital:** Fox Chase Cancer Ctr (page 95); **Address:** Fox Chase Cancer Ctr, Dept Radiation Oncology, 333 Cottman Ave, Philadelphia, PA 19111; **Phone:** 215-728-2916; **Board Cert:** Radiation Oncology 00; **Med School:** NY Med Coll 84; **Resid:** Radiation Oncology, Stong Meml/Genesee Hosp 88

Kuettel, Michael MD/PhD [RadRO] - **Spec Exp:** Prostate Cancer; **Hospital:** Roswell Park Cancer Inst (page 107); **Address:** Elm and Carlton St, Buffalo, NY 14263; **Phone:** 716-845-1562; **Board Cert:** Radiation Oncology 92; **Med School:** Med Coll Wisc ; **Resid:** Internal Medicine, Northwestern Hosp; Radiation Oncology, Johns Hopkins Hosp; **Fac Appt:** Prof Med, SUNY Buffalo

Lepanto, Philip Bliss MD [RadRO] - **Hospital:** St Mary's Hosp - Huntington, WV; **Address:** St Mary's Hosp, Dept Radiation Oncology, 2900 First Ave, Huntington, WV 25702; **Phone:** 304-526-1143; **Board Cert:** Therapeutic Radiology 75; **Med School:** Univ Louisville Sch Med 70; **Resid:** Radiology, Hosp Univ Penn 72; Radium Therapy, Hosp Univ Penn 75; **Fac Appt:** Clin Prof Rad, Marshall Univ

Machtay, Mitchell MD [RadRO] - **Spec Exp:** Head & Neck Cancer; Brain Tumors; Eye Tumors/Cancer; **Hospital:** Thomas Jefferson Univ Hosp (page 110); **Address:** Bodine Ctr for Cancer Treatment, Dept Rad Onc, 111 S 11 St, Philadelphia, PA 19107-5097; **Phone:** 215-955-6706; **Board Cert:** Radiation Oncology 94; **Med School:** NYU Sch Med 89; **Resid:** Radiation Oncology, Hosp Univ Penn 93

McCormick, Beryl MD [RadRO] - **Spec Exp:** Breast Cancer; Eye Tumors/Cancer; **Hospital:** Meml Sloan Kettering Cancer Ctr (page 100); **Address:** Meml Sloan Kettering, Div Radiation Oncology, 1275 York Ave, rm SM 04, New York, NY 10021-6007; **Phone:** 212-639-6828; **Board Cert:** Therapeutic Radiology 77; **Med School:** UMDNJ-NJ Med Sch, Newark 73; **Resid:** Therapeutic Radiology, Meml Sloan Kettering Cancer Ctr 77; **Fac Appt:** Prof RadRO, Cornell Univ-Weill Med Coll

McKenna, W Gillies MD/PhD [RadRO] - **Spec Exp:** Lung Cancer; Head & Neck Cancer; Skin Cancer; **Hospital:** Hosp Univ Penn - UPHS (page 113); **Address:** Hosp Univ Penn - Dept Radiation Oncology, 3400 Spruce St, 2 Donner, Philadelphia, PA 19104; **Phone:** 215-662-3147; **Board Cert:** Therapeutic Radiology 85; **Med School:** Albert Einstein Coll Med 81; **Resid:** Radiation Therapy, Natl Cancer Inst 85; **Fac Appt:** Clin Prof RadRO, Univ Pennsylvania

Minsky, Bruce MD [RadRO] - **Spec Exp:** Colon & Rectal Cancer; Esophageal Cancer; Gastrointestinal Cancer; **Hospital:** Meml Sloan Kettering Cancer Ctr (page 100); **Address:** Meml Sloan Kettering Cancer Ctr, Dept Rad Onc, 1275 York Ave, New York, NY 10021-6007; **Phone:** 212-639-6817; **Board Cert:** Radiation Oncology 87; **Med School:** Univ Mass Sch Med 82; **Resid:** Radiation Oncology, Harvard Jt Ctr Rad Ther 86

Nori, Dattatreyudu MD [RadRO] - **Spec Exp:** Breast Cancer; Prostate Cancer; Gynecologic Cancer; **Hospital:** NY-Presby Hosp - NY Weill Cornell Med Ctr (page 103); **Address:** 525 E 68th St, Box 575, New York, NY 10021-4870; **Phone:** 212-746-3679; **Board Cert:** Therapeutic Radiology 79; **Med School:** India 70; **Resid:** Radiation Oncology, Meml Sloan Kettering Cancer Ctr 75; **Fellow:** Radiation Oncology, Meml Sloan Kettering Cancer Ctr 78; **Fac Appt:** Prof RadRO, Cornell Univ-Weill Med Coll

Pollack, Alan MD/PhD **[RadRO]** - **Spec Exp:** Prostate Cancer; Genitourinary Cancer; Sarcoma; **Hospital:** Fox Chase Cancer Ctr (page 95); **Address:** Fox Chase Cancer Ctr, Dept Radiation Oncology, 333 Cottman Ave, Philadelphia, PA 19111; **Phone:** 215-728-2940; **Board Cert:** Radiation Oncology 93; **Med School:** Univ Miami Sch Med 87; **Resid:** Radiation Therapy, MD Anderson Cancer Ctr 92; **Fac Appt:** Prof RadRO, Temple Univ

Pollack, Jed MD **[RadRO]** - **Spec Exp:** Head & Neck Cancer; Prostate Cancer; Brain Tumors; **Hospital:** Long Island Jewish Med Ctr; **Address:** 270-05 76th Ave, Dept Rad Onc, New Hyde Park, NY 11040; **Phone:** 718-470-7192; **Board Cert:** Therapeutic Radiology 85; **Med School:** Univ New Mexico 81; **Resid:** Therapeutic Radiology, Mem Sloan-Kettering Cancer Ctr; **Fac Appt:** Asst Clin Prof RadRO, Albert Einstein Coll Med

Regine, William F MD **[RadRO]** - **Spec Exp:** Stereotactic Radiosurgery; Brain & Spinal Tumors; Gastrointestinal Cancer; **Hospital:** Univ of MD Med Sys; **Address:** Greenbaum Cancer Ctr, Gudelsky Bldg, Ground Fl, 22 S Green St, Baltimore, MD 21201; **Phone:** 410-328-6080; **Board Cert:** Radiation Oncology 92; **Med School:** SUNY Upstate Med Univ 87; **Resid:** Radiation Oncology, Thomas Jefferson Univ Hosp 91; **Fellow:** Radiation Oncology, Thomas Jefferson Univ Hosp 92; **Fac Appt:** Prof RadRO, Univ MD Sch Med

Rotman, Marvin MD **[RadRO]** - **Spec Exp:** Bladder & Prostate Cancer; Gynecologic Cancer; Breast Cancer; **Hospital:** SUNY Downstate Med Ctr; **Address:** 450 Clarkson Ave, Box 1211, Brooklyn, NY 11203-2056; **Phone:** 718-270-2181; **Board Cert:** Radiology 66; Radiation Oncology 99; **Med School:** Jefferson Med Coll 58; **Resid:** Internal Medicine, Albert Einstein Med Ctr 60; Radiation Oncology, Montefiore Hosp Med Ctr 65; **Fac Appt:** Prof RadRO, SUNY Downstate

Schiff, Peter B MD/PhD **[RadRO]** - **Spec Exp:** Prostate Cancer; Gynecologic Cancer; Breast Cancer; **Hospital:** NY-Presby Hosp - Columbia Presby Med Ctr (page 103); **Address:** Columbia Presby Med Ctr, Dept Rad Oncology, 622 W 168th St, New York, NY 10032-3720; **Phone:** 212-305-2991; **Board Cert:** Radiation Oncology 90; **Med School:** Albert Einstein Coll Med 84; **Resid:** Radiation Oncology, Meml Sloan Kettering Cancer Ctr 88; **Fac Appt:** Prof RadRO, Columbia P&S

Solin, Lawrence J MD **[RadRO]** - **Spec Exp:** Breast Cancer; **Hospital:** Hosp Univ Penn - UPHS (page 113); **Address:** Univ Penn Med Ctr, Dept Rad Onc, 3400 Spruce St, 2 Donner Bldg, Philadelphia, PA 19104; **Phone:** 215-662-7267; **Board Cert:** Radiation Oncology 99; **Med School:** Brown Univ 78; **Resid:** Surgery, Jefferson Univ Hosp 81; Radiation Oncology, Jefferson Univ Hosp/Hosp Univ Penn 84; **Fac Appt:** Prof RadRO, Univ Pennsylvania

Stock, Richard MD **[RadRO]** - **Spec Exp:** Prostate Cancer; **Hospital:** Mount Sinai Med Ctr (page 101); **Address:** 1184 5th Ave, Ste P134, New York, NY 10029; **Phone:** 212-241-7502; **Board Cert:** Radiation Oncology 93; **Med School:** Mount Sinai Sch Med 88; **Resid:** Radiation Oncology, Meml Sloan Kettering Cancer Ctr 92; **Fac Appt:** Prof Rad, Mount Sinai Sch Med

Wharam Jr, Moody D MD **[RadRO]** - **Spec Exp:** Pediatric Cancers; Brain Tumors; Rhabdomyosarcoma; **Hospital:** Johns Hopkins Hosp - Baltimore (page 97); **Address:** Sidney Kimmel Cancer Ctr at Johns Hopkins Hosp, Dept Rad Onc, 401 N Broadway St, Ste 1440, Baltimore, MD 21231; **Phone:** 410-955-7312; **Board Cert:** Therapeutic Radiology 74; **Med School:** Univ VA Sch Med 69; **Resid:** Radiation Oncology, UCSF Medical Ctr 73; **Fac Appt:** Prof RadRO, Johns Hopkins Univ

Yahalom, Joachim MD [RadRO] - **Spec Exp:** Lymphoma; Hodgkin's Disease; Multiple Myeloma; **Hospital:** Meml Sloan Kettering Cancer Ctr (page 100); **Address:** Meml Sloan Kettering Cancer Ctr, Dept Rad Oncology, 1275 York Ave, New York, NY 10021-6007; **Phone:** 212-639-5999; **Board Cert:** Radiation Oncology 88; **Med School:** Israel 76; **Resid:** Internal Medicine, Hadassah Hosp 79; Radiation Oncology, Hadassah Hosp 84; **Fellow:** Radiation Oncology, Meml Sloan Kettering Canc Ctr 86; **Fac Appt:** Prof RadRO, Cornell Univ-Weill Med Coll

Zelefsky, Michael J. MD [RadRO] - **Spec Exp:** Prostate Cancer; Brachytherapy; Genitourinary Cancer; **Hospital:** Meml Sloan Kettering Cancer Ctr (page 100); **Address:** Meml Sloan-Kettering Cancer Ctr, 1275 York Ave, New York, NY 10021-6094; **Phone:** 212-639-6802; **Board Cert:** Radiation Oncology 91; **Med School:** Albert Einstein Coll Med 86; **Resid:** Radiation Oncology, Meml Sloan Kettering Cancer Ctr 90; **Fac Appt:** Prof RadRO, Cornell Univ-Weill Med Coll

Southeast

Anscher, Mitchell MD [RadRO] - **Spec Exp:** Prostate Cancer; Brachytherapy; **Hospital:** Duke Univ Med Ctr (page 94); **Address:** Duke University Med Ctr, Dept Radiation Oncology, Box 3085, Durham, NC 27710; **Phone:** 919-668-5637; **Board Cert:** Radiation Oncology 87; Internal Medicine 84; **Med School:** Med Coll VA 81; **Resid:** Internal Medicine, St Marys Hosp 84; Radiation Oncology, Duke Univ Med Ctr 87; **Fac Appt:** Prof RadRO, Duke Univ

Brizel, David M MD [RadRO] - **Spec Exp:** Head & Neck Cancer; **Hospital:** Duke Univ Med Ctr (page 94); **Address:** Duke Univ Med Ctr, Dept Rad Onc, Box 3085, Durham, NC 27710-0001; **Phone:** 919-668-5637; **Board Cert:** Radiation Oncology 87; **Med School:** Northwestern Univ 83; **Resid:** Radiation Oncology, Harvard Joint Center 87; **Fac Appt:** Prof RadRO, Duke Univ

Chakravarthy, Anuradha MD [RadRO] - **Spec Exp:** Breast Cancer; Gastrointestinal Cancer; **Hospital:** Vanderbilt Univ Med Ctr (page 116); **Address:** Vanderbilt Univ Med Ctr-Dept of Radiation Onc, 1301 22nd Ave S, Nashville, TN 37232; **Phone:** 615-322-2555; **Board Cert:** Radiation Oncology 94; Internal Medicine 86; Medical Oncology 89; **Med School:** Geo Wash Univ 83; **Resid:** Internal Medicine, Mayo Clinic 86; Medical Oncology, Univ MD Cancer Ctr 89; **Fellow:** Radiation Oncology, Johns Hopkins Hosp; **Fac Appt:** Asst Prof RadRO, Vanderbilt Univ

Crocker, Ian MD [RadRO] - **Spec Exp:** Brain Tumors; **Hospital:** Emory Univ Hosp; **Address:** Emory Univ Hosp - Dept Radiation Oncology, 1365 Clifton Rd NE, T Ste 104, Atlanta, GA 30322; **Phone:** 404-778-3473; **Board Cert:** Therapeutic Radiology 99; Internal Medicine 80; **Med School:** Canada 76; **Resid:** Internal Medicine, Univ Hosp-Univ West Ontario 80; **Fellow:** Radiation Oncology, Princess Margaret Hosp-Univ Toronto 83; **Fac Appt:** Prof RadRO, Emory Univ

Ferree, Carolyn Ruth Black MD [RadRO] - **Spec Exp:** Breast Cancer; Lymphoma; Pediatric Cancers; **Hospital:** Wake Forest Univ Baptist Med Ctr (page 117); **Address:** Wake Forest Univ Baptist Med Ctr, Medical Center Blvd, Winston Salem, NC 27157-0001; **Phone:** 336-713-3600; **Board Cert:** Therapeutic Radiology 74; **Med School:** Wake Forest Univ 70; **Resid:** Therapeutic Radiology, NC Baptist Hosp 74; **Fac Appt:** Prof RadRO, Wake Forest Univ

Halle, Jan MD [RadRO] - **Spec Exp:** Breast Cancer; Lung Cancer; **Hospital:** Univ NC Hosps (page 112); **Address:** Univ North Carolina Sch Med, Dept Rad Onc, CB 7512, Chapel Hill, NC 27599; **Phone:** 919-966-7700; **Board Cert:** Therapeutic Radiology 82; **Med School:** Tufts Univ 75; **Resid:** Radiation Oncology, North Carolina Meml-UNC 81

Kelly, Maria MD **[RadRO]** - **Spec Exp:** Breast Cancer; Brachytherapy-HDR; Intensity Modulated Radiotherapy (IMRT); **Hospital:** Univ Virginia Med Ctr; **Address:** Moser Radiation Therapy Ctr, 2871 Ivy Rd, Charlottesville, VA 22903; **Phone:** 434-982-0777; **Board Cert:** Radiation Oncology 92; **Med School:** Ireland 83; **Resid:** Radiation Oncology, Univ Virginia Medical Ctr 89; **Fellow:** Radiation Oncology, Univ Virginia Medical Ctr 90; **Fac Appt:** Assoc Prof RadRO, Univ VA Sch Med

Kun, Larry E MD **[RadRO]** - **Spec Exp:** Brain Tumors; **Hospital:** St Jude Children's Research Hosp; **Address:** St Jude Chldns Research Hosp-Dept Rad Onc, 332 N Lauderdale St, rm C2002F, MS 220, Memphis, TN 38105; **Phone:** 901-495-3565; **Board Cert:** Therapeutic Radiology 73; **Med School:** Jefferson Med Coll 68; **Resid:** Therapeutic Radiology, Penrose Cancer Hosp 72; **Fac Appt:** Prof Rad, Univ Tenn Coll Med, Memphis

Lee, W Robert MD **[RadRO]** - **Spec Exp:** Prostate Cancer; Prostate Brachytherapy; **Hospital:** Wake Forest Univ Baptist Med Ctr (page 117); **Address:** Wake Forest Univ Baptist Med Ctr - Dept Rad Onc, Medical Center Blvd, 1st Fl Outpatient Cancer Ctr, Winston-Salem, NC 27157; **Phone:** 336-713-3600; **Board Cert:** Radiation Oncology 94; **Med School:** Univ VA Sch Med 89; **Resid:** Radiation Oncology, Univ Florida 93; **Fac Appt:** Prof RadRO, Wake Forest Univ

Lewin, Alan A MD **[RadRO]** - **Spec Exp:** Breast Cancer; Lung Cancer; Brain & Spinal Cord Tumors; **Hospital:** Baptist Hosp of Miami; **Address:** Baptist Hospital Cancer Treatment Ctr, Dept Rad Onc, 8900 N Kendall Drive, Miami, FL 33176-2118; **Phone:** 786-596-6566; **Board Cert:** Therapeutic Radiology 82; Medical Oncology 81; Hematology 78; Internal Medicine 76; **Med School:** Geo Wash Univ 73; **Resid:** Internal Medicine, Mt Sinai Hosp 76; **Fellow:** Hematology and Oncology, Beth Israel Med Ctr 78; Radiation Oncology, Joint Ctr Radiation Therapy 80

Marcus Jr, Robert B MD **[RadRO]** - **Spec Exp:** Pediatric Radiation Oncology; Sarcoma; Bone Cancer; **Hospital:** Emory Univ Hosp; **Address:** Emory Clinic, 1365 Clifton Rd NE, Atlanta, GA 30322; **Phone:** 404-778-5323; **Board Cert:** Therapeutic Radiology 80; **Med School:** Univ Fla Coll Med 75; **Resid:** Radiation Oncology, Shands Hosp 79; **Fac Appt:** Prof RadRO, Emory Univ

Marks, Lawrence MD **[RadRO]** - **Spec Exp:** Breast Cancer; Lung Cancer; **Hospital:** Duke Univ Med Ctr (page 94); **Address:** Duke University Medical Center, Box 3085, Durham, NC 27710; **Phone:** 919-668-5640; **Board Cert:** Radiation Oncology 89; **Med School:** Univ Rochester 85; **Resid:** Radiation Oncology, Mass Genl Hosp 89; **Fac Appt:** Prof RadRO, Duke Univ

Mendenhall, Nancy P MD **[RadRO]** - **Spec Exp:** Breast Cancer; Lymphoma; Hodgkin's Disease; **Hospital:** Shands Hlthcre at Univ of FL (page 109); **Address:** University of Florida, Dept Radiation Oncology, 2000 SW Archer Rd, Box 100385, Gainesville, FL 32610-0385; **Phone:** 352-265-0287; **Board Cert:** Therapeutic Radiology 85; **Med School:** Univ Fla Coll Med 80; **Resid:** Radiology, Shands-Univ of Florida 84; **Fac Appt:** Prof RadRO, Univ Fla Coll Med

Mendenhall, William M MD **[RadRO]** - **Spec Exp:** Head & Neck Cancer; Stereotactic Radiosurgery; Colon Cancer; **Hospital:** Shands Hlthcre at Univ of FL (page 109); **Address:** University of Florida, Dept Radiation Oncology, 2000 SW Archer Rd, Box 100385, Gainesville, FL 32610-0385; **Phone:** 352-265-0287; **Board Cert:** Therapeutic Radiology 83; **Med School:** Univ S Fla Coll Med 78; **Resid:** Radiation Oncology, University of Florida 83; **Fac Appt:** Prof RadRO, Univ Fla Coll Med

Merchant, Thomas DO **[RadRO]** - **Spec Exp:** Brain Tumors-Pediatric; **Hospital:** St Jude Children's Research Hosp; **Address:** St Jude Children's Research Hosp, 332 N Lauderdale, Memphis, TN 38105; **Phone:** 901-495-3604; **Board Cert:** Radiation Oncology 95; **Med School:** Chicago Coll Osteo Med 89; **Resid:** Radiation Oncology, Meml Sloan Kettering Cancer Ctr 94

Meredith, Ruby F MD **[RadRO]** - **Spec Exp:** Multiple Myeloma; **Hospital:** Univ of Ala Hosp at Birmingham; **Address:** U Ala Hosps-Rad Onc, 619 19th St S, Birmingham, AL 35233; **Phone:** 205-934-4763; **Board Cert:** Radiation Oncology 87; **Med School:** Ohio State Univ 83; **Resid:** Radiation Oncology, Med Coll Va 87; **Fac Appt:** Prof RadRO, Univ Ala

Prosnitz, Leonard MD **[RadRO]** - **Spec Exp:** Lymphoma; Breast Cancer; Hyperthermia Treatment of Cancer; **Hospital:** Duke Univ Med Ctr (page 94); **Address:** Duke Univ Med Ctr, Dept Rad Onc, Box 3085, Durham, NC 27710; **Phone:** 919-668-5640; **Board Cert:** Therapeutic Radiology 70; **Med School:** SUNY Downstate 61; **Resid:** Internal Medicine, Dartmouth Affil Hosps 63; Radiation Oncology, Yale-New Haven Hosp 69; **Fellow:** Hematology and Oncology, Yale-New Haven Hosp 67; **Fac Appt:** Prof RadRO, Duke Univ

Randall, Marcus MD **[RadRO]** - **Spec Exp:** Gynecologic Cancer; **Hospital:** Pitt Cty Mem Hosp - Univ Med Ctr East Carolina; **Address:** Leo W. Jenkins Cancer Center, 600 Moye Blvd, Greenville, NC 27835; **Phone:** 252-847-5215; **Board Cert:** Therapeutic Radiology 86; **Med School:** Univ NC Sch Med 82; **Resid:** Radiation Oncology, Univ Va Med Ctr 86; **Fellow:** Radiation Oncology, Univ Va Med Ctr 86; **Fac Appt:** Prof RadRO, E Carolina Univ

Rich, Tyvin Andrew MD **[RadRO]** - **Spec Exp:** Colon & Rectal Cancer; Chemo-Radiation Combined Therapy; Esophageal Cancer; **Hospital:** Univ Virginia Med Ctr; **Address:** Univ Va Hlth Sys, Dept Rad Onc, Box 800383, Charlottesville, VA 22908; **Phone:** 434-924-5191; **Board Cert:** Radiation Oncology 78; **Med School:** Univ VA Sch Med 73; **Resid:** Radiation Therapy, Mass Genl Hosp 78; **Fellow:** Radiation Oncology, Mt Vernon Hosp/Gray Lab; **Fac Appt:** Prof RadRO, Univ VA Sch Med

Rosenman, Julian MD **[RadRO]** - **Spec Exp:** Lung Cancer; Breast Cancer; Prostate Cancer; **Hospital:** Univ NC Hosps (page 112); **Address:** University N Carolina, Dept Radiology, Box 7512, Chapel Hill, NC 27514-9722; **Phone:** 919-966-7700; **Board Cert:** Therapeutic Radiology 81; **Med School:** Univ Tex SW, Dallas 77; **Resid:** Therapeutic Radiology, Mass Genl Hosp 81; **Fac Appt:** Prof RadRO, Univ NC Sch Med

Sailer, Scott MD **[RadRO]** - **Spec Exp:** Head & Neck Cancer; Genitourinary Cancer; Pediatric Cancer; **Hospital:** WakeMed Cary; **Address:** 300 Ashville Ave, Ste 110, Cary, NC 27511; **Phone:** 919-854-4588; **Board Cert:** Radiation Oncology 88; **Med School:** Harvard Med Sch 84; **Resid:** Radiation Therapy, Mass Genl Hosp 88

Shaw, Edward Gus MD **[RadRO]** - **Spec Exp:** Stereotactic Radiosurgery; Brain Tumors; **Hospital:** Wake Forest Univ Baptist Med Ctr (page 117); **Address:** Wake Forest Baptist Med Ctr, Comp Cancer Ctr - Dept Rad Oncology, Medical Center Blvd, Winston Salem, NC 27157-1029; **Phone:** 336-713-3600; **Board Cert:** Radiation Oncology 87; **Med School:** Rush Med Coll 83; **Resid:** Radiation Oncology, Mayo Grad Sch Med 87; **Fac Appt:** Prof RadRO, Wake Forest Univ

Spencer, Sharon MD **[RadRO]** - **Spec Exp:** Head & Neck Cancer; **Hospital:** Univ of Ala Hosp at Birmingham; **Address:** UAB, Dept Rad Onc, 1824 6th Ave S, Birmingham, AL 35233; **Phone:** 205-934-2762; **Board Cert:** Radiation Oncology 88; **Med School:** Univ Ala 83; **Resid:** Radiation Oncology, Univ of Ala Hosp at Birmingham 87; **Fac Appt:** Assoc Prof RadRO, Univ Ala

Tepper, Joel MD **[RadRO]** - **Spec Exp:** Gastrointestinal Cancer; Sarcoma; Colon Cancer; **Hospital:** Univ NC Hosps (page 112); **Address:** North Carolina Clin Cancer Ctr, Dept Rad Onc - CB#7512, Chapel Hill, NC 27599-7512; **Phone:** 919-966-0400; **Board Cert:** Therapeutic Radiology 76; **Med School:** Washington Univ, St Louis 72; **Resid:** Therapeutic Radiology, Mass Genl Hosp 76; **Fellow:** Therapeutic Radiology, Mass Genl Hosp 77; **Fac Appt:** Prof RadRO, Univ NC Sch Med

Toonkel, Leonard M MD [RadRO] - **Spec Exp:** Prostate Cancer; Breast Cancer; Brachytherapy; **Hospital:** Mount Sinai Med Ctr - Miami; **Address:** Dept Rad Onc, 4300 Alton Rd, Miami Beach, FL 33140; **Phone:** 305-535-3400; **Board Cert:** Therapeutic Radiology 79; **Med School:** Univ Miami Sch Med 75; **Resid:** Radium Therapy, Jackson Meml Hosp 77; Radiology, MD Anderson Hosp 78; **Fellow:** Radiation Oncology, MD Anderson Hosp 79; **Fac Appt:** Assoc Clin Prof Rad, Univ Miami Sch Med

Trotti III, Andrea MD [RadRO] - **Spec Exp:** Head & Neck Cancer; Gastrointestinal Cancer; Skin Cancer; **Hospital:** H Lee Moffitt Cancer Ctr & Research Inst; **Address:** HL Moffitt Cancer Ctr, Rad Onc, 12902 Magnolia, Tampa, FL 33612-9416; **Phone:** 813-972-8424; **Board Cert:** Radiation Oncology 88; **Med School:** Univ Fla Coll Med 84; **Resid:** Radiation Oncology, Univ Alabama 88; **Fac Appt:** Prof RadRO, Univ S Fla Coll Med

Willett, Chris MD [RadRO] - **Spec Exp:** Gastrointestinal Cancer; **Hospital:** Duke Univ Med Ctr (page 94); **Address:** Duke Univ Med Ctr, PO Box 3085, Durham, NC 27710; **Phone:** 919-668-5640; **Board Cert:** Therapeutic Radiology 85; **Med School:** Tufts Univ 81; **Resid:** Radiation Oncology, Mass Genl Hosp 86; **Fac Appt:** Prof Rad, Duke Univ

Midwest

Abrams, Ross A MD [RadRO] - **Spec Exp:** Gastrointestinal Cancer; **Hospital:** Rush Univ Med Ctr; **Address:** Rush Univ Med Ctr, Dept Radiation Oncology, 1653 W Congress Pkwy, Chicago, IL 60612; **Phone:** 312-942-5751; **Board Cert:** Internal Medicine 76; Medical Oncology 79; Hematology 82; Radiation Oncology 87; **Med School:** Univ Pennsylvania 73; **Resid:** Internal Medicine, Pennsylvania Hosp 75; Hematology and Oncology, Univ Penn Hosp 76; **Fellow:** Hematology and Oncology, Natl Cancer Inst 78; Radiation Oncology, Med Coll Wisconsin 87; **Fac Appt:** Prof RadRO, Rush Med Coll

Charboneau, J William MD [RadRO] - **Spec Exp:** Radiofrequency Tumor Ablation; Liver Cancer; Thyroid Cancer; **Hospital:** Mayo Med Ctr & Clin - Rochester; **Address:** 200 First St SW, Rochester, MN 55905-0002; **Phone:** 507-284-2097; **Board Cert:** Diagnostic Radiology 80; **Med School:** Univ Wisc 76; **Resid:** Radiology, Mayo Clinic 80; **Fac Appt:** Prof Rad, Mayo Med Sch

Emami, Bahman MD [RadRO] - **Spec Exp:** Head & Neck Cancer; Lung Cancer; **Hospital:** Loyola Univ Med Ctr (page 98); **Address:** Loyola Univ Med Ctr, Dept Rad Onc, 2160 S First Ave Bldg 105 - rm 2932, Maywood, IL 60153-5590; **Phone:** 708-216-2555; **Board Cert:** Therapeutic Radiology 76; **Med School:** Iran 68; **Resid:** Radium Therapy, Tufts Univ-New Eng Med Ctr 76; **Fellow:** Radium Therapy, Tufts Univ-New England Med Ctr 77; **Fac Appt:** Prof RadRO, Loyola Univ-Stritch Sch Med

Forman, Jeffrey D MD [RadRO] - **Spec Exp:** Prostate Cancer; Genitourinary Cancer; **Hospital:** Harper Univ Hosp; **Address:** Harper Hosp, Dept Radiation Oncology, 3990 John R St, Detroit, MI 48021-2097; **Phone:** 313-745-2593; **Board Cert:** Radiation Oncology 86; **Med School:** NYU Sch Med 82; **Resid:** Radiation Oncology, Johns Hopkins Hosp 86; **Fellow:** Therapeutic Radiology, Johns Hopkins Hosp 87; **Fac Appt:** Prof RadRO, Wayne State Univ

Grigsby, Perry W MD [RadRO] - **Spec Exp:** Gynecologic Cancer; Thyroid Cancer; **Hospital:** Barnes-Jewish Hosp (page 85); **Address:** Washington University Achool of Medicine, 660 S Euclid Ave, Box 8224, St Louis, MO 63110; **Phone:** 314-747-7236; **Board Cert:** Radiation Oncology 87; **Med School:** Univ KY Coll Med 82; **Resid:** Radiation Oncology, Barnes Jewish Hosp 85; **Fac Appt:** Prof Rad, Washington Univ, St Louis

Halpern, Howard MD/PhD [RadRO] - **Spec Exp:** Breast Cancer; Esophageal Cancer; Gynecologic Cancer; **Hospital:** Univ of Chicago Hosps; **Address:** 1801 W Taylor St, rm C400, MC-933, Chicago, IL 60612; **Phone:** 312-996-3630; **Board Cert:** Therapeutic Radiology 84; **Med School:** Univ Miami Sch Med 80; **Resid:** Therapeutic Radiology, Jnt Ctr Rad Ther Harvard 84; **Fellow:** Therapeutic Radiology, Jnt Ctr Rad Ther Harvard 85; **Fac Appt:** Prof Rad, Univ Chicago-Pritzker Sch Med

Haraf, Daniel MD [RadRO] - **Spec Exp:** Head & Neck Cancer; Lung Cancer; Prostate Cancer; **Hospital:** Univ of Chicago Hosps; **Address:** U Chicago Hospitals, Dept Radiation Oncology, 5758 S Maryland, MS 9006, Chicago, IL 60637; **Phone:** 773-702-2630; **Board Cert:** Internal Medicine 85; Radiation Oncology 90; **Med School:** Univ Hlth Sci/Chicago Med Sch 82; **Resid:** Internal Medicine, Michael Reese Hosp 85; **Fellow:** Radiation Oncology, Michael Reese Hosp/Univ Chicago 88; **Fac Appt:** Clin Prof RadRO, Univ Chicago-Pritzker Sch Med

Hellman, Samuel MD [RadRO] - **Spec Exp:** Breast Cancer; Prostate Cancer; **Hospital:** Univ of Chicago Hosps; **Address:** Univ Chicago, 5758 S Maryland Ave, MC-9006, Chicago, IL 60637-1470; **Phone:** 773-702-4346; **Board Cert:** Therapeutic Radiology 64; **Med School:** SUNY Upstate Med Univ 59; **Resid:** Radiology, Grace New Haven Comm Hosp 62; **Fellow:** Radiology, Yale-New Haven Hosp 64; **Fac Appt:** Prof Rad, Univ Chicago-Pritzker Sch Med

Kiel, Krystyna D MD [RadRO] - **Spec Exp:** Breast Cancer-Breast Brachytherapy; Sarcoma; Gastrointestinal Cancer; **Hospital:** Northwestern Meml Hosp; **Address:** Northwestern Meml Hosp, Radiation Oncology, 251 E Huron St, Ste L178, Chicago, IL 60611-2914; **Phone:** 312-926-2520; **Board Cert:** Therapeutic Radiology 00; **Med School:** Univ Mass Sch Med 77; **Resid:** Radiation Oncology, Mass Genl Hosp 82; **Fac Appt:** Assoc Prof Rad, Northwestern Univ

Kim, Jae Ho MD [RadRO] - **Spec Exp:** Brain Tumors; Spinal Cord Tumors; Breast Cancer; **Hospital:** Henry Ford Hosp; **Address:** Dept. Rad/Onc, 2799 W Grand Blvd, Detroit, MI 48202; **Phone:** 313-916-1029; **Board Cert:** Therapeutic Radiology 73; **Med School:** Korea 59; **Resid:** Therapeutic Radiology, Meml-Sloan-Kettering 72; **Fellow:** Radiology, Meml-Sloan-Kettering 68; **Fac Appt:** Prof RadRO, Wayne State Univ

Kinsella, Timothy James MD [RadRO] - **Spec Exp:** Brain Tumors; Sarcoma; Gastrointestinal Cancer; **Hospital:** Univ Hosps of Cleveland; **Address:** Univ Hosp Cleveland- Dept Radiation Oncology, 11100 Euclid Ave Fl BSMT - rm B181, MC LT6068, Cleveland, OH 44106-6068; **Phone:** 216-844-2530; **Board Cert:** Internal Medicine 77; Medical Oncology 79; Therapeutic Radiology 80; **Med School:** Univ Rochester 74; **Resid:** Internal Medicine, Mayo Clinic 76; Radiation Oncology, Joint Ctr for Rad Therapy 80; **Fellow:** Medical Oncology, Dana Farber Cancer Ctr 77; **Fac Appt:** Prof RadRO, Case West Res Univ

Lawrence, Theodore S MD/PhD [RadRO] - **Spec Exp:** Gastrointestinal Cancer; Liver Cancer; Pancreatic Cancer; **Hospital:** Univ Michigan Hlth Sys; **Address:** Univ Hosp, Dept Radiation Oncology, 1500 E Med Ctr Dr, B2C502, Box 0010, Ann Arbor, MI 48109-0010; **Phone:** 734-936-4300; **Board Cert:** Internal Medicine 83; Medical Oncology 85; Radiation Oncology 87; **Med School:** Cornell Univ-Weill Med Coll 80; **Resid:** Internal Medicine, Stanford Univ Hosp 83; Radiation Oncology, Natl Cancer Inst 87; **Fellow:** Medical Oncology, Natl Cancer Inst 86; **Fac Appt:** Prof Rad, Univ Mich Med Sch

Lee, Chung K MD [RadRO] - **Spec Exp:** Head & Neck Cancer; Breast Cancer; Lymphoma; **Hospital:** Fairview-Univ Med Ctr - Univ Campus; **Address:** Dept of Therapeutic Radiology-Radiation Oncology, 420 Delaware St SE, MC 494, Minneapolis, MN 55455; **Phone:** 612-273-6700; **Board Cert:** Therapeutic Radiology 76; **Med School:** Korea 65; **Resid:** Therapeutic Radiology, Univ of Minn Hosp 76; Therapeutic Radiology, Yonsei Univ Hosp 71; **Fac Appt:** Prof Rad TR, Univ Minn

443

Lin, Hsiu-San MD/PhD [RadRO] - **Spec Exp:** Melanoma-Choroidal (eye); Lymphoma; Sarcoma-Soft Tissue; **Hospital:** Barnes-Jewish Hosp (page 85); **Address:** Center for Advanced Medicine Bldg, Lower Level, Dept Radiation Oncology, 4921 Parkview Pl, St Louis, MO 63110; **Phone:** 314-747-7236; **Board Cert:** Therapeutic Radiology 82; **Med School:** Taiwan 60; **Resid:** Internal Medicine, Cook County Hosp 64; Radiation Oncology, Mallinckrodt Inst Radiology/Washington Univ Med Ct 81; **Fellow:** Virology, Univ of Chicago; Medical Biophysics, Univ of Toronto; **Fac Appt:** Prof RadRO, Washington Univ, St Louis

Macklis, Roger M MD [RadRO] - **Spec Exp:** Pediatric Abdominal Tumors; Brain Tumors; Lymphoma; **Hospital:** Cleveland Clin Fdn (page 92); **Address:** Cleveland Cin Fdn, Dept Rad Onc T18, 9500 Euclid Ave, Cleveland, OH 44195; **Phone:** 216-444-5576; **Board Cert:** Radiation Oncology 89; **Med School:** Harvard Med Sch 83; **Resid:** Radiation Oncology, Joint Ctr Radiotherapy Inst 87; **Fellow:** Research, Dana Farber Cancer Inst 87; **Fac Appt:** Prof RadRO, Case West Res Univ

Martenson Jr, James A MD [RadRO] - **Spec Exp:** Mucositis; Esophageal Cancer; **Hospital:** Mayo Med Ctr & Clin - Rochester; **Address:** Mayo Clinic, Dept Rad/Onc, 200 First St SW, Rochester, MN 55905; **Phone:** 507-284-4561; **Board Cert:** Therapeutic Radiology 85; **Med School:** Univ Wash 81; **Resid:** Radiation Oncology, Mayo Clinic 85; **Fac Appt:** Assoc Prof Rad, Mayo Med Sch

Mehta, Minesh P MD [RadRO] - **Spec Exp:** Brain Tumors; Lung Cancer; Pediatric Radiation Oncology; **Hospital:** Univ WI Hosp & Clins; **Address:** Univ Wisconsin, Dept Rad Onc, 600 Highland Ave, K4B-100, Madison, WI 53792; **Phone:** 608-263-8500; **Board Cert:** Radiation Oncology 88; **Med School:** Zambia 81; **Resid:** Ndola Central Hosp/Univ Wisc 83; Ndola Central Hosp/Univ Wisc 88; **Fac Appt:** Prof RadRO, Univ Wisc

Michalski, Jeff M MD [RadRO] - **Spec Exp:** Prostate Cancer; Sarcoma; Pediatric Cancers; **Hospital:** Barnes-Jewish Hosp (page 85); **Address:** Washington University School of Medicine, Dept Radiation Oncology, 660 S Euclid Ave, Box 8224, St Louis, MO 63110; **Phone:** 314-362-8566; **Board Cert:** Radiation Oncology 91; **Med School:** Med Coll Wisc 86; **Resid:** Radiation Oncology, Columbia Presbyterian Med Ctr 88; Radiation Oncology, Mallinckrodt Inst of Radiology 90; **Fellow:** Radiation Oncology, Mallinckrodt Inst of Radiology 91; **Fac Appt:** Assoc Prof RadRO, Washington Univ, St Louis

Mittal, Bharat MD [RadRO] - **Spec Exp:** Head & Neck Cancer; Lymphoma; Skin Cancer; **Hospital:** Northwestern Meml Hosp; **Address:** 251 E Huron St, Bldg LC-178, Chicago, IL 60611; **Phone:** 312-926-2520; **Board Cert:** Radiation Oncology 81; **Med School:** India 75; **Resid:** Internal Medicine, Christian Med Coll 76; Radiation Oncology, Northwestern Meml Hosp 80; **Fellow:** Radiation Oncology, Mallinckrodt Inst 81; **Fac Appt:** Prof Rad, Northwestern Univ

Movsas, Benjamin MD [RadRO] - **Spec Exp:** Lung Cancer; Brain Cancer; Prostate Cancer; **Hospital:** Henry Ford Hosp; **Address:** Henry Ford Health System, Dept Radiation Oncology, 2799 W Grand Blvd, Detroit, MI 48202; **Phone:** 313-916-5188; **Board Cert:** Radiation Oncology 99; **Med School:** Washington Univ, St Louis 90; **Resid:** Radiation Oncology, National Cancer Inst 95

Mundt, Arno J MD [RadRO] - **Spec Exp:** Gynecologic Cancer; Intensity Modulated Radiotherapy (IMRT); **Hospital:** Univ of Chicago Hosps; **Address:** University of Chicago Hospitals, 5841 S Maryland Ave, MC 9006, Chicago, IL 60637; **Phone:** 773-702-6870; **Board Cert:** Radiation Oncology 94; **Med School:** Univ Mich Med Sch 87; **Resid:** Physical Medicine & Rehabilitation, George Washington Univ Hosp 90; Radiation Oncology, Univ Chicago Hosps 93; **Fellow:** Univ Chicago Hosps 94; **Fac Appt:** Assoc Prof RadRO, Univ Chicago-Pritzker Sch Med

Myerson, Robert J MD **[RadRO]** - **Spec Exp:** Gastrointestinal Cancer; Breast Cancer; Hyperthermia Treatment of Cancer; **Hospital:** Barnes-Jewish Hosp (page 85); **Address:** Ctr for Advanced Med-Siteman Cancer Ctr, 4921 Parkview Pl, LL, St. Louis, MO 63110; **Phone:** 314-747-7236; **Board Cert:** Therapeutic Radiology 85; **Med School:** Univ Miami Sch Med 80; **Resid:** Radiation Therapy, Hosp Univ Penn 84; **Fac Appt:** Prof RadRO, Washington Univ, St Louis

Pierce, Lori J MD **[RadRO]** - **Spec Exp:** Breast Cancer; **Hospital:** Univ Michigan Hlth Sys; **Address:** Univ Hosp, Dept Rad Onc, 1500 E Med Ctr Dr, rm B2C440, Box 0010, Ann Arbor, MI 48109-0999; **Phone:** 734-936-4319; **Board Cert:** Radiation Oncology 89; **Med School:** Duke Univ 85; **Resid:** Radiation Oncology, Hosp Univ Penn 89; **Fac Appt:** Assoc Prof RadRO, Univ Mich Med Sch

Sandler, Howard M MD **[RadRO]** - **Spec Exp:** Prostate Cancer; Genitourinary Cancer; Brain Tumors; **Hospital:** Univ Michigan Hlth Sys; **Address:** Univ Michigan Med Ctr, Dept Rad Onc, 1500 E Medical Ctr Dr. UH B2C502, Box 0010, Ann Arbor, MI 48109-0010; **Phone:** 734-936-9338; **Board Cert:** Radiation Oncology 89; **Med School:** Univ Conn 85; **Resid:** Radiation Oncology, Hosp Univ Penn 89; **Fac Appt:** Prof RadRO, Univ Mich Med Sch

Schomberg, Paula J MD **[RadRO]** - **Spec Exp:** Brain Tumors; Pediatric Cancers; **Hospital:** Mayo Med Ctr & Clin - Rochester; **Address:** Mayo Clinic - Charlton Bldg, Desk R, 200 1st St SW, Rochester, MN 55905; **Phone:** 507-284-3551; **Board Cert:** Therapeutic Radiology 84; **Med School:** Med Coll Wisc 79; **Resid:** Radium Therapy, Mayo Clinic 83; **Fac Appt:** Prof RadRO, Mayo Med Sch

Small, William MD **[RadRO]** - **Spec Exp:** Gynecologic Cancer; **Hospital:** Northwestern Meml Hosp; **Address:** 251 E Huron St, Galter Pav LC-178, Chicago, IL 60611; **Phone:** 312-926-2520; **Board Cert:** Radiation Oncology 95; **Med School:** Northwestern Univ 90; **Resid:** Radiation Oncology, Northwestern Univ 94; **Fac Appt:** Asst Prof Rad, Northwestern Univ

Suh, John H MD **[RadRO]** - **Spec Exp:** Brain Tumors-Adult & Pediatric; Clinical Trials; Gamma Knife Surgery; **Hospital:** Cleveland Clin Fdn (page 92); **Address:** Cleveland Clinic, Dept Rad/Onc, Desk T28, 9500 Euclid Ave, Cleveland, OH 44195; **Phone:** 216-444-5574; **Board Cert:** Radiation Oncology 00; **Med School:** Univ Miami Sch Med 90; **Resid:** Radiation Oncology, Cleveland Clinic 94; **Fellow:** Radiation Oncology, Cleveland Clinic 95

Taylor, Marie E MD **[RadRO]** - **Spec Exp:** Breast Cancer; **Hospital:** Barnes-Jewish Hosp (page 85); **Address:** Center for Advanced Med-Siteman Cancer Ctr, 4921 Parkview Pl Fl LL, St Louis, MO 63110; **Phone:** 314-747-7236; **Board Cert:** Radiation Oncology 87; **Med School:** Univ Wash 82; **Resid:** Radiation Oncology, Univ Wash Med Ctr 86

Thornton Jr, Allan F MD **[RadRO]** - **Spec Exp:** Proton Beam Therapy; **Address:** Midwest Proton Radiotherapy Institute, 2425 N Milo Sampson Ln, Bloomington, IN 47408; **Phone:** 812-856-6774; **Board Cert:** Radiation Oncology 99; **Med School:** Univ VA Sch Med 81; **Resid:** Radiation Oncology, Princess Margaret Hosp 86

Turrisi III, Andrew Thomas MD **[RadRO]** - **Spec Exp:** Lung Cancer; Genitourinary Cancer-Male; Gastrointestinal Cancer; **Hospital:** Harper Univ Hosp; **Address:** Gershenson Radiation-Oncology Ctr, 3990 John R St, Detroit, MI 48201; **Phone:** 313-966-2274; **Board Cert:** Internal Medicine 77; Medical Oncology 81; Therapeutic Radiology 00; **Med School:** Georgetown Univ 74; **Resid:** Internal Medicine, Georgetown Univ Hosp 77; Radiation Oncology, Univ Penn Hosp 82; **Fellow:** Medical Oncology, Natl Cancer Inst-NIH 80; **Fac Appt:** Prof RadRO, Wayne State Univ

Vicini, Frank A MD [RadRO] - **Spec Exp:** Breast Cancer; Prostate Cancer; Brachytherapy; **Hospital:** William Beaumont Hosp; **Address:** William Beaumont Hospital, 3601 W 13 Mile Rd, Royal Oak, MI 48073; **Phone:** 248-551-1219; **Board Cert:** Radiation Oncology 99; **Med School:** Wayne State Univ 85; **Resid:** Radiation Oncology, William Beaumont Hosp 89; **Fellow:** Radiation Oncology, Harvard Med Sch/Joint Ctr for Rad Ther 90; **Fac Appt:** Assoc Clin Prof RadRO, Univ Mich Med Sch

Weichselbaum, Ralph R MD [RadRO] - **Spec Exp:** Gene Targeted Radiotherapy; Head & Neck Cancer; Esophageal Cancer; **Hospital:** Univ of Chicago Hosps; **Address:** Univ Chicago, Dept Rad Onc, 5758 S Maryland Ave, MC-9006-DCAM, Chicago, IL 60637; **Phone:** 773-702-0817; **Board Cert:** Therapeutic Radiology 75; **Med School:** Univ IL Coll Med 71; **Resid:** Therapeutic Radiology, Harvard Jt Ctr Rad Therapy 75; **Fellow:** Radiology, Harvard Med Sch 76; **Fac Appt:** Prof Rad, Univ Chicago-Pritzker Sch Med

Wilson, J Frank MD [RadRO] - **Spec Exp:** Breast Cancer; Skin Cancer; **Hospital:** Froedtert Meml Lutheran Hosp; **Address:** Dept Radiation Oncology, 9200 W Wisconsin Ave, Milwaukee, WI 53226; **Phone:** 414-805-4400; **Board Cert:** Therapeutic Radiology 71; **Med School:** Univ MO-Columbia Sch Med 65; **Resid:** Radiation Oncology, Penrose Cancer Hosp 69; **Fellow:** Radiation Oncology, NCI/NIH 71; **Fac Appt:** Prof RadRO, Med Coll Wisc

Great Plains and Mountains

Gaffney, David K MD/PhD [RadRO] - **Spec Exp:** Breast Cancer; Gynecologic Cancer; **Hospital:** Univ Utah Hosps and Clins; **Address:** Huntsman Cancer Inst, Dept Rad Onc, 1950 Circle of Hope, Ste 1440, Salt Lake City, UT 84112; **Phone:** 801-581-2396; **Board Cert:** Radiation Oncology 97; **Med School:** Med Coll Wisc 92; **Resid:** Radiation Oncology, Univ Utah Hosps 96; **Fac Appt:** Assoc Prof Rad, Univ Utah

Rabinovitch, Rachel A MD [RadRO] - **Spec Exp:** Breast Cancer; Lymphoma; **Hospital:** Univ Colorado Hosp; **Address:** Anschutz Cancer Pavilion, Dept Rad, 1665 N Ursula St, Box F-706, Aurora, CO 80010-0510; **Phone:** 720-848-0116; **Board Cert:** Radiation Oncology 94; **Med School:** Albert Einstein Coll Med 89; **Resid:** Radiation Oncology, Meml Sloan Kettering Cancer Ctr 93; **Fac Appt:** Assoc Prof RadRO, Univ Colorado

Shrieve, Dennis C MD [RadRO] - **Spec Exp:** Brain Tumor-Adult & Pediatric; Genitourinary Cancer; Gastrointestinal Cancer; **Hospital:** Univ Utah Hosps and Clins; **Address:** Huntsman Cancer Institute, 2000 Circle of Hope, Salt Lake City, UT 84112; **Phone:** 801-585-0100; **Board Cert:** Radiation Oncology 93; **Med School:** Univ Miami Sch Med ; **Resid:** Radiation Oncology, UCSF Med Ctr; **Fac Appt:** Prof RadRO, Univ Utah

Smalley, Stephen R MD [RadRO] - **Spec Exp:** Colon Cancer; Gastrointestinal Cancer; **Hospital:** Olathe Med Ctr; **Address:** Olathe Med Ctr, 20375 W 151st St, Doctors Bldg, Ste 180, Olathe, KS 66061-4575; **Phone:** 913-768-7200; **Board Cert:** Internal Medicine 82; Radiation Oncology 87; Medical Oncology 85; **Med School:** Univ MO-Kansas City 79; **Resid:** Internal Medicine, Mayo Clinic 82; Radiation Oncology, Mayo Clinic 86; **Fellow:** Medical Oncology, Mayo Clinic 84; **Fac Appt:** Prof RadRO, Univ Kans

Southwest

Ang, Kie-Kian MD/PhD [RadRO] - **Spec Exp:** Head & Neck Cancer; **Hospital:** UT MD Anderson Cancer Ctr, The (page 115); **Address:** UT MD Anderson Cancer Ctr, 1515 Holcombe Blvd, Box 97, Houston, TX 77030; **Phone:** 713-563-2300; **Board Cert:** Radiation Oncology 87; **Med School:** Belgium 75; **Resid:** Radiation Oncology, Univ Hosp Louvian 80; **Fac Appt:** Prof Rad, Univ Tex, Houston

Buchholz, Thomas A MD [RadRO] - **Spec Exp:** Breast Cancer; **Hospital:** UT MD Anderson Cancer Ctr, The (page 115); **Address:** Univ Texas MD Anderson Cancer Ctr, 1515 Holcombe Blvd, Box 97, Houston, TX 77030; **Phone:** 713-794-4892; **Board Cert:** Radiation Oncology 93; **Med School:** Tufts Univ 88; **Resid:** Radiation Oncology, Univ Washington Med Ctr 93; **Fellow:** Research, Univ Washington Med Ctr 94; **Fac Appt:** Assoc Prof Rad, Univ Tex, Houston

Choy, Hak MD [RadRO] - **Spec Exp:** Lung Cancer; **Hospital:** UTSW Med Ctr - Dallas; **Address:** UT SW Med Ctr - Dallas, Dept Rad-Onc, 5801 Forest Park Rd, Dallas, TX 75390; **Phone:** 214-645-7600; **Board Cert:** Radiation Oncology 93; **Med School:** Univ Tex Med Br, Galveston 87; **Resid:** Radiation Oncology, Ohio State Univ Hosp 89; Radiation Oncology, Univ of Texas Health Science Ctr 91; **Fac Appt:** Prof RadRO, Univ Tex SW, Dallas

Cox, James D MD [RadRO] - **Spec Exp:** Lymphoma; Lung Cancer; Gynecologic Cancer; **Hospital:** UT MD Anderson Cancer Ctr, The (page 115); **Address:** Univ Tex MD Anderson Cancer Ctr, 1515 Holcombe Blvd, Unit 97, Houston, TX 77030; **Phone:** 713-563-2316; **Board Cert:** Radiation Oncology 99; **Med School:** Univ Rochester 65; **Resid:** Radiology, Penrose Cancer Hosp 69; **Fellow:** Therapeutic Radiology, Inst Gustave-Roussy 70; **Fac Appt:** Prof RadRO, Univ Tex, Houston

Eifel, Patricia J MD [RadRO] - **Spec Exp:** Gynecologic Cancer; Cervical, Vulvar, Vaginal Cancers; Uterine Cancer; **Hospital:** UT MD Anderson Cancer Ctr, The (page 115); **Address:** MD Anderson Cancer Ctr, Dept Rad Onc, 1515 Holcombe Blvd, Box 97, Houston, TX 77030-4009; **Phone:** 713-563-2343; **Board Cert:** Therapeutic Radiology 83; **Med School:** Stanford Univ 77; **Resid:** Radiation Oncology, Stanford Univ Med Ctr 81; **Fellow:** Therapeutic Radiology, Stanford Univ Med Ctr 82; **Fac Appt:** Prof RadRO, Univ Tex, Houston

Grado, Gordon L MD [RadRO] - **Spec Exp:** Prostate Cancer; Brachytherapy; **Hospital:** Scottsdale Hlthcare - Osborn; **Address:** 2926 N Civic Center Plaza, Scottsdale, AZ 85251; **Phone:** 480-614-6300; **Board Cert:** Therapeutic Radiology 81; Radiation Oncology 99; **Med School:** Southern IL Univ 77; **Resid:** Therapeutic Radiology, Mayo Clinic 81

Gunderson, Leonard MD [RadRO] - **Spec Exp:** Gastrointestinal Cancer; Brachytherapy; Sarcoma; **Hospital:** Mayo Clin Hosp - Scottsdale; **Address:** Mayo Clinic Scottsdale, Dept Radiation Oncology, 13400 E Shea Blvd, Scottsdale, AZ 85259-5404; **Phone:** 480-301-7351; **Board Cert:** Therapeutic Radiology 75; **Med School:** Univ KY Coll Med 69; **Resid:** Radiation Oncology, Latter Day Saints Hosp 74; **Fac Appt:** Prof RadRO, Mayo Med Sch

Herman, Terence Spencer MD [RadRO] - **Spec Exp:** Breast Cancer; Sarcoma; Brain Tumors; **Hospital:** UTSA - Univ Hosp; **Address:** 7703 Floyd Curl Drive, MC 7889, San Antonio, TX 78229-3901; **Phone:** 210-616-5648; **Board Cert:** Internal Medicine 75; Medical Oncology 77; Therapeutic Radiology 85; **Med School:** Univ Conn 72; **Resid:** Internal Medicine, Univ Arizona 75; Radiation Oncology, Stanford Univ 85; **Fellow:** Medical Oncology, Univ Arizona 77; **Fac Appt:** Prof RadRO, Univ Tex, San Antonio

Komaki, Ritsuko MD [RadRO] - **Spec Exp:** Lung Cancer; Thymoma; Esophageal Cancer; **Hospital:** UT MD Anderson Cancer Ctr, The (page 115); **Address:** UT-MD Anderson Cancer Ctr, Dept Rad Onc, 1515 Holcombe Blvd, Unit 97, Houston, TX 77030; **Phone:** 713-563-2300; **Board Cert:** Therapeutic Radiology 01; **Med School:** Japan 69; **Resid:** Radiation Oncology, Med Coll Wisc 78; **Fac Appt:** Prof Rad TR, Univ Tex, Houston

Kuske, Robert R MD [RadRO] - **Spec Exp:** Breast Cancer; Breast Cancer-Breast Brachytherapy; **Hospital:** Scottsdale Hlthcare - Shea; **Address:** 8994 E Desert Cove Ave, Ste 100, Scottsdale, AZ 85260; **Phone:** 602-274-4484; **Board Cert:** Therapeutic Radiology 85; **Med School:** Univ Cincinnati 80; **Resid:** Radiation Oncology, Univ Cincinnati Med Ctr 84

McNeese, Marsha MD [RadRO] - **Spec Exp:** Breast Cancer; **Hospital:** UT MD Anderson Cancer Ctr, The (page 115); **Address:** MD Anderson Cancer Ctr, Rad Oncology, 1515 Holcombe Blvd. Unit 97, Houston, TX 77030-4009; **Phone:** 713-563-2300; **Board Cert:** Therapeutic Radiology 78; **Med School:** Louisiana State Univ 74; **Resid:** Radiation Oncology, Univ Texas/MD Anderson Cancer Ctr 77; **Fac Appt:** Prof RadRO, Univ Tex, Houston

Medbery, Clinton A MD [RadRO] - **Spec Exp:** Breast Cancer; Gynecologic Cancer; **Hospital:** St Anthony Hosp; **Address:** Frank C Love Cancer Institute, 1000 N Lee St, Oklahoma City, OK 73102; **Phone:** 405-272-7311; **Board Cert:** Internal Medicine 80; Medical Oncology 83; Radiation Oncology 87; **Med School:** Med Univ SC 76; **Resid:** Internal Medicine, Naval Hosp 80; Radiation Oncology, Natl Cancer Inst 87; **Fellow:** Medical Oncology, Naval Hosp 82

Pistenmaa, David A MD/PhD [RadRO] - **Spec Exp:** Stereotactic Radiosurgery; Prostate Cancer; Breast Cancer; **Hospital:** St Paul Univ Hosp; **Address:** UTSW Med Ctr, Dept Rad Onc, 5801 Forest Park Rd, Dallas, TX 75390; **Phone:** 214-645-8525; **Board Cert:** Therapeutic Radiology 74; **Med School:** Stanford Univ 69; **Resid:** Radiation Oncology, Stanford Univ Med Ctr 73; **Fac Appt:** Prof RadRO, Univ Tex SW, Dallas

Senzer, Neil N MD [RadRO] - **Spec Exp:** Developmental Therapeutics; Gene Targeted Radiotherapy; **Hospital:** Baylor Univ Medical Ctr (page 86); **Address:** Baylor Univ Med Ctr, Dept Radiation Oncology, 3535 Worth St, Dallas, TX 75246-2044; **Phone:** 214-370-1400; **Board Cert:** Pediatrics 76; Pediatric Hematology-Oncology 78; Therapeutic Radiology 85; **Med School:** SUNY Buffalo 71; **Resid:** Pediatrics, Johns Hopkins Hosp 74; Radiation Oncology, St Barnabas Med Ctr 85; **Fellow:** Pediatric Hematology-Oncology, St Jude Chldns Rsch Hosp 78

Shina, Donald C MD [RadRO] - **Spec Exp:** Breast Cancer; **Hospital:** St Vincent Hosp - Santa Fe; **Address:** Santa Fe Cancer Ctr at St Vincent Hosp, 455 Saint Michael's Drive, Santa Fe, NM 87505; **Phone:** 505-820-5233; **Board Cert:** Internal Medicine 77; Medical Oncology 79; Therapeutic Radiology 81; **Med School:** Case West Res Univ 74; **Resid:** Internal Medicine, Univ Hosps 77; **Fellow:** Radiation Oncology, Univ Hosps 80; Medical Oncology, Univ Hosps 80

Strom, Eric Alan MD [RadRO] - **Spec Exp:** Breast Cancer; Intensity Modulated Radiotherapy (IMRT); **Hospital:** UT MD Anderson Cancer Ctr, The (page 115); **Address:** MD Anderson Cancer Ctr, Clin Rad Onc, 1515 Holcombe Blvd, Box 0097, Houston, TX 77030; **Phone:** 713-563-2300; **Board Cert:** Internal Medicine 85; Radiation Oncology 90; **Med School:** Northwestern Univ 82; **Resid:** Internal Medicine, Univ Kentucky 85; Radiation Oncology, UT-MD Anderson Cancer Ctr 90; **Fac Appt:** Assoc Prof RadRO, Univ Tex, Houston

West Coast and Pacific

Blasko, John C MD [RadRO] - **Spec Exp:** Prostate Cancer; **Hospital:** Swedish Med Ctr - Seattle; **Address:** 1101 Madison, Ste 1101, Seattle, WA 98104; **Phone:** 206-215-2480; **Board Cert:** Therapeutic Radiology 76; **Med School:** Univ MD Sch Med 69; **Resid:** Diagnostic Radiology, Maine Med Ctr 74; Radium Therapy, Univ Wash 76; **Fac Appt:** Prof Rad, Univ Wash

Donaldson, Sarah S MD [RadRO] - **Spec Exp:** Pediatric Cancers; Hodgkin's Disease; **Hospital:** Stanford Univ Med Ctr; **Address:** 875 Blake Wilbur Drive, CC Bldg Fl G - rm 226, MC 5847, Stanford, CA 94305-5847; **Phone:** 650-723-6195; **Board Cert:** Therapeutic Radiology 74; **Med School:** Harvard Med Sch 68; **Resid:** Radiation Oncology, Stanford Univ Med Ctr 72; **Fellow:** Pediatric Hematology-Oncology, Inst Gustave-Roussy 73; Pediatric Hematology-Oncology, MD Anderson Cancer Ctr; **Fac Appt:** Prof RadRO, Stanford Univ

Douglas, James G MD [RadRO] - **Spec Exp:** Pediatric Cancers; Head & Neck Cancer; **Hospital:** Univ Wash Med Ctr; **Address:** Univ Washington Medical Ctr, Dept Radiation Onc, 1959 NE Pacific St, Box 356043, Seattle, WA 98195-6043; **Phone:** 206-598-4100; **Board Cert:** Pediatrics 86; Radiation Oncology 97; **Med School:** Case West Res Univ 80; **Resid:** Pediatrics, Children's Hosp Med Ctr 83; Radiation Oncology, Univ Washington Med Ctr 96; **Fellow:** Pediatric Hematology-Oncology, Natl Inst Hlth 86; **Fac Appt:** Assoc Prof Ped, Univ Wash

Goffinet, Don R MD [RadRO] - **Spec Exp:** Breast Cancer; Head & Neck Cancer; **Hospital:** Stanford Univ Med Ctr; **Address:** 875 Blake Wilbur Drive, MC 5847, Stanford, CA 94305; **Phone:** 650-723-5714; **Board Cert:** Therapeutic Radiology 73; **Med School:** Stanford Univ 64; **Resid:** Surgery, Stanford Univ 66; Radiation Therapy, Stanford Univ 72; **Fac Appt:** Prof Rad TR, Stanford Univ

Halberg, Francine MD [RadRO] - **Spec Exp:** Breast Cancer; **Hospital:** Marin Genl Hosp; **Address:** Marin Cancer Inst-Dept of Rad.Oncology, 1350 S Eliseo Drive, Greenbrae, CA 94904-2011; **Phone:** 415-925-7326; **Board Cert:** Internal Medicine 81; Therapeutic Radiology 84; **Med School:** Cornell Univ-Weill Med Coll 78; **Resid:** Internal Medicine, USPHS Hosp 81; **Fellow:** Radiation Oncology, Stanford Univ Med Ctr 84; **Fac Appt:** Assoc Prof RadRO, UCSF

Hancock, Steven MD [RadRO] - **Spec Exp:** Prostate Cancer; Breast Cancer; Cancer Survivors-Late Effects of Therapy; **Hospital:** Stanford Univ Med Ctr; **Address:** Stanford Cancer Center-Dept Rad Onc, 875 Blake Wilber Drive, MC 5847, Stanford, CA 94305; **Phone:** 650-723-6440; **Board Cert:** Therapeutic Radiology 82; Internal Medicine 80; **Med School:** Stanford Univ 76; **Resid:** Radium Therapy, Stanford Univ Med Ctr 81; Internal Medicine, Stanford Univ Med Ctr 79; **Fac Appt:** Prof RadRO, Stanford Univ

Hoppe, Richard T MD [RadRO] - **Spec Exp:** Lymphoma; Hodgkin's Disease; **Hospital:** Stanford Univ Med Ctr; **Address:** Stanford Med Ctr, Dept Rad Onc, 875 Blake Wilbur, rm G224, MC 5847, Stanford, CA 94305-5847; **Phone:** 650-723-5510; **Board Cert:** Therapeutic Radiology 76; **Med School:** Cornell Univ-Weill Med Coll 71; **Resid:** Radium Therapy, Stanford Univ 76; **Fac Appt:** Prof Rad, Stanford Univ

Juillard, Guy J F MD [RadRO] - **Spec Exp:** Head & Neck Cancer; Breast Cancer; Gynecologic Cancer; **Hospital:** UCLA Med Ctr (page 111); **Address:** 200 UCLA Med Plz, Ste B-265, Los Angeles, CA 90095; **Phone:** 310-825-7145; **Board Cert:** Radiation Oncology 91; **Med School:** France 63; **Resid:** Radium Therapy, Inst Gustave Roussy 63; **Fac Appt:** Prof RadRO, UCLA

Larson, David Andrew MD/PhD [RadRO] - **Spec Exp:** Neuro-Oncology; Brain Cancer; **Hospital:** UCSF Med Ctr; **Address:** UCSF Med Ctr, Dept Rad Onc, 505 Parnassus Ave, rm L-75, San Francisco, CA 94143-0226; **Phone:** 415-353-8900; **Board Cert:** Radiology 86; Neuroradiology 96; **Med School:** Univ Miami Sch Med 81; **Resid:** Radium Therapy, Joint Ctr RadTherapy 85; **Fac Appt:** Prof RadRO, UCSF

Leibel, Steven A MD [RadRO] - **Spec Exp:** Prostate Cancer; **Hospital:** Stanford Univ Med Ctr; **Address:** Stanford University Medical Center, 875 Blake Wilber Dr, MC5827, Stanford, CA 94305-5827; **Phone:** 650-736-9069; **Board Cert:** Therapeutic Radiology 76; Radiation Oncology 99; **Med School:** UCSF 72; **Resid:** Radiation Oncology, UCSF Med Ctr 76; **Fac Appt:** Prof RadRO, Stanford Univ

Pezner, Richard D MD [RadRO] - **Spec Exp:** Brain Tumors; Gastrointestinal Cancer; Stereotactic Radiosurgery; **Hospital:** City of Hope Natl Med Ctr & Beckman Rsch (page 89); **Address:** 1500 E Duarte Rd, City Hope Comprehensive Cancer Ctr, Duarte, CA 91010-3012; **Phone:** 626-359-8111; **Board Cert:** Radiology 79; **Med School:** Northwestern Univ 75; **Resid:** Radiation Oncology, Oregon Health Sci Ctr 79; **Fac Appt:** Assoc Clin Prof Rad, UC Irvine

Phillips, Theodore Locke MD [RadRO] - **Spec Exp:** Brain Tumors; Head & Neck Cancer; **Hospital:** UCSF Med Ctr; **Address:** UCSF Med Ctr, Rad Oncology, 505 Parnassus Ave, rm L-08, San Francisco, CA 94143-0226; **Phone:** 415-353-8900; **Board Cert:** Therapeutic Radiology 65; **Med School:** Univ Pennsylvania 59; **Resid:** Radiation Oncology, UCSF Med Ctr 63; **Fac Appt:** Prof RadRO, UCSF

Quivey, Jeanne Marie MD [RadRO] - **Spec Exp:** Breast Cancer; Eye Tumors/Uveal Melanoma; Head & Neck Cancer/IMRT; **Hospital:** UCSF Med Ctr; **Address:** 1600 Divisadero St, Ste H1031, San Francisco, CA 94115; **Phone:** 415-353-7175; **Board Cert:** Therapeutic Radiology 74; **Med School:** UCSF 70; **Resid:** Radiation Therapy, UCSF Med Ctr 74; **Fac Appt:** Prof RadRO, UCSF

Roach III, Mack MD [RadRO] - **Spec Exp:** Prostate Cancer; Genitourinary Cancer; Lung Cancer; **Hospital:** UCSF - Mt Zion Med Ctr; **Address:** UCSF Mt Zion Cancer Center, 1600 Divisadero St, Ste H1031, San Francisco, CA 94115; **Phone:** 415-353-7175; **Board Cert:** Medical Oncology 85; Radiation Oncology 87; Internal Medicine 84; **Med School:** Stanford Univ 79; **Resid:** Internal Medicine, ML King Genl Hosp 81; Radiation Oncology, Stanford Univ Med Ctr 87; **Fellow:** Medical Oncology, UCSF Med Ctr 83; **Fac Appt:** Prof RadRO, UCSF

Rose, Christopher Marshall MD [RadRO] - **Spec Exp:** Prostate Cancer; Breast Cancer; Intensity Modulated Radiotherapy (IMRT); **Hospital:** Providence St Joseph Med Ctr; **Address:** St Joseph Med Ctr, Dept Radiation Therapy, 501 S Buena Vista St, Burbank, CA 91505-4866; **Phone:** 818-847-3440; **Board Cert:** Radiation Oncology 99; **Med School:** Harvard Med Sch 74; **Resid:** Internal Medicine, Beth Israel Deaconess 76; Radiation Oncology, Joint Ctr Rad Therapy 79; **Fellow:** Research, British Inst Cancer Rsch 79; **Fac Appt:** Assoc Clin Prof RadRO, UCLA

Rossi, Carl John MD [RadRO] - **Spec Exp:** Prostate Cancer; Proton Beam Therapy; **Hospital:** Loma Linda Univ Med Ctr; **Address:** Loma Linda Univ Med Ctr, 11234 Anderson St, Ste B121, Loma Linda, CA 92354; **Phone:** 909-558-4280; **Board Cert:** Radiation Oncology 94; **Med School:** Loyola Univ-Stritch Sch Med 88; **Resid:** Radiation Oncology, Loma Linda Univ Med Ctr 92; **Fac Appt:** Asst Prof RadRO, Loma Linda Univ

Russell, Kenneth J MD [RadRO] - **Spec Exp:** Prostate Cancer; Lymphoma; Genitourinary Cancer; **Hospital:** Univ Wash Med Ctr; **Address:** Seattle Cancer Care Alliance, G1101, 825 Eastlake Ave E, Seattle, WA 98109; **Phone:** 206-288-7100; **Board Cert:** Therapeutic Radiology 84; **Med School:** Harvard Med Sch 79; **Resid:** Radiation Therapy, Stanford Univ Med Ctr 83; **Fellow:** Radiological Biology, Stanford Univ Med Ctr 85; **Fac Appt:** Prof Rad, Univ Wash

Seagren, Stephen L MD [RadRO] - **Spec Exp:** Lung Cancer; Head & Neck Cancer; Prostate Cancer; **Hospital:** UCSD Med Ctr; **Address:** UCSD Med Ctr, Dept Rad Onc, 200 W Arbor Dr, San Diego, CA 92103-8757; **Phone:** 619-543-5303; **Board Cert:** Internal Medicine 72; Therapeutic Radiology 77; Medical Oncology 77; **Med School:** Northwestern Univ 67; **Resid:** Radiation Oncology, USCD 77; Internal Medicine, Univ Minn, Hennepin Co Genl Hosp 71; **Fellow:** Medical Oncology, LA Co-USC Med Ctr 75; Harob Genl Hosp 76; **Fac Appt:** Prof Rad, UCSD

Shank, Brenda MD/PhD [RadRO] - **Spec Exp:** Breast Cancer; Lung Cancer; Anal & Rectal Cancer; **Hospital:** Doctors Med Ctr; **Address:** 2000 Vale Rd, San Pablo, CA 94806; **Phone:** 510-970-5239; **Board Cert:** Therapeutic Radiology 80; **Med School:** UMDNJ-RW Johnson Med Sch 76; **Resid:** Radiation Therapy, Mem Sloan Kettering Cancer Ctr 79; **Fellow:** Radiation Oncology, Mem Sloan Kettering Cancer Ctr 80; **Fac Appt:** Clin Prof RadRO, UCSF

Streeter Jr, Oscar E MD [RadRO] - **Spec Exp:** Lung Cancer; Head & Neck Cancer; **Hospital:** USC Norris Canc Comp Ctr; **Address:** 1441 Eastlake Ave, Ste G338, Los Angeles, CA 90033; **Phone:** 323-865-3051; **Board Cert:** Radiation Oncology 89; **Med School:** Howard Univ 82; **Resid:** Radiation Oncology, Howard Univ 86; **Fac Appt:** Assoc Prof RadRO, USC Sch Med

Tripuraneni, Prabhakar MD [RadRO] - **Spec Exp:** Prostate Brachytherapy; Head & Neck Cancer; Lymphoma; **Hospital:** Scripps Meml Hosp - La Jolla; **Address:** Scripps Clinic, Div Radiation Oncology, 10666 N Torrey Pines Rd, MSB 1, La Jolla, CA 92037; **Phone:** 858-554-2000; **Board Cert:** Therapeutic Radiology 83; **Med School:** India 76; **Resid:** Radiation Oncology, Univ Alberta 81; Radiation Oncology, UCSF Med Ctr 83; **Fac Appt:** Clin Prof Rad, UCSD

Vijayakumar, Srinivasan MD [RadRO] - **Spec Exp:** Brachytherapy; Prostate Cancer; Conformal Radiotherapy; **Hospital:** UC Davis Med Ctr; **Address:** UC Davis Med Ctr, Cancer Ctr, 4671 X St, Sacramento, CA 95817; **Phone:** 916-734-8252; **Board Cert:** Therapeutic Radiology 86; **Med School:** India 78; **Resid:** Radiation Oncology, Madras Univ Med Ctr 81; Radiation Oncology, Michael Reese Hosp 84; **Fellow:** Brachytherapy, Univ Chicago Hosps 85; **Fac Appt:** Prof Rad, UC Davis

Wong, Jeffrey Y C MD [RadRO] - **Spec Exp:** Radioimmunotherapy; Prostate Cancer; **Hospital:** City of Hope Natl Med Ctr & Beckman Rsch (page 89); **Address:** City of Hope National edical Ctr, Dept Radiation Oncology, 1500 E Duarte Rd, Duarte, CA 91768; **Phone:** 626-359-8111 x62969; **Board Cert:** Therapeutic Radiology 85; **Med School:** Johns Hopkins Univ 81; **Resid:** Radiation Oncology, UCSF Med Ctr 85; **Fac Appt:** Clin Prof Rad, UC Irvine

DIAGNOSTIC RADIOLOGY

New England

Kopans, Daniel B MD [DR] - **Spec Exp:** Breast Imaging; **Hospital:** Mass Genl Hosp; **Address:** Mass Genl Hosp - Avon Comprehensive Breast Ctr, 15 Parkman St, WAC 240, Boston, MA 02114-3117; **Phone:** 617-726-3093; **Board Cert:** Diagnostic Radiology 77; **Med School:** Harvard Med Sch 73; **Resid:** Diagnostic Radiology, Mass Genl Hosp 77; **Fac Appt:** Prof Rad, Harvard Med Sch

McCarthy, Shirley M MD/PhD [DR] - **Spec Exp:** Infertility; Gynecologic Cancer; Pelvic MRI; **Hospital:** Yale - New Haven Hosp; **Address:** Yale-New Haven Hosp, Tompkins East-2, 789 Howard Ave, New Haven, CT 06519; **Phone:** 203-785-5251; **Board Cert:** Diagnostic Radiology 83; **Med School:** Yale Univ 79; **Resid:** Radiology, Yale-New Haven Hosp 83; **Fellow:** Cross Sectional Imaging, UCSF Med Ctr 84; **Fac Appt:** Prof DR, Yale Univ

Schepps, Barbara MD [DR] - **Spec Exp:** Breast Imaging; **Hospital:** Rhode Island Hosp; **Address:** RI Hosp, Dept Radiology, 593 Eddy St, Providence, RI 02903; **Phone:** 401-444-6266; **Board Cert:** Radiology 73; **Med School:** Hahnemann Univ 68; **Resid:** Radiology, Boston City Hosp 72; **Fac Appt:** Clin Prof Rad, Brown Univ

Weinreb, Jeffrey C MD [DR] - **Spec Exp:** MRI; Breast Cancer MRI; Abdominal Imaging; **Hospital:** Yale - New Haven Hosp; **Address:** Yale University School of Medicine, Dept Radiology, 333 Cedar St, rm MRC147, New Haven, CT 06520; **Phone:** 203-785-5913; **Board Cert:** Diagnostic Radiology 83; **Med School:** Mount Sinai Sch Med 78; **Resid:** Diagnostic Radiology, LI Jewish Med Ctr 82; **Fellow:** Ultrasound/CT, Hosp U Penn 83; **Fac Appt:** Prof Rad, Yale Univ

Mid Atlantic

Austin, John H M MD [DR] - **Spec Exp:** Lung Cancer; **Hospital:** NY-Presby Hosp - Columbia Presby Med Ctr (page 103); **Address:** Columbia Presby Hosp, Dept Radiology, 622 W 168th St, MHB 3-202C, New York, NY 10032-3784; **Phone:** 212-305-2986; **Board Cert:** Diagnostic Radiology 70; **Med School:** Yale Univ 65; **Resid:** Radiology, UCSF Med Ctr 68; **Fellow:** Radiology, UCSF Med Ctr 70; **Fac Appt:** Prof Rad, Columbia P&S

Berg, Wendie A MD/PhD [DR] - **Spec Exp:** Breast Imaging; Breast Cancer; **Hospital:** Johns Hopkins Hosp - Baltimore (page 97); **Address:** Johns Hopkins - Greenspring Station Breast Ctr, 10755 Falls Rd, Pav 1, Ste 440, Lutherville, MD 21093; **Phone:** 410-583-2888; **Board Cert:** Diagnostic Radiology 92; **Med School:** Johns Hopkins Univ 87; **Resid:** Diagnostic Radiology, Johns Hopkins Hosp 92; **Fellow:** Abdominal Imaging, Johns Hopkins Univ 92

Conant, Emily F MD [DR] - **Spec Exp:** Breast Cancer; **Hospital:** Hosp Univ Penn - UPHS (page 113); **Address:** Hosp Univ Penn - Dept Radiology, 3400 Spruce St, 1 Silverstein, Philadelphia, PA 19104; **Phone:** 215-662-4032; **Board Cert:** Diagnostic Radiology 89; **Med School:** Univ Pennsylvania 83; **Resid:** Radiology, Hosp Univ Penn 86; **Fellow:** Breast Imaging, Hosp Univ Penn 89; **Fac Appt:** Assoc Prof Rad, Univ Pennsylvania

Dershaw, D David MD [DR] - **Spec Exp:** Breast Imaging; Breast Cancer; **Hospital:** Meml Sloan Kettering Cancer Ctr (page 100); **Address:** 1275 York Ave, New York, NY 10021-6007; **Phone:** 212-639-7295; **Board Cert:** Diagnostic Radiology 78; **Med School:** Jefferson Med Coll 74; **Resid:** Diagnostic Radiology, New York Hosp 78; **Fellow:** Ultrasound, Thomas Jefferson Univ Hosp 79; **Fac Appt:** Prof Rad, Cornell Univ-Weill Med Coll

Edelstein, Barbara A MD **[DR]** - **Spec Exp:** Breast Cancer; Women's Imaging; **Address:** 1045 Park Ave, New York, NY 10028; **Phone:** 212-860-7700; **Board Cert:** Diagnostic Radiology 83; **Med School:** NY Med Coll 77; **Resid:** Diagnostic Radiology, Montefiore Hosp 82

Evers, Kathryn MD **[DR]** - **Spec Exp:** Breast Cancer; Mammography; **Hospital:** Fox Chase Cancer Ctr (page 95); **Address:** Fox Chase Cancer Center, Dept Radiology, 333 Cottman Ave, Philadelphia, PA 19111; **Phone:** 215-728-3024; **Board Cert:** Diagnostic Radiology 80; **Med School:** NYU Sch Med 75; **Resid:** Radiology, Hosp Univ Penn 80; **Fellow:** Neurodevelopmental Disabilities, Hosp Univ Penn 81; **Fac Appt:** Assoc Prof Rad, Hahnemann Univ

Fishman, Elliot MD **[DR]** - **Spec Exp:** CT Scan-Body; Abdominal Imaging; Cancer Imaging; **Hospital:** Johns Hopkins Hosp - Baltimore (page 97); **Address:** Johns Hopkins Hosp, Dept Radiology, 601 N Caroline St, JHOC 3254, Baltimore, MD 21287; **Phone:** 410-955-5173; **Board Cert:** Diagnostic Radiology 81; **Med School:** Univ MD Sch Med 77; **Resid:** Diagnostic Radiology, Sinai Hosp 80; **Fellow:** Computerized Tomography, Johns Hopkins Hosp 81; **Fac Appt:** Prof Rad, Johns Hopkins Univ

Hann, Lucy MD **[DR]** - **Spec Exp:** Ultrasound of Liver & Bile Duct Tumors; Uterine Ultrasound in Tamoxifen Patients; Ovarian Cancer Ultrasound Diagnosis; **Hospital:** Meml Sloan Kettering Cancer Ctr (page 100); **Address:** Memorial Sloan-Kettering Cancer Ctr, 1275 York Ave, rm C278, New York, NY 10021; **Phone:** 212-639-2179; **Board Cert:** Diagnostic Radiology 77; **Med School:** Harvard Med Sch 71; **Resid:** Diagnostic Radiology, Hosp U Penn 74; Diagnostic Radiology, Mass General 77; **Fellow:** Body Imaging, Mass General 78; **Fac Appt:** Prof Rad, Cornell Univ-Weill Med Coll

Hricak, Hedvig MD/PhD **[DR]** - **Spec Exp:** Prostate Cancer-MR Spectroscopy (MRSI); Breast Imaging; **Hospital:** Meml Sloan Kettering Cancer Ctr (page 100); **Address:** Meml Sloan Kettering Cancer Ctr, Dept Radiology, 1275 York Ave, New York, NY 10021; **Phone:** 212-639-7284; **Board Cert:** Diagnostic Radiology 78; **Med School:** Yugoslavia 70; **Resid:** Radiology, Hosp M Stojanovic 73; Diagnostic Radiology, St Joseph Mercy Hosp 77; **Fellow:** Radiation Oncology, Henry Ford Hosp 78

Mitnick, Julie MD **[DR]** - **Spec Exp:** Mammography; Breast Cancer; **Address:** 650 1st Ave Fl 2, New York, NY 10016; **Phone:** 212-686-4440; **Board Cert:** Diagnostic Radiology 77; **Med School:** NYU Sch Med 73; **Resid:** Diagnostic Radiology, NYU Med Ctr 77; **Fellow:** Pediatric Radiology, NYU Med Ctr 78; **Fac Appt:** Assoc Clin Prof DR, NYU Sch Med

Orel, Susan G MD **[DR]** - **Spec Exp:** Breast Imaging; Breast Cancer; **Hospital:** Hosp Univ Penn - UPHS (page 113); **Address:** Hospital of University Pennsylvania, Dept Radiology, 3400 Spruce St, 1 Silverstein, Philadelphia, PA 19104; **Phone:** 215-662-3016; **Board Cert:** Diagnostic Radiology 89; **Med School:** Univ Pennsylvania 86; **Resid:** Diagnostic Radiology, Johns Hopkins Hosp 89; **Fac Appt:** Prof Rad, Univ Pennsylvania

Panicek, David MD **[DR]** - **Spec Exp:** Bone Cancer; Soft Tissue Tumors; **Hospital:** Meml Sloan Kettering Cancer Ctr (page 100); **Address:** Memorial Hosp - Dept Radiology, 1275 York Ave, rm C276G, New York, NY 10021; **Phone:** 212-639-5825; **Board Cert:** Diagnostic Radiology 84; **Med School:** Cornell Univ-Weill Med Coll 80; **Resid:** Radiology, New York Hosp-Cornell 84; **Fac Appt:** Prof Rad, Cornell Univ-Weill Med Coll

Rao, Vijay M MD **[DR]** - **Spec Exp:** Head & Neck Tumors Imaging; TMJ Imaging; ENT Imaging; **Hospital:** Thomas Jefferson Univ Hosp (page 110); **Address:** 111 S 11th St, Gibbon Bldg, rm 3350, Philadelphia, PA 19107; **Phone:** 215-955-4804; **Board Cert:** Diagnostic Radiology 78; Neuroradiology 97; **Med School:** India 73; **Resid:** Diagnostic Radiology, Thos Jefferson Univ Hosp 78; **Fac Appt:** Prof Rad, Thomas Jefferson Univ

453

Southeast

Abbitt, Patricia L MD [DR] - **Spec Exp:** Ultrasound; Interventional Radiology; Breast Imaging; **Hospital:** Shands Hlthcre at Univ of FL (page 109); **Address:** 1600 SW Archer Rd, PO Box 100374, Shands Healthcare, Dept Radiology, Gainesville, FL 32612; **Phone:** 352-265-0291; **Board Cert:** Diagnostic Radiology 86; **Med School:** Tufts Univ 81; **Resid:** Diagnostic Radiology, Univ VA Med Ctr 86; **Fellow:** Breast Imaging, Univ VA Med Ctr 87; **Fac Appt:** Prof Rad, Univ Fla Coll Med

Cardenosa, Gilda MD [DR] - **Spec Exp:** Breast Imaging; **Hospital:** Moses H Cone Mem Hosp; **Address:** 1002 N Church St, Ste 100, Greensboro, NC 27401; **Phone:** 336-271-4999; **Board Cert:** Diagnostic Radiology 89; **Med School:** Columbia P&S 84; **Resid:** Radiology, Mass Genl Hosp 89

Patz, Edward F MD [DR] - **Spec Exp:** Thoracic Imaging; PET Imaging; Lung Cancer; **Hospital:** Duke Univ Med Ctr (page 94); **Address:** Duke Univ Med Ctr, Dept Radiology, Box 3808, Durham, NC 27710; **Phone:** 919-684-2711; **Board Cert:** Diagnostic Radiology 90; **Med School:** Univ MD Sch Med 85; **Resid:** Radiology, Brigham & Womens Hosp 90; **Fellow:** Thoracic Radiology, Brigham & Womens Hosp 90; **Fac Appt:** Prof Rad, Duke Univ

Pisano, Etta D MD [DR] - **Spec Exp:** Breast Imaging; **Hospital:** Univ NC Hosps (page 112); **Address:** UNC Health Care, 101 Manning Dr, Box 7510, Chapel Hill, NC 27299-7510; **Phone:** 919-966-1081; **Board Cert:** Diagnostic Radiology 88; **Med School:** Duke Univ 83; **Resid:** Diagnostic Radiology, Beth Israel Hosp 88; **Fac Appt:** Prof Rad, Univ NC Sch Med

Midwest

Helvie, Mark A MD [DR] - **Spec Exp:** Breast Imaging; Breast Cancer; Mammography; **Hospital:** Univ Michigan Hlth Sys; **Address:** 2910N Taubman Univ Michigan Health Ctr, 1500 E Medical Ctr Drive, Ann Arbor, MI 48109-0326; **Phone:** 734-936-4367; **Board Cert:** Internal Medicine 83; Diagnostic Radiology 86; **Med School:** Univ NC Sch Med 80; **Resid:** Internal Medicine, Univ Michigan Hosps 83; Radiology, Univ Michigan Hosps 86; **Fellow:** Ultrasound/CT, Univ Michigan Hosps 87; **Fac Appt:** Prof Rad, Univ Mich Med Sch

Jackson, Valerie P MD [DR] - **Spec Exp:** Breast Imaging; **Hospital:** Indiana Univ Hosp (page 90); **Address:** Indiana Univ Hosp, Dept Radiology, 550 N University Blvd, #0663, Indianapolis, IN 46202; **Phone:** 317-274-1866; **Board Cert:** Diagnostic Radiology 82; **Med School:** Indiana Univ 78; **Resid:** Radiology, Indiana Univ Med Ctr 82; **Fac Appt:** Prof Rad, Indiana Univ

Mendelson, Ellen B MD [DR] - **Spec Exp:** Women's Imaging; Breast Cancer; **Hospital:** Northwestern Meml Hosp; **Address:** Lynn Sage Breast Ctr, 675 N St Clair, 13-Galter, Chicago, IL 60611; **Phone:** 312-926-6120; **Board Cert:** Diagnostic Radiology 84; **Med School:** Northwestern Univ 80; **Resid:** Diagnostic Radiology, Northwestern Meml Hosp 84; **Fellow:** Angiography, Northwestern Meml Hosp 85; **Fac Appt:** Assoc Clin Prof Rad, Northwestern Univ

Monsees, Barbara MD [DR] - **Spec Exp:** Mammography; Breast Cancer; **Hospital:** Barnes-Jewish Hosp (page 85); **Address:** Mallinckrodt Inst Radiology, 510 S Kingshighway Blvd, St Louis, MO 63110; **Phone:** 314-454-7500; **Board Cert:** Diagnostic Radiology 80; **Med School:** Washington Univ, St Louis 75; **Resid:** Pediatrics, St Louis Chldns Hosp 77; Diagnostic Radiology, Mallinckrodt Inst Radiology 80; **Fac Appt:** Prof Rad, Washington Univ, St Louis

Sagel, Stuart Steven MD **[DR]** - **Spec Exp:** Lung Cancer; Occupational Lung Disease; Pulmonary Embolism; **Hospital:** Barnes-Jewish Hosp (page 85); **Address:** Mallinckrodt Inst Rad-Barnes Hosp, 510 S Kingshighway Blvd, Box 8131, St Louis, MO 63110-1016; **Phone:** 314-362-2927; **Board Cert:** Diagnostic Radiology 70; **Med School:** Temple Univ 65; **Resid:** Diagnostic Radiology, Yale New Haven Hosp 68; Diagnostic Radiology, UCSF Med Ctr 70; **Fac Appt:** Prof Rad, Washington Univ, St Louis

Swensen, Stephen J MD **[DR]** - **Spec Exp:** Lung Cancer; **Hospital:** Mayo Med Ctr & Clin - Rochester; **Address:** Mayo Clinic - Diagnostic Radiology, 200 1st St SW, Rochester, MN 55905; **Phone:** 507-284-3207; **Board Cert:** Diagnostic Radiology 86; **Med School:** Univ Wisc 81; **Resid:** Diagnostic Radiology, Mayo Clinic 86; **Fellow:** Pulmonary Radiology, Brigham & Womens Hosp 87; **Fac Appt:** Prof Rad, Mayo Med Sch

Southwest

Huynh, Phan Tuong MD **[DR]** - **Spec Exp:** Mammography; Breast Cancer; **Hospital:** St Luke's Episcopal Hosp - Houston; **Address:** 6624 Fannin St, St Luke's Twr Fl 10-Womens Ctr, Houston, TX 77030; **Phone:** 832-355-8130; **Board Cert:** Diagnostic Radiology 94; **Med School:** Univ VA Sch Med 89; **Resid:** Radiology, Univ Va 94; **Fellow:** Mammography, Unv Va 95; **Fac Appt:** Assoc Clin Prof Rad, Baylor Coll Med

Otto, Pamela MD **[DR]** - **Spec Exp:** Mammography; **Hospital:** UTSA - Univ Hosp; **Address:** 7703 Floyd Curl Drive, MC 7800, San Antonio, TX 78229-3900; **Phone:** 210-567-6470; **Board Cert:** Diagnostic Radiology 93; **Med School:** Univ MO-Columbia Sch Med 88; **Resid:** Radiology, Univ Texas Hlth Sci Ctr 93; **Fellow:** Radiology, Univ Texas Hlth Sci Ctr; **Fac Appt:** Assoc Prof Rad, Univ Tex, San Antonio

West Coast and Pacific

Bassett, Lawrence W MD **[DR]** - **Spec Exp:** Breast Imaging; **Hospital:** UCLA Med Ctr (page 111); **Address:** 200 UCLA Med Plaza, rm 165-47, Box 956952, Los Angeles, CA 90095-6952; **Phone:** 310-206-9608; **Board Cert:** Diagnostic Radiology 75; **Med School:** UC Irvine 68; **Resid:** Radiology, UCLA Med Ctr 72; **Fac Appt:** Prof Rad, UCLA

NEURORADIOLOGY

Mid Atlantic

Koeller, Kelly K MD **[NRad]** - **Spec Exp:** Brain Tumor Imaging; **Hospital:** Armed Forces Inst of Path; **Address:** Armed Forces Inst of Pathology, 14th St-Alaska Ave, rm M121, Washington, DC 20306; **Phone:** 202-782-2166; **Board Cert:** Diagnostic Radiology 90; Neuroradiology 04; **Med School:** Univ Tenn Coll Med, Memphis 82; **Resid:** Radiology, Naval Hosp 90; **Fellow:** Neuroradiology, UCSF Med Ctr 92; **Fac Appt:** Prof NRad, Uniformed Srvs Univ, Bethesda

Vezina, L Gilbert MD **[NRad]** - **Spec Exp:** Pediatric Neuroradiology; Brain Tumors; Neurofibromatosis; **Hospital:** Chldns Natl Med Ctr; **Address:** Chldns Natl Med Ctr, Dept Radiology, 111 Michigan Ave NW, rm 2400, Washington, DC 20010-2970; **Phone:** 202-884-3651; **Board Cert:** Diagnostic Radiology 87; Neuroradiology 98; **Med School:** McGill Univ 83; **Resid:** Diagnostic Radiology, Mass Genl Hosp 87; **Fellow:** Neurological Radiology, Mass Genl Hosp 87; **Fac Appt:** Prof Rad, Geo Wash Univ

Southeast

Murtagh, F Reed MD **[NRad]** - **Spec Exp:** Brain & Spinal Imaging; Neuro-Oncology; **Hospital:** H Lee Moffitt Cancer Ctr & Research Inst; **Address:** Univ Diagnostic Institute-USF, 3301 Alumni Drive, Tampa, FL 33612; **Phone:** 813-975-0725; **Board Cert:** Diagnostic Radiology 78; Neuroradiology 95; **Med School:** Temple Univ 71; **Resid:** Diagnostic Radiology, Jackson Meml Hosp 78; **Fellow:** Neurological Radiology, Univ Miami; **Fac Appt:** Prof NRad, Univ S Fla Coll Med

Provenzale, James M MD **[NRad]** - **Spec Exp:** Brain Tumor Imaging; Multiple Sclerosis Imaging; Pediatric Brain Disorder Imaging; **Hospital:** Duke Univ Med Ctr (page 94); **Address:** Duke University Medical Ctr, Dept Radiology, Box 3808, Durham, NC 27710; **Phone:** 919-684-7218; **Board Cert:** Neurology 88; Diagnostic Radiology 91; Neuroradiology 01; **Med School:** Albany Med Coll 83; **Resid:** Neurology, NC Memorial Hosp 87; Radiology, Mass General Hosp 91; **Fellow:** Neuroradiology, Mass General Hosp 92; **Fac Appt:** Prof Rad, Duke Univ

West Coast and Pacific

Atlas, Scott W MD **[NRad]** - **Spec Exp:** Stroke; MRI; Brain Tumors; **Hospital:** Stanford Univ Med Ctr; **Address:** Stanford Univ Med Ctr, Dept Rad, 300 Pasteur Drive, rm S-047, Stanford, CA 94304-2204; **Phone:** 650-498-7152; **Board Cert:** Diagnostic Radiology 85; Neuroradiology 95; **Med School:** Univ Chicago-Pritzker Sch Med 81; **Resid:** Radiology, Northwestern Univ Med Ctr 85; **Fellow:** Neuroradiology, Hosp Univ Penn 87; **Fac Appt:** Prof Rad, Stanford Univ

Dillon, William P MD **[NRad]** - **Spec Exp:** Brain Tumors; **Hospital:** UCSF Med Ctr; **Address:** 505 Parnassus Ave, rm L 371, San Francisco, CA 94143-0628; **Phone:** 415-353-1668; **Board Cert:** Diagnostic Radiology 82; Neuroradiology 96; **Med School:** Loyola Univ-Stritch Sch Med 78; **Resid:** Diagnostic Radiology, Univ Utah Hosp 82; **Fellow:** Neuroradiology, UCSF Med Ctr 83; **Fac Appt:** Prof Rad, UCSF

VASCULAR & INTERVENTIONAL RADIOLOGY

New England

Hallisey, Michael J MD **[VIR]** - **Spec Exp:** Uterine Fibroid Embolization; Liver Tumors Cryoablation; Chemoembolization; **Hospital:** Hartford Hosp; **Address:** 85 Seymour St, Ste 911, Hartford, CT 06106; **Phone:** 860-522-4158; **Board Cert:** Diagnostic Radiology 91; Vascular & Interventional Radiology 98; **Med School:** Univ Conn 87; **Resid:** Diagnostic Radiology, Hospital of St Raphael 91

Mid Atlantic

Geschwind, Jean-Francois H MD **[VIR]** - **Spec Exp:** Liver Cancer; Cancer Chemoembolization; Cancer Radiotherapy; **Hospital:** Johns Hopkins Hosp - Baltimore (page 97); **Address:** Johns Hopkins Hosp, 600 N Wolfe St, Cardiovascular Rad-Blalock 545, Baltimore, MD 21287; **Phone:** 410-614-2237; **Board Cert:** Diagnostic Radiology 98; **Med School:** Boston Univ 91; **Resid:** Diagnostic Radiology, UCSF Med Ctr 96; **Fellow:** Interventional Radiology, Johns Hopkins Hosp 98; **Fac Appt:** Assoc Prof Rad, Johns Hopkins Univ

Haskal, Ziv MD **[VIR]** - **Spec Exp:** Uterine Fibroid Embolization; Vascular Disease; Liver Cancer Chemoembolization; **Hospital:** NY-Presby Hosp - Columbia Presby Med Ctr (page 103); **Address:** Director, Div Interventional Radiology, 177 Fort Washington Ave, Ste 4-100, New York, NY 10032; **Phone:** 212-305-8070; **Board Cert:** Diagnostic Radiology 91; Vascular & Interventional Radiology 99; **Med School:** Boston Univ 86; **Resid:** Diagnostic Radiology, UCSF Med Ctr 91; **Fellow:** Vascular & Interventional Radiology, UCSF Med Ctr 92; **Fac Appt:** Prof Rad, Columbia P&S

Soulen, Michael C MD **[VIR]** - **Spec Exp:** Cancer Radiotherapy; Cancer Chemoembolization; Radiofrequency Tumor Ablation; **Hospital:** Hosp Univ Penn - UPHS (page 113); **Address:** Hosp Univ Penn, Dept Interventional Radiology, 3400 Spruce St, Philadelphia, PA 19104; **Phone:** 215-662-4034; **Board Cert:** Diagnostic Radiology 89; Vascular & Interventional Radiology 95; **Med School:** Univ Pennsylvania 84; **Resid:** Radiology, Johns Hopkins Med Inst 89; **Fellow:** Vascular & Interventional Radiology, Thomas Jefferson Univ Hosp 91; **Fac Appt:** Assoc Prof Rad, Univ Pennsylvania

Southeast

Coldwell, Douglas M MD **[VIR]** - **Spec Exp:** Inoperable Cancer Treatment; Brachytherapy & Theraspheres; Radiofrequency Tumor Ablation; **Hospital:** Univ Hosps & Clins - Jackson; **Address:** Univ Mississippi Med Ctr, Dept Radiology, 2500 N State St, Jackson, MS 39216; **Phone:** 601-815-3983; **Board Cert:** Diagnostic Radiology 86; Vascular & Interventional Radiology 95; **Med School:** Univ Tex Med Br, Galveston 80; **Resid:** Diagnostic Radiology, Hershey Med Ctr-Penn St Univ 83; **Fellow:** Vascular & Interventional Radiology, MD Anderson Hosp-Tumor Inst 84; **Fac Appt:** Prof Rad, Univ Miss

Mauro, Matthew MD **[VIR]** - **Spec Exp:** Cancer Chemoembolization; Cancer Radiotherapy; Gastrointestinal Cancer; **Hospital:** Univ NC Hosps (page 112); **Address:** University NC Hosps, Dept Radiology, CB 7510, 2006 Old Clinic Bldg, Chapel Hill, NC 27599-7510; **Phone:** 919-966-4400; **Board Cert:** Diagnostic Radiology 81; Vascular & Interventional Radiology 03; **Med School:** Cornell Univ-Weill Med Coll 77; **Resid:** Radiology, Univ NC Hosps 81; **Fellow:** Interventional Radiology, Mallinckrodt Inst 82; **Fac Appt:** Prof Rad, Univ NC Sch Med

Midwest

Rilling, William S MD [VIR] - **Spec Exp:** Liver Cancer Chemoembolization; Arteriovenous Malformations; Uterine Fibroid Embolization; **Hospital:** Froedtert Meml Lutheran Hosp; **Address:** Froedtert & Medical College Clinics, Dept Interventional Radiology, 9200 W Wisconsin Ave, Milwaukee, WI 53226; **Phone:** 414-805-3728; **Board Cert:** Diagnostic Radiology 95; Vascular & Interventional Radiology 97; **Med School:** Univ Wisc 90; **Resid:** Diagnostic Radiology, Univ Wisc Affil Hosps 95; **Fellow:** Vascular & Interventional Radiology, Northwestern Meml Hosp 96; **Fac Appt:** Assoc Prof Rad, Univ Wisc

Salem, Riad MD [VIR] - **Spec Exp:** Cancer Radiotherapy; Cancer Chemoembolization; Liver Cancer; **Hospital:** Northwestern Meml Hosp; **Address:** Northwestern Univ Med Sch - Dept Radiology, 676 N St Clair St, Ste 800, Chicago, IL 60611; **Phone:** 312-695-0517; **Board Cert:** Diagnostic Radiology 97; Vascular & Interventional Radiology 99; **Med School:** McGill Univ 93; **Resid:** Diagnostic Radiology, Geo Washington Univ Hosp 97; **Fellow:** Childrens Hosp; Hosp Univ Penn; **Fac Appt:** Asst Prof Rad, Northwestern Univ

West Coast and Pacific

Goodwin, Scott Craig MD [VIR] - **Spec Exp:** Uterine Fibroid Embolization; Chemoembolization/Liver Tumors; **Hospital:** VA Med Ctr - W Los Angeles; **Address:** Dept of Veterans Affairs Greater LA Health Care System, 11301 Willshire Blvd Bldg 500 - rm 0608, Los Angeles, CA 90073; **Phone:** 310-268-3478; **Board Cert:** Diagnostic Radiology 89; Vascular & Interventional Radiology 96; **Med School:** Harvard Med Sch 84; **Resid:** Diagnostic Radiology, UCLA Medical Ctr 88; **Fellow:** Vascular & Interventional Radiology, UCLA Medical Ctr 89; **Fac Appt:** Prof Rad, UCLA

NUCLEAR MEDICINE

Mid Atlantic

Alavi, Abass MD [NuM] - **Spec Exp:** Brain Cancer; Pulmonary Imaging; PET Imaging; **Hospital:** Hosp Univ Penn - UPHS (page 113); **Address:** Hosp Univ Penn, Div Nuclear Med, 3400 Spruce St, Donner Bldg rm 110, Philadelphia, PA 19104; **Phone:** 215-662-3014; **Board Cert:** Nuclear Medicine 73; Internal Medicine 72; **Med School:** Iran 64; **Resid:** Internal Medicine, Albert Einstein Med Ctr/Phila VA Hosp 69; Hematology, Hosp Univ Penn 70; **Fellow:** Nuclear Medicine, Hosp Univ Penn 73; **Fac Appt:** Prof Rad, Univ Pennsylvania

Goldsmith, Stanley J MD [NuM] - **Spec Exp:** Thyroid Cancer; Neuroendocrine Tumors & Disorders; PET Imaging; **Hospital:** NY-Presby Hosp - NY Weill Cornell Med Ctr (page 103); **Address:** 520 E 70th St Bldg Starr - rm 221, New York, NY 10021-9800; **Phone:** 212-746-4588; **Board Cert:** Internal Medicine 69; Nuclear Medicine 72; Endocrinology 72; **Med School:** SUNY Downstate 62; **Resid:** Internal Medicine, Kings Co Hosp 67; **Fellow:** Endocrinology, Diabetes & Metabolism, Mt Sinai Hosp 68; Nuclear Medicine, Bronx VA Hosp 69; **Fac Appt:** Prof Rad, Cornell Univ-Weill Med Coll

Kramer, Elissa MD [NuM] - **Spec Exp:** Cancer Detection & Staging/PET; Lymphedema Imaging; Radioimmunotherapy of Cancer; **Hospital:** NYU Med Ctr (page 104); **Address:** 560 1st Ave, rm HW231, New York, NY 10016-6402; **Phone:** 212-263-7410; **Board Cert:** Nuclear Medicine 82; Diagnostic Radiology 82; **Med School:** NYU Sch Med 77; **Resid:** Radiology, Bellevue Hosp/NYU 80; **Fellow:** Nuclear Medicine, Bellevue Hosp/NYU 82; **Fac Appt:** Prof Rad, NYU Sch Med

Larson, Steven M MD [NuM] - **Spec Exp:** Thyroid Cancer; PET Imaging; **Hospital:** Meml Sloan Kettering Cancer Ctr (page 100); **Address:** Meml Sloan Kettering Cancer Ctr, Nuclear Med, 1275 York Ave, Box 77, New York, NY 10021; **Phone:** 212-639-7373; **Board Cert:** Nuclear Medicine 72; Internal Medicine 73; **Med School:** Univ Wash 65; **Resid:** Internal Medicine, Virginia Mason Hosp 70; Nuclear Medicine, Natl Inst Hlth 72; **Fac Appt:** Prof NuM, Cornell Univ-Weill Med Coll

Strauss, H William MD [NuM] - **Spec Exp:** Cardiac Imaging in Cancer Therapy; Thyroid Disorders; **Hospital:** Meml Sloan Kettering Cancer Ctr (page 100); **Address:** Meml Sloan Kettering Cancer Ctr, 1275 York Ave, S-212, Box 77, Nw York, NY 10021; **Phone:** 212-639-7238; **Board Cert:** Nuclear Medicine 72; **Med School:** SUNY Downstate 65; **Resid:** Internal Medicine, Downstate Med Ctr 67; Internal Medicine, Bellevue Hosp 68; **Fellow:** Nuclear Medicine, Johns Hopkins Hosp 70; **Fac Appt:** Prof Rad, Cornell Univ-Weill Med Coll

Southeast

Alazraki, Naomi P MD [NuM] - **Spec Exp:** Nuclear Oncology; **Hospital:** VA Med Ctr - Atlanta; **Address:** VA Medical Ctr - Atlanta, 1670 Clairmont Rd, MC 115, Decatur, GA 30033; **Phone:** 404-728-7629; **Board Cert:** Nuclear Medicine 72; Diagnostic Radiology 72; **Med School:** Albert Einstein Coll Med 66; **Resid:** Radiology, Univ Hospital 71; **Fac Appt:** Prof Rad, Emory Univ

Coleman, Ralph Edward MD [NuM] - **Spec Exp:** PET Imaging; SPECT Imaging; Tumor Imaging; **Hospital:** Duke Univ Med Ctr (page 94); **Address:** Duke Univ Med Ctr, Erwin Rd, Box 3949, Durham, NC 27710; **Phone:** 919-684-7244; **Board Cert:** Nuclear Medicine 74; Internal Medicine 73; **Med School:** Washington Univ, St Louis 68; **Resid:** Internal Medicine, Royal Victoria Hosp 70; **Fellow:** Nuclear Medicine, Mallinckrodt Inst Radiology 74; **Fac Appt:** Prof Rad, Duke Univ

Midwest

Dillehay, Gary MD [NuM] - **Spec Exp:** Lymphoma; Bone Densitometry; **Hospital:** Loyola Univ Med Ctr (page 98); **Address:** Loyola Univ Med Ctr - Nuclear Medicine, 2160 S 1st Ave, Bldg 107 - rm 0846, Maywood, IL 60153; **Phone:** 708-216-3559; **Board Cert:** Nuclear Medicine 85; Nuclear Radiology 87; **Med School:** Mayo Med Sch 79; **Resid:** Diagnostic Radiology, Northwestern Meml Hosp 83; Nuclear Medicine, Northwestern Meml Hosp 84; **Fac Appt:** Assoc Prof Rad, Loyola Univ-Stritch Sch Med

Neumann, Donald R MD [NuM] - **Spec Exp:** Nuclear Oncology; Nuclear Cardiology; **Hospital:** Cleveland Clin Fdn (page 92); **Address:** Cleveland Clinic, MFI Dept, 9500 Euclid Ave, MS Gb3, Cleveland, OH 44195; **Phone:** 216-444-2193; **Board Cert:** Diagnostic Radiology 87; Nuclear Radiology 90; **Med School:** Wright State Univ 80; **Resid:** Diagnostic Radiology, Mount Sinai Med Ctr 87; **Fellow:** Magnetic Resonance Imaging, Mount Sinai Med Ctr

Siegel, Barry MD [NuM] - **Spec Exp:** Cancer Detection & Staging; PET Imaging; **Hospital:** Barnes-Jewish Hosp (page 85); **Address:** Mallinckrodt Inst of Radiology, 510 S Kingshighway Blvd, St Louis, MO 63110-1016; **Phone:** 314-362-2809; **Board Cert:** Diagnostic Radiology 77; Nuclear Medicine 73; Nuclear Radiology 81; **Med School:** Washington Univ, St Louis 69; **Resid:** Diagnostic Radiology, Mallinckrodt Inst of Rad 73; **Fellow:** Nuclear Medicine, Mallinckrodt Inst of Rad 73; **Fac Appt:** Prof Rad, Washington Univ, St Louis

Silberstein, Edward B MD [NuM] - **Spec Exp:** Thyroid Cancer; Prostate Cancer Pain; Lymphoma; **Hospital:** Univ Hosp - Cincinnati; **Address:** Univ Hosp, 234 Goodman Ave, G026 Mont Reid Pav, Cincinnati, OH 45219-2364; **Phone:** 513-584-9032; **Board Cert:** Internal Medicine 80; Nuclear Medicine 72; Hematology 72; Medical Oncology 81; **Med School:** Harvard Med Sch 62; **Resid:** Internal Medicine, Univ Cincinnati Hosp 64; Internal Medicine, Univ Hosps-Case Western Reserve 67; **Fellow:** Hematology, New England Med Ctr 68; **Fac Appt:** Prof Emeritus Med, Univ Cincinnati

Wiseman, Gregory MD [NuM] - **Spec Exp:** Lymphoma, Non-Hodgkin's; Multiple Myeloma; Radioimmunotherapy of Cancer; **Hospital:** Mayo Med Ctr & Clin - Rochester; **Address:** Mayo Clinic, Dept Nuc Med, 200 First St SW, Charlton Bldg, Rochester, MN 55905; **Phone:** 507-284-9599; **Board Cert:** Internal Medicine 86; Hematology 88; Nuclear Medicine 02; **Med School:** Univ Utah 83; **Resid:** Internal Medicine, Mayo Clinic 86; Nuclear Medicine, Univ Washington Med Ctr 92; **Fellow:** Hematology, Mayo Clinic 89; Medical Oncology, Univ Washington 91; **Fac Appt:** Asst Prof Rad, Mayo Med Sch

Southwest

Podoloff, Donald MD [NuM] - **Spec Exp:** Prostate Cancer; Breast Cancer; **Hospital:** UT MD Anderson Cancer Ctr, The (page 115); **Address:** UT MD Anderson Cancer Ctr, 1515 Holcombe Blvd, Box 57, Houston, TX 77030; **Phone:** 713-745-1160; **Board Cert:** Diagnostic Radiology 73; Nuclear Medicine 75; Nuclear Radiology 75; **Med School:** SUNY Downstate 64; **Resid:** Internal Medicine, Beth Israel Med Ctr 68; Radiology, Wilford Hall USAF Med Ctr 73; **Fac Appt:** Prof NR, Univ Tex, Houston

West Coast and Pacific

Scheff, Alice M MD [NuM] - **Spec Exp:** Breast Imaging; Thyroid Imaging; Neurologic Imaging; **Hospital:** Santa Clara Vly Med Ctr; **Address:** 751 S Bascom Ave, San Jose, CA 95128; **Phone:** 408-885-6970; **Board Cert:** Nuclear Medicine 82; Nuclear Radiology 83; **Med School:** Penn State Univ-Hershey Med Ctr 78; **Resid:** Diagnostic Radiology, Penn State-Hershey Med Ctr 82; Nuclear Medicine, Penn State-Hershey Med Ctr 82; **Fellow:** Magnetic Resonance Imaging, Long Beach Meml Med Ctr

Waxman, Alan D MD [NuM] - **Spec Exp:** PET Imaging-Brain; Thyroid Cancer; Cancer Detection & Staging; **Hospital:** Cedars-Sinai Med Ctr (page 88); **Address:** Cedars-Sinai Med Ctr, Taper Imaging, 870 Beverly Blvd, rm 1251, Los Angeles, CA 90048-1804; **Phone:** 310-423-4216; **Board Cert:** Nuclear Medicine 72; **Med School:** USC Sch Med 63; **Resid:** Nuclear Medicine, Wadsworth VA Hosp 65; **Fellow:** Internal Medicine, Natl Inst Hlth 67; **Fac Appt:** Clin Prof Rad, USC Sch Med

SURGERY

A surgeon manages a broad spectrum of surgical conditions affecting almost any area of the body. The surgeon establishes the diagnosis and provides the preoperative, operative and postoperative care to surgical patients and is usually responsible for the comprehensive management of the trauma victim and the critically ill surgical patient.

The surgeon uses a variety of diagnostic techniques, including endoscopy, for observing internal structures and may use specialized instruments during operative procedures. A general surgeon is expected to be familiar with the salient features of other surgical specialties in order to recognize problems in those areas and to know when to refer a patient to another specialist.

Training required: Five years

PHYSICIAN LISTINGS

SURGICAL ONCOLOGY
FOX CHASE CANCER CENTER

333 Cottman Avenue
Philadelphia, Pennsylvania 19111-2497
Phone: 1-888-FOX CHASE • Fax: 215-728-2702 • www.fccc.edu

The most experienced surgical oncologists have the best treatment outcomes. Fox Chase surgeons are highly specialized and focus solely on cancer. The comprehensive surgical oncology program at Fox Chase encompasses the following surgical subspecialties: breast surgical oncology; gastrointestinal surgical oncology; gynecologic surgical oncology; head and neck surgical oncology; orthopedic surgical oncology; plastic surgery and reconstruction; thoracic surgical oncology; and urologic surgical oncology.

Surgical oncologists at Fox Chase Cancer Center use the latest technologies available for each form of adult cancer. A major focus of surgical oncology at Fox Chase is preserving organs and their function, including breast-conserving surgery and removal of colon or rectal tumors while preserving the bowel and anal sphincter. Techniques include minimally invasive procedures that permit organ preservation and shorten recovery time. The staff includes specialists in plastic, reconstructive and endoscopic surgery.

Our gastrointestinal surgeons have extensive experience with pancreatic cancer, advanced and recurrent cancer in the gastrointestinal tract and rare tumors such as sarcomas.

Our urologic surgical oncologists have broad expertise in the care of patients with cancers of the prostate, bladder, kidney, ureter, adrenal gland, testes and penis. Fox Chase urologists annually perform hundreds of complex open and laparoscopic surgeries for cancer. These services include minimally invasive surgery, organ-sparing resections, urinary diversions, laparoscopic urologic surgery and cryosurgical ablation.

Fox Chase experts in gynecologic cancer offer the most advanced treatments for women with cancers of the uterus, ovary and cervix. We also have a comprehensive research program to develop new treatments for ovarian cancer.

The head and neck cancer center at Fox Chase provides patients with one-stop consultations with surgeons, radiation oncologists and medical oncologists. Our surgical team offers expertise not only in surgical oncology but also in otolaryngology, plastic surgery and microvascular reconstruction.

Surgical oncology staff members also conduct research on improving surgical techniques and in several areas of multidisciplinary care. Among the innovative approaches are cryosurgery and laser surgery.

BREAST CANCER

If the diagnosis is breast cancer, patients have the option of meeting one-on-one with a surgeon or meeting with a panel of experts at Fox Chase's multidisciplinary Breast Evaluation Center.

At the Breast Evaluation Center, patients with newly diagnosed breast cancers receive a multidisciplinary review and treatment recommendations from a panel of specialists in medical, surgical and radiation oncology, diagnostic radiology, pathology and reconstructive surgery, when appropriate. The panel reaches a consensus during the initial appointment and recommends a state-of-the-art treatment plan.

Diagnostic techniques include stereotactic breast biopsy and, at the time of surgery, sentinel lymph-node biopsy. Treatment options include breast-preserving surgery (lumpectomy) with radiation therapy as well as mastectomy with reconstructive surgery. Women who choose mastectomy have several options for breast reconstruction. Fox Chase surgeons can perform a skin-sparing mastectomy to ease this process.

SURGERY

The NYU Medical Center's Department of Surgery performs more than 5,000 outpatient and inpatient procedures each year. Use of minimally invasive techniques, such as laparoscopic and endoscopic surgery, speed recovery and improve patient outcome. Cancer patients receive truly multidisciplinary care at the newly-opened NYU Clinical Cancer Center where oncologists work with surgeons to provide comprehensive treatment in a convenient, central location. All surgeons are board-certified by the American Board of Surgery and serve on the faculty of New York University School of Medicine.

GENERAL SURGERY – State-of-the-art care by top surgeons providing diagnostic laparoscopy, appendectomy, hernia repair, cholecystectomy, colon resection, splenectomy, and other corrective procedures

BREAST SURGERY – Surgeons at NYU are expert in the full range of surgical reconstructive techniques

COLON – More than 80 percent of colectomies are performed using laparoscopic surgery; small incisions reduce the need for pain medication and dramatically speed recovery

ESOPHAGEAL AND GASTRIC – Radiologist and medical oncologists work with surgeons to tailor treatment for tumor reduction and removal

PANCREATIC – Nationally recognized for an exceptional 98 percent surgical survival rate; laparoscopic surgery improves the outcome for elderly patients

LIVER – Radio frequency ablation uses targeted probes to destroy tumors and heal lesions

VIRTUAL COLONOSCOPY – A noninvasive method of cancer screening that uses painless imaging similar to a CT scan

THORACIC – Video-assisted thoracoscopy for the diagnosis and treatment of a variety of benign and malignant conditions of the lung and chest cavity

Specialists at the NCI-designated NYU Cancer Institute seek to enhance and coordinate the extensive resources of NYU Medical Center to optimize research, treatment, and the ultimate control of cancer.

Our new NYU Clinical Cancer Center is located at 160 East 34th Street. This state-of-the-art 13-level, 85,000-square-foot building serves as "home base" for patients, by providing the latest cancer prevention, screening, diagnostic treatment, genetic counseling, and support services in one central location. The NYU Clinical Cancer Center stands to dramatically improve the lives of people with cancer. As part of NYU Medical Center, patients can access a variety of other non-cancer services throughout the institution.

PHYSICIAN REFERRAL
1-888-7-NYU-MED
(1-888-769-8633)
www.nyumc.org
www.nyuci.org

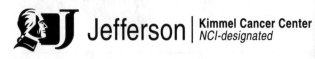

SURGICAL ONCOLOGY PROGRAM
UCLA HEALTHCARE

1-800-UCLA-MD1 (825-2631)
www.healthcare.ucla.edu

Using the latest in surgical technologies — including minimally invasive surgery and robotics — UCLA's surgical oncology program offers a multidisciplinary approach to modern cancer therapy for solid tumors of the breast, lung, colon, liver and pancreas; soft-tissue and bone sarcomas; and melanoma.

Sophisticated diagnostic and therapeutic services, some only available at select medical centers, offer adults and children the accurate staging of cancers and the latest cancer surgery approaches. Post-operative treatments may include the latest the field has to offer in chemotherapy, radiation, biological therapy and gene therapy.

The Center for Advanced Surgical and Interventional Technology (CASIT), a UCLA-based collaboration among surgery, engineering, and industry, is taking surgery to the next step by exploring innovative surgical approaches for the future, including robotics to perform minimally invasive procedures.

UCLA'S JONSSON CANCER CENTER

Designated by the National Cancer Institute as one of only 38 comprehensive cancer centers in the United States, UCLA's Jonsson Cancer Center has earned an international reputation for developing new cancer therapies, providing the best in experimental and traditional treatments, and expertly guiding and training the next generation of medical researchers. The center's 250 physicians and scientists treat upwards of 20,000 patient visits per year and offer hundreds of clinical trials that provide the latest in experimental cancer treatments (www.cancer.mednet.ucla.edu). The center also offers patients and families psychological and support services.

UCLA's Jonsson Cancer Center has been ranked the best cancer center in the western United States by U.S. News & World Report's Annual Best Hospitals survey for the past five years. UCLA Medical Center, of which the Cancer Center is a part, has ranked best in the West for the past 15 years.

**Call 1-800-UCLA-MD1 (825-2631)
for a referral to a UCLA doctor.**

U C L A Healthcare

UCLA'S SURGICAL ONCOLOGY PROGRAM OFFERS TREATMENTS FOR CANCERS OF THE:

- **Breast**
- **Lung**
- **Colon**
- **Liver**
- **Pancreas**
- **Bowel**
- **Skin (Melanoma)**

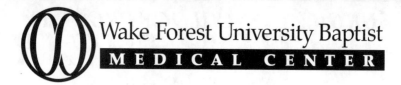

Wake Forest University Baptist
MEDICAL CENTER

BREAST CANCER CENTER OF EXCELLENCE
COMPREHENSIVE CANCER CENTER

Medical Center Boulevard • Winston-Salem, NC 27157
Health On-Call® (Patient Access) 1-800-446-2255
PAL® (Physician-to-physician calls) 1-800-277-7654
www.wfubmc.edu/cancer

OVERVIEW

In 1996, the cross-programmatic nature of breast cancer research at Wake Forest Baptist was formally recognized, and the Breast Cancer Center of Excellence was established to facilitate collaboration among the Cancer Center's four programs.

RESEARCH

The Breast Cancer Center of Excellence takes a multidisciplinary, comprehensive approach involving all basic scientists, public health scientists and clinicians. Areas of emphasis at the Center include breast carcinogenesis (what causes cells to mutate into cancer cells), breat cancer risk assessment and prevention, novel modes of breast imaging and quality of life issues for breast cancer patients. The clinical arm is mediated via the Breast Care Center, which has enabled us to initiate a variety of translational research projects.

MULTIDISCIPLINARY CARE

Breast Care Center—As the area's only truly multidisciplinary breast care program, the Center consolidates the services of a multidisciplinary team in a central location so the patient can be seen by multiple specialists during a single visit. With a pathology laboratory located in the clinic, they can provide "on the spot" diagnosis.

The team includes surgical oncologists, radiologists, medical and radiation oncologists, plastic surgeons, pathologists, specialty nurses and genetic counselors.

In most cases, by the end of the day the patient leaves with a comprehensive treatment plan in place, thus reducing the stressful period between the diagnosis of breast cancer and the beginning of treatment. This also decreases the number of visits to the medical center required to set up complex multimodality care.

In addition to receiving the latest advances in treatment such as sentinel lymph node mapping, breast conserving surgery, immediate breast reconstruction and radiation implants, patients have access to the latest clinical trials on breast cancer treatment and prevention.

The Center's extensive laboratory research programs in breast cancer allow for rapid translation of research from the lab to the clinic. Patients benefit from clinical trials assessing the most up-to-date approaches in the prevention, diagnosis, treatment, and follow-up of breast cancer, so both doctors and their patients make informed decisions.

Genetic screening is available for those who are concerned about hereditary risk factors. Patients who are at high risk may elect to participate in breast cancer prevention trials.

SURGERY

New England

Becker, James MD [S] - **Spec Exp:** Inflammatory Bowel Disease; Gastrointestinal Cancer; Gastrointestinal Disorders; **Hospital:** Boston Med Ctr; **Address:** Boston Med Ctr, Dept Surg, 88 E Newton St, rm C500, Boston, MA 02118-2393; **Phone:** 617-638-8600; **Board Cert:** Surgery 99; **Med School:** Case West Res Univ 75; **Resid:** Surgery, Univ Utah Med Ctr 80; **Fellow:** Research, Mayo Clinic 82; **Fac Appt:** Prof S, Boston Univ

Cady, Blake MD [S] - **Spec Exp:** Breast Cancer; Thyroid Cancer; **Hospital:** Rhode Island Hosp; **Address:** 503 Eddy St, APC 435, Providence, RI 02903; **Phone:** 401-444-6158; **Board Cert:** Surgery 66; **Med School:** Cornell Univ-Weill Med Coll 57; **Resid:** Surgery, Boston City Hosp 65; Surgery; **Fellow:** Surgery, NY Meml Cancer Hosp 67; **Fac Appt:** Prof S, Brown Univ

Cioffi, William MD [S] - **Spec Exp:** Trauma; Cancer Surgery; **Hospital:** Rhode Island Hosp; **Address:** Rhode Island Hosp, Dept Surg, 2 Dudley St, Ste 470, Providence, RI 02905; **Phone:** 401-553-8348; **Board Cert:** Surgery 95; Surgical Critical Care 97; **Med School:** Univ VT Coll Med 81; **Resid:** Surgery, Med Ctr Hosp VT 86; **Fac Appt:** Prof S, Brown Univ

Eisenberg, Burton L. MD [S] - **Spec Exp:** Breast Cancer; Melanoma; Sarcoma; **Hospital:** Dartmouth - Hitchcock Med Ctr; **Address:** Dartmouth-Hitchcock Med Ctr, Dept Surgery, One Medical Center Drive, Lebanon, NH 03756; **Phone:** 603-653-3614; **Board Cert:** Surgery 99; **Med School:** Univ Tenn Coll Med, Memphis 74; **Resid:** Surgery, Wilford Hall USAF Med Ctr 79; **Fellow:** Surgical Oncology, Meml Sloan-Kettering Cancer Ctr 81

Hughes, Kevin S MD [S] - **Spec Exp:** Breast Cancer; Ovarian Cancer; **Hospital:** Mass Genl Hosp; **Address:** Massachusetts General Hospital, Wang Bldg Fl 2 - rm 240, Boston, MA 02114; **Phone:** 617-724-4800; **Board Cert:** Surgery 93; **Med School:** Dartmouth Med Sch 79; **Resid:** Surgery, Mercy Hosp 84; **Fellow:** Surgical Oncology, National Cancer Inst 85; **Fac Appt:** Assoc Prof S, Harvard Med Sch

Iglehart, J Dirk MD [S] - **Spec Exp:** Breast Cancer; **Hospital:** Brigham & Women's Hosp (page 87); **Address:** Brigham & Women's Hosp, Dept Surg, 75 Francis St, Boston, MA 02115; **Phone:** 617-632-5178; **Board Cert:** Surgery 95; **Med School:** Harvard Med Sch 75; **Resid:** Surgery, Duke Univ Med Ctr 81; Thoracic Surgery, Duke Univ Med Ctr 84; **Fac Appt:** Prof S, Harvard Med Sch

Jenkins, Roger L MD [S] - **Spec Exp:** Transplant-Liver; Liver Cancer; Bile Duct Reconstruction; **Hospital:** Lahey Clin; **Address:** Lahey Clin, Dept Hepatobiliary, 41 Mall Rd, Burlington, MA 01805; **Phone:** 781-744-2500; **Board Cert:** Surgery 93; **Med School:** Univ VT Coll Med 77; **Resid:** Surgery, New Eng Deaconess Hosp 82; **Fellow:** Cardiovascular Surgery, Deaconess Hosp 83; Transplant Surgery, Univ Pittsburgh Hosp; **Fac Appt:** Prof S, Tufts Univ

Kavanah, Maureen MD [S] - **Spec Exp:** Breast Cancer; Gynecologic Cancer; Melanoma; **Hospital:** Boston Med Ctr; **Address:** Boston Medical Ctr, 720 Harrison Ave, Ste 700, Boston, MA 02118; **Phone:** 617-638-8473; **Board Cert:** Surgery 99; **Med School:** Tufts Univ 75; **Resid:** Surgery, St Elizabeths Hosp 79; **Fellow:** Surgical Oncology, Boston Univ Med Ctr 81; **Fac Appt:** Assoc Prof S, Boston Univ

Kern, Kenneth A MD [S] - **Spec Exp:** Breast Cancer; **Hospital:** Hartford Hosp; **Address:** 85 Seymour St, Ste 1011, Hartford, CT 06106; **Phone:** 860-525-5656; **Board Cert:** Surgery 03; **Med School:** Harvard Med Sch 78; **Resid:** Surgery, Johns Hopkins Hosp 85; **Fellow:** Surgical Oncology, National Cancer Inst 87; **Fac Appt:** Assoc Prof S, Univ Conn

Krag, David MD [S] - **Spec Exp:** Sentinel Node Surgery; Breast Cancer; **Hospital:** FAHC - UHC Campus; **Address:** Vermont Coll Med, Surgery Given Bldg, #E309C, Burlington, VT 05405; **Phone:** 802-656-5830; **Board Cert:** Surgery 96; **Med School:** Loyola Univ-Stritch Sch Med 80; **Resid:** Surgery, UC Davis Med Ctr 83; **Fellow:** Surgical Oncology, UCLA Med Ctr 84; **Fac Appt:** Assoc Prof S, Univ VT Coll Med

Osteen, Robert T MD [S] - **Spec Exp:** Breast Cancer; Colon & Rectal Cancer; Melanoma & Sarcoma; **Hospital:** Brigham & Women's Hosp (page 87); **Address:** Brigham & Women's Hosp, Dept Surg, 75 Francis St, Boston, MA 02115; **Phone:** 617-732-6718; **Board Cert:** Surgery 95; **Med School:** Duke Univ 66; **Resid:** Surgery, Duke Univ Med Ctr 68; Surgery, PB Brigham 75; **Fac Appt:** Assoc Prof S, Harvard Med Sch

Ponn, Teresa MD [S] - **Spec Exp:** Breast Cancer; **Hospital:** Yale - New Haven Hosp; **Address:** Yale-New Haven Breast Ctr, 800 Howard Ave, Lower Level, PO Box 208062, New Haven, CT 06520-8062; **Phone:** 203-785-2328; **Board Cert:** Surgery 00; **Med School:** Univ Fla Coll Med 76; **Resid:** Surgery, Stanford Univ Med Ctr 82; **Fac Appt:** Asst Prof S, Yale Univ

Salem, Ronald R MD [S] - **Spec Exp:** Cancer Surgery; **Hospital:** Yale - New Haven Hosp; **Address:** Yale Univ Sch Med, Dept Surg, 333 Cedar St, Box 208062, New Haven, CT 06520-8062; **Phone:** 203-785-3577; **Board Cert:** Surgery 00; **Med School:** Zimbabwe 78; **Resid:** Surgery, Hammersmith Hosp 85; Surgery, New Eng-Deaconess Hosp 89; **Fac Appt:** Assoc Prof S, Yale Univ

Shamberger, Robert MD [S] - **Spec Exp:** Pediatric Cancers; **Hospital:** Children's Hospital - Boston; **Address:** Children's Hosp-Dept Surgery, 300 Longwood Ave, Fegan - 3, Boston, MA 02115; **Phone:** 617-355-8326; **Board Cert:** Surgery 02; Surgical Critical Care 99; Pediatric Surgery 03; **Med School:** Harvard Med Sch 75; **Resid:** Surgery, Massachusetts Genl Hosp 78; Pediatric Surgery, Children's Hosp Boston 85; **Fellow:** Surgical Oncology, NCI-Surgical Branch 80; **Fac Appt:** Prof S, Harvard Med Sch

Smith, Barbara Lynn MD/PhD [S] - **Spec Exp:** Breast Cancer; **Hospital:** Mass Genl Hosp; **Address:** Mass Genl Hosp-Gillette Ctr, 100 Blossom St, Cox Bldg, Fl 1, Boston, MA 02114; **Phone:** 617-724-4800; **Board Cert:** Surgery 00; **Med School:** Harvard Med Sch 83; **Resid:** Surgery, Brigham & Women's Hosp 89; **Fac Appt:** Asst Prof S, Harvard Med Sch

Sutton, John E. MD [S] - **Spec Exp:** Esophageal Cancer; Liver & Biliary Surgery; Pancreatic Cancer; **Hospital:** Dartmouth - Hitchcock Med Ctr; **Address:** One Medical Center Drive, Lebanon, NH 03756; **Phone:** 603-650-8022; **Board Cert:** Surgery 01; Surgical Critical Care 95; **Med School:** Georgetown Univ 74; **Resid:** Surgery, Dartmouth-Hitchcock Med Ctr 81; **Fellow:** Critical Care Medicine, Dartmouth-Hitchcock Med Ctr 83; **Fac Appt:** Prof S, Dartmouth Med Sch

Swanson, Richard MD [S] - **Spec Exp:** Pancreatic Cancer; Gastrointestinal Cancer; Liver Cancer; **Hospital:** Brigham & Women's Hosp (page 87); **Address:** Brigham & Women's Hospital, Dept Surgical Oncology, 75 Francis St, Boston, MA 02115; **Phone:** 617-732-8818; **Board Cert:** Surgery 99; **Med School:** Harvard Med Sch 80; **Resid:** Surgery, Mass Genl Hosp 87; **Fellow:** Surgical Oncology, MD Anderson Cancer Ctr 89; **Fac Appt:** Assoc Prof S, Harvard Med Sch

Tanabe, Kenneth K MD [S] - **Spec Exp:** Liver Cancer; Colon & Rectal Cancer; Melanoma; **Hospital:** Mass Genl Hosp; **Address:** Mass General Hosp, Div Surgical Oncology, 100 Blossom St, Bldg Cox - rm 626, Boston, MA 02114; **Phone:** 617-724-3868; **Board Cert:** Surgery 00; **Med School:** UCSD 85; **Resid:** Surgery, NY Hosp-Cornell 90; **Fellow:** Surgical Oncology, MD Anderson Cancer Ctr; **Fac Appt:** Assoc Prof S, Harvard Med Sch

Udelsman, Robert MD [S] - **Spec Exp:** Parathyroid Cancer; Adrenal Minimally Invasive Surgery; Thyroid Cancer & Surgery; **Hospital:** Yale - New Haven Hosp; **Address:** Yale Sch Med, Rm FMB102, 330 Cedar St, Box 208062, New Haven, CT 06520-3218; **Phone:** 203-785-2697; **Board Cert:** Surgery 99; **Med School:** Geo Wash Univ 81; **Resid:** Surgery, Natl Inst Hlth 86; Surgery, Johns Hopkins Hosp 89; **Fellow:** Gastrointestinal Surgery, Johns Hopkins Hosp 90; **Fac Appt:** Prof S, Yale Univ

Ward, Barbara MD [S] - **Spec Exp:** Breast Cancer; Breast Disease; **Hospital:** Greenwich Hosp; **Address:** 77 Lafayette Pl, Ste 301, Greenwich, CT 06830-5426; **Phone:** 203-863-4300; **Board Cert:** Surgery 02; **Med School:** Temple Univ 83; **Resid:** Surgery, Yale-New Haven Hosp 90; **Fellow:** Surgical Oncology, Natl Cancer Inst 87; **Fac Appt:** Assoc Clin Prof S, Yale Univ

Warshaw, Andrew L MD [S] - **Spec Exp:** Pancreatic Cancer; Pancreatic Surgery; Liver Cancer; **Hospital:** Mass Genl Hosp; **Address:** Mass Genl Hosp, Dept Surg, 55 Fruit St White Bldg - rm 506, Boston, MA 02114-2696; **Phone:** 617-726-8254; **Board Cert:** Surgery 71; Surgical Critical Care 86; **Med School:** Harvard Med Sch 63; **Resid:** Surgery, Mass Genl Hosp 71; **Fellow:** Internal Medicine, Mass Genl Hosp; **Fac Appt:** Prof S, Harvard Med Sch

Zinner, Michael MD [S] - **Spec Exp:** Colon & Rectal Cancer; Gastrointestinal Surgery; Pancreatic Cancer; **Hospital:** Brigham & Women's Hosp (page 87); **Address:** Brigham & Women's Hosp, Dept Surg, 75 Francis St, Twr 1, Ste 220, Boston, MA 02115; **Phone:** 617-732-8181; **Board Cert:** Surgery 00; **Med School:** Univ Fla Coll Med 71; **Resid:** Surgery, Johns Hopkins Hosp 74; Surgery, Johns Hopkins Hosp 79; **Fac Appt:** Prof S, Harvard Med Sch

Mid Atlantic

Alfonso, Antonio MD [S] - **Spec Exp:** Breast Cancer; Head & Neck Surgery; **Hospital:** Long Island Coll Hosp (page 93); **Address:** Long Island Coll Hosp, 339 Hicks St, Brooklyn, NY 11201-6005; **Phone:** 718-875-3244; **Board Cert:** Surgery 73; **Med School:** Philippines 68; **Resid:** Surgery, Temple Univ Hosp 72; **Fellow:** Surgical Oncology, Meml Sloan Kettering Cancer Ctr 74; **Fac Appt:** Prof S, SUNY Downstate

August, David MD [S] - **Spec Exp:** Cancer Surgery; Gastrointestinal Cancer; Breast Cancer; **Hospital:** Robert Wood Johnson Univ Hosp - New Brunswick (page 106); **Address:** Canc Inst NJ, 195 Little Albany St, New Brunswick, NJ 08903-1914; **Phone:** 732-235-7701; **Board Cert:** Surgery 95; **Med School:** Yale Univ 80; **Resid:** Surgery, Yale-New Haven Hosp 86; **Fellow:** Surgical Oncology, Natl Cancer Inst 84; **Fac Appt:** Assoc Prof S, UMDNJ-RW Johnson Med Sch

Axelrod, Deborah MD [S] - **Spec Exp:** Breast Cancer; Breast Disease; **Hospital:** NYU Med Ctr (page 104); **Address:** NYU Clinical Cancer Ctr, 160 E 34th St, New York, NY 10016; **Phone:** 212-731-5366; **Board Cert:** Surgery 98; **Med School:** Israel 82; **Resid:** Surgery, Beth Israel Med Ctr 88; **Fellow:** Surgical Oncology, Meml Sloan Kettering Cancer Ctr 86; **Fac Appt:** Assoc Prof S, NYU Sch Med

Ballantyne, Garth MD [S] - **Spec Exp:** Laparoscopic Abdominal Surgery; Gastroesophageal Reflux Disease (GERD); Colon Cancer; **Hospital:** Hackensack Univ Med Ctr (page 96); **Address:** 20 Prospect Ave, Ste 901, Hackensack, NJ 07601-1974; **Phone:** 201-996-2959; **Board Cert:** Surgery 84; Colon & Rectal Surgery 85; **Med School:** Columbia P&S 77; **Resid:** Surgery, UCLA Med Ctr 80; Surgery, Northwestern Univ 82; **Fellow:** Colon & Rectal Surgery, Mayo Clinic 84; **Fac Appt:** Prof S, UMDNJ-NJ Med Sch, Newark

Bartlett, David L MD **[S]** - **Spec Exp:** Peritoneal Carcinomatosis; Pancreatic Cancer; Liver Cancer; **Hospital:** UPMC Shadyside (page 114); **Address:** UPMC Cancer Ctr, 5150 Centre Ave, rm 415, Pittsburgh, PA 15232; **Phone:** 412-692-2852; **Board Cert:** Surgery 94; **Med School:** Univ Tex, Houston 87; **Resid:** Surgery, Hosp Univ Penn 93; **Fellow:** Surgical Oncology, Meml Sloan-Kettering Cancer Ctr 95; **Fac Appt:** Assoc Prof S, Univ Pittsburgh

Bass, Barbara MD **[S]** - **Spec Exp:** Breast Cancer; Endocrine Tumors; **Hospital:** Univ of MD Med Sys; **Address:** 22 S Greene St, Ste S4B10, Baltimore, MD 21201; **Phone:** 410-328-6187; **Board Cert:** Surgery 96; **Med School:** Univ VA Sch Med 79; **Resid:** Surgery, Geo Wash Univ 82; Surgery, Geo Wash Univ 86; **Fellow:** Surgery, Walter Reed Inst 84; **Fac Appt:** Prof S, Univ MD Sch Med

Borgen, Patrick I MD **[S]** - **Spec Exp:** Breast Cancer; **Hospital:** Meml Sloan Kettering Cancer Ctr (page 100); **Address:** 205 E 64th St, New York, NY 10021-6635; **Phone:** 212-639-5248; **Board Cert:** Surgery 91; **Med School:** Louisiana State Univ 84; **Resid:** Surgery, Ochsner Fdn Hosp 89; **Fellow:** Surgical Oncology, Meml Sloan Kettering Canc Ctr 90; **Fac Appt:** Prof S, Cornell Univ-Weill Med Coll

Brennan, Murray MD **[S]** - **Spec Exp:** Sarcoma; Pancreatic Cancer; Tumor Surgery; **Hospital:** Meml Sloan Kettering Cancer Ctr (page 100); **Address:** 1275 York Ave, rm C1265, New York, NY 10021; **Phone:** 212-639-6586; **Board Cert:** Surgery 75; **Med School:** New Zealand 64; **Resid:** Surgery, Univ Otago Hosp 69; **Fellow:** Surgery, Harvard Med Sch 72; Surgery, Peter Bent Brigham Hosp 75; **Fac Appt:** Prof S, Cornell Univ-Weill Med Coll

Cameron, John MD **[S]** - **Spec Exp:** Pancreatic Cancer; Pancreatic Surgery; Biliary Cancer; **Hospital:** Johns Hopkins Hosp - Baltimore (page 97); **Address:** 600 North Wolfe St Bldg Blalock - Ste 679, Baltimore, MD 21287; **Phone:** 410-955-5166; **Board Cert:** Surgery 70; Thoracic Surgery 71; **Med School:** Johns Hopkins Univ 62; **Resid:** Surgery, Johns Hopkins Hosp 70; **Fellow:** Thoracic Surgery, Johns Hopkins Hosp 71; **Fac Appt:** Prof S, Johns Hopkins Univ

Chabot, John A MD **[S]** - **Spec Exp:** Liver & Biliary Surgery; Pancreatic Cancer & Surgery; Thyroid & Parathyroid Surgery; **Hospital:** NY-Presby Hosp - Columbia Presby Med Ctr (page 103); **Address:** 161 Ft Washington Ave, Fl 8, New York, NY 10032; **Phone:** 212-305-9468; **Board Cert:** Surgery 00; **Med School:** Dartmouth Med Sch 83; **Resid:** Surgery, Columbia-Presby Med Ctr 90; **Fac Appt:** Assoc Prof S, Columbia P&S

Choti, Michael A MD **[S]** - **Spec Exp:** Gastrointestinal Cancer; Colon & Rectal Cancer; Carcinoid Tumors; **Hospital:** Johns Hopkins Hosp - Baltimore (page 97); **Address:** Johns Hopkins Hosp., 600 N Wolfe St, Bldg Halsted - rm 614, Baltimore, MD 21287; **Phone:** 410-955-7113; **Board Cert:** Surgery 91; **Med School:** Yale Univ 83; **Resid:** Surgery, Hosp Univ Penn 90; **Fellow:** Surgical Oncology, Meml Sloan -Kettering Cancer Ctr. 92; **Fac Appt:** Assoc Prof S, Johns Hopkins Univ

Coit, Daniel G MD **[S]** - **Spec Exp:** Melanoma; Pancreatic Cancer; Stomach Cancer; **Hospital:** Meml Sloan Kettering Cancer Ctr (page 100); **Address:** 1275 York Ave, New York, NY 10021-6007; **Phone:** 212-639-8411; **Board Cert:** Surgery 94; **Med School:** Univ Cincinnati 76; **Resid:** Internal Medicine, New England Deaconess Hosp 78; Surgery, New England Deaconess Hosp 83; **Fellow:** Surgical Oncology, Meml Sloan Kettering Canc Ctr 85; **Fac Appt:** Assoc Prof S, Cornell Univ-Weill Med Coll

Edge, Stephen B MD **[S]** - **Spec Exp:** Breast Cancer; **Hospital:** Roswell Park Cancer Inst (page 107); **Address:** Roswell Park Cancer Inst, Dept Surgical Oncology, Elm & Carlton Streets, Buffalo, NY 14263; **Phone:** 716-845-5789; **Board Cert:** Surgery 96; **Med School:** Case West Res Univ 79; **Resid:** Surgery, Univ Hosp 86; **Fellow:** Surgical Oncology, Natl Cancer Inst 84; **Fac Appt:** Prof S, SUNY Buffalo

Edington, Howard D MD [S] - **Spec Exp:** Breast Cancer & Surgery; Melanoma; Reconstructive Surgery; **Hospital:** UPMC Presby, Pittsburgh (page 114); **Address:** Magee-Women's Hospital, Dept Surgery, 300 Halket St, Ste 2601, Oakland, PA 15213; **Phone:** 412-641-1342; **Board Cert:** Surgery 98; Plastic Surgery 93; Hand Surgery 94; **Med School:** Temple Univ 83; **Resid:** Surgery, Univ Pittsburgh Med Ctr 89; **Fellow:** Hand Surgery, Univ Pittsburgh Med Ctr 91; National Cancer Inst 93

Emond, Jean C MD [S] - **Spec Exp:** Transplant-Liver; Liver Cancer; **Hospital:** NY-Presby Hosp - Columbia Presby Med Ctr (page 103); **Address:** 622 W 168th St, PH - Fl 14, New York, NY 10032; **Phone:** 212-305-0914; **Board Cert:** Surgery 94; **Med School:** Univ Chicago-Pritzker Sch Med 79; **Resid:** Surgery, Cook Cty Hosp 84; **Fellow:** Surgery, Hopital P Brousse/Univ de Paris Sud 85; Transplant Surgery, Univ Chicago Hosps 87; **Fac Appt:** Prof S, Columbia P&S

Eng, Kenneth MD [S] - **Spec Exp:** Colon & Rectal Cancer & Surgery; Pancreatic Cancer & Surgery; Inflammatory Bowel Disease; **Hospital:** NYU Med Ctr (page 104); **Address:** 530 1st Ave, Ste 6B, New York, NY 10016-6402; **Phone:** 212-263-7301; **Board Cert:** Surgery 82; **Med School:** NYU Sch Med 67; **Resid:** Surgery, NYU Med Ctr 72; **Fac Appt:** Prof S, NYU Sch Med

Enker, Warren MD [S] - **Spec Exp:** Gastrointestinal Cancer & Surgery; Colon & Rectal Cancer & Surgery; Liver Tumor-Radio Frequency Ablation; **Hospital:** Beth Israel Med Ctr - Petrie Division (page 93); **Address:** 350 E 17th St Bldg Baird - Ste 1622, New York, NY 10003; **Phone:** 212-420-3960; **Board Cert:** Surgery 73; **Med School:** SUNY Downstate 67; **Resid:** Surgery, Univ Chicago Hosps 72; **Fellow:** Cancer Immunology, Univ Chicago Hosps 73; Cancer Immunology, Univ Minnesota Med Ctr 74; **Fac Appt:** Prof S, Albert Einstein Coll Med

Estabrook, Alison MD [S] - **Spec Exp:** Breast Cancer; Breast Disease-Benign; Breast Cancer-High Risk Women; **Hospital:** St Luke's - Roosevelt Hosp Ctr - Roosevelt Div (page 93); **Address:** 425 W 59th St, Ste 7A, New York, NY 10019-1104; **Phone:** 212-523-7500; **Board Cert:** Surgery 94; **Med School:** NYU Sch Med 78; **Resid:** Surgery, Columbia Presby Med Ctr 84; **Fellow:** Surgical Oncology, Columbia Presby Med Ctr 82; **Fac Appt:** Prof S, Columbia P&S

Fong, Yuman MD [S] - **Spec Exp:** Pancreatic Cancer; Liver Cancer & Gallbladder Cancer; Stomach Cancer; **Hospital:** Meml Sloan Kettering Cancer Ctr (page 100); **Address:** Memorial Sloan-Kettering Cancer Ctr, 1275 York Ave, New York, NY 10021; **Phone:** 212-639-2016; **Board Cert:** Surgery 02; **Med School:** Cornell Univ-Weill Med Coll 86; **Resid:** Surgery, NY-Cornell Med Ctr 92; **Fellow:** Surgical Oncology, Meml Sloan-Kettering Cancer Ctr 94; **Fac Appt:** Prof S, Cornell Univ-Weill Med Coll

Fraker, Douglas L MD [S] - **Spec Exp:** Melanoma & Sarcoma; Endocrine Surgery; Liver Cancer; **Hospital:** Hosp Univ Penn - UPHS (page 113); **Address:** Hosp Univ Penn, Dept Surgery, 3400 Spruce St, 4 Silverstein Pavilion, Philadelphia, PA 19104; **Phone:** 215-662-7866; **Board Cert:** Surgery 02; **Med School:** Harvard Med Sch 83; **Resid:** Surgery, UCSF Med Ctr 86; Surgery, UCSF Med Ctr 91; **Fellow:** Surgical Oncology, National Cancer Inst 89; **Fac Appt:** Prof S, Univ Pennsylvania

Frazier, Thomas MD [S] - **Spec Exp:** Breast Cancer; **Hospital:** Bryn Mawr Hosp; **Address:** 101 S Bryn Mawr Ave, Ste 201, Bryn Mawr, PA 19010; **Phone:** 610-520-0700; **Board Cert:** Surgery 04; **Med School:** Univ Pennsylvania 68; **Resid:** Surgery, Hosp Univ Penn 75; **Fellow:** Surgical Oncology, MD Anderson Cancer Ctr 76; **Fac Appt:** Clin Prof S, Jefferson Med Coll

Gibbs, John F MD [S] - **Spec Exp:** Liver Cancer; Liver & Biliary Surgery; Pancreatic Cancer; **Hospital:** Roswell Park Cancer Inst (page 107); **Address:** Roswell Park Cancer Inst, Dept Surg Onc, Elm & Carlton Sts, Buffalo, NY 14263-0001; **Phone:** 716-845-5807; **Board Cert:** Surgery 00; **Med School:** UCSD 85; **Resid:** Surgery, Rush Presby-St Luke's Med Ctr 90; **Fellow:** Transplant Surgery, Baylor Univ Med Ctr 92; Surgical Oncology, Roswell Park Cancer Inst 96; **Fac Appt:** Assoc Prof S, SUNY Buffalo

Hoffman, John P MD **[S]** - **Spec Exp:** Pancreatic Cancer; Gastrointestinal Cancer; Breast Cancer; **Hospital:** Fox Chase Cancer Ctr (page 95); **Address:** Fox Chase Cancer Ctr, 333 Cottman Ave, Philadelphia, PA 19111-2497; **Phone:** 215-728-3518; **Board Cert:** Surgery 98; **Med School:** Case West Res Univ 70; **Resid:** Surgery, Virginia Mason Hosp 77; **Fellow:** Surgical Oncology, Meml Sloan Kettering Cancer Ctr 80; **Fac Appt:** Prof S, Temple Univ

Jaques, David P MD **[S]** - **Spec Exp:** Stomach & Pancreatic Cancer; Sarcoma; Melanoma; **Hospital:** Meml Sloan Kettering Cancer Ctr (page 100); **Address:** Memorial Sloan Kattering Cancer Ctr, Dept Surgery, 1275 York Ave, New York, NY 10021; **Phone:** 212-639-6743; **Board Cert:** Surgery 94; **Med School:** Univ Mich Med Sch 78; **Resid:** Surgery, Walter Reed AMC 83; **Fellow:** Surgical Oncology, Memorial Sloan Kettering Cancer Ctr 85

Johnson, Ronald R MD **[S]** - **Spec Exp:** Breast Cancer & Surgery; **Hospital:** Magee-Womens Hosp - UPMC (page 114); **Address:** Magee-Womens Hosp - UPMC, 300 Halket St, Ste 2601, Pittsburgh, PA 15213; **Phone:** 412-641-1225; **Board Cert:** Surgery 99; **Med School:** Univ Pittsburgh 83; **Resid:** Surgery, Univ Pittsburgh Med Ctr 89

Karpeh Jr, Martin S MD **[S]** - **Spec Exp:** Gastrointestinal Cancer; Esophageal Cancer; Colon & Rectal Cancer; **Hospital:** Stony Brook Univ Hosp; **Address:** Stony Brook Univ Hosp, Hlth Science Ctr, Fl T18 - rm 060, Stony Brook, NY 11794-8191; **Phone:** 631-444-1793; **Board Cert:** Surgery 98; **Med School:** Penn State Univ-Hershey Med Ctr 83; **Resid:** Surgery, Hosp Univ Penn 89; **Fellow:** Surgical Oncology, Memorial Sloan Kettering Cancer Ctr 91; **Fac Appt:** Prof S, SUNY Stony Brook

Kaufman, Howard L MD **[S]** - **Spec Exp:** Cancer Surgery; Vaccine Therapy; Melanoma; **Hospital:** NY-Presby Hosp - Columbia Presby Med Ctr (page 103); **Address:** Columbia University, MHB-7SK, 177 Fort Washington Ave, New York, NY 10032; **Phone:** 212-342-6042; **Board Cert:** Surgery 96; **Med School:** Loyola Univ-Stritch Sch Med 86; **Resid:** Surgery, Boston Univ Hosp 95; **Fellow:** Surgical Oncology, Natl Cancer Inst 96; **Fac Appt:** Assoc Prof S, Columbia P&S

Kraybill Jr, William G MD **[S]** - **Spec Exp:** Sarcoma-Soft Tissue; Melanoma; Skin Cancer-Advanced; **Hospital:** Roswell Park Cancer Inst (page 107); **Address:** Roswell Park Cancer Inst, Dept Surgical Oncology, Elm & Carlton Sts, Buffalo, NY 14263; **Phone:** 716-845-3284; **Board Cert:** Surgery 95; **Med School:** Univ Cincinnati 69; **Resid:** Surgery, Univ Oregon Hlth Sci Ctr 78; **Fellow:** Surgical Oncology, Meml Sloan Kettering Cancer Ctr 80; **Fac Appt:** Prof S, SUNY Buffalo

Lee, Kenneth KW MD **[S]** - **Spec Exp:** Pancreatic Cancer & Surgery; Gastrointestinal Cancer & Surgery; **Hospital:** UPMC Presby, Pittsburgh (page 114); **Address:** Univ Pittsburgh, 497 Scaife Hall, Pittsburgh, PA 15261; **Phone:** 412-647-0457; **Board Cert:** Surgery 98; **Med School:** Univ Chicago-Pritzker Sch Med 81; **Resid:** Surgery, Univ Chicago Hosps 88; **Fac Appt:** Assoc Prof S, Univ Pittsburgh

Leffall Jr, LaSalle D MD **[S]** - **Spec Exp:** Breast Cancer; Head & Neck Surgery; **Hospital:** Howard Univ Hosp; **Address:** 2041 Georgia Ave NW, Ste 4000, Washington, DC 20060; **Phone:** 202-865-6237; **Board Cert:** Surgery 58; **Med School:** Howard Univ 52; **Resid:** Surgery, Freedmens Hosp 56; Surgery, DC Genl Hosp 55; **Fellow:** Surgery, New York Meml Hosp Ctr 59; **Fac Appt:** Prof S, Howard Univ

Libutti, Steven K MD **[S]** - **Spec Exp:** Liver Cancer; Pancreatic & Gastrointestinal Cancer; Endocrine Tumors; **Hospital:** Natl Inst of Hlth - Clin Ctr; **Address:** National Cancer Institute, Surgery Branch, Bldg 10, 10 Center Drive, rm 2B07, Bethesda, MD 20892; **Phone:** 301-496-5049; **Board Cert:** Surgery 96; **Med School:** Columbia P&S 90; **Resid:** Surgery, Columbia Presby Med Ctr 95; **Fellow:** Surgical Oncology, Natl Cancer Inst 96

Lotze, Michael T MD/PhD [S] - Spec Exp: Melanoma; Gene Therapy; Immunotherapy & Cytokine Biology; **Hospital:** UPMC Presby, Pittsburgh (page 114); **Address:** Center for Biotechnology & Bioengineering, 300 Technology Drive, Pittsburgh, PA 15219; **Phone:** 412-624-8121; **Board Cert:** Surgery 83; **Med School:** Northwestern Univ 74; **Resid:** Surgery, Strong Meml Hosp 77; **Fellow:** Surgical Oncology, Natl Cancer Institute 80; **Fac Appt:** Prof S, Univ Pittsburgh

Marsh Jr, James Wallis MD [S] - Spec Exp: Transplant-Liver; Liver Cancer; **Hospital:** UPMC Presby, Pittsburgh (page 114); **Address:** UPMC Liver Cancer Ctr, 3459 Fifth Ave 7 South, Pittsburgh, PA 15213; **Phone:** 412-692-2001; **Board Cert:** Sports Medicine 03; **Med School:** Univ Ark 79; **Resid:** Surgery, St Paul Hosp 84; **Fellow:** Transplant Surgery, Mayo Clinic 85; Transplant Surgery, Univ Pittsburgh Hosps 86; **Fac Appt:** Assoc Prof S, Univ Pittsburgh

Michelassi, Fabrizio MD [S] - Spec Exp: Stomach Cancer; Inflammatory Bowel Disease/Crohn's; Pancreatic Cancer; **Hospital:** NY-Presby Hosp - NY Weill Cornell Med Ctr (page 103); **Address:** Weill Med Ctr, 525 E 68 St, Rm E739, New York, NY 10021; **Phone:** 212-746-6006; **Board Cert:** Surgery 02; **Med School:** Italy 75; **Resid:** Surgery, NYU Med Ctr 84; **Fellow:** Research, Mass Genl Hosp 83; **Fac Appt:** Prof S, Cornell Univ-Weill Med Coll

Morrow, Monica MD [S] - Spec Exp: Breast Cancer; **Hospital:** Fox Chase Cancer Ctr (page 95); **Address:** Fox Chase Cancer Ctr, Dept Surgical Oncology, 333 Cottman Ave, Philadelphia, PA 19111-2497; **Phone:** 215-728-3096; **Board Cert:** Surgery 01; **Med School:** Jefferson Med Coll 76; **Resid:** Surgery, Med Ctr Hosp Vermont 81; **Fellow:** Surgical Oncology, Meml Sloan Kettering Cancer Ctr 83; **Fac Appt:** Prof S, Temple Univ

Nava-Villarreal, Hector MD [S] - Spec Exp: Esophageal Cancer; Stomach Cancer; Barrett's Esophagus; **Hospital:** Roswell Park Cancer Inst (page 107); **Address:** Roswell Park Cancer Inst, Elm & Carlton Sts, Buffalo, NY 14263; **Phone:** 716-845-5915; **Board Cert:** Surgery 01; **Med School:** Mexico 67; **Resid:** Surgery, Buffalo Genl Hosp 74; **Fellow:** Surgical Oncology, Roswell Park Cancer Inst 76; **Fac Appt:** Assoc Prof S, SUNY Buffalo

Numann, Patricia MD [S] - Spec Exp: Breast Cancer; Thyroid Surgery; **Hospital:** Univ. Hosp.-SUNY Upstate; **Address:** SUNY Hlth Sci Ctr, Dept Surg, 750 E Adams Street, rm 8140, Syracuse, NY 13210; **Phone:** 315-464-4603; **Board Cert:** Surgery 94; **Med School:** SUNY Upstate Med Univ 65; **Resid:** Surgery, SUNY Upstate Med Ctr 70; **Fac Appt:** Prof S, SUNY Upstate Med Univ

O'Hea, Brian MD [S] - Spec Exp: Breast Cancer; Sentinel Node Surgery; **Hospital:** Stony Brook Univ Hosp; **Address:** SUNY Stony Brook, Dept Surg, HSC T-18, Rm 060, Stony Brook, NY 11794-8191; **Phone:** 631-444-1795; **Board Cert:** Surgery 92; **Med School:** Georgetown Univ 86; **Resid:** Surgery, St Vincent Hosp 91; **Fellow:** Breast Disease, Meml Sloan-Kettering Cancer Ctr 96; **Fac Appt:** Asst Prof S, SUNY Stony Brook

Osborne, Michael P MD [S] - Spec Exp: Breast Cancer; Breast Cancer-High Risk Women; **Hospital:** NY-Presby Hosp - NY Weill Cornell Med Ctr (page 103); **Address:** 425 E 61 St Fl 8, New York, NY 10021-8722; **Phone:** 212-821-0828; **Med School:** England 70; **Resid:** Surgery, Charing Cross Hosp 77; Surgery, Royal Marsden Hosp 80; **Fellow:** Surgical Oncology, Meml Sloan-Kettering Canc Ctr 81; **Fac Appt:** Prof S, Cornell Univ-Weill Med Coll

Petrelli, Nicholas J MD [S] - Spec Exp: Cancer Surgery; Gastrointestinal Cancer; **Hospital:** Christiana Care Hlth Svs; **Address:** Helen F Graham Cancer Ctr, 4701 Ogletown-Stanton Rd, Ste 1213, Newark, DE 19713; **Phone:** 302-623-4550; **Board Cert:** Surgery 97; **Med School:** Tulane Univ 73; **Resid:** Surgery, St Mary's Hosp-Med Ctr 78; **Fellow:** Surgical Oncology, Roswell Park Cancer Inst 80; **Fac Appt:** Prof S, Thomas Jefferson Univ

Ridge, John A MD/PhD **[S]** - **Spec Exp:** Head & Neck Cancer & Surgery; Thyroid & Parathyroid Cancer & Tumors; Adrenal Tumors; **Hospital:** Fox Chase Cancer Ctr (page 95); **Address:** Fox Chase Cancer Center, Dept Surgical Oncology, 7701 Burholme Ave, Philadelphia, PA 19111; **Phone:** 215-728-3517; **Board Cert:** Surgery 97; **Med School:** Stanford Univ 81; **Resid:** Surgery, Univ Colorado Med Ctr 87; **Fellow:** Surgical Oncology, Meml Sloan-Kettering Cancer Ctr 89

Roh, Mark S MD **[S]** - **Spec Exp:** Liver Cancer; **Hospital:** Allegheny General Hosp; **Address:** Allegheny General Hospital, Dept Surgery, 320 E North Ave, Pittsburgh, PA 15212; **Phone:** 412-359-6738; **Board Cert:** Surgery 96; **Med School:** Ohio State Univ 79; **Resid:** Surgery, Univ of Pitt Med Ctr 86; **Fellow:** Surgical Oncology, Meml Sloan-Kettering Cancer Ctr 87; **Fac Appt:** Prof S, Drexel Univ Coll Med

Rosato, Ernest F MD **[S]** - **Spec Exp:** Gastrointestinal Cancer & Surgery; Esophageal Cancer; Pancreatic Cancer; **Hospital:** Hosp Univ Penn - UPHS (page 113); **Address:** Hosp Univ Penn, Dept Surg, 3400 Spruce St, 4 Silverstein, Philadelphia, PA 19104; **Phone:** 215-662-2033; **Board Cert:** Surgery 69; **Med School:** Univ Pennsylvania 62; **Resid:** Surgery, Hosp Univ Penn 68; **Fac Appt:** Prof S, Univ Pennsylvania

Rosenberg, Steven MD **[S]** - **Spec Exp:** Melanoma; Kidney Cancer; **Hospital:** Natl Inst of Hlth - Clin Ctr; **Address:** National Cancer Institute, 9000 Rockville Pike Bldg 10 - rm 2-B-42, Bethesda, MD 20892; **Phone:** 301-496-4164; **Board Cert:** Surgery 75; **Med School:** Jefferson Med Coll 64; **Resid:** Surgery, Peter Bent Brigham Hosp 74

Roses, Daniel F MD **[S]** - **Spec Exp:** Breast Cancer; Melanoma; Thyroid & Parathyroid Cancer & Surgery; **Hospital:** NYU Med Ctr (page 104); **Address:** 530 First Ave, Ste 6E, New York, NY 10016-6402; **Phone:** 212-263-7329; **Board Cert:** Surgery 75; **Med School:** NYU Sch Med 69; **Resid:** Surgery, NYU-Bellevue Hosp 74; **Fellow:** Surgical Oncology, NYU-Bellevue Hosp 78; **Fac Appt:** Prof Surg & Onc, NYU Sch Med

Schnabel, Freya MD **[S]** - **Spec Exp:** Breast Cancer; Breast Cancer-High Risk Women; **Hospital:** NY-Presby Hosp - Columbia Presby Med Ctr (page 103); **Address:** 161 Fort Washington Ave, Ste 1011, New York, NY 10032; **Phone:** 212-305-1534; **Board Cert:** Surgery 98; **Med School:** NYU Sch Med 82; **Resid:** Surgery, NYU Med Ctr 87; **Fellow:** Research, SUNY Hlth Sci Ctr 88; **Fac Appt:** Assoc Clin Prof S, Columbia P&S

Schraut, Wolfgang H MD **[S]** - **Spec Exp:** Inflammatory Bowel Disease; Gastrointestinal Surgery; Colon & Rectal Cancer & Surgery; **Hospital:** UPMC Presby, Pittsburgh (page 114); **Address:** Univ Pittsburgh Medical Ctr, Dept Surgery, 497 Scaife Hall, Pittsburgh, PA 15261; **Phone:** 412-647-0311; **Board Cert:** Surgery 99; **Med School:** Germany 70; **Resid:** Surgery, Univ Chicago Hosps 78; **Fac Appt:** Prof S, Univ Pittsburgh

Schwartz, Gordon F MD **[S]** - **Spec Exp:** Breast Cancer; Cancer Surgery; **Hospital:** Thomas Jefferson Univ Hosp (page 110); **Address:** 1015 Chestnut St, Ste 510, Philadelphia, PA 19107-4305; **Phone:** 215-627-8487; **Board Cert:** Surgery 70; **Med School:** Harvard Med Sch 60; **Resid:** Surgery, Columbia-Presby Med Ctr 68; **Fellow:** Oncology, Univ Penn 69; **Fac Appt:** Prof S, Jefferson Med Coll

Shah, Jatin P MD **[S]** - **Spec Exp:** Head & Neck Cancer; Thyroid Cancer; Skull Base Tumors; **Hospital:** Meml Sloan Kettering Cancer Ctr (page 100); **Address:** 1275 York Ave, Ste C1061, New York, NY 10021-6007; **Phone:** 212-639-7604; **Board Cert:** Surgery 75; **Med School:** India 64; **Resid:** Surgery, SSG Hosp 67; Surgery, New York Infirm 74; **Fellow:** Head & Neck Surgical Oncology, Meml Sloan-Kettering Hosp 72; **Fac Appt:** Prof S, Cornell Univ-Weill Med Coll

Shaha, Ashok MD [S] - **Spec Exp:** Head & Neck Cancer; Thyroid Cancer & Surgery; Parathyroid Surgery; **Hospital:** Meml Sloan Kettering Cancer Ctr (page 100); **Address:** 1275 York Ave, New York, NY 10021-6007; **Phone:** 212-639-7649; **Board Cert:** Surgery 92; **Med School:** India 70; **Resid:** Surgery, Downstate Med Ctr 81; **Fellow:** Surgical Oncology, Meml Sloan Kettering Cancer Ctr 76; Head and Neck Surgery, Meml Sloan Kettering Cancer Ctr 82; **Fac Appt:** Prof S, Cornell Univ-Weill Med Coll

Sigurdson, Elin Ruth MD [S] - **Spec Exp:** Breast Cancer; Colon & Rectal Cancer; Melanoma; **Hospital:** Fox Chase Cancer Ctr (page 95); **Address:** 7701 Burholme Ave, Philadelphia, PA 19111-2412; **Phone:** 215-728-3519; **Board Cert:** Surgery 97; **Med School:** Canada 80; **Resid:** Surgery, Univ Toronto Med Ctr 84; **Fellow:** Surgical Oncology, Meml Sloan-Kettering Cancer Ctr 87; **Fac Appt:** Assoc Prof S

Singer, Samuel MD [S] - **Spec Exp:** Sarcoma-Soft Tissue; **Hospital:** Meml Sloan Kettering Cancer Ctr (page 100); **Address:** Meml Sloan Kettering Cancer Ctr, 1275 York Ave, rm 1210, New York, NY 10021; **Phone:** 212-639-2940; **Board Cert:** Surgery 98; **Med School:** Harvard Med Sch 82; **Resid:** Surgery, Brigham & Women's Hosp 88; **Fellow:** Surgical Oncology, Dana Farber Cancer Inst 90; **Fac Appt:** Assoc Prof S, Cornell Univ-Weill Med Coll

Skinner, Kristin A MD [S] - **Spec Exp:** Breast Cancer; Gastrointestinal Cancer; Melanoma; **Hospital:** NYU Med Ctr (page 104); **Address:** NYU Clinical Cancer, 160 E 35th St Fl 3, New York, NY 10016; **Phone:** 212-731-5367; **Board Cert:** Surgery 96; **Med School:** Johns Hopkins Univ 88; **Resid:** Surgery, UCLA Med Ctr 95; **Fellow:** Surgical Oncology, UCLA Med Ctr 94; **Fac Appt:** Assoc Prof S, NYU Sch Med

Sugarbaker, Paul H MD [S] - **Spec Exp:** Peritoneal Carcinomatosis; Cystadenocarcinoma; Ovarian Cancer; **Hospital:** Washington Hosp Ctr; **Address:** Washington Hosp Ctr, 106 Irving St NW, Ste 3900N, Washington, DC 20010; **Phone:** 202-877-3908; **Board Cert:** Surgery 73; **Med School:** Cornell Univ-Weill Med Coll 67; **Resid:** Surgery, Peter Bent Brigham Hosp 73; **Fellow:** Surgery, Mass Genl Hosp 76; **Fac Appt:** Prof S, Univ Wash

Tartter, Paul MD [S] - **Spec Exp:** Breast Cancer; Breast Cancer in Elderly; Sentinel Node Surgery; **Hospital:** St Luke's - Roosevelt Hosp Ctr - Roosevelt Div (page 93); **Address:** 425 W 59th St, Ste 7A, New York, NY 10019; **Phone:** 212-523-7500; **Board Cert:** Surgery 91; **Med School:** Brown Univ 77; **Resid:** Surgery, Mount Sinai Hosp 82; **Fac Appt:** Assoc Prof S, Columbia P&S

Tsangaris, Theodore N MD [S] - **Spec Exp:** Breast Cancer; **Hospital:** Johns Hopkins Hosp - Baltimore (page 97); **Address:** Breast Center, Johns Hopkins Hospital, 600 N Wolfe St, Baltimore, MD 21287; **Phone:** 410-955-2615; **Board Cert:** Surgery 91; **Med School:** Geo Wash Univ 83; **Resid:** Surgery, George Washington Univ Med Ctr 89; **Fellow:** Surgical Oncology, Baylor Univ Med Ctr 90; **Fac Appt:** Assoc Prof S, Johns Hopkins Univ

Weigel, Ronald J MD/PhD [S] - **Spec Exp:** Breast Cancer; **Hospital:** Thomas Jefferson Univ Hosp (page 110); **Address:** 1025 Walnut St, Ste 605, Philadelphia, PA 19107; **Phone:** 215-955-0526; **Board Cert:** Surgery 01; **Med School:** Yale Univ 86; **Resid:** Surgery, Duke Univ Med Ctr 92; **Fellow:** Immunology, Duke Univ Med Ctr; **Fac Appt:** Prof S, Jefferson Med Coll

Yang, James C MD [S] - **Spec Exp:** Kidney Cancer; Kidney Cancer Clinical Trials; Immunotherapy; **Hospital:** Natl Inst of Hlth - Clin Ctr; **Address:** National Cancer Institute, CRC Bldg, Rm 35952, 9000 Rockville Pike, Bethesda, MD 20892; **Phone:** 301-496-2132; **Board Cert:** Surgery 95; **Med School:** UCSD 78; **Resid:** Surgery, UCSD Med Ctr 84; **Fellow:** Surgical Oncology, Natl Cancer Inst 86

Southeast

Balch, Charles MD [S] - **Spec Exp:** Sentinel Node Surgery; Melanoma; Cancer Surgery; **Hospital:** Johns Hopkins Hosp - Baltimore (page 97); **Address:** 1900 Duke St, Ste 200, Alexandria, VA 22314; **Phone:** 410-614-1022; **Board Cert:** Surgery 97; **Med School:** Columbia P&S 67; **Resid:** Surgery, Univ Alabama Med Ctr 71; Surgery, Univ Alabama Med Ctr 75; **Fellow:** Immunology, Scripps Clin-Rsch Fdn 73; **Fac Appt:** Prof Surg & Onc, Johns Hopkins Univ

Beauchamp, Robert D MD [S] - **Spec Exp:** Breast Cancer; Colon & Rectal Cancer; Pancreatic Cancer; **Hospital:** Vanderbilt Univ Med Ctr (page 116); **Address:** Medical Center North, rm D4316, 1161 21St Ave S, Nashville, TN 37232-2730; **Phone:** 615-322-2363; **Board Cert:** Surgery 97; Surgical Critical Care 93; **Med School:** Univ Tex Med Br, Galveston 82; **Resid:** Surgery, Univ Tex Med Br 87; **Fellow:** Cellular Molecular Biology, Vanderbilt Univ 89; **Fac Appt:** Prof S, Vanderbilt Univ

Behrns, Kevin E MD [S] - **Spec Exp:** Pancreatic Cancer; **Hospital:** Univ NC Hosps (page 112); **Address:** Univ North Carolina, Div GI Surgery, 320 Med Wing E Campus Box 7081, Chapel Hill, NC 27599-7210; **Phone:** 919-966-8436; **Board Cert:** Surgery 96; **Med School:** Mayo Med Sch 88; **Resid:** Surgery, Mayo Clinic 95; **Fac Appt:** Assoc Prof S, Univ NC Sch Med

Bland, Kirby MD [S] - **Spec Exp:** Breast Cancer; Colon Cancer; Thyroid & Parathyroid Surgery; **Hospital:** Univ of Ala Hosp at Birmingham; **Address:** University of Alabama, Dept Surgery, 2000 6th Ave S, Birmingham, AL 35233; **Phone:** 205-975-2193; **Board Cert:** Surgery 00; **Med School:** Univ Ala 68; **Resid:** Surgery, Univ Fla Hosp 70; Surgery, Univ Fla Hosp 76; **Fellow:** Surgical Oncology, Univ Tex/Anderson Hosp 77; **Fac Appt:** Prof S, Univ Ala

Calvo, Benjamin MD [S] - **Spec Exp:** Pancreatic Cancer; Endocrine Cancer; Breast Cancer; **Hospital:** Univ NC Hosps (page 112); **Address:** Dept Surg CB 7213, Chapel Hill, NC 27599; **Phone:** 919-966-5221; **Board Cert:** Surgery 99; **Med School:** Univ MD Sch Med 81; **Resid:** Surgery, G Washington Univ Hosp 88; Surgery, Natl Inst Hlth 91; **Fellow:** Surgery, Meml Sloan Kettering Cancer Ctr 93; **Fac Appt:** Assoc Prof S, Univ NC Sch Med

Cance, William George MD [S] - **Spec Exp:** Pancreatic Cancer; Colon & Rectal Cancer; Endocrine Cancer; **Hospital:** Shands Hlthcre at Univ of FL (page 109); **Address:** Shands at the University of Florida, PO Box 100286, 1600 SW Archer Rd, Gainesville, FL 32610-0286; **Phone:** 352-265-0622; **Board Cert:** Surgery 98; **Med School:** Duke Univ 82; **Resid:** Surgery, Barnes Hosp-Wash Univ 88; **Fellow:** Surgical Oncology, Meml Sloan Kettering Canc Ctr 90; **Fac Appt:** Assoc Prof S, Univ NC Sch Med

Carey, Larry C MD [S] - **Spec Exp:** Pancreatic Cancer; Biliary Cancer; **Hospital:** Tampa Genl Hosp; **Address:** 4 Columbia Drive, Box 650, Tampa, FL 33606; **Phone:** 813-259-0935; **Board Cert:** Surgery 65; Critical Care Medicine 87; **Med School:** Ohio State Univ 59; **Resid:** Surgery, Milwaukee Co Genl Hosp 65; **Fac Appt:** Prof S, Univ S Fla Coll Med

Chari, Ravi S MD [S] - **Spec Exp:** Liver Cancer; Biliary Cancer; Transplant-Liver; **Hospital:** Vanderbilt Univ Med Ctr (page 116); **Address:** Vanderbilt Univ Med Ctr-Div Hepatobillary Surgery, 1313 21st Ave S, Ste 801 Oxford House, Nashville, TN 37232-4753; **Phone:** 615-936-2573; **Board Cert:** Surgery 97; **Med School:** Canada 89; **Resid:** Surgery, Duke Univ Med Ctr 96; **Fellow:** Transplant Surgery, Univ Toronto-Toronto Hosp 98; **Fac Appt:** Assoc Prof S, Vanderbilt Univ

Copeland III, Edward M MD [S] - **Spec Exp:** Breast Cancer; Colon & Rectal Cancer; Melanoma; **Hospital:** Shands Hlthcre at Univ of FL (page 109); **Address:** Univ Florida Coll Medicine, Dept Surgery, 1600 SW Archer Rd, Box 100286, Gainesville, FL 32610; **Phone:** 352-265-0378; **Board Cert:** Surgery 71; **Med School:** Cornell Univ-Weill Med Coll 63; **Resid:** Surgery, Hosp Univ Penn 69; Surgical Oncology, Univ TX MD Anderson Cancer Ctr 72; **Fellow:** Research, HospUniv Penn 67; **Fac Appt:** Prof S, Univ Fla Coll Med

Flynn, Michael B MD [S] - **Spec Exp:** Head & Neck Cancer; Head & Neck Surgery; **Hospital:** Univ of Louisville Hosp; **Address:** Univ Surgical Assoc - Children's Hospital Fdn Bldg, 601 S Floyd St, Ste 700, Louisville, KY 40202-1845; **Phone:** 502-583-8303; **Board Cert:** Surgery 72; **Med School:** Ireland 62; **Resid:** Surgery, Univ Maryland Hosp 69; **Fellow:** Surgical Oncology, MD Anderson Hosp 71; **Fac Appt:** Prof S, Univ Louisville Sch Med

Hanks, John B MD [S] - **Spec Exp:** Endocrine Cancer & Surgery; Breast Cancer & Surgery; Thyroid Cancer & Surgery; **Hospital:** Univ Virginia Med Ctr; **Address:** Univ VA Hlth Sys, Dept Surg, PO Box 800709, Charlottesville, VA 22908-0709; **Phone:** 434-924-0376; **Board Cert:** Surgery 01; **Med School:** Univ Rochester 73; **Resid:** Surgery, Duke Univ Med Ctr 82; **Fac Appt:** Prof S, Univ VA Sch Med

Hemming, Alan W MD [S] - **Spec Exp:** Liver & Pancreatic Cancer; Transplant-Liver; Hepatobiliary Surgery; **Hospital:** Shands Hlthcre at Univ of FL (page 109); **Address:** University of Florida, Dept Surgery, 1600 SW Archer Rd, rm 6142, Box 100286, Gainsville, FL 32610; **Phone:** 352-265-0606; **Board Cert:** Surgery 04; **Med School:** Canada 87; **Resid:** Surgery, Univ British Columbia Med Ctr 93; **Fellow:** Transplant Surgery, Univ of Toronto/Hosp for Sick Children 95; Hepatobiliary Surgery, Univ of Toronto 96; **Fac Appt:** Assoc Prof S, Univ Fla Coll Med

Herrmann, Virginia M MD [S] - **Spec Exp:** Breast Cancer; Endocrine Cancers; **Hospital:** Meml Med Ctr - Savannah; **Address:** Center for Breast Care, 4700 Waters Ave, Ste 405, Savannah, GA 31404; **Phone:** 912-350-2700; **Board Cert:** Surgery 00; Surgical Critical Care 91; **Med School:** St Louis Univ 74; **Resid:** Surgery, St Louis U Hosps 79; **Fellow:** Surgery, Harvard-Brigham Hosp 80; **Fac Appt:** Prof S, Med Coll GA

Hinder, Ronald A MD [S] - **Spec Exp:** Gastroesophageal Reflux Disease (GERD); Endoscopic Surgery; Gastrointestinal Cancer; **Hospital:** St Luke's Hosp - Jacksonville; **Address:** Mayo Clinic - General Surgery, 4500 San Pablo Rd, Jacksonville, FL 32224; **Phone:** 904-953-2523; **Med School:** South Africa 65; **Resid:** Surgery, Johannesberg Hosp 72; **Fellow:** Gastrointestinal Surgery, Mayo Clinic 78; **Fac Appt:** Prof S, Mayo Med Sch

Israel, Philip Z MD [S] - **Spec Exp:** Breast Cancer; **Hospital:** WellStar Kennestone Hosp; **Address:** 702 Canton Rd, Marietta, GA 30060; **Phone:** 770-428-4486; **Board Cert:** Surgery 67; **Med School:** Emory Univ 61; **Resid:** Surgery, Emory Univ Hosp 66; **Fac Appt:** Prof S, Univ Tenn Coll Med,Chattanooga

Kelley, Mark C MD [S] - **Spec Exp:** Breast Cancer; Melanoma; **Hospital:** Vanderbilt Univ Med Ctr (page 116); **Address:** Vanderbilt Univ Med Ctr, Div Surg Oncology, 2220 Pierce Ave, 597 Preston Rsch Bldg, Nashville, TN 37232; **Phone:** 615-322-2391; **Board Cert:** Surgery 96; **Med School:** Univ Fla Coll Med 89; **Resid:** Surgery, Univ Fla-Shands Hosp 95; **Fellow:** Surgical Oncology, John Wayne Cancer Inst-St Johns Hosp 97

Leight, George MD [S] - **Spec Exp:** Breast Cancer; Thyroid Cancer; Parathyroid Cancer & Surgery; **Hospital:** Duke Univ Med Ctr (page 94); **Address:** Duke Univ Med Ctr, Dept Surg, DUMC 3513, Durham, NC 27710; **Phone:** 919-684-6849; **Board Cert:** Surgery 99; **Med School:** Duke Univ 72; **Resid:** Surgery, Duke Univ Med Ctr 78; **Fac Appt:** Prof S, Duke Univ

Levine, Edward A MD [S] - **Spec Exp:** Mesothelioma; Esophageal Cancer; Peritoneal Carcinomatosis; **Hospital:** Wake Forest Univ Baptist Med Ctr (page 117); **Address:** Wake Forest Univ Baptist Med Ctr, Dept Surg, Medical Center Blvd, Winston-Salem, NC 27157; **Phone:** 336-716-4276; **Board Cert:** Surgery 99; **Med School:** Univ Hlth Sci/Chicago Med Sch 85; **Resid:** Surgery, Michael Reese Hosp 90; **Fellow:** Surgical Oncology, Univ Illinois 92; **Fac Appt:** Prof S, Wake Forest Univ

Lyerly, H Kim MD [S] - **Spec Exp:** Breast Cancer; Cancer Immune Therapy; **Hospital:** Duke Univ Med Ctr (page 94); **Address:** Duke Univ Med Ctr, Box 3843, Durham, NC 27710; **Phone:** 919-681-8350; **Board Cert:** Surgery 01; **Med School:** UCLA 83; **Resid:** Surgery, Duke Univ Med Ctr 90; **Fac Appt:** Prof S, Duke Univ

McGrath, Patrick C MD [S] - **Spec Exp:** Breast Cancer; Cancer Surgery; **Hospital:** Univ Kentucky Med Ctr; **Address:** Univ Kentucky Med Ctr, Dept Surgery, 800 Rose St, rm C212, Lexington, KY 40536-0293; **Phone:** 859-323-6346; **Board Cert:** Surgery 96; **Med School:** Univ IL Coll Med 80; **Resid:** Surgery, Med Coll Virginia 86; **Fellow:** Surgical Oncology, Med Coll Virginia 88; **Fac Appt:** Prof S, Univ KY Coll Med

McMasters, Kelly M MD [S] - **Spec Exp:** Melanoma; Breast Cancer; Liver Cancer; **Hospital:** Univ of Louisville Hosp; **Address:** Univ Surgical Associates, 601 S. Floyd St. Ste 700, Louisville, KY 40202; **Phone:** 502-583-8303; **Board Cert:** Surgery 95; **Med School:** UMDNJ-RW Johnson Med Sch ; **Resid:** Surgery, Univ Louisville Sch Med 94; **Fellow:** Surgical Oncology, Texas-MD Anderson Cancer Ctr 95; **Fac Appt:** Prof S, Univ Louisville Sch Med

Neifeld, James MD [S] - **Spec Exp:** Melanoma; Head & Neck Cancer; Gastrointestinal Cancer; **Hospital:** Med Coll of VA Hosp; **Address:** Medical College of Virginia Hospital, PO Box 980645, Richmond, VA 23298-0645; **Phone:** 804-828-9325; **Board Cert:** Surgery 98; **Med School:** Med Coll VA 72; **Resid:** Surgery, Med Coll VA Hosp 78; **Fac Appt:** Prof S, Med Coll VA

Pappas, Theodore N MD [S] - **Spec Exp:** Pancreatic Surgery; **Hospital:** Duke Univ Med Ctr (page 94); **Address:** Duke Univ Med Ctr, Box 3479, Durham, NC 27710-0001; **Phone:** 919-681-3442; **Board Cert:** Surgery 97; **Med School:** Ohio State Univ 81; **Resid:** Surgery, Brigham & Womens Hosp 88; **Fellow:** Gastroenterology, Wadworth VA Med Ctr 85; **Fac Appt:** Prof S, Duke Univ

Pinson, C Wright MD [S] - **Spec Exp:** Transplant- Liver; Liver & Billary Cancer & Surgery; Pancreatic Cancer & Surgery; **Hospital:** Vanderbilt Univ Med Ctr (page 116); **Address:** Vanderbilt Transplant Ctr, TVC 3810A, 1312 21st Ave S, Nashville, TN 37232-5545; **Phone:** 615-343-9324; **Board Cert:** Surgery 96; Surgical Critical Care 97; **Med School:** Vanderbilt Univ 80; **Resid:** Surgery, Oregon Health Sci Ctr 86; **Fellow:** Gastrointestinal Surgery, Lahey Clinic 87; Transplant Surgery, Deaconess Hosp 88; **Fac Appt:** Prof S, Vanderbilt Univ

Polk Jr, Hiram C MD [S] - **Spec Exp:** Melanoma; Colon Cancer; **Hospital:** Univ of Louisville Hosp; **Address:** 601 S Floyd St, Ste 700, Louisville, KY 40292-0001; **Phone:** 502-583-8303; **Board Cert:** Surgery 66; **Med School:** Harvard Med Sch 60; **Resid:** Surgery, Barnes Hosp 65; **Fac Appt:** Prof S, Univ Louisville Sch Med

Reintgen, Douglas Scott MD [S] - **Spec Exp:** Melanoma-Sentinel Node; Breast Cancer-Sentinel Node; Cancer Surgery; **Hospital:** Lakeland Regl Med Ctr; **Address:** 3525 Lakeland Hills Blvd, Lakeland, FL 33805; **Phone:** 863-603-6565; **Board Cert:** Surgery 97; **Med School:** Duke Univ 79; **Resid:** Surgery, Duke Univ Med Ctr 87; **Fac Appt:** Prof S, Univ S Fla Coll Med

Robinson, David S MD [S] - **Spec Exp:** Breast Cancer; Head & Neck Cancer; Gastrointestinal Cancer; **Hospital:** University Hosp and Med Ctr -Tamarac; **Address:** 1283 University Drive, Coral Springs, FL 33071; **Phone:** 954-345-2718; **Board Cert:** Surgery 93; **Med School:** Univ Kans 72; **Resid:** Surgery, Univ Va Med Ctr 74; Surgery, Univ Va Med Ctr 78; **Fellow:** Oncology Research, UCLA Med Ctr 77; Surgical Oncology, Meml Sloan-Kettering Cancer Ctr 82

Rosemurgy, Alexander S MD [S] - **Spec Exp:** Pancreatic Cancer; Gastrointestinal Surgery; **Hospital:** Tampa Genl Hosp; **Address:** Digestive Disorders Ctr at Tampa General Hospital, 2 Columbia Drive, Box 1289, Tampa, FL 33601; **Phone:** 813-844-7393; **Board Cert:** Surgery 95; Surgical Critical Care 03; **Med School:** Univ Mich Med Sch 79; **Resid:** Surgery, Univ Chicago 84; **Fac Appt:** Prof S, Univ S Fla Coll Med

Sondak, Vernon K MD [S] - **Spec Exp:** Cancer Surgery; Melanoma; Sarcoma; **Hospital:** H Lee Moffitt Cancer Ctr & Research Inst; **Address:** MCC Cutaneous Prog- # 3057, 12902 Magnolia Drive, Tampa, FL 33612; **Phone:** 813-745-1968; **Board Cert:** Surgery 96; **Med School:** Boston Univ 80; **Resid:** Surgery, UCLA Med Ctr 87; **Fellow:** Surgical Oncology, UCLA Med Ctr 84; **Fac Appt:** Prof S, Univ Fla Coll Med

Urist, Marshall M MD [S] - **Spec Exp:** Cancer Surgery; Breast Cancer; Melanoma; **Hospital:** Univ of Ala Hosp at Birmingham; **Address:** Univ Alabama Sch Med, Dept Surgery, 1922 7th Ave S, Kracke Bldg, Ste 321, Birmingham, AL 35294; **Phone:** 205-934-3065; **Board Cert:** Surgery 00; **Med School:** Univ Chicago-Pritzker Sch Med 71; **Resid:** Surgery, Johns Hopkins Hosp 78; **Fellow:** Surgical Oncology, Johns Hopkins Hosp 76; **Fac Appt:** Prof S, Univ Ala

Vickers, Selwyn M MD [S] - **Spec Exp:** Pancreatic Cancer; Liver Tumors; Gastrointestinal Surgery; **Hospital:** Univ of Ala Hosp at Birmingham; **Address:** University of Alabama, 406 Kracke Bldg, 1922 7th Ave S, Birmingham, AL 35294; **Phone:** 205-975-8710; **Board Cert:** Surgery 03; **Med School:** Johns Hopkins Univ 86; **Resid:** Surgery, Johns Hopkins Hosp 92; **Fellow:** Surgical Oncology, Johns Hopkins 93; **Fac Appt:** Prof S, Johns Hopkins Univ

Vogel, Stephen Burton MD [S] - **Spec Exp:** Esophageal Cancer; Liver Cancer; **Hospital:** Shands Hlthcre at Univ of FL (page 109); **Address:** University of Florida, Dept Surgery, PO Box 100286, Gainesville, FL 32610-0286; **Phone:** 352-265-0604; **Board Cert:** Surgery 76; **Med School:** Univ Fla Coll Med 67; **Resid:** Surgery, Univ Minn Hosp 75; **Fac Appt:** Prof S, Univ Fla Coll Med

Willis, Irvin MD [S] - **Spec Exp:** Pancreatic Surgery; Cancer Surgery; Laparoscopic Surgery; **Hospital:** Mount Sinai Med Ctr - Miami; **Address:** 4302 Alton Rd, Ste 630, Miami Beach, FL 33140-2876; **Phone:** 305-534-6050; **Board Cert:** Surgery 70; **Med School:** Univ Cincinnati 64; **Resid:** Surgery, Univ Miami-Jackson Meml 69

Wood, William C MD [S] - **Spec Exp:** Breast Cancer; **Hospital:** Emory Univ Hosp; **Address:** Emory Univ Hosp, Dept Surgery, 1364 Clifton Rd NE, Ste B206, Atlanta, GA 30322; **Phone:** 404-727-5800; **Board Cert:** Surgery 74; **Med School:** Harvard Med Sch 66; **Resid:** Surgery, Mass Genl Hosp 73; **Fac Appt:** Prof S, Emory Univ

Yeatman, Timothy MD [S] - **Spec Exp:** Colon Cancer; Gastrointestinal Cancer; **Hospital:** H Lee Moffitt Cancer Ctr & Research Inst; **Address:** 12902 Magnolia, Tampa, FL 33612-9416; **Phone:** 813-979-7292; **Board Cert:** Surgery 00; **Med School:** Emory Univ 84; **Resid:** Surgery, Univ Florida 90; **Fellow:** Surgical Oncology, MD Anderson Cancer Ctr 92; **Fac Appt:** Prof S, Univ S Fla Coll Med

Midwest

Aranha, Gerard MD [S] - **Spec Exp:** Pancreatic & Biliary Surgery; Stomach Cancer; Esophageal Cancer; **Hospital:** Loyola Univ Med Ctr (page 98); **Address:** Loyola Univ Med Ctr, Dept Surg, 2160 S First Ave Bldg 110 - rm 3236, Maywood, IL 60153-5590; **Phone:** 708-327-3430; **Board Cert:** Surgery 96; **Med School:** India 69; **Resid:** Surgery, Loyola Univ Med Ctr 75; **Fellow:** Surgical Oncology, Univ Minn Hosp 77; **Fac Appt:** Prof S, Loyola Univ-Stritch Sch Med

Bouwman, David L MD [S] - **Spec Exp:** Breast Cancer; **Hospital:** Harper Univ Hosp; **Address:** Harper Univ Hosp, Dept Surg, 3990 John R, Detroit, MI 48201; **Phone:** 800-527-6266; **Board Cert:** Surgery 99; **Med School:** Johns Hopkins Univ 71; **Resid:** Surgery, Johns Hopkins Hosp 73; Surgery, Wayne State Univ Hosp 78; **Fac Appt:** Prof S

Brems, John MD [S] - **Spec Exp:** Transplant-Liver; Pancreatic Cancer & Surgery; Cancer Surgery; **Hospital:** Loyola Univ Med Ctr (page 98); **Address:** 2160 S 1st Ave, MC-EMS-3268, Maywood, IL 60153-3304; **Phone:** 708-327-2539; **Board Cert:** Surgery 95; Surgical Critical Care 00; **Med School:** St Louis Univ 81; **Resid:** Surgery, St Louis Univ 86; **Fellow:** Transplant Surgery, UCLA Med Ctr 87; **Fac Appt:** Prof S, Loyola Univ-Stritch Sch Med

Brunt, L Michael MD [S] - **Spec Exp:** Endocrine Cancer; Adrenal Surgery; Gastrointestinal Cancer; **Hospital:** Barnes-Jewish Hosp (page 85); **Address:** Washington Univ Sch Medicine, Dept Surg, 660 S Euclid Ave, Box 8109, St Louis, MO 63110; **Phone:** 314-454-7194; **Board Cert:** Surgery 96; **Med School:** Johns Hopkins Univ 80; **Resid:** Surgery, Barnes Hosp 87; **Fellow:** Surgery, Barnes Hosp 84; **Fac Appt:** Assoc Prof S, Washington Univ, St Louis

Chang, Alfred Edward MD [S] - **Spec Exp:** Breast Cancer; Gastrointestinal Cancer; Melanoma & Sarcoma; **Hospital:** Univ Michigan Hlth Sys; **Address:** Univ Mich Comp Cancer Ctr & Geriatric Ctr, 1500 E Med Ctr Dr 3302 CGC, Ann Arbor, MI 48109-0932; **Phone:** 734-936-4392; **Board Cert:** Surgery 01; **Med School:** Harvard Med Sch 74; **Resid:** Surgery, Hosp Univ Penn 82; Surgery, Duke Univ Med Ctr 76; **Fellow:** Surgical Oncology, Natl Cancer Inst 79; **Fac Appt:** Prof S, Univ Mich Med Sch

Chapman, William C MD [S] - **Spec Exp:** Transplant-Liver-Adult & Pediatric; Liver Cancer & Surgery; Biliary Surgery; **Hospital:** Barnes-Jewish Hosp (page 85); **Address:** Washington Univ Sch Med, 660 S Euclid Ave, Box 8604, St Louis, MO 63110; **Phone:** 314-747-3969; **Board Cert:** Surgery 01; Surgical Critical Care 01; **Med School:** Med Univ SC 84; **Resid:** Surgery, Vanderbilt Univ Med Ctr 91; **Fellow:** Hepatobiliary Surgery, Kings College Hosp 92; **Fac Appt:** Prof S, Washington Univ, St Louis

Crowe Jr, Joseph P MD [S] - **Spec Exp:** Breast Cancer; Tumor Surgery; **Hospital:** Cleveland Clin Fdn (page 92); **Address:** Cleveland Clinic, Dept Surg, 9500 Euclid Ave, Desk A80, Cleveland, OH 44195; **Phone:** 216-444-3024; **Board Cert:** Surgery 04; **Med School:** Case West Res Univ 78; **Resid:** Surgery, Univ Hosp-Case West Res 83; **Fellow:** Surgical Oncology, Meml Sloan Kettering Cancer Ctr 85

Donohue, John H MD [S] - **Spec Exp:** Gastrointestinal Cancer; Breast Cancer; Stomach Cancer; **Hospital:** Mayo Med Ctr & Clin - Rochester; **Address:** Mayo Clinic, Dept Surg, 200 First St SW, Rochester, MN 55905; **Phone:** 507-284-0362; **Board Cert:** Surgery 95; **Med School:** Harvard Med Sch 78; **Resid:** Surgery, UCSF Med Ctr 81; Surgery, UCSF Med Ctr 85; **Fellow:** Surgery, Natl Inst Hlth 83; Surgical Oncology, Meml Sloan-Kettering Canc Ctr 87; **Fac Appt:** Prof S, Mayo Med Sch

Eberlein, Timothy J MD [S] - **Spec Exp:** Breast Cancer; Melanoma; Tumor Immune Therapies; **Hospital:** Barnes-Jewish Hosp (page 85); **Address:** Wash Univ School of Medicine, Dept Surgery, 660 S Euclid Ave, Box 8109, St Louis, MO 63110-1093; **Phone:** 314-362-8020; **Board Cert:** Surgery 95; **Med School:** Univ Pittsburgh 77; **Resid:** Surgery, Peter Bent Brigham Hosp 79; Surgery, Brigham-Womens Hosp 85; **Fellow:** Allergy & Immunology, Natl Inst Hlth 82; **Fac Appt:** Prof S, Washington Univ, St Louis

Ellison, E Christopher MD [S] - **Spec Exp:** Biliary Surgery; Pancreatic Cancer; **Hospital:** Ohio St Univ Med Ctr (page 105); **Address:** 1654 Upham Drive, Ste 327 Means Hall, Columbus, OH 43210-1236; **Phone:** 614-293-9722; **Board Cert:** Surgery 01; **Med School:** Univ Wisc 75; **Resid:** Surgery, Ohio State Univ 81; **Fac Appt:** Prof S, Ohio State Univ

Farrar, William B MD [S] - **Spec Exp:** Breast Cancer; Thyroid Cancer; **Hospital:** Arthur G James Cancer Hosp & Research Inst (page 105); **Address:** 410 W 10th Ave, N924 Doan Hall, Columbus, OH 43010; **Phone:** 614-293-8890; **Board Cert:** Surgery 00; **Med School:** Univ VA Sch Med 75; **Resid:** Surgery, Ohio State Univ Hosps 80; **Fellow:** Surgical Oncology, Meml Sloan-Kettering Cancer Ctr 82; **Fac Appt:** Prof S, Ohio State Univ

Fung, John J MD/PhD [S] - **Spec Exp:** Transplant-Liver; Transplant-Kidney; Liver & Biliary Cancer & Surgery; **Hospital:** Cleveland Clin Fdn (page 92); **Address:** Cleveland Clinic, Dept Surgery, Desk A80, 9500 Euclid Ave, Cleveland, OH 44195; **Phone:** 216-444-3776; **Board Cert:** Surgery 97; **Med School:** Univ Chicago-Pritzker Sch Med 82; **Resid:** Surgery, Strong Memorial Hosp 88; **Fellow:** Transplant Surgery, Univ Pittsburgh 86; **Fac Appt:** Prof S, Cleveland Cl Coll Med/Case West Res

Gabram, Sheryl MD [S] - **Spec Exp:** Breast Cancer; Breast Disease-Benign; **Hospital:** Loyola Univ Med Ctr (page 98); **Address:** 2160 S First Ave, Bldg 110 - rm 3232, Maywood, IL 60153-3304; **Phone:** 708-216-8563; **Board Cert:** Surgery 96; Surgical Critical Care 89; **Med School:** Georgetown Univ 82; **Resid:** Surgery, Washington Hosp Ctr 87; **Fellow:** Trauma, Hartford Hosp 88; **Fac Appt:** Prof S, Loyola Univ-Stritch Sch Med

Goulet Jr, Robert J MD [S] - **Spec Exp:** Breast Cancer; **Hospital:** Indiana Univ Hosp (page 90); **Address:** Indiana Univ Hosp, Cancer Pavilion, 535 Barnhill Drive, rm 431, Indianapolis, IN 46202-5112; **Phone:** 317-274-3616; **Board Cert:** Surgery 95; **Med School:** SUNY Downstate 79; **Resid:** Surgery, SUNY-Downstate Med Ctr 86; **Fac Appt:** Assoc Clin Prof S

Grant, Clive S MD [S] - **Spec Exp:** Thyroid & Parathyroid Cancer & Surgery; Adrenal Surgery; Breast Cancer; **Hospital:** Mayo Med Ctr & Clin - Rochester; **Address:** Mayo Clinic, Dept Surg, 200 First St SW, Rochester, MN 55905-0001; **Phone:** 507-284-2644; **Board Cert:** Surgery 01; **Med School:** Univ Colorado 74; **Resid:** Surgery, Mayo Clinic 80; **Fac Appt:** Prof S, Mayo Med Sch

Harkema, James M MD [S] - **Spec Exp:** Breast Cancer; Thyroid Cancer; Parathyroid Cancer; **Hospital:** Sparrow Hosp; **Address:** Sparrow Professional Bldg, Breast Hlth Clinic, 1200 E Michigan Ave, Ste 655, Lansing, MI 48912; **Phone:** 517-267-2461; **Board Cert:** Surgery 75; **Med School:** Univ Mich Med Sch 68; **Resid:** Surgery, Univ Mich Hosp 74; **Fac Appt:** Prof S, Mich State Univ

Howe, James MD [S] - **Spec Exp:** Endocrine Surgery; Gastrointestinal Cancer; Colon & Rectal Cancer; **Hospital:** Univ Iowa Hosp & Clinics; **Address:** Univ Iowa, Dept Surg, 200 Hawkins Drive, 1504 John Colloton Pavilion, Iowa City, IA 52242-1086; **Phone:** 319-356-1727; **Board Cert:** Surgery 95; **Med School:** Univ VT Coll Med 87; **Resid:** Surgery, Barnes Hosp-Wash Univ 94; **Fellow:** Research, Wash Univ-NCI 91; Surgical Oncology, Meml Sloan Kettering Cancer Ctr 96; **Fac Appt:** Assoc Prof S, Univ Iowa Coll Med

Lillemoe, Keith Douglas MD [S] - **Spec Exp:** Pancreatic Cancer; Colon Cancer & Surgery; **Hospital:** Indiana Univ Hosp (page 90); **Address:** Indiana Univ, Dept Surgery, 545 Barnhill Drive, EH 203, Indianapolis, IN 46202; **Phone:** 317-274-5707; **Board Cert:** Surgery 95; **Med School:** Johns Hopkins Univ 78; **Resid:** Surgery, Johns Hopkins Hosp 85; **Fac Appt:** Prof S, Indiana Univ

Mamounas, Eleftherios P MD [S] - **Spec Exp:** Breast Cancer; **Hospital:** Aultman Hosp; **Address:** Aultman Cancer Ctr, 2600 6th St SW, Canton, OH 44710; **Phone:** 330-363-6281; **Board Cert:** Surgery 99; **Med School:** Greece 83; **Resid:** Surgery, McKeesport Hosp 89; **Fellow:** Clinical Oncology, Univ Pittsburgh 91; Surgical Oncology, Roswell Park Cancer Inst 92; **Fac Appt:** Asst Clin Prof S, Case West Res Univ

Melvin, W Scott MD [S] - **Spec Exp:** Liver & Biliary Surgery; Pancreatic Cancer; Laparoscopic Abdominal Surgery; **Hospital:** Ohio St Univ Med Ctr (page 105); **Address:** 410 W 10th Ave, Ste N729 Doan Hall, Columbus, OH 43210; **Phone:** 614-293-4499; **Board Cert:** Surgery 93; **Med School:** Med Coll OH 87; **Resid:** Surgery, Univ Maryland 92; **Fellow:** Gastrointestinal Surgery, Grant Med Ctr 93; **Fac Appt:** Assoc Prof S, Ohio State Univ

Millis, J Michael MD [S] - **Spec Exp:** Transplant-Liver-Adult & Pediatric; Liver Cancer; Transplant-Pancreas; **Hospital:** Univ of Chicago Hosps; **Address:** Univ Chicago, Dept Surgery, 5841 S Maryland Ave, MS 5027, Chicago, IL 60637; **Phone:** 773-702-6319; **Board Cert:** Surgery 01; Surgical Critical Care 01; **Med School:** Univ Tenn Coll Med, Memphis 85; **Resid:** Surgery, UCLA Med Ctr 92; **Fellow:** Transplant Surgery, UCLA Med Ctr 94; **Fac Appt:** Prof S, Univ Chicago-Pritzker Sch Med

Moley, Jeffrey F MD [S] - **Spec Exp:** Thyroid Cancer & Disorders; Endocrine Cancers & Surgery; Melanoma; **Hospital:** Barnes-Jewish Hosp (page 85); **Address:** Washington University School of Medicine, Dept Surgery, 660 S Euclid Ave, Box 8109, St. Louis, MO 63110; **Phone:** 314-362-2280; **Board Cert:** Surgery 98; **Med School:** Columbia P&S 80; **Resid:** Surgery, Yale-New Haven Hosp 85; **Fellow:** Surgical Oncology, National Cancer Inst 87; **Fac Appt:** Prof S, Washington Univ, St Louis

Nathanson, S David MD [S] - **Spec Exp:** Breast Cancer & Risk Assessment; Melanoma; Sarcoma; **Hospital:** Henry Ford Hosp; **Address:** 2799 W Grand Blvd, Detroit, MI 48202; **Phone:** 313-916-3149; **Board Cert:** Surgery 02; **Med School:** South Africa 66; **Resid:** Surgery, Univ Witwaterstrand 74; Surgical Oncology, UCLA 80; **Fellow:** Surgery, Univ Calif Davis 82; **Fac Appt:** Clin Prof S, Case West Res Univ

Newman, Lisa A MD [S] - **Spec Exp:** Breast Cancer; **Hospital:** Univ Michigan Hlth Sys; **Address:** Cancer Center, 1500 E Medical Center Drive, rm 3308-CGC, Ann Arbor, MI 48109; **Phone:** 734-936-8771; **Board Cert:** Surgery 01; Surgical Critical Care 94; **Med School:** SUNY Downstate 85; **Resid:** Surgery, Downstate Med Ctr 90; **Fac Appt:** Assoc Prof S, Univ Mich Med Sch

Niederhuber, John E MD [S] - **Spec Exp:** Breast Cancer; Liver & Pancreatic Cancer; Esophageal Cancer; **Hospital:** Univ WI Hosp & Clins; **Address:** Univ Wisconsin Clin Sci Ctr, 600 Highland Ave, rm H4-752, Madison, WI 53792-6164; **Phone:** 608-265-5212; **Board Cert:** Surgery 74; **Med School:** Ohio State Univ 64; **Resid:** Surgery, Univ Mich Hosp 73; **Fellow:** Immunology, Karolinska Inst 71; **Fac Appt:** Prof Surg & Onc, Univ Wisc

Onders, Raymond P MD [S] - **Spec Exp:** Laparoscopic Surgery; Diaphragm Pacing via Laparoscopy; Gastrointestinal Cancer; **Hospital:** Univ Hosps of Cleveland; **Address:** University Hospitals of Cleveland, Lakeside Bldg, 11100 Euclid Ave Fl 7 - rm 7002, Cleveland, OH 44106; **Phone:** 216-844-5797; **Board Cert:** Surgery 01; **Med School:** NE Ohio Univ 88; **Resid:** Surgery, Case Western Reserve Univ 93; **Fac Appt:** Asst Prof S, Case West Res Univ

Pass, Helen MD [S] - **Spec Exp:** Cancer Surgery; Breast Cancer; **Hospital:** William Beaumont Hosp; **Address:** Breast Care Ctr - WBH, 3601 W 13 Mile Rd, Royal Oak, MI 48073; **Phone:** 248-551-3300; **Board Cert:** Surgery 03; **Med School:** Univ Mich Med Sch 87; **Resid:** Surgery, Univ Tex Hlth Sci Ctr/MD Anderson Cancer Ctr 89; Surgery, Georgetown Univ Hosp 94; **Fellow:** Surgery, NCI/NIH 92

Posner, Mitchell C MD [S] - **Spec Exp:** Pancreatic Cancer; Gastrointestinal Cancer; Esophageal Cancer; **Hospital:** Univ of Chicago Hosps; **Address:** Univ of Chicago Hospitals, 5841 S Maryland Ave, Ste G204, MC 5031, Chicago, IL 60637; **Phone:** 773-834-0156; **Board Cert:** Surgery 97; **Med School:** SUNY Buffalo 81; **Resid:** Surgery, Univ Colorado Sch Med 86; **Fellow:** Surgical Oncology, Meml Sloan Kettering 88; **Fac Appt:** Prof S, Univ Chicago-Pritzker Sch Med

Rikkers, Layton F MD [S] - **Spec Exp:** Liver & Biliary Surgery/Cancer; Pancreatic Cancer; **Hospital:** Univ WI Hosp & Clins; **Address:** 600 Highland Ave, rm H4-710D, Madison, WI 53792; **Phone:** 608-265-8854; **Board Cert:** Surgery 96; **Med School:** Stanford Univ 70; **Resid:** Surgery, Univ Utah Hosp 73; Surgery, Univ Utah Hosp 76; **Fellow:** Hepatology, Royal Free Hosp 74; **Fac Appt:** Prof S, Univ Wisc

Saha, Sukamal MD [S] - **Spec Exp:** Sentinel Node Surgery; Colon Cancer; **Hospital:** McLaren Reg Med Ctr; **Address:** 3500 Calkins Rd, Ste A, Flint, MI 48532; **Phone:** 810-230-9600; **Board Cert:** Surgery 00; **Med School:** India 77; **Resid:** Surgery, Hahnemann Univ Hosp 85; Surgery, Easton Hosp 87; **Fellow:** Surgical Oncology, Tulane Univ Med Ctr 89; Head and Neck Surgery, Roswell Park Meml Hosp; **Fac Appt:** Asst Prof S, Mich State Univ

Sarr, Michael G MD [S] - **Spec Exp:** Pancreatic Cancer; Gastrointestinal Cancer; Obesity/Bariatric Surgery; **Hospital:** Mayo Med Ctr & Clin - Rochester; **Address:** Mayo Clinic, Dept Surg, Desk West 6, Rochester, MN 55905; **Phone:** 507-284-2644; **Board Cert:** Surgery 01; **Med School:** Johns Hopkins Univ 76; **Resid:** Surgery, Johns Hopkins Hosp 82; **Fellow:** Surgery, Mayo Clinic 84; Surgery, Johns Hopkins Hosp 85; **Fac Appt:** Prof S, Mayo Med Sch

Scott-Conner, Carol E.H. MD/PhD [S] - **Spec Exp:** Cancer Surgery; Laparoscopic Surgery; Critical Care; **Hospital:** Univ Iowa Hosp & Clinics; **Address:** Univ Iowa, Dept Surg, 200 Hawkins Drive, rm 4601-JCP, Iowa City, IA 52242-1086; **Phone:** 319-356-0330; **Board Cert:** Surgery 00; Surgical Critical Care 98; **Med School:** NYU Sch Med 76; **Resid:** Surgery, NYU Med Ctr 81; **Fac Appt:** Prof S, Univ Iowa Coll Med

Sener, Stephen MD [S] - **Spec Exp:** Breast Cancer; Pancreatic Cancer; Lymphedema; **Hospital:** Evanston Hosp; **Address:** 2650 Ridge Ave, Birch Bldg, rm 106, Evanston, IL 60201-1718; **Phone:** 847-570-1328; **Board Cert:** Surgery 01; **Med School:** Northwestern Univ 77; **Resid:** Surgery, Northwestern Univ 82; **Fellow:** Surgery, Meml Sloan Kettering Cancer Ctr 84; **Fac Appt:** Prof S, Northwestern Univ

Siperstein, Allan E MD [S] - **Spec Exp:** Laparoscopic Surgery; Endocrine Tumors & Surgery; Thyroid & Parathyroid Cancer & Surgery; **Hospital:** Cleveland Clin Fdn (page 92); **Address:** Cleveland Clinic Fdn, Dept Genl Surg, 9500 Euclid Ave, Desk A80, Cleveland, OH 44195; **Phone:** 216-444-5664; **Board Cert:** Surgery 97; **Med School:** Univ Tex SW, Dallas 83; **Resid:** Surgery, UCSF Med Ctr 90; **Fellow:** Research, UCSF Med Ctr 88

Strasberg, Steven M MD [S] - **Spec Exp:** Liver & Biliary Cancer & Surgery; Pancreatic Cancer & Surgery; Gastrointestinal Cancer & Surgery; **Hospital:** Barnes-Jewish Hosp (page 85); **Address:** Washington University School of Medicine, Dept Surgery, 660 S Euclid Ave, Box 8109, Saint Louis, MO 63110; **Phone:** 314-362-7147; **Med School:** Canada 63; **Resid:** Surgery, Toronto General Hosp 69; **Fellow:** Surgical Research, Toronto General Hosp 71; **Fac Appt:** Prof S, Washington Univ, St Louis

Tuttle, Todd M MD [S] - **Spec Exp:** Breast Cancer; Minimally Invasive Cancer Surgery; Cancer Surgery; **Hospital:** Fairview-Univ Med Ctr - Univ Campus; **Address:** Univ Minn, Dept Surgery, 420 Delaware St SE, MMC 195, Minneapolis, MN 55455; **Phone:** 612-625-2991; **Board Cert:** Surgery 95; **Med School:** Johns Hopkins Univ 88; **Resid:** Surgery, Med Coll Virginia Hosps 94; **Fellow:** Surgical Oncology, MD Anderson Cancer Ctr 96; **Fac Appt:** Assoc Prof S

Walker, Alonzo P MD [S] - **Spec Exp:** Breast Cancer; **Hospital:** Froedtert Meml Lutheran Hosp; **Address:** Dept Surgery, 9200 W Wisconsin Ave, Milwaukee, WI 53226-3522; **Phone:** 414-805-5737; **Board Cert:** Surgery 04; **Med School:** Univ Fla Coll Med 76; **Resid:** Surgery, Univ Md Hosps 83; **Fac Appt:** Prof S, Med Coll Wisc

Walsh, R Matthew MD [S] - **Spec Exp:** Pancreatic Cancer; Gastrointestinal Surgery; Hepatobiliary Surgery; **Hospital:** Cleveland Clin Fdn (page 92); **Address:** Cleveland Clinic, Dept Surgery, Desk A80, 9500 Euclid Ave, Cleveland, OH 44195; **Phone:** 216-445-7576; **Board Cert:** Surgery 99; **Med School:** Med Coll Wisc 85; **Resid:** Surgery, Loyola Univ Hosp 90; **Fellow:** Endoscopy, Mass General Hosp 91; Hepatopancreatobiliary Surgery, Cleveland Clinic; **Fac Appt:** Assoc Prof S, Cleveland Cl Coll Med/Case West Res

Witt, Thomas MD [S] - **Spec Exp:** Breast Cancer; Breast Disease; **Hospital:** Rush Univ Med Ctr; **Address:** 1725 W Harrison St, Ste 409, Chicago, IL 60612-3828; **Phone:** 312-942-2302; **Board Cert:** Surgery 00; **Med School:** Northwestern Univ 75; **Resid:** Surgery, Rush Presby-St Lukes Med Ctr 80; **Fellow:** Surgical Oncology, Meml Sloan Kettering Cancer Ctr 82; **Fac Appt:** Assoc Prof S, Rush Med Coll

Great Plains and Mountains

Edney, James A MD [S] - **Spec Exp:** Breast Cancer; Thyroid & Parathyroid Cancer & Surgery; Cancer Surgery; **Hospital:** Nebraska Med Ctr; **Address:** Univ Nebraska Med Ctr, Dept Surgery, 984030 Nebraska Medical Ctr, Omaha, NE 68198-4030; **Phone:** 402-559-7272; **Board Cert:** Surgery 01; **Med School:** Univ Nebr Coll Med 75; **Resid:** Surgery, Univ Nebraska Med Ctr 80; **Fellow:** Surgical Oncology, Univ Colorado Med Ctr 81; **Fac Appt:** Prof S, Univ Nebr Coll Med

Mulvihill, Sean J MD [S] - **Spec Exp:** Gastrointestinal Surgery; Liver & Biliary Cancer & Surgery; Pancreatic Cancer & Surgery; **Hospital:** Univ Utah Hosps and Clins; **Address:** Univ Utah, Dept Surgery, 30 N 1900 E, rm 3B110, Salt Lake City, UT 84132; **Phone:** 801-581-7304; **Board Cert:** Surgery 99; **Med School:** USC Sch Med 81; **Resid:** Surgery, UCLA Med Ctr 87; **Fac Appt:** Prof S, Univ Utah

Nelson, Edward W MD [S] - **Spec Exp:** Breast Cancer; **Hospital:** Univ Utah Hosps and Clins; **Address:** University Utah Medical Ctr, Dept Surgery, 50 N Medical Drive, Salt Lake City, UT 84132; **Phone:** 801-581-7738; **Board Cert:** Surgery 99; **Med School:** Univ Utah 74; **Resid:** Surgery, Univ Utah Medical Ctr 79; **Fac Appt:** Prof S, Univ Utah

Pearlman, Nathan W MD [S] - **Spec Exp:** Gastrointestinal Cancer; Melanoma; Head & Neck Cancer; **Hospital:** Univ Colorado Hosp; **Address:** C313, University Hosp, 4200 E 9th Ave, Denver, CO 80262; **Phone:** 720-848-0168; **Board Cert:** Surgery 74; **Med School:** Univ IL Coll Med 66; **Resid:** Surgery, Univ Colorado Med Ctr 73; **Fellow:** Surgical Oncology, Sloan-Kettering Cancer Ctr 75; **Fac Appt:** Prof S, Univ Colorado

Southwest

Ames, Frederick C MD [S] - **Spec Exp:** Breast Cancer; **Hospital:** UT MD Anderson Cancer Ctr, The (page 115); **Address:** MD Anderson Cancer Ctr, Dept Surgery, 1515 Holcombe Blvd, Box 444, Houston, TX 77030-4009; **Phone:** 713-792-6929; **Board Cert:** Surgery 75; **Med School:** Univ Tex Med Br, Galveston 69; **Resid:** Surgery, St Joseph Hosp 74; **Fellow:** Surgical Oncology, MD Anderson Cancer Ctr 75; **Fac Appt:** Prof S, Univ Tex, Houston

Brunicardi, F Charles MD [S] - **Spec Exp:** Islet Cell Transplant; Pancreatic Cancer; Gastroesophageal Reflux Disease (GERD); **Hospital:** St Luke's Episcopal Hosp - Houston; **Address:** 6550 Fannin St, Ste 1661, Houston, TX 77030; **Phone:** 713-798-8070; **Board Cert:** Surgery 98; **Med School:** Rutgers Univ 80; **Resid:** Surgery, SUNY Brooklyn Hlth Sci Ctr 89; **Fellow:** SUNY Brooklyn Hlth Sci Ctr 86; **Fac Appt:** Prof S, Baylor Coll Med

Curley, Steven A MD [S] - **Spec Exp:** Colon & Rectal Cancer; Liver Cancer; Hepatobiliary Surgery; **Hospital:** UT MD Anderson Cancer Ctr, The (page 115); **Address:** MD Anderson Cancer Ctr, Dept Surg Onc, Unit 444, PO Box 301402, Houston, TX 77230-1402; **Phone:** 713-794-4957; **Board Cert:** Surgery 97; **Med School:** Univ Tex, Houston 82; **Resid:** Surgery, Univ New Mexico Hosps 88; **Fellow:** Surgical Oncology, MD Anderson Cancer Ctr 90; **Fac Appt:** Prof S, Univ Tex, Houston

Dooley, William C MD [S] - **Spec Exp:** Breast Cancer; Metastatic Disease Management; Tumors-Rare & Multiple; **Hospital:** OU Med Ctr; **Address:** 825 NE 10th St, Ste 5200, Oklahoma City, OK 73104; **Phone:** 405-271-7867; **Board Cert:** Surgery 97; **Med School:** Vanderbilt Univ 82; **Resid:** Surgery, Oxford Univ; Surgery, Johns Hopkins 87; **Fellow:** Medical Oncology, Johns Hopkins 88; **Fac Appt:** Prof S, Univ Okla Coll Med

Edwards, Michael J MD [S] - **Spec Exp:** Cancer Surgery; Breast Cancer; Melanoma; **Hospital:** UAMS Med Ctr; **Address:** 4301 W Markham St, Slot 520, Shorey -Ste S706, Little Rock, AR 72205; **Phone:** 501-686-7874; **Board Cert:** Surgery 96; **Med School:** Emory Univ 81; **Resid:** Surgery, Univ Louisville Hosp 86; **Fellow:** Surgical Oncology, MD Anderson Cancer Ctr 87; **Fac Appt:** Prof S, Univ Ark

Euhus, David M MD [S] - **Spec Exp:** Breast Cancer; **Hospital:** UTSW Med Ctr - Dallas; **Address:** Univ Texas SW Med Ctr - Div Surg Oncology, 5323 Harry Hines Blvd, Dallas, TX 75390-9155; **Phone:** 214-648-6467; **Board Cert:** Surgery 01; **Med School:** St Louis Univ 84; **Resid:** Surgery, UCLA Med Ctr 91; **Fellow:** Surgical Oncology, UCLA Med Ctr 88; Breast Disease, Queens Med Ctr; **Fac Appt:** Assoc Prof S, Univ Tex SW, Dallas

Evans, Douglas B MD [S] - **Spec Exp:** Pancreatic Cancer; Thyroid Cancer; Endocrine Cancers; **Hospital:** UT MD Anderson Cancer Ctr, The (page 115); **Address:** Dept Surg/Onc, Unit 444, P.O. Box 301402, Houston, TX 77030-4095; **Phone:** 713-794-4324; **Board Cert:** Surgery 96; **Med School:** Boston Univ 83; **Resid:** Surgery, Dartmouth-Hitchcock Med Ctr 88; **Fellow:** Surgical Oncology, MD Anderson Cancer Ctr 90; **Fac Appt:** Prof S, Univ Tex, Houston

Feig, Barry W MD [S] - **Spec Exp:** Gastrointestinal Cancer; Sarcoma; Breast Cancer; **Hospital:** UT MD Anderson Cancer Ctr, The (page 115); **Address:** University of Texas MD Anderson Cancer Ctr, 1515 Holcombe Blvd, Box 444, Houston, TX 77030; **Phone:** 713-794-1002; **Board Cert:** Surgery 98; Surgical Critical Care 96; **Med School:** SUNY Upstate Med Univ 84; **Resid:** Surgery, NW Univ Med School 90; **Fellow:** Trauma, Univ of Minn 91; Surgical Oncology, UT MD Anderson 94; **Fac Appt:** Assoc Prof S, Univ Tex, Houston

Fisher, William E MD [S] - Spec Exp: Pancreatic Cancer; **Hospital:** St Luke's Episcopal Hosp - Houston; **Address:** Baylor College of Medicine, Dept Surgery, 6550 Fannin St, Ste 1661, Houston, TX 77030; **Phone:** 713-798-8070; **Board Cert:** Surgery 99; **Med School:** Univ Cincinnati 90; **Resid:** Surgery, Ohio State U Hosps 96; **Fellow:** Cancer Research, Ohio State U Hosps 98; **Fac Appt:** Asst Prof S, Baylor Coll Med

Grant, Michael MD [S] - Spec Exp: Breast Cancer; **Hospital:** Baylor Univ Medical Ctr (page 86); **Address:** 3409 Worth St, Ste 300, Dallas, TX 75246; **Phone:** 214-826-7300; **Board Cert:** Surgery 01; **Med School:** Univ Tex, Houston 87; **Resid:** Surgery, Baylor Univ Med Ctr 92; **Fellow:** Breast Cancer, Baylor Univ Med Ctr 93

Hunt, Kelly K MD [S] - Spec Exp: Breast Cancer; Colon & Rectal Cancer; Gene Therapy; **Hospital:** UT MD Anderson Cancer Ctr, The (page 115); **Address:** MD Anderson Cancer Ctr, 1515 Holcombe Blvd, Box 444, Houston, TX 77030; **Phone:** 713-792-7216; **Board Cert:** Surgery 01; **Med School:** Univ Tenn Coll Med, Memphis 86; **Resid:** Surgery, UCLA Med Ctr 93; **Fellow:** Surgical Oncology, MD Anderson Cancer Ctr 96; **Fac Appt:** Assoc Prof S, Univ Tex, Houston

Jackson, Gilchrist MD [S] - Spec Exp: Laparoscopic Surgery-Abdominal; Cancer Surgery; Head & Neck Surgery; **Hospital:** St Luke's Episcopal Hosp - Houston; **Address:** 2727 W Holcombe Blvd, MC 3, Houston, TX 77025; **Phone:** 713-442-1132; **Board Cert:** Surgery 98; **Med School:** Univ Louisville Sch Med 74; **Resid:** Surgery, Parkland Hosp 79; **Fellow:** Surgical Oncology, MD Anderson Hosp 80; **Fac Appt:** Assoc Clin Prof S, Baylor Coll Med

Klimberg, V Suzanne MD [S] - Spec Exp: Breast Cancer; **Hospital:** UAMS Med Ctr; **Address:** Univ Arkansas Medical Sciences, 4301 W Markham, MS 725, Little Rock, AR 72205; **Phone:** 501-686-6504; **Board Cert:** Surgery 99; **Med School:** Univ Fla Coll Med 84; **Resid:** Surgery, Univ Fla 90; **Fellow:** Clinical Oncology, Univ Fla 91; Clinical Oncology, Univ Arkansas for Med Scis 91; **Fac Appt:** Prof S, Univ Ark

Krouse, Robert S MD [S] - Spec Exp: Cancer Surgery; Gastrointestinal Cancer; Palliative Care; **Hospital:** VA Medical Center - Tucson; **Address:** SAVAHCS-Surg Care Line, 2-112, 3601 S 6th Ave, Tucson, AZ 85723; **Phone:** 520-792-1450 x6145; **Board Cert:** Surgery 98; **Med School:** Hahnemann Univ 91; **Resid:** Surgery, Univ Hawaii Integrated Surg Prog 93; Immunotherapy - Natl Cancer Inst 94; **Fellow:** Surgery, W Virginia Univ Sch Med 97; Surgical Oncology, City of Hope Natl Med Ctr 00; **Fac Appt:** Asst Prof S, Univ Ariz Coll Med

Kuhn, Joseph A MD [S] - Spec Exp: Liver Cancer; Head & Neck Cancer; Cancer Surgery; **Hospital:** Baylor Univ Medical Ctr (page 86); **Address:** 3409 Worth St, Ste 420, Dallas, TX 75246; **Phone:** 214-824-9963; **Board Cert:** Surgery 99; Surgical Critical Care 93; **Med School:** Univ Tex Med Br, Galveston 84; **Resid:** Surgery, Baylor Univ Med 89; **Fellow:** Surgical Oncology, City Hosp Natl Med Ctr 92

Lee, Jeffrey E MD [S] - Spec Exp: Melanoma; Pancreatic Cancer; Endocrine Tumors; **Hospital:** UT MD Anderson Cancer Ctr, The (page 115); **Address:** UT MD Anderson Cancer Ctr, 1400 Holcombe Blvd, Unit 444 Fl 12, Houston, TX 77030-4009; **Phone:** 713-792-7218; **Board Cert:** Surgery 99; **Med School:** Stanford Univ 84; **Resid:** Surgery, Stanford Univ Hosp 87; Surgery, Stanford Univ Hosp 91; **Fellow:** Immunology, Stanford Univ Sch Med 89; Surgical Oncology, Univ Tex-MD Anderson Cancer Ctr 93; **Fac Appt:** Prof S, Univ Tex, Houston

Leitch, A Marilyn MD [S] - Spec Exp: Breast Cancer; **Hospital:** Zale Lipshy Univ Hosp - Dallas; **Address:** Univ Teas SW Med Ctr - Dept Surgery, 5323 Harry Hines Blvd, Dallas, TX 75390-9155; **Phone:** 214-648-3039; **Board Cert:** Surgery 03; **Med School:** Univ Tex SW, Dallas 78; **Resid:** Surgery, UCLA Med Ctr 84; **Fellow:** Surgical Oncology, MD Anderson Cancer Ctr 85; **Fac Appt:** Prof S, Univ Tex SW, Dallas

Li, Benjamin D L MD [S] - **Spec Exp:** Gastrointestinal Cancer; Sarcoma; Breast Cancer; **Hospital:** Louisiana State Univ Hosp; **Address:** LSU Hlth Scis Ctr, Dept Surg, 1501 Kings Hwy, Shreveport, LA 71130; **Phone:** 318-675-6123; **Board Cert:** Surgery 02; **Med School:** Yale Univ 86; **Resid:** Surgery, Northwestern Univ-McGraw Med Ctr 92; **Fellow:** Surgical Oncology, Roswell Park Cancer Inst 95; **Fac Appt:** Prof S, Louisiana State Univ

Pisters, Peter MD [S] - **Spec Exp:** Pancreatic Cancer; Sarcoma-Soft Tissue; Gastrointestinal Cancer; **Hospital:** UT MD Anderson Cancer Ctr, The (page 115); **Address:** MD Anderson Cancer Ctr, PO Box 301402, Houston, TX 77230; **Phone:** 713-794-1572; **Board Cert:** Surgery 01; **Med School:** Canada 85; **Resid:** Surgery, NYU/Bellevue Hosp 92; **Fellow:** Surgical Research, Meml Sloan-Kettering Cancer Ctr 89; Surgical Oncology, Meml Sloan-Kettering Cancer Ctr 94; **Fac Appt:** Assoc Prof S, Univ Tex, Houston

Pockaj, Barbara A MD [S] - **Spec Exp:** Melanoma; Breast Cancer; Clinical Trials; **Hospital:** Mayo Clin Hosp - Scottsdale; **Address:** Mayo Clinic - Scottsdale, Dept Surgery, 13400 E Shea Blvd, Scottsdale, AZ 85259; **Phone:** 480-301-6551; **Board Cert:** Surgery 96; **Med School:** Vanderbilt Univ 87; **Resid:** Surgery, Case Western Res Univ Affil Hosps 95; **Fellow:** Surgical Oncology, Natl Inst Hlth 92; **Fac Appt:** Assoc Prof S, Mayo Med Sch

Pollock, Raphael MD/PhD [S] - **Spec Exp:** Sarcoma; **Hospital:** UT MD Anderson Cancer Ctr, The (page 115); **Address:** Surgical Oncology Dept, 1400 Holcombe Blvd FC12.3044, Box 301402, Houston, TX 77230-1240; **Phone:** 713-792-8850; **Board Cert:** Surgery 03; **Med School:** St Louis Univ 77; **Resid:** Surgery, Univ Chicago 79; Surgery, Rush Presby-St Lukes Hosp 82; **Fellow:** Surgical Oncology, MD Anderson Cancer Ctr 84; **Fac Appt:** Prof S, Univ Tex, Houston

Ross, Merrick I MD [S] - **Spec Exp:** Sentinel Node Surgery; Breast Cancer; Melanoma; **Hospital:** UT MD Anderson Cancer Ctr, The (page 115); **Address:** UT MD Anderson Cancer Ctr, Dept Surg, PO Box 301402, Houston, TX 77230; **Phone:** 713-792-7217; **Board Cert:** Surgery 97; **Med School:** Univ IL Coll Med 80; **Resid:** Surgery, Univ Illinois Hosp & Clin 82; Surgery, Univ Illinois Hosp & Clin 87; **Fellow:** Research, Scripps Clin & Rsch 84; Surgical Oncology, Univ TX-MD Anderson Cancer Ctr 89; **Fac Appt:** Prof S, Univ Tex, Houston

Singletary, S Eva MD [S] - **Spec Exp:** Breast Cancer; **Hospital:** UT MD Anderson Cancer Ctr, The (page 115); **Address:** Univ Tex MD Anderson Canc Ctr, 1515 Holcombe Blvd, Box 444, Houston, TX 77030-4009; **Phone:** 713-792-6937; **Board Cert:** Surgery 94; **Med School:** Med Univ SC 77; **Resid:** Surgery, Shands Hosp-Univ Florida 83; **Fellow:** Surgery, MD Anderson Hosp 85; **Fac Appt:** Prof S, Univ Tex, Houston

Skibber, John M MD [S] - **Spec Exp:** Rectal Cancer; Anal & Perianal Cancer; Colon & Rectal Cancer-Familial; **Hospital:** UT MD Anderson Cancer Ctr, The (page 115); **Address:** UT MD Anderson Cancer Ctr, Dept of Surgical Oncology - Unit 444 PO Box 301402, Houston, TX 77230-1402; **Phone:** 713-792-5165; **Board Cert:** Surgery 98; **Med School:** Jefferson Med Coll 81; **Resid:** Surgery, NYU Med Ctr 89; **Fellow:** Surgical Oncology, Univ Texas-MD Anderson 89; **Fac Appt:** Prof S, Univ Tex, Houston

Stolier, Alan J MD [S] - **Spec Exp:** Breast Cancer; **Hospital:** Meml Med Ctr - Baptist Campus; **Address:** 2820 Napoleon Ave, Ste 110B, New Orleans, LA 70115; **Phone:** 504-897-4223; **Board Cert:** Surgery 94; **Med School:** Louisiana State Univ 70; **Resid:** Surgery, Charity Hosp 74; **Fellow:** Surgical Oncology, MD Anderson Hosp 76

Vauthey, Jean Nicolas MD [S] - **Spec Exp:** Hepatobiliary Surgery; Liver Cancer; Gallbladder & Bile Duct Cancer; **Hospital:** UT MD Anderson Cancer Ctr, The (page 115); **Address:** UT MD Anderson Cancer Ctr -Surgical Oncology, 1515 Holcombe Blvd, Box 444, Houston, TX 77030; **Phone:** 713-792-2022; **Board Cert:** Surgery 00; **Med School:** Switzerland 79; **Resid:** Surgery, Ochsner Med Fdn 89; **Fellow:** Hepatobiliary Surgery, Med Fac Univ Bern 91; Surgical Oncology, Meml Sloan-Kettering Cancer Ctr 93; **Fac Appt:** Prof S, Univ Tex, Houston

Woltering, Eugene MD [S] - **Spec Exp:** Carcinoid Tumors; **Hospital:** Louisiana State Univ Hosp; **Address:** LSUHSC-Dept Surg, 1542 Tulane Ave, rm 701, New Orleans, LA 70112; **Phone:** 504-568-2279; **Board Cert:** Surgery 02; **Med School:** Ohio State Univ 75; **Resid:** Surgery, Vanderbilt Med Ctr 82; Surgical Oncology, Natl Inst Hlth 79; **Fellow:** Surgical Oncology, Ohio State 84

Wood, R Patrick MD [S] - **Spec Exp:** Transplant-Liver; Liver Cancer & Surgery; **Hospital:** St Luke's Episcopal Hosp - Houston; **Address:** 6624 Fannin St, Ste 1200, Houston, TX 77030; **Phone:** 713-795-8994; **Board Cert:** Surgery 95; Surgical Critical Care 92; **Med School:** Univ Rochester 79; **Resid:** Surgery, NYU/Bellevue Hosp Ctr 84; **Fellow:** Transplant Surgery, Univ Pittsburgh 85; **Fac Appt:** Clin Prof S, Univ Tex, Houston

West Coast and Pacific

Anderson, Benjamin O MD [S] - **Spec Exp:** Breast Cancer; Breast Reconstruction; **Hospital:** Univ Wash Med Ctr; **Address:** Univ Washington Dept Surg, 1959 NE Pacific St, Box 356410, Seattle, WA 98195-6410; **Phone:** 206-288-2166; **Board Cert:** Surgery 02; **Med School:** Albert Einstein Coll Med 85; **Resid:** Surgery, Univ Colorado 92; **Fellow:** Surgical Oncology, Meml Sloan Kettering Cancer Ctr 94; **Fac Appt:** Prof S, Univ Wash

Bilchik, Anton J MD [S] - **Spec Exp:** Gastrointestinal Cancer; Laparoscopic Surgery; **Hospital:** St John's Hlth Ctr, Santa Monica; **Address:** John Wayne Cancer Institute, 2200 Santa Monica Blvd, Santa Monica, CA 90404-2302; **Phone:** 310-449-5206; **Board Cert:** Surgery 97; **Med School:** South Africa 85; **Resid:** Surgery, UCLA Med Ctr 96; **Fellow:** John Wayne Cancer Inst. 98; **Fac Appt:** Asst Clin Prof S, UCLA

Byrd, David MD [S] - **Spec Exp:** Tumor Surgery; Breast Cancer; Melanoma; **Hospital:** Univ Wash Med Ctr; **Address:** UWMC, Dept Surgery, 1959 NE Pacific St, Box 356165, Seattle, WA 98195; **Phone:** 206-598-4477; **Board Cert:** Surgery 98; **Med School:** Tulane Univ 82; **Resid:** Surgery, Univ Wash Med Ctr 87; **Fellow:** Surgical Oncology, Univ Tex-MD Anderson Cancer Ctr 92; **Fac Appt:** Assoc Prof S, Univ Wash

Chang, Helena MD [S] - **Spec Exp:** Breast Cancer; **Hospital:** UCLA Med Ctr (page 111); **Address:** 200 UCLA Medical Plaza, Ste B265-1, Revlon Breast Clinic, Los Angeles, CA 90095-8344; **Phone:** 310-825-2144; **Board Cert:** Surgery 97; **Med School:** Temple Univ 81; **Resid:** Surgery, Epis Hosp 86; **Fellow:** Surgical Oncology, Meml Sloan-Kettering 88; **Fac Appt:** Prof S, UCLA

Clark, Orlo H MD [S] - **Spec Exp:** Thyroid Cancer; Pancreatic Cancer; Parathyroid Cancer; **Hospital:** UCSF - Mt Zion Med Ctr; **Address:** Cancer Ctr, 1600 Divisadero St 3rd Fl, San Francisco, CA 94115; **Phone:** 415-353-7687; **Board Cert:** Surgery 74; **Med School:** Cornell Univ-Weill Med Coll 67; **Resid:** Surgery, UCSF Med Ctr 70; Surgery, UCSF Med Ctr 73; **Fellow:** Surgery, Royal Med Sch London 71; **Fac Appt:** Prof S, UCSF

Eilber, Frederick Richard MD [S] - **Spec Exp:** Tumor Surgery; Sarcoma; **Hospital:** UCLA Med Ctr (page 111); **Address:** 200 Medical Plaza, Ste 120, Los Angeles, CA 90095-1718; **Phone:** 310-825-7086; **Board Cert:** Surgery 73; **Med School:** Univ Mich Med Sch 65; **Resid:** Surgery, Univ Maryland Hosp 72; **Fellow:** Surgery, Univ Tex-MD Anderson Hosp 73; **Fac Appt:** Prof S, UCLA

Ellenhorn, Joshua MD [S] - **Spec Exp:** Gastrointestinal Cancer; Head & Neck Cancer; **Hospital:** City of Hope Natl Med Ctr & Beckman Rsch (page 89); **Address:** 1500 Duarte Rd, Duarte, CA 91010; **Phone:** 626-359-8111 x65342; **Board Cert:** Surgery 00; **Med School:** Boston Univ 84; **Resid:** Surgery, Univ Cincinnati Hosp 91; **Fellow:** Surgical Oncology, Meml Sloan-Kettering Cancer Ctr 93

Esserman, Laura J MD [S] - **Spec Exp:** Breast Cancer; **Hospital:** UCSF - Mt Zion Med Ctr; **Address:** UCSF-Mt Zion Hosp, Clin Cancer Ctr, 1600 Divisadero St Fl 2, San Francisco, CA 94115; **Phone:** 415-353-7070; **Board Cert:** Surgery 01; **Med School:** Stanford Univ 83; **Resid:** Surgery, Stanford Univ Med Ctr 91; **Fellow:** Oncology, Stanford Univ Med Ctr 88; **Fac Appt:** Assoc Prof S, UCSF

Essner, Richard MD [S] - **Spec Exp:** Sentinel Node Surgery; Melanoma; Gastrointestinal Surgery; **Hospital:** St John's Hlth Ctr, Santa Monica; **Address:** 2200 Santa Monica Blvd, Santa Monica, CA 90404-2302; **Phone:** 310-998-3906; **Board Cert:** Surgery 94; **Med School:** Emory Univ 85; **Resid:** Surgery, Univ NC Hosps 92; **Fac Appt:** Asst Clin Prof S, USC Sch Med

Giuliano, Armando E MD [S] - **Spec Exp:** Breast Cancer; **Hospital:** St John's Hlth Ctr, Santa Monica; **Address:** 2200 Santa Monica Blvd, Santa Monica, CA 90404; **Phone:** 310-829-8089; **Board Cert:** Surgery 99; **Med School:** Univ Chicago-Pritzker Sch Med 73; **Resid:** Surgery, UCSF Med Ctr 80; **Fellow:** Surgical Oncology, UCLA Med Ctr 80; **Fac Appt:** Prof S, UCLA

Goodnight, James E MD [S] - **Spec Exp:** Melanoma; Breast Cancer; Bone & Soft Tissue Cancers; **Hospital:** UC Davis Med Ctr; **Address:** UC Davis Med Ctr, Dept Surgery, 2221 Stockton Blvd, rm 3112, Sacramento, CA 95817; **Phone:** 916-734-3190; **Board Cert:** Surgery 97; **Med School:** Baylor Coll Med 68; **Resid:** Surgery, Univ Utah Hosp 76; **Fellow:** Surgical Oncology, UCLA Med Ctr 78; **Fac Appt:** Prof S, UC Davis

Hoque, Laura W MD [S] - **Spec Exp:** Breast Cancer; Breast Disease; **Hospital:** Kapiolani Med Ctr for Women & Chldn; **Address:** Kapi'olani Womens Ctr, 1907 S Beretania St, Ste 501, Honolulu, HI 96826; **Phone:** 808-949-3444; **Board Cert:** Surgery 99; **Med School:** Boston Univ 93; **Resid:** Surgery, St Vincents Hosp 98; **Fellow:** Breast Surgery, Meml Sloan Kettering Cancer Ctr 99; **Fac Appt:** Assoc Clin Prof S, Univ Hawaii JA Burns Sch Med

Jeffrey, Stefanie S MD [S] - **Spec Exp:** Breast Cancer; **Hospital:** Stanford Univ Med Ctr; **Address:** Stanford University Medical Ctr, Chief of Breast Surgery, 1201 Welch Rd Bldg MSLS - rm P214, MC 5494, Stanford, CA 94305-5494; **Phone:** 650-723-5461; **Board Cert:** Surgery 04; **Med School:** UCSF 78; **Resid:** Surgery, UCSF Medical Ctr 84; **Fac Appt:** Assoc Prof S, Stanford Univ

Johnson, Denise L MD [S] - **Spec Exp:** Melanoma; Breast Cancer; **Hospital:** Stanford Univ Med Ctr; **Address:** Stanford Univ Med Ctr-Dept Surg, 300 Pasteur Drive, Ste H3680, MC 5655, Stanford, CA 94305; **Phone:** 650-723-5672; **Board Cert:** Surgery 01; **Med School:** Washington Univ, St Louis 78; **Resid:** Surgery, Univ Illinois 86; Immunology, Univ Texas 82; **Fellow:** Surgical Oncology, City of Hope 89; **Fac Appt:** Assoc Prof S, Stanford Univ

Kaufman, Cary MD [S] - **Spec Exp:** Breast Cancer; Breast Disease; **Hospital:** St Joseph Hosp - Bellingham; **Address:** 2940 Squalicum Pkwy, Ste 101, Bellingham, WA 98225; **Phone:** 360-671-9877; **Board Cert:** Surgery 00; **Med School:** UCLA 73; **Resid:** Surgery, Univ Wash 75; Surgery, Haarbor-UCLA Med Ctr 79; **Fac Appt:** Asst Clin Prof S, Univ Wash

Klein, Andrew S MD [S] - **Spec Exp:** Transplant-Liver; Liver Cancer; Liver Failure; **Hospital:** Cedars-Sinai Med Ctr (page 88); **Address:** Cedars-Sinai Medical Center, 8635 W Third St, Ste 590W, Los Angeles, CA 90048; **Phone:** 310-423-2641; **Board Cert:** Surgery 96; **Med School:** Johns Hopkins Univ 79; **Resid:** Surgery, Johns Hopkins Hosp 82; Surgery, Johns Hopkins Hosp 86; **Fellow:** Transplant Surgery, UCLA-CHS 88

Knudson, Mary Margaret MD [S] - **Spec Exp:** Breast Cancer; Trauma; **Hospital:** UCSF Med Ctr; **Address:** 1001 Potrero Ave, Ward 3A, San Francisco, CA 94110; **Phone:** 415-206-8814; **Board Cert:** Surgery 92; Surgical Critical Care 98; **Med School:** Univ Mich Med Sch 76; **Resid:** Surgery, Beth Israel Hosp 79; Surgery, Univ Mich Med Ctr 82; **Fellow:** Pediatric Surgery, Stanford Univ Hosps; **Fac Appt:** Assoc Prof S, UCSF

Norton, Jeffrey A MD [S] - **Spec Exp:** Pancreatic Cancer; Gastrointestinal Cancer & Surgery; Endocrine Surgery; **Hospital:** Stanford Univ Med Ctr; **Address:** 875 Blake Wilbur Drive, Clinic F, MS 5820, Stanford, CA 94305; **Phone:** 650-723-5461; **Board Cert:** Surgery 01; **Med School:** SUNY Upstate Med Univ 73; **Resid:** Surgery, Duke Univ Med Ctr 78; **Fellow:** Research, Natl Cancer Inst 82; **Fac Appt:** Prof S, Stanford Univ

Pellegrini, Carlos MD [S] - **Spec Exp:** Esophageal Cancer & Surgery; **Hospital:** Univ Wash Med Ctr; **Address:** Univ Washington, Dept Surg, 1959 NE Pacific St, Box 356410, Seattle, WA 98195; **Phone:** 206-543-3106; **Board Cert:** Surgery 98; **Med School:** Argentina 71; **Resid:** Surgery, Granadero Hosp 75; Surgery, Univ Chicago Hosps 79; **Fac Appt:** Prof S, Univ Wash

Reber, Howard A MD [S] - **Spec Exp:** Pancreatic Cancer; Pancreatitis; Gastrointestinal Cancer; **Hospital:** UCLA Med Ctr (page 111); **Address:** UCLA Medical Ctr, Dept Surgery, 10833 Le Conte Ave, Box 956904, Los Angeles, CA 90095-6904; **Phone:** 310-825-4976; **Board Cert:** Surgery 71; **Med School:** Univ Pennsylvania 64; **Resid:** Surgery, Hosp Univ Penn 70; **Fac Appt:** Prof S, UCLA

Schneider, Philip D MD/PhD [S] - **Spec Exp:** Cancer Surgery; Minimally Invasive Surgery; **Hospital:** UC Davis Med Ctr; **Address:** UC Davis, Div Surg Oncology, 4501 X St, Ste 3010, Sacramento, CA 95817; **Phone:** 916-734-7280; **Board Cert:** Surgery 02; **Med School:** St Louis Univ 72; **Resid:** Surgery, Univ Minn Hosps 81; Surgical Oncology, Meml Hosp 76; **Fac Appt:** Prof S, UC Davis

Silverstein, Melvin J MD [S] - **Spec Exp:** Breast Cancer; **Hospital:** USC Norris Canc Comp Ctr; **Address:** USC Norris Cancer Center, 1441 Eastlake Ave, rm 7415, Los Angeles, CA 90033; **Phone:** 323-865-3535; **Board Cert:** Surgery 71; **Med School:** Albany Med Coll 65; **Resid:** Surgery, Boston City Hosp-Tufts Univ 70; **Fellow:** Surgical Oncology, UCLA Med Ctr 75; **Fac Appt:** Prof S, USC Sch Med

Traverso, L William MD [S] - **Spec Exp:** Pancreatic Cancer; Laparoscopic Surgery; **Hospital:** Virginia Mason Med Ctr; **Address:** Virginia Mason Med Ctr, Dept Surg, 1100 9th Ave, Seattle, WA 98101; **Phone:** 206-223-8855; **Board Cert:** Surgery 98; **Med School:** UCLA 73; **Resid:** Surgery, UCLA Med Ctr 78; **Fac Appt:** Clin Prof S, Univ Wash

Vargas, Hernan I MD [S] - **Spec Exp:** Breast Cancer; **Hospital:** UCLA Med Ctr (page 111); **Address:** 1000 W Carson St, Harbor UCLA Med Ctr—Box 25, Torrance, CA 90509; **Phone:** 310-222-6715; **Board Cert:** Surgery 02; **Med School:** Peru 86; **Resid:** Surgery, Harbor/UCLA Med Ctr 93; **Fellow:** Surgical Oncology, NIH/NCI/Surgery Branch 96; **Fac Appt:** Assoc Prof S, UCLA

Wagman, Lawrence D MD [S] - **Spec Exp:** Liver Cancer; Gastrointestinal Cancer; Breast Cancer; **Hospital:** City of Hope Natl Med Ctr & Beckman Rsch (page 89); **Address:** City of Hope National Cancer Ctr, Dept Surgery, 1500 Duarte Rd, Duarte, CA 91010; **Phone:** 626-359-8111 x63058; **Board Cert:** Surgery 95; **Med School:** Columbia P&S 78; **Resid:** Surgery, Univ Virginia Med Ctr 83; **Fellow:** Surgical Oncology, NIH/NCI 85; **Fac Appt:** Assoc Clin Prof S, UCSD

Warren, Robert S MD [S] - **Spec Exp:** Liver Cancer; **Hospital:** UCSF Med Ctr; **Address:** 1600 Divisadero St, rm A710, San Francisco, CA 94143-1932; **Phone:** 415-353-9846; **Board Cert:** Surgery 98; **Med School:** Univ Minn 80; **Resid:** Surgery, Univ Minn Hosps 88; **Fellow:** Surgical Oncology, Meml Sloan-Kettering Cancer Ctr 86; **Fac Appt:** Prof S, UCSF

THORACIC SURGERY

A *thoracic surgeon provides the operative, perioperative care and critical care of patients with pathologic conditions within the chest. Included is the surgical care of coronary artery disease, cancers of the lung, esophagus and chest wall, abnormalities of the trachea, abnormalities of the great vessels and heart valves, congenital anomalies, tumors of the mediastinum and diseases of the diaphragm. The management of the airway and injuries of the chest is within the scope of the specialty.*

Thoracic surgeons have the knowledge, experience and technical skills to accurately diagnose, operate upon safely and effectively manage patients with thoracic diseases of the chest. This requires substantial knowledge of cardiorespiratory physiology and oncology, as well as capability in the use of heart assist devices, management of abnormal heart rhythms and drainage of the chest cavity, respiratory support systems, endoscopy and invasive and noninvasive diagnostic techniques.

Training required: *Seven to eight years*

PHYSICIAN LISTINGS

497

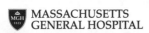
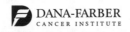
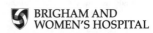

THE MOUNT SINAI MEDICAL CENTER
THORACIC SURGERY

One Gustave L. Levy Place (Fifth Avenue and 100th Street)
New York, NY 10029-6574   Phone: (212) 241-6500
Physician Referral: 1-800-MD-SINAI (637-4624)
www.mountsinai.org

Thoracic Surgery at Mount Sinai is famed for its advancements in the application of minimally invasive techniques, its focus on state-of-the-art multidisciplinary treatment of difficult tumors, and its commitment to treating patients whose conditions others believe to be incurable.

Successful care of a patient with lung or esophageal cancer and ultimately cure of these diseases is based on a multi-modality, fully–integrated and comprehensive thoracic oncology program.

Clinical care at Mount Sinai may also draw upon its expertise in behavioral medicine, genetic testing, and environmental medicine.

LUNG CANCER
Mount Sinai offers the widest possible spectrum of screening and diagnostic tests, including:

- CT screenings for the early detection of lung cancer.
- Advanced endoscopic techniques designed to detect early lesions and survey for early recurrence.
- Advanced CT and PET capabilities, as well as innovative MRI technology with ultrasensitive resolution.

In addition to radiation, chemotherapy, and surgical treatments to combat cancers in every stage; Mount Sinai offers:

- Minimally invasive lung cancer surgery: with faculty who have led national trials in VATS lobectomy, Mount Sinai is the leader in minimally invasive approaches in the New York tri-state area. Advances in this area include robotic techniques using the *daVinci Surgical System®* .

- Photodynamic therapy (PDT): for individuals with unresectable tumors of the airway and esophagus, especially those experiencing difficulty in breathing or swallowing.

- Laser therapy and stenting for esophageal and lung cancer: Laser therapy can be used to burn away portions of an unresectable tumor that blocks the esophagus or airway, while stenting may be recommended either following laser therapy to make its effects more durable or when laser therapy cannot be used.

- Access to Mount Sinai-led clinical trials, including those designed to carefully stage cancer and those employing cutting-edge biologic therapies.

ESOPHAGEAL CANCER
Mount Sinai offers the widest possible spectrum of screening and diagnostic tests. Treatment involves minimally invasive surgery with or without chemotherapy and radiation.

THE MOUNT SINAI MEDICAL CENTER

Coordinated Care
One of the strengths of Mount Sinai's Thoracic Oncology Program is the teamwork that its multidisciplinary experts bring to patient care. This team includes:

- Thoracic surgeons
- Medical oncologists
- Radiation oncologists
- Pathologists
- Radiologists
- Pulmonologists
- Gastroenterologists
- Plastic surgeons
- Oncology-dedicated nurses
- Respiratory therapists
- Physical and occupational therapists
- Nutritionists
- Social workers
- Psychiatrists and psychologists

Coordinating information among team members to ensure seamless care for the patient is one of the program's highest priorities.

Our team also provides a seamless approach to the diagnosis, treatment and follow up of patients who are affected by swallowing and reflux disorders. This includes:

- Gastroenterology
- Otolaryngology
- Speech and swallowing therapy
- Thoracic surgery
- Medical and Radiation oncology
- Radiology

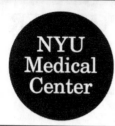

550 First Avenue (at 31st Street)
New York, NY 10016
Physician Referral:
1-888-7-NYU-MED
www.nyumc.org

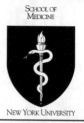

SCHOOL OF
MEDICINE

NEW YORK UNIVERSITY

NYU MEDICAL CENTER
A LEADER IN MINIMALLY
INVASIVE THORACIC SURGERY

On the technological forefront of minimally invasive techniques, the Division of Thoracic Surgery at NYU Medical Center dedicates itself to the diagnosis and treatment of abdominal, lung, mediastinal, and chest wall problems. At NYU Hospitals Center, the majority of thoracic procedures are performed utilizing video-assisted equipment, which benefits surgeon and patient alike.

Use of video-assisted equipment means not only a more accurate and safe surgery, but it also means smaller incisions, an indispensable benefit to the patient, reducing discomfort, recovery time, and length of stay. Moving away from the traditional method of long incisions through the muscular abdominal wall, NYU's thoracic surgeons perform the same procedures through much smaller openings, with better results.

The Division of Thoracic Surgery at NYU Hospitals Center uses minimally invasive techniques to provide its patients maximum comfort and accuracy of diagnosis and treatment. Below are just some of the latest interventions performed by its doctors:

VIDEO-ASSISTED THORACOSCOPY

- Sympathectomy for Hyperhydrosis
- Pleural Biopsy
- Pleurectomy
- Pleurodesis
- Mediastinal Evaluation
- Lung Resection
- Lung Volume Reduction Procedures
- Esophageal Procedures

VIDEO-ASSISTED BRONCHOSCOPY

- Diagnostic Evaluation
- Laser Resection of Tumor
- Endobronchial Stent Insertion

VIDEO-ASSISTED MEDIASTINOSCOPY

- Staging Procedures
- Diagnostic Evaluations

The burgeoning field of minimally invasive thoracic surgery is constantly growing in leaps and bounds. In terms of its importance to the medical field, it has been compared to open-heart surgery, or even to anesthesia. Doctors at NYU Hospitals Center dedicate their time not only to unsurpassed clinical care, but also to contributions through research. For example, its surgeons have performed more minimally invasive port-access cardiac surgeries than any other hospital in the world, and their expertise in unparalleled.

PHYSICIAN REFERRAL
1-888-7-NYU-MED
(1-888-769-8633)
www.nyumc.org

THORACIC ONCOLOGY PROGRAM
UCLA HEALTHCARE

1-800-UCLA-MD1 (825-2631)
www.healthcare.ucla.edu

UCLA's Thoracic Oncology Program provides highly integrated medical, surgical and radiation oncology services to patients with benign and malignant tumors of the lung, esophagus, pleura, mediastinum, chest wall, and all other areas of the thoracic cavity.

UCLA's program partners scientists specializing in cell signaling, angiogenesis inhibition, immunotherapy and gene therapy with experts in molecular imaging, epidemiology, pathology, biostatistics and patient care.

The Lung Cancer Program at UCLA's Jonsson Cancer Center has been designated a Specialized Program of Research Excellence (SPORE) by the National Cancer Institute, making it one of a handful of programs nationwide to receive national recognition and substantial research funding to improve prevention, detection and treatment of lung cancer. The goal is to translate basic research from the lab into patient care much more quickly and effectively.

UCLA'S JONSSON CANCER CENTER

Designated by the National Cancer Institute as one of only 38 comprehensive cancer centers in the United States, UCLA's Jonsson Cancer Center has earned an international reputation for developing new cancer therapies, providing the best in experimental and traditional treatments, and expertly guiding and training the next generation of medical researchers. The center's 250 physicians and scientists treat upwards of 20,000 patient visits per year and offer hundreds of clinical trials that provide the latest in experimental cancer treatments (www.cancer.mednet.ucla.edu). The center also offers patients and families psychological and support services.

UCLA's Jonsson Cancer Center has been ranked the best cancer center in the western United States by U.S. News & World Report's Annual Best Hospitals survey for the past five years. UCLA Medical Center, of which the Cancer Center is a part, has ranked best in the West for the past 15 years.

**Call 1-800-UCLA-MD1 (825-2631)
for a referral to a UCLA doctor.**

UCLA Healthcare

UCLA'S THORACIC ONCOLOGY PROGRAM OFFERS TREATMENTS FOR TUMORS OF THE:

- Lung
- Esophagus
- Pleura
- Mediastinum
- Chest Wall
- All other areas of the thoracic cavity

THE UNIVERSITY OF TEXAS
MD ANDERSON
CANCER CENTER
Making Cancer History™

1515 Holcombe Blvd.
Houston, Texas 77030-4095
Tel. 713-792-6161
Toll Free 800-392-1611
www.mdanderson.org

THORACIC ONCOLOGY

The M. D. Anderson Thoracic Center services include consultation, evaluation, and treatment of patients with tumors originating in the chest. Investigational treatment of thoracic malignancies, including multimodality treatments, innovative chemotherapy, gene therapy, chemoprevention, and performance of minor thoracic procedures.

Diseases treated include lung and esophageal cancer, tracheal tumors, thymoma, mesothelioma, cardiovascular diseases, pulmonary metastases, mediastinal tumors, chest wall and sternal tumors, and pleural and pericardial diseases and effusions.

Center features include:

- Expertise and novel approaches to the administration of chemotherapy plus radiation for patients with inoperable tumors

- Neoadjuvant chemotherapy protocols for locally advanced tumors that can be reduced to facilitate subsequent operations

- Endoscopic surgery, including laser resections to reestablish an airway

- Surgical techniques that permit en bloc resections and reconstruction of the vertebral bodies for lung cancers that invade the spinal column-locations historically considered untouchable

- Detailed preoperative testing for redefining the lower physiologic limits for patients considered medically inoperable

- Pulmonary-sparing techniques and close postoperative monitoring in intensive care and step-down telemetry units to allow safe recovery for those with advanced emphysema or cardiac disease

- High-level experience in managing malignant pleural effusions utilizing the Pleurx-Denver catheter, a method that avoids hospital admission and prolonged chest tube drainage

- Availability of three-dimensional conformal radiotherapy and brachytherapy for respectable lesions

- Photodynamic therapy for endobronchial tumors

- High dose rate endobronchial brachytherapy, which boosts tumors dose and relieves obstruction of airway quickly

M. D. Anderson is one of the largest cancer centers in the world. We've been working to eliminate cancer for more than six decades. Our depth of experience informs every aspect of your care.

We focus exclusively on cancer and have seen cases of every kind. Our doctors treat more rare cancers in a single day than most physicians see in a lifetime. That means you receive expert care no matter what your diagnosis.

We are the top-ranked cancer hospital in the United States according to the 2004 *U.S.News & World Report* annual survey of hospitals.

M. D. Anderson ranks first in the number and amount of research grants awarded by the National Cancer Institute. By studying how cancer begins and responds to various treatments, we can help patients overcome disease and prevent recurrence.

At M. D. Anderson, we understand that cancer is not just a physical disease. To help you cope with every aspect of cancer, we provide a number of support programs.

THORACIC SURGERY

New England

Mathisen, Douglas MD [TS] - **Spec Exp:** Tracheal Surgery; Lung Cancer; Esophageal Cancer;
Hospital: Mass Genl Hosp; **Address:** Mass Genl Hosp, Dept Thor Surg, 55 Fruit St, Blake 1570,
Boston, MA 02114; **Phone:** 617-726-6826; **Board Cert:** Surgery 82; Thoracic Surgery 92; **Med School:**
Univ IL Coll Med 74; **Resid:** Surgery, Mass Genl Hosp 81; Thoracic Surgery, Mass Genl Hosp 82;
Fellow: Surgical Oncology, Natl Cancer Inst 79; **Fac Appt:** Prof S, Harvard Med Sch

Shahian, David MD [TS] - **Spec Exp:** Coronary Artery Surgery; Heart Valve Surgery; Lung Cancer;
Hospital: St Elizabeth's Med Ctr; **Address:** St Elizabeth's Hosp, Dept Surgery, 736 Cambridge St,
Boston, MA 02135; **Phone:** 617-789-5004; **Board Cert:** Thoracic Surgery 00; **Med School:** Harvard
Med Sch 73; **Resid:** Surgery, Mass Genl Hosp 78; **Fellow:** Thoracic Surgery, Rush Presby-St Lukes
Hosp 80; **Fac Appt:** Assoc Clin Prof S, Harvard Med Sch

Sugarbaker, David J MD [TS] - **Spec Exp:** Mesothelioma; Transplant-Lung; Esophageal Cancer;
Hospital: Brigham & Women's Hosp (page 87); **Address:** Brigham & Women's Hosp, Div Thoracic Surg,
75 Francis St, Boston, MA 02115-6110; **Phone:** 617-732-5004; **Board Cert:** Surgery 87; Thoracic
Surgery 99; **Med School:** Cornell Univ-Weill Med Coll 79; **Resid:** Surgery, Brigham & Women's Hosp
82; Surgery, Brigham & Women's Hosp 86; **Fellow:** Thoracic Surgery, Toronto Genl Hosp 88; **Fac Appt:**
Prof S, Harvard Med Sch

Wain, John MD [TS] - **Spec Exp:** Transplant-Lung; Lung Cancer; Esophageal Cancer; **Hospital:** Mass
Genl Hosp; **Address:** Mass Genl Hosp, Dept Thor Surg, 55 Fruit St, Blake 1570, Boston, MA 02114;
Phone: 617-726-5200; **Board Cert:** Thoracic Surgery 00; **Med School:** Jefferson Med Coll 80; **Resid:**
Surgery, Mass Genl Hosp 85; Medical Oncology, City Hope Med Ctr 86; **Fellow:** Cardiothoracic Surgery,
Mass Genl Hosp 88; **Fac Appt:** Asst Prof TS, Harvard Med Sch

Wright, Cameron D MD [TS] - **Spec Exp:** Lung Cancer; Esophageal Cancer; Tracheal Surgery;
Hospital: Mass Genl Hosp; **Address:** Division of Surgery, 55 Fruit St, Blake 1570, Boston, MA 02114-
2696; **Phone:** 617-726-5801; **Board Cert:** Surgery 95; Thoracic Surgery 97; **Med School:** Univ Mich
Med Sch 80; **Resid:** Surgery, Mass Genl Hosp 86; Thoracic Surgery, Mass Genl Hosp 88; **Fac Appt:**
Assoc Prof S, Harvard Med Sch

Mid Atlantic

Altorki, Nasser MD [TS] - **Spec Exp:** Esophageal Cancer; Lung Cancer; Gastroesophageal Reflux
Disease (GERD); **Hospital:** NY-Presby Hosp - NY Weill Cornell Med Ctr (page 103); **Address:** 525 E
68th St, New York, NY 10021-4870; **Phone:** 212-746-5156; **Board Cert:** Surgery 96; Thoracic Surgery
98; **Med School:** Egypt 78; **Resid:** Surgery, Univ Chicago Hosps 85; **Fellow:** Cardiothoracic Surgery,
Univ Chicago Hosps 87; **Fac Appt:** Prof S, Cornell Univ-Weill Med Coll

Bains, Manjit MD [TS] - **Spec Exp:** Cardiothoracic Surgery; Esophageal Cancer; Lung Cancer;
Hospital: Meml Sloan Kettering Cancer Ctr (page 100); **Address:** 1275 York Ave, rm C-861, New York,
NY 10021; **Phone:** 212-639-7450; **Board Cert:** Surgery 71; Thoracic Surgery 72; **Med School:** India
63; **Resid:** Surgery, Rochester Genl Hosp 70; **Fellow:** Thoracic Surgery, Sloan Kettering Cancer Ctr 72;
Fac Appt: Clin Prof S, Cornell Univ-Weill Med Coll

Demmy, Todd L MD [TS] - **Spec Exp:** Lung Cancer; Thoracic Cancers; Esophageal Cancer; **Hospital:** Roswell Park Cancer Inst (page 107); **Address:** Roswell Park Cancer Inst, Carlton Bldg, Elm & Carlton Sts, rm 243, Buffalo, NY 14263; **Phone:** 716-845-5873; **Board Cert:** Surgical Critical Care 92; Surgery 97; Thoracic Surgery 00; **Med School:** Jefferson Med Coll 83; **Resid:** Surgery, Baylor Univ Medical Ctr 88; Thoracic Surgery, Allegheny Genl Hosp 91; **Fac Appt:** Assoc Prof S, SUNY Buffalo

Friedberg, Joseph MD [TS] - **Spec Exp:** Lung Cancer; Mesothelioma; Minimally Invasive Thoracic Surgery; **Hospital:** Univ Penn Med Ctr - Presbyterian; **Address:** Presbyterian Medical Ctr, 51 N 39th St, rm W266, Philadelphia, PA 19104; **Phone:** 215-662-9195; **Board Cert:** Surgery 96; Thoracic Surgery 97; **Med School:** Harvard Med Sch 86; **Resid:** Surgery, Mass General Hosp 94; **Fellow:** Cardiothoracic Surgery, Brigham & Womens Hosp 96

Gharagozloo, Farid MD [TS] - **Spec Exp:** Video Assisted Thoracic Surgery (VATS); Lung Cancer; **Hospital:** G Washington Univ Hosp; **Address:** 2175 K St NW, Ste 300, Washington, DC 20037; **Phone:** 202-775-8600; **Board Cert:** Surgery 90; Thoracic Surgery 93; **Med School:** Johns Hopkins Univ 83; **Resid:** Surgery, Mayo Clinic 89; Research, Harvard Med Sch 86; **Fellow:** Cardiothoracic Surgery, Mayo Clinic 92; **Fac Appt:** Prof S, Geo Wash Univ

Goldberg, Melvyn MD [TS] - **Spec Exp:** Lung Cancer; Esophageal Cancer; Barrett's Esophagus; **Hospital:** Fox Chase Cancer Ctr (page 95); **Address:** Fox Chase Cancer Center, 7701 Burholme Ave, Philadelphia, PA 19111; **Phone:** 215-728-6900 x2570; **Med School:** Canada 65; **Resid:** Surgery, Totonto General Hosp 72; Thoracic Surgery, The London Chest Hosp 73; **Fellow:** Cardiothoracic Surgery, Univ Toronto Med Ctr 74

Heitmiller, Richard F MD [TS] - **Spec Exp:** Esophageal Surgery; Esophageal Cancer; Lung Cancer; **Hospital:** Union Meml Hosp - Baltimore; **Address:** 3333 N Calvert St, Ste 610, Baltimore, MD 21218; **Phone:** 410-554-2063; **Board Cert:** Surgery 97; Thoracic Surgery 99; **Med School:** Johns Hopkins Univ 79; **Resid:** Surgery, Mass Genl Hosp 85; **Fellow:** Thoracic Surgery, Mass Genl Hosp 87

Kaiser, Larry R MD [TS] - **Spec Exp:** Lung Cancer; Esophageal Cancer; Mediastinal Tumors; **Hospital:** Hosp Univ Penn - UPHS (page 113); **Address:** Hosp Univ Pennsylvania, Dept Surgery, 3400 Spruce St, 4 Silverstein, Philadelphia, PA 19104-4219; **Phone:** 215-662-7538; **Board Cert:** Thoracic Surgery 96; **Med School:** Tulane Univ 77; **Resid:** Surgery, UCLA Med Ctr 83; Cardiothoracic Surgery, Univ Toronto Hosps 85; **Fellow:** Surgical Oncology, UCLA Med Ctr 81; **Fac Appt:** Prof S, Univ Pennsylvania

Keenan, Robert J. MD [TS] - **Spec Exp:** Lung Cancer; Esophageal Cancer; Mediastinal Tumors; **Hospital:** Allegheny General Hosp; **Address:** Allegheny Genl Hosp, 14th Fl, 320 E North Ave, Pittsburgh, PA 15212; **Phone:** 412-359-6137; **Board Cert:** Surgery 00; **Med School:** Canada 84; **Resid:** Surgery, Univ Toronto Med Ctr 89; **Fellow:** Thoracic Surgery, Univ Pittsburgh Med Ctr 90; Thoracic Surgery, Univ Toronto Med Ctr 91; **Fac Appt:** Prof TS, Drexel Univ Coll Med

Keller, Steven M MD [TS] - **Spec Exp:** Lung Cancer; Esophageal Cancer; Palmar Hyperhidrosis; **Hospital:** Montefiore Med Ctr; **Address:** Greene Medical Arts Pavilion, 3400 Bainbridge Ave, Ste 5B, Bronx, NY 10467-2404; **Phone:** 718-920-7580; **Board Cert:** Surgery 96; Thoracic Surgery 96; **Med School:** Albany Med Coll 77; **Resid:** Surgery, Mount Sinai Hosp 85; Thoracic Surgery, Mem Sloan Kettering Cancer Ctr 87; **Fellow:** Surgical Oncology, NIH/National Cancer Inst 83; **Fac Appt:** Prof TS, Albert Einstein Coll Med

Krasna, Mark MD [TS] - **Spec Exp:** Esophageal Cancer; Lung Tumors; Mesothelioma; **Hospital:** Univ of MD Med Sys; **Address:** 22 S Green St, Rm N4E35, Baltimore, MD 21201; **Phone:** 410-328-6366; **Board Cert:** Surgery 90; Thoracic Surgery 00; **Med School:** Israel 82; **Resid:** Surgery, CMDNJ-Rutgers Med Sch 88; **Fellow:** Cardiothoracic Surgery, New England Deaconess-Harvard 90; **Fac Appt:** Prof S, Univ MD Sch Med

Krellenstein, Daniel J MD [TS] - **Spec Exp:** Lung Tumors; **Hospital:** Mount Sinai Med Ctr (page 101); **Address:** 16 E 98th St, Ste 1F, New York, NY 10029-6545; **Phone:** 212-423-9311; **Board Cert:** Surgery 74; Thoracic Surgery 77; **Med School:** SUNY Buffalo 64; **Resid:** Surgery, SUNY Downstate Med Ctr 72; **Fac Appt:** Assoc Clin Prof TS, Mount Sinai Sch Med

Landreneau, Rodney MD [TS] - **Spec Exp:** Lung Cancer; Esophageal Cancer; Gastroesophageal Reflux Disease (GERD); **Hospital:** UPMC Shadyside (page 114); **Address:** UPMC Cancer Ctr - Shadyside, 5200 Centre Ave, Ste 715, Pittsburgh, PA 15232; **Phone:** 412-623-2025; **Board Cert:** Thoracic Surgery 94; **Med School:** Louisiana State Univ 65; **Resid:** Surgery, Parkland Meml Hosp 83; **Fellow:** Cardiothoracic Surgery, Univ Mich Med Ctr 85; **Fac Appt:** Prof S, Univ Pittsburgh

Pierson III, Richard N MD [TS] - **Spec Exp:** Transplant-Lung; Lung Cancer; Transplant-Heart; **Hospital:** Univ of MD Med Sys; **Address:** Univ Maryland Med Ctr, Dept Cardiothoracic Surg, 22 S Greene St, rm N4W94, Baltimore, MD 21201; **Phone:** 410-328-5842; **Board Cert:** Surgery 00; Thoracic Surgery 02; **Med School:** Columbia P&S 83; **Resid:** Surgery, Univ Mich Med Ctr 90; **Fellow:** Cardiothoracic Surgery, Mass General Hosp 92; **Fac Appt:** Assoc Prof TS, Univ MD Sch Med

Steinglass, Kenneth MD [TS] - **Spec Exp:** Lung Cancer; Esophageal Cancer; Chest Surgery; **Hospital:** NY-Presby Hosp - Columbia Presby Med Ctr (page 103); **Address:** 161 Fort Washington Ave Fl 3 - Ste 322, New York, NY 10032-3713; **Phone:** 212-305-3408; **Board Cert:** Thoracic Surgery 00; Vascular Surgery 96; **Med School:** Harvard Med Sch 72; **Resid:** Surgery, Columbia-Presby 77; **Fellow:** Thoracic Surgery, Mayo Clinic 79; **Fac Appt:** Clin Prof S, Columbia P&S

Swanson, Scott J MD [TS] - **Spec Exp:** Lung Cancer. Transplant-Lung; Video Assisted Thoracic Surgery (VATS); Esophageal & Swallowing Disorders; **Hospital:** Mount Sinai Med Ctr (page 101); **Address:** 1190 Fifth Ave GP2W Box 1028, New York, NY 10029-6503; **Phone:** 212-659-6800; **Board Cert:** Surgery 91; Thoracic Surgery 96; **Med School:** Harvard Med Sch 85; **Resid:** Surgery, Brigham & Women's Hosp 90; Brigham & Women's Hosp 94

Yang, Stephen C MD [TS] - **Spec Exp:** Mesothelioma; Lung Cancer; **Hospital:** Johns Hopkins Hosp - Baltimore (page 99); **Address:** Johns Hopkins Hosp, 600 N Wolfe St Bldg Osler - rm 624, Baltimore, MD 21287-5674; **Phone:** 410-614-3891; **Board Cert:** Surgery 95; Thoracic Surgery 96; **Med School:** Med Coll VA 84; **Resid:** Surgery, Univ Tex Hlth Sci Ctr 90; **Fellow:** Thoracic Surgery, MD Anderson Cancer Ctr 92; **Fac Appt:** Assoc Prof TS, Johns Hopkins Univ

Southeast

D'Amico, Thomas MD [TS] - **Spec Exp:** Lung Cancer; Esophageal Cancer; **Hospital:** Duke Univ Med Ctr (page 94); **Address:** Duke Univ Med Ctr, Box 3496, Durham, NC 27710; **Phone:** 919-684-4891; **Board Cert:** Surgery 95; Thoracic Surgery 98; **Med School:** Columbia P&S 87; **Resid:** Surgery, Duke Univ Med Ctr 89; Cardiothoracic Surgery, Duke Univ Med Ctr 96; **Fellow:** Thoracic Oncology, Meml Sloan Kettering Cancer Ctr; **Fac Appt:** Assoc Prof S, Duke Univ

Daniel, Thomas M MD **[TS]** - **Spec Exp:** Esophageal Cancer; Thoracoscopic Lung Cancer Surgery; Thoracoscopic Sympathectomy; **Hospital:** Univ Virginia Med Ctr; **Address:** Univ Virginia Hlth System, Dept Surg, Box 800679, Charlottesville, VA 22908-0679; **Phone:** 434-924-5052; **Board Cert:** Surgery 75; Thoracic Surgery 94; Vascular Surgery 94; **Med School:** Univ VA Sch Med 64; **Resid:** Internal Medicine, Grady Meml Hosp-Emory Univ 66; Surgery, Duke Univ Med Ctr 75; **Fac Appt:** Prof S, Univ VA Sch Med

Detterbeck, Frank C MD **[TS]** - **Spec Exp:** Lung Cancer; Mediastinal Tumors; Esophageal Cancer; **Hospital:** Univ NC Hosps (page 112); **Address:** Univ North Carolina, Div Cardiothoracic Surg, Med Sch Wing C, rm 354, CB 7065, Chapel Hill, NC 27599-7065; **Phone:** 919-966-3381; **Board Cert:** Thoracic Surgery 01; **Med School:** Northwestern Univ 83; **Resid:** Surgery, Virginia Mason Hosp 88; **Fellow:** Cardiothoracic Surgery, Univ North Carolina Hosps 91; **Fac Appt:** Prof S, Univ NC Sch Med

Egan, Thomas MD **[TS]** - **Spec Exp:** Transplant-Lung; Thoracic Cancers; **Hospital:** Univ NC Hosps (page 112); **Address:** University of N Carolina Hospitals at Chapel Hill, CB 7065, Chapel Hill, NC 27599-7065; **Phone:** 919-966-3381; **Board Cert:** Thoracic Surgery 99; **Med School:** Univ Toronto 76; **Resid:** Surgery, Univ Toronto 86; Thoracic Surgery, Univ Toronto 88; **Fellow:** Transplant Surgery, Washington Univ 89; **Fac Appt:** Prof S, Univ NC Sch Med

Kiernan, Paul D MD **[TS]** - **Spec Exp:** Lung Cancer; Esophageal Cancer; Mediastinal Masses; **Hospital:** Inova Fairfax Hosp; **Address:** 3301 Woodburn Rd, Ste 301, Annandale, VA 22003; **Phone:** 703-280-5858; **Board Cert:** Thoracic Surgery 03; **Med School:** Georgetown Univ 74; **Resid:** Surgery, Mayo Clinic 79; Cardiothoracic Surgery, Mayo Clinic 81; **Fellow:** Vascular Surgery, Mayo Clinic 82; **Fac Appt:** Assoc Clin Prof S, Georgetown Univ

Miller, Joseph MD **[TS]** - **Spec Exp:** Lung Cancer; Empyema; **Hospital:** Emory Univ Hosp; **Address:** 550 Peachtree St NE, MOT-6th Fl, Atlanta, GA 30308-2225; **Phone:** 404-686-2515; **Board Cert:** Surgery 73; Thoracic Surgery 75; **Med School:** Emory Univ 65; **Resid:** Surgery, Mayo Clin 72; Thoracic Surgery, Emory Univ Hosp 74; **Fac Appt:** Prof S, Emory Univ

Nesbitt, Jonathan C MD **[TS]** - **Spec Exp:** Lung Cancer; Esophageal Cancer; Chest Diseases-Benign; **Hospital:** St Thomas Hosp - Nashville; **Address:** Cardiovascular Surgical Assocs, Saint Thomas Medical Bldg, 4230 Harding Rd, Ste 450, Nashville, TN 37205; **Phone:** 615-385-4781; **Board Cert:** Surgical Critical Care 93; Surgery 98; Thoracic Surgery 98; **Med School:** Georgetown Univ 81; **Resid:** Surgery, Vanderbilt Univ Medical Ctr 87; Thoracic Surgery, Albany Medical Ctr 89; **Fac Appt:** Asst Clin Prof S, Vanderbilt Univ

Ninan, Mathew MD **[TS]** - **Spec Exp:** Lung Cancer; Transplant-Lung; Esophageal Cancer; **Hospital:** Vanderbilt Univ Med Ctr (page 116); **Address:** Vanderbilt-Ingram Cancer Ctr, 2986 The Vanderbilt Clinic, Nashville, TN 37232-5734; **Phone:** 615-322-0064; **Med School:** India 88; **Resid:** Surgery, University of London 94; **Fellow:** Cardiothoracic Surgery, University of Pittsburgh 98; **Fac Appt:** Asst Prof TS, Vanderbilt Univ

Putnam Jr, Joe B MD **[TS]** - **Spec Exp:** Lung Cancer; Esophageal Cancer; Sarcoma-Soft Tissue; **Hospital:** Vanderbilt Univ Med Ctr (page 116); **Address:** Vanderbilt Univ Med Ctr - Thoracic Surgery, 1301 22nd Ave S, TVC-Ste 2986, Nashville, TN 37232-5734; **Phone:** 615-343-9202; **Board Cert:** Thoracic Surgery 97; **Med School:** Univ NC Sch Med 79; **Resid:** Surgery, Univ Rochester 86; Thoracic Surgery, Univ Mich Med Ctr 88; **Fellow:** Surgical Oncology, NCI/NIH-Surg Branch 84; **Fac Appt:** Prof TS, Vanderbilt Univ

Reed, Carolyn MD [TS] - **Spec Exp:** Esophageal Cancer; Lung Cancer; **Hospital:** MUSC Med Ctr; **Address:** Medical Universityof S Carolina, Hollings Cancer Ctr, 96 Jonathan-Lucas St, Ste 418, Charleston, SC 29425; **Phone:** 843-792-3362; **Board Cert:** Surgery 93; Thoracic Surgery 05; **Med School:** Univ Rochester 77; **Resid:** Surgery, NY Hosp-Cornell Med Ctr 82; Thoracic Surgery, NY Hosp-Cornell Med Ctr 85; **Fellow:** Surgical Oncology, Memorial Sloan Kettering Cancer Ctr 83; **Fac Appt:** Prof S, Univ SC Sch Med

Robinson, Lary A MD [TS] - **Spec Exp:** Lung Cancer; Mesothelioma; **Hospital:** H Lee Moffitt Cancer Ctr & Research Inst; **Address:** 12902 Magnolia Drive, Tampa, FL 33612-9497; **Phone:** 813-979-7282; **Board Cert:** Thoracic Surgery 03; Surgery 02; Surgical Critical Care 00; **Med School:** Washington Univ, St Louis 72; **Resid:** Surgery, Duke Univ Med Ctr 74; Thoracic Surgery, Duke Univ Med Ctr 81; **Fellow:** Cardiothoracic Surgery, St Thomas Hosp 82; Cardiothoracic Surgery, Duke Univ Med Ctr 83; **Fac Appt:** Prof S, Univ S Fla Coll Med

Zorn, George L MD [TS] - **Spec Exp:** Transplant-Lung; Lung Cancer; **Hospital:** Univ of Ala Hosp at Birmingham; **Address:** Univ Ala at Birmingham - Bldg 720THT, 1900 Univ Blvd, Birmingham, AL 35294; **Phone:** 205-934-2536; **Board Cert:** Surgery 74; Thoracic Surgery 87; **Med School:** Emory Univ 68; **Resid:** Surgery, Columbia - Presby Hosp 73; Thoracic Surgery, Univ Alabama 77; **Fac Appt:** Assoc Prof S, Univ Ala

Midwest

Deschamps, Claude MD [TS] - **Spec Exp:** Gastroesophageal Reflux Disease (GERD); Esophageal Cancer; Lung Cancer; **Hospital:** St Mary's Hosp - Rochester; **Address:** Mayo Clinic, Div Thoracic Surg, 200 First St SW, Rochester, MN 55905; **Phone:** 507-284-8462; **Board Cert:** Surgery 94; **Med School:** Univ Montreal 79; **Resid:** Surgery, Univ Montreal Hosps 84; Thoracic Surgery, Univ Montreal Hosp 85; **Fellow:** Thoracic Surgery, Mayo Clinic 87; **Fac Appt:** Prof S, Mayo Med Sch

Faber, L. Penfield MD [TS] - **Spec Exp:** Lung Cancer; Esophageal Cancer; Thoracic Cancers; **Hospital:** Rush Univ Med Ctr; **Address:** 1725 W Harrison St, Ste 218, Chicago, IL 60612-3817; **Phone:** 312-738-3732; **Board Cert:** Surgery 62; Thoracic Surgery 63; **Med School:** Northwestern Univ 56; **Resid:** Surgery, Presby-St Luke's Hosp 61; Thoracic Surgery, Hines VA Hosp 63; **Fac Appt:** Prof TS, Rush Med Coll

Ferguson, Mark MD [TS] - **Spec Exp:** Barrett's Esophagus; Esophageal Cancer; Lung Cancer; **Hospital:** Univ of Chicago Hosps; **Address:** 5841 S Maryland Ave, MC 5035, Chicago, IL 60637-1470; **Phone:** 773-702-3551; **Board Cert:** Surgery 93; Thoracic Surgery 03; **Med School:** Univ Chicago-Pritzker Sch Med 77; **Resid:** Surgery, Univ Chicago Hosps 82; **Fellow:** Cardiothoracic Surgery, Univ Chicago Hosps 84; **Fac Appt:** Prof S, Univ Chicago-Pritzker Sch Med

Iannettoni, Mark D MD [TS] - **Spec Exp:** Transplant-Lung; Lung Cancer; Esophageal Cancer; **Hospital:** Univ Iowa Hosp & Clinics; **Address:** Univ Iowa Hosp & Clinics, 200 Hawkins Dr, 1602-ICP, Iowa City, IA 52242; **Phone:** 319-356-1133; **Board Cert:** Surgery 02; Thoracic Surgery 02; **Med School:** SUNY Upstate Med Univ 85; **Resid:** Surgery, SUNY Upstate Med Ctr 91; Thoracic Surgery, Univ Mich Med Ctr 93; **Fellow:** Thoracic Surgery, Univ Mich Med Sch 94; **Fac Appt:** Prof S, Univ Iowa Coll Med

Maddaus, Michael A MD [TS] - **Spec Exp:** Esophageal Cancer; Lung Cancer; Minimally Invasive Thoracic Surgery; **Hospital:** Fairview-Univ Med Ctr - Univ Campus; **Address:** Univ Minn Hosps, 420 Delaware St, Box 207 UMHC, Minneapolis, MN 55455; **Phone:** 612-624-9461; **Board Cert:** Surgery 00; Thoracic Surgery 93; **Med School:** Univ Minn 82; **Resid:** Surgery, Univ Minn 90; Thoracic Surgery, Univ Toronto 91; **Fellow:** Cardiac Surgery, St Michael's Hosp/Hosp Sich Chldn 92; Thoracic Oncology, Meml Sloan Kettering Cancer Ctr 92; **Fac Appt:** Prof S, Univ Minn

Meyers, Bryan MD [TS] - **Spec Exp:** Lung Cancer; Esophageal Cancer; Transplant-Lung; **Hospital:** Barnes-Jewish Hosp (page 85); **Address:** 3108 Queeny Tower, St Louis, MO 63110; **Phone:** 314-362-8598; **Board Cert:** Surgery 98; Thoracic Surgery 99; **Med School:** Univ Chicago-Pritzker Sch Med 86; **Resid:** Surgery, Mass Genl Hosp 96; **Fellow:** Cardiothoracic Surgery, Barnes Hosp-Wash Univ 98; **Fac Appt:** Assoc Prof S, Washington Univ, St Louis

Orringer, Mark B MD [TS] - **Spec Exp:** Esophageal Cancer; Esophageal Disorders, Benign; Cardiothoracic Surgery; **Hospital:** Univ Michigan Hlth Sys; **Address:** Univ Mich, Taubman Ctr, 1500 E Med Ctr Drive, rm TC 2120, Box 0344, Ann Arbor, MI 48109-0344; **Phone:** 734-936-4975; **Board Cert:** Surgery 73; Thoracic Surgery 74; **Med School:** Univ Pittsburgh 67; **Resid:** Thoracic Surgery, Johns Hopkins Hosp 73; **Fac Appt:** Prof S, Univ Mich Med Sch

Pairolero, Peter MD [TS] - **Spec Exp:** Chest Wall Tumors; **Hospital:** Mayo Med Ctr & Clin - Rochester; **Address:** Mayo Clinic, Div Genl Thoracic Surg, 200 First St SW, Rochester, MN 55905-4317; **Phone:** 507-284-2808; **Board Cert:** Surgery 72; Thoracic Surgery 74; **Med School:** Univ Mich Med Sch 63; **Resid:** Surgery, Mayo Clinic 71; Thoracic Surgery, Mayo Clinic 73; **Fellow:** Cerebrovascular Disease, Mayo Clinic 69

Pass, Harvey MD [TS] - **Spec Exp:** Lung Cancer; Mesothelioma; Clinical Trials; **Hospital:** Harper Univ Hosp; **Address:** Harper Hosp - Wayne State Univ, 3990 John R St, Ste 2102, Detroit, MI 48201-2018; **Phone:** 313-745-1413; **Board Cert:** Thoracic Surgery 01; **Med School:** Duke Univ 73; **Resid:** Surgery, Duke Univ Med Ctr 75; Surgery, Univ Miss Med Ctr 80; **Fellow:** Cardiothoracic Surgery, MUSC Med Ctr 82; **Fac Appt:** Prof S, Wayne State Univ

Patterson, G Alexander MD [TS] - **Spec Exp:** Transplant-Lung, Heart & Lung; Lung Cancer; Esophageal Cancer; **Hospital:** Barnes-Jewish Hosp (page 85); **Address:** One Barnes Jewish Hospital Plaza, Queeny Tower, Ste 3108, St Louis, MO 63110; **Phone:** 314-362-6025; **Board Cert:** Surgery 78; Thoracic Surgery 81; Vascular Surgery 82; **Med School:** Canada 74; **Resid:** Surgery, Queens Univ Med Ctr 78; Vascular Surgery, Univ Toronto Med Ctr 79; **Fellow:** Research, Toronto Genl Hosp 81; Surgical Critical Care, Johns Hopkins Hosp 82; **Fac Appt:** Prof S, Washington Univ, St Louis

Raman, Jai MD [TS] - **Spec Exp:** Atrial Fibrillation; Heart Failure & Ventricular Containment; Mesothelioma; **Hospital:** Univ of Chicago Hosps; **Address:** University of Chicago Hosps, 5841 S Maryland Ave, Ste E500, MC 5040, Chicago, IL 60637; **Phone:** 773-702-2500; **Med School:** India 75; **Resid:** St Vincent's Hosp 80; **Fellow:** Thoracic Surgery, Austin Hosp 83; Pediatric Cardiac Surgery, Royal Children's Hosp 85; **Fac Appt:** Assoc Prof S, Univ Chicago-Pritzker Sch Med

Great Plains and Mountains

Bull, David A MD [TS] - **Spec Exp:** Cardiothoracic Surgery; Esophageal Cancer; **Hospital:** Univ Utah Hosps and Clins; **Address:** University Utah School of Medicine, 30 N 1900 East, rm 3C127, Salt Lake City, UT 84132; **Phone:** 801-581-5311; **Board Cert:** Thoracic Surgery 95; Vascular Surgery 94; Surgery 99; Surgical Critical Care 99; **Med School:** UCSF 85; **Resid:** Surgery, UCSF Medical Ctr 87; Surgery, Univ Arizona Hosps 90; **Fellow:** Vascular Surgery, Univ Arizona Hosps 92; Cardiothoracic Surgery, Univ Arizona Hosps 94; **Fac Appt:** Assoc Prof TS, Univ Utah

Karwande, Shreekanth V MD [TS] - **Spec Exp:** Thoracic Cancers; Lung Cancer; **Hospital:** Univ Utah Hosps and Clins; **Address:** Univ Utah Med Ctr, Cardiothoracic Surg, 30 N 1900 E, Ste 3C127, Salt Lake City, UT 84132; **Phone:** 801-581-5311; **Board Cert:** Thoracic Surgery 03; **Med School:** India 73; **Resid:** Surgery, Erie Co Med Ctr 81; Cardiothoracic Surgery, New York Hosp 85; **Fellow:** Cardiothoracic Surgery, Meml Sloan Kettering Cancer Ctr; **Fac Appt:** Prof S, Univ Utah

Southwest

Harrison, Lynn MD [TS] - **Spec Exp:** Coronary Revascularization; Lung Cancer; Mitral Valve Repair; **Hospital:** L Boggs Med Ctr; **Address:** 3535 Bienville St, Ste E325, New Orleans, LA 70119; **Phone:** 504-412-1606; **Board Cert:** Thoracic Surgery 00; **Med School:** Univ Okla Coll Med 70; **Resid:** Surgery, Duke Univ Hosp 72; Thoracic Surgery, Duke Univ Hosp 79; **Fellow:** Cardiothoracic Surgery, Duke Univ 79; **Fac Appt:** Prof S, Louisiana State Univ

Roth, Jack MD [TS] - **Spec Exp:** Esophageal Cancer; Lung Cancer; Gene Therapy; **Hospital:** UT MD Anderson Cancer Ctr, The (page 115); **Address:** Dept of Thoracic & Cardiovascular Surgery Unit 445, 1515 Holcombe Blvd, Houston, TX 77030-1402; **Phone:** 713-792-7664; **Board Cert:** Thoracic Surgery 02; **Med School:** Johns Hopkins Univ 71; **Resid:** Surgery, Johns Hopkins Hosp 73; Thoracic Surgery, UCLA Ctr Hlth Sci 79; **Fellow:** Surgical Oncology, UCLA 75; **Fac Appt:** Prof TS, Univ Tex, Houston

West Coast and Pacific

De Meester, Tom R MD [TS] - **Spec Exp:** Gastric Disorders & Cancer; Esophageal Disorders & Cancer; Tracheal & Lung Disorders & Cancer; **Hospital:** USC Univ Hosp - R K Eamer Med Plz; **Address:** 1510 San Pablo St, Ste 514, Los Angeles, CA 90033; **Phone:** 323-442-5925; **Board Cert:** Surgery 71; Thoracic Surgery 71; **Med School:** Univ Mich Med Sch 63; **Resid:** Surgery, Univ Mich Hosp 65; Surgery, Johns Hopkins Hosp 66; **Fellow:** Thoracic Surgery, Johns Hopkins Hosp 68; **Fac Appt:** Prof S, USC Sch Med

Holmes, E Carmack MD [TS] - **Spec Exp:** Lung Cancer; **Hospital:** UCLA Med Ctr (page 111); **Address:** UCLA Med Ctr, Dept Surg, 10833 Le Conte Ave, rm 64-140 CHS, Los Angeles, CA 90095-7313; **Phone:** 310-206-2105; **Board Cert:** Surgery 73; Thoracic Surgery 74; **Med School:** Univ NC Sch Med 64; **Resid:** Surgery, Johns Hopkins Hosp 73; Surgery, Natl Cancer Inst 69; **Fac Appt:** Prof S, UCLA

Jablons, David M MD [TS] - **Spec Exp:** Esophageal Surgery; Lung Cancer; Mesothelioma; **Hospital:** UCSF - Mt Zion Med Ctr; **Address:** 2330 Post St, Ste 420, San Francisco, CA 94115; **Phone:** 415-353-1607; **Board Cert:** Thoracic Surgery 02; **Med School:** Albany Med Coll 84; **Resid:** Surgery, New Eng Med Ctr-Tufts Univ 86; Surgery, New Eng Med Ctr-Tufts Univ 91; **Fellow:** Surgical Oncology, Natl Cancer Inst-NIH 89; Cardiothoracic Surgery, New York Hosp-Cornell 93; **Fac Appt:** Assoc Prof S, UCSF

Kernstine, Kemp H MD/PhD [TS] - **Spec Exp:** Lung Cancer & Disease; Esophageal Cancer & Surgery; Tracheal Surgery; **Hospital:** City of Hope Natl Med Ctr & Beckman Rsch (page 89); **Address:** City of Hope Comprehensive Cancer Ctr, 1500 E Duarte Rd, Duarte, CA 91010; **Phone:** 626-359-8111 x68845; **Board Cert:** Thoracic Surgery 96; Surgery 01; **Med School:** Duke Univ 82; **Resid:** Surgery, Univ Minn Med Ctr 88; **Fellow:** Cardiothoracic Surgery, Brigham & Women's Hosp 94; **Fac Appt:** Assoc Prof S, Univ Iowa Coll Med

McKenna Jr, Robert J MD [TS] - **Spec Exp:** Lung Cancer; Gastroesophageal Reflux Disease (GERD); Video Assisted Thoracic Surgery (VATS); **Hospital:** Cedars-Sinai Med Ctr (page 88); **Address:** 8635 W 3rd St, Ste 975W, Los Angeles, CA 90048-6101; **Phone:** 310-652-0530; **Board Cert:** Thoracic Surgery 97; **Med School:** USC Sch Med 77; **Resid:** Surgery, Stanford Univ Hosp 82; Cardiothoracic Surgery, Good Samaritan Hosp 87; **Fellow:** Thoracic Surgery, MD Anderson Tumor Inst 83; **Fac Appt:** Clin Prof TS, UCLA

Morton, Donald L MD **[TS]** - **Spec Exp:** Melanoma; Sarcoma; Breast Cancer; **Hospital:** St John's Hlth Ctr, Santa Monica; **Address:** John Wayne Cancer Inst, 2200 Santa Monica Blvd, Santa Monica, CA 90404; **Phone:** 310-829-8363; **Board Cert:** Surgery 67; Thoracic Surgery 69; **Med School:** UCSF 58; **Resid:** Surgery, Natl Cancer Inst-NIH 62; Thoracic Surgery, UCSF Med Ctr 66; **Fellow:** Surgery, Cancer Rsch Inst-UCSF 66; **Fac Appt:** Prof Emeritus S, UCLA

Vallieres, Eric MD **[TS]** - **Spec Exp:** Lung Cancer; Mesothelioma; Mediastinal & Thoracic Cancers; **Hospital:** Swedish Med Ctr - Seattle; **Address:** 1221 Madison St, Ste 400, Seattle, WA 98104; **Phone:** 206-215-6800; **Med School:** Canada 82; **Resid:** Surgery, Univ of Toronto 88; Thoracic Surgery, Univ of Toronto 89; **Fellow:** Cardiovascular Surgery, Univ of Montreal 90

Whyte, Richard MD **[TS]** - **Spec Exp:** Lung Cancer; Esophageal Cancer; **Hospital:** Stanford Univ Med Ctr; **Address:** Stanford Univ Sch Med, Div Thor Surg, 300 Pasteur Dr, Bldg CVRB - rm 205, Stanford, CA 94305-5407; **Phone:** 650-723-6649; **Board Cert:** Surgery 91; Thoracic Surgery 93; **Med School:** Univ Pittsburgh 83; **Resid:** Surgery, Mass Genl Hosp 90; Thoracic Surgery, Univ Michigan Hosp 92; **Fac Appt:** Assoc Prof TS, Stanford Univ

Wood, Douglas E MD **[TS]** - **Spec Exp:** Lung & Esophageal Cancer; Tracheal Tumors/Tracheal Stenosis; Mesothelioma; **Hospital:** Univ Wash Med Ctr; **Address:** Univ Washington, Div Cardiothoracic Surg, 1959 Pacific NE Bldg AA - rm 115, Box 356310, Seattle, WA 98195-6310; **Phone:** 206-685-3228; **Board Cert:** Surgery 99; Thoracic Surgery 01; Surgical Critical Care 93; **Med School:** Harvard Med Sch 83; **Resid:** Surgery, Mass Genl Hosp 89; Thoracic Surgery, Mass Genl Hosp 91; **Fellow:** Surgical Critical Care, Mass Genl Hosp 91; **Fac Appt:** Prof S, Univ Wash

UROLOGY

A urologist manages benign and malignant medical and surgical disorders of the genitourinary system and the adrenal gland. This specialist has comprehensive knowledge of, and skills in, endoscopic, percutaneous and open surgery of congenital and acquired conditions of the urinary and reproductive systems and their contiguous structures.

Training required: *Five years*

PHYSICIAN LISTINGS

DANA-FARBER/BRIGHAM AND WOMEN'S
CANCER CENTER

GENITOURINARY ONCOLOGY TREATMENT CENTER

75 Francis Street • 44 Binney Street
Boston, MA 02115
1-877-DFCI-BWH • www.dfbwcancer.org

TRUSTED EXPERTISE

The Genitourinary Oncology Treatment Center is a specialized center of Dana-Farber/Brigham and Women's Cancer Center, combining the clinical expertise, focus, and innovation of Dana-Farber Cancer Institute, one of the nation's leading cancer centers, with the world-class care and services of Brigham and Women's Hospital, one of the nation's leading teaching hospitals. Dana-Farber Cancer Institute and Brigham and Women's Hospital are teaching affiliates of Harvard Medical School.

DISEASES TREATED

Our physicians provide innovative treatment for all genitourinary cancers, including prostate, testicular, renal, bladder, penile, and kidney cancers.

ADVANCED TREATMENT

Staffed by medical, urologic, and radiation oncologists, the Genitourinary Oncology Treatment Center is a leading multidisciplinary and multispecialty evaluation and treatment center, as well as an innovative research center. We provide expert, compassionate, and state-of-the-art care. A tailored treatment plan is developed for each patient based on the latest surgical, chemotherapy, and radiation treatment approaches, including access to National Cancer Institute clinical trials. Experts in the Center have pioneered new approaches in the assessment and treatment of prostate, kidney, and other genitourinary cancers, leading to better outcomes and quality-of-life for patients. The Center offers one of the world's only MRI-guided brachytherapy programs for prostate cancer and is one of only a handful of centers providing treatment for patients with testis cancer. The Center also provides less invasive surgical treatment and cutting-edge immunotherapy for the treatment of kidney cancer.

INNOVATIVE CLINICAL TRIALS

Patients have access to innovative clinical trials, many supported by the National Institutes of Health, through Dana-Farber/Harvard Cancer Center, a National Cancer Institute-designated Comprehensive Cancer Center. Our research faculty includes international leaders in molecular genetics, image-guided radiotherapy, tumor markers, and surgical robotics.

COMPREHENSIVE SUPPORT SERVICES

Dana-Farber/Brigham and Women's Cancer Center also provides a wide array of support services and complementary therapies for patients with genitourinary cancer, including counseling and support groups, services for international patients, interpreter services, patient education, pastoral care, nutrition counseling, and specialized nursing.

Call **1-877-DFCI-BWH** for more information, or to make an appointment with a specialist at Dana-Farber/Brigham and Women's Cancer Center.

DANA-FARBER/PARTNERS CANCERCARE

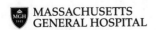 MASSACHUSETTS GENERAL HOSPITAL

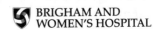 DANA-FARBER CANCER INSTITUTE

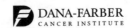 BRIGHAM AND WOMEN'S HOSPITAL

UROLOGY & UROLOGIC ONCOLOGY CENTER
CITY OF HOPE CANCER CENTER

City of Hope®

Where the Power of Knowledge Saves Lives®

1500 East Duarte Road
Duarte, California 91010
Tel. 800-826-HOPE (4673)
www.cityofhope.org

The department of Urology at City of Hope is recognized for its extensive expertise in urinary reconstruction and laparoscopic cystectomy, and is a leader in laparoscopic radical prostatectomy (LRP) including robotic-assisted LRP. All offer significant advances in improving patient quality of life. The center also treats urologic problems resulting from treatment of non-urologic cancers.

LAPAROSCOPIC AND ROBOTIC-ASSISTED TREATMENT METHODS

City of Hope was one of the first centers in the United States to offer laparoscopic radical prostatectomy (LRP) and now uses the *da Vinci®* Surgical System to perform robotic-assisted radical prostatectomies, significantly reducing recovery time and side effects. City of Hope is the leader in the Western United States in total robotic-assisted LRPs and one of only a few centers nationally offering both laparoscopic and robotic-assisted radical prostatectomies.

City of Hope also offers radiation therapy options including Ultrasound Guided Prostate Seed Implants as well as Hormone Therapy and Chemotherapy for advanced stages of prostate cancer.

It is one of the few institutions in the world routinely performing complete urinary bladder removals (radical cystoprostatectomy) using minimally invasive laparoscopic surgery.

URINARY DIVERSIONS

In addition to doing the oldest and simplest form of urinary diversion—Ileal Conduit Urinary Diversion—City of Hope is a leader in offering the Indiana Pouch Reservoir method and also performs orthotopic neobladder reconstruction.

RESEARCH AND CLINICAL TRIALS

The Department's Kaplan Clinical Research Laboratory is actively engaged in research in the diagnosis and treatment of urologic cancers such as prostate, bladder and kidney. The laboratory focuses on diagnosis using molecular tools, and the use of bionanotechnology for the production of smart devices for therapy and diagnosis.

CITY OF HOPE is a National Cancer Institute (NCI)-designated Comprehensive Cancer Center–the highest accolade given by the NCI.

Other distinctions include:

- Founding member of the National Comprehensive Cancer Network, setting national standards of care for cancer;

- Scoring in the top 1 percent of hospitals surveyed by the Joint Commission on Accreditation of Healthcare Organizations (JCAHO); and

- Receiving the highest score possible in all applicable categories in the California Hospital Experience Survey (formerly known as PEP-C).

Helford Clinical Research Hospital, opened in 2005, continues City of Hope's tradition of progress and further substantiates City of Hope's ranking by U.S. News & World Report as one of America's 50 best cancer hospitals.

For more information, call 800-826-4673.

INDIANA UNIVERSITY HOSPITAL
A CLARIAN HEALTH PARTNER
550 University Boulevard • Indianapolis, Indiana 46202
317-274-5000 • www.clarian.org

One of the oldest urology departments in the nation, the Department of Urology at the Indiana University School of Medicine is one of the leading centers for the treatment of urologic cancers. Our physicians possess considerable experience in all methods of surgical, non-surgical and investigational treatment of all forms of urological cancer. Working closely with medical oncologists at the Indiana University Cancer Center, our program provides a true multidisciplinary approach individualized for the needs and diagnosis of each patient.

WORLD-CLASS CANCER CARE

Indiana University Hosptial's Urologic Oncology Program is a leader in cancer diagnosis and treatment, making it one of the most widely recognized cancer programs in the U.S. and the world. The program brings together the talents, strengths and resources of a diverse group of individuals and organizations with a single focus: to reduce cancer incidence, suffering and mortality in Indiana and beyond. This program is most well known for setting the standard of care for the treatment of testicular cancer worldwide. While this program is known for this contribution, there are active programs in the study and treatment of all forms of urologic cancer.

AMONG AN ELITE GROUP

Based on its record of ground breaking research and superior clinical patient care, the IU Cancer Center is a National Cancer Institute-designated Cancer Center, the only such center providing patient care in Indiana. This designation places it among an elite group of centers focusing on excellent clinical care and the rapid implementation of new discoveries into the treatment of cancer. Such a designation ensures patients will have access to all of the newest cancer treatment modalities available from the National Cancer Institute.

FIRST IN INDIANA OFFERING MINIMALLY INVASIVE TREATMENT OPTIONS

The Department of Urology has always been at the forefront of cancer care and performed the first minimally invasive surgeries for kidney cancer and prostate cancer in the state of Indiana. The first laparoscopic radical prostatectomies in Indiana, with and without robotic assistance, were performed by IU surgeons. In 2005, over 100 patients will choose to have a laparoscopic radical prostatectomy at Indiana University Hospital. A wide variety of advanced urologic laparoscopic surgeries are now routinely performed on a daily basis. Our surgeons are part of the national and international academic laparoscopic community, which ensures the latest advances in laparoscopy are immediately available to our patients.

COMPREHENSIVE CARE IN ONE LOCATION

IU Hospital and the IU Cancer Center offer interdisciplinary clinical programs that allow patients to see—in one simple visit—a variety of specialists who work as a team to provide complete cancer care. The IU Cancer Center was the first cancer center in Indiana to truly operate as a multidisciplinary center. IU Hospital and IU Cancer Center have full representation of all medical and surgical specialties, giving patients access to the range of services they may need throughout their course of treatment.

518   Sponsored Page

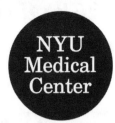
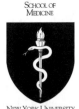

GENITOURINARY ONCOLOGY PROGRAM
UCLA HEALTHCARE

1-800-UCLA-MD1 (825-2631)
www.healthcare.ucla.edu

UCLA's Genitourinary Oncology Program specializes in the management of localized and advanced urologic cancers of the:

Prostate • Kidney • Bladder

UCLA's Prostate Cancer Program brings together a multidisciplinary team to treat benign prostate hyperplasia (BPH) and prostate cancer. At UCLA, more than 100 prostatectomies are performed for prostate cancer annually, and potency-sparing surgery is performed in appropriate cases with good results. Other options include external beam radiation therapy, radioactive seed implantation for localized disease, cryosurgery for localized or minimally invasive disease, hormonal and chemotherapeutic treatment of advanced disease, and clinical trials of new drugs for hormone-refractory metastatic prostate cancer.

The UCLA Kidney Cancer Program provides expertise in developing individualized treatment plans, using both standard and innovative experimental therapies, including immunotherapy, gene therapy, chemotherapy and tumor vaccines. The program has achieved a more than 35 percent response rate with a combination of surgery and immunotherapy, while the average in the country remains between 12 and 15 percent.

UCLA'S JONSSON CANCER CENTER

Designated by the National Cancer Institute as one of only 38 comprehensive cancer centers in the United States, UCLA's Jonsson Cancer Center has earned an international reputation for developing new cancer therapies, providing the best in experimental and traditional treatments, and expertly guiding and training the next generation of medical researchers. The center's 250 physicians and scientists treat upwards of 20,000 patient visits per year and offer hundreds of clinical trials that provide the latest in experimental cancer treatments (www.cancer.mednet.ucla.edu). The center also offers patients and families psychological and support services.

UCLA's Jonsson Cancer Center has been ranked the best cancer center in the western United States by U.S. News & World Report's Annual Best Hospitals survey for the past five years. UCLA Medical Center, of which the Cancer Center is a part, has ranked best in the West for the past 15 years.

Call 1-800-UCLA-MD1 (825-2631)
for a referral to a UCLA doctor.

UCLA Healthcare

THE END OF CANCER BEGINS WITH RESEARCH

In 2002, the Prostate Cancer Program at UCLA's Jonsson Cancer Center was designated by the National Cancer Institute as a site of research excellence, making it one of the few institutions nationwide tapped to improve prevention, detection and treatment of prostate cancer. The designation as a Specialized Program of Research (SPORE) comes with a five-year $11.5 million grant to further expand UCLA's renowned prostate cancer program. Researchers are focusing on two major areas: new molecular targets for therapies, and investigating nutritional strategies to prevent the disease and impede tumor growth.

GENITOURINARY ONCOLOGY

M. D. Anderson's Genitourinary Center diagnoses, treats and manages cancers of the genitourinary system. This center sees more than 21,600 patient visits in the last year. This multi-disciplinary center has specialized teams of oncologists to handle malignancies of the prostate, bladder, kidney, testis, penis and extragonadal germ cell tumors. The multi-disciplinary care model allows patients to review and evaluate multiple treatment modlities in a single visit and partner with their physician in choosing the most appropriate treatment for them, as individuals.

Standard treatment available from our Genitourinary Oncologists include:

- Evaluation of patients with elevated or problematic prostate-specific antigen levels
- Treatment plans tailored for the individual patient
- Management of complex, high-risk, and salvage clinical presentations
- Management of rare genitourinary tumors such as penile and urachal carcinoma
- Innovative and novel therapies arriving from clinical research, including multiple options for androgen-independent prostate cancer

Technological advantages include IMRT (Intensity Modulated Radiation Therapy), X Knife, Cryoablation, nerve grafts and nerve-sparing procedures that help retain sexual function and enhance quality of life, as well as other state-of-the-art laparoscopic and minimally invasvie surgeries. A Proton Therapy Center will open at the hospital in early 2006, providing an additional treatment modality available for many GU centers.

CLINICAL TRIALS

The Gastrointestinal Oncology Center offers an extensive array of clinical trials. A clinical trial is one of the most advanced stages of a long careful research process. Clinical trials are designed to test the effectiveness of new treatment, including novel drugs, surgical procedures, or combinations of therapy.

New and Innovative therapies generally are available at M.D. Anderson several years before they become standard in the community. Our clinical trials incorporate state-of-the-art patient care, while evaluating the most recent developments in cancer medicine. They also offer treatment opportunities for difficult or aggressive tumors.

M. D. Anderson is one of the largest cancer centers in the world. We've been working to eliminate cancer for more than six decades. Our depth of experience informs every aspect of your care.

We focus exclusively on cancer and have seen cases of every kind. Our doctors treat more rare cancers in a single day than most physicians see in a lifetime. That means you receive expert care no matter what your diagnosis.

We are the top-ranked cancer hospital in the United States according to the 2004 *U.S.News & World Report* annual survey of hospitals.

M. D. Anderson ranks first in the number and amount of research grants awarded by the National Cancer Institute. By studying how cancer begins and responds to various treatments, we can help patients overcome disease and prevent recurrence.

At M. D. Anderson, we understand that cancer is not just a physical disease. To help you cope with every aspect of cancer, we provide a number of support programs.

Wake Forest University Baptist
MEDICAL CENTER

PROSTATE CANCER CENTER OF EXCELLENCE
COMPREHENSIVE CANCER CENTER

Medical Center Boulevard • Winston-Salem, NC 27157
Health On-Call® (Patient Access) 1-800-446-2255
PAL® (Physician-to-physician calls) 1-800-277-7654
www.wfubmc.edu/cancer

OVERVIEW

The Prostate Cancer Center of Excellence was established in 1999 as a center for innovative research and treatment of this common but complex cancer. The Prostate Cancer Center of Excellence has three broad areas of emphasis: chemoprevention, molecular epidemiology and novel therapies.

RESEARCH

Because the optimal treatment for many prostate cancers is still uncertain, the greatest impact on reducing mortality and morbidity from prostate cancer can be achieved by research focused on chemoprevention, on identifying men at high risk for the disease or its recurrence, and on the development of new therapies for men with existing prostate cancer.

In chemoprevention, studies are being conducted on soy protein with isoflavones and vitamin D as preventive agents. Risk factor research is examining aberrations at the cellular and molecular level that contribute to increased risk for the disease. Among the new therapies being explored are the use of dendritic (immune) cells and vitamin D to fight off prostate cancer.

MULTIDISCIPLINARY CARE

In clinical treatment, Wake Forest Baptist has brought together experts in genitourinary medical oncology, radiation oncology, urologic oncology, pathology and radiology in a unique and comprehensive multidisciplinary clinic. Through a weekly clinic, the Genitourinary Oncology Group provides assessment of all new patients to determine the most effective treatment program including initial treatment, long-term follow-up and quality of life issues. The clinic sees patients with prostate, bladder, testicular, adrenal and other related cancers.

THE LATEST TREATMENT MODALITIES

3D Conformal and Intensity Modulated Radiation Therapy — Among the newer treatment options for cancer of the prostate, brain, lung, and head and neck are two methods of focusing radiation on the tumor and surrounding at-risk tissues while optimally sparing nearby normal tissues: 3-dimensional (3D) conformal radiation therapy, and intensity modulated radiation therapy (IMRT). This approach uses anatomic computed tomographic and/or magnetic resonance images of the patient, computer-generated radiation dose calculations, and a computer-controlled linear accelerator to conform or "paint" the radiation dose very precisely to match the shape of the tumor to be treated, avoiding critical structures that may be only millimeters away.

The linear accelerator radiation beam intensity is varied, or modulated, over space and time during the patient's treatment, hence the term "Intensity Modulated" radiation therapy. In combination with advanced imaging techniques like magnetic resonance spectroscopy and positron emission tomography that image both tumor anatomy and biology, IMRT holds great promise for improving local tumor control and survival, even in the most resistant and aggressive human cancers.

Brachytherapy— involves the implantation of radioactive sources in or near a tumor. A full range of brachytherapy treatment options are available for treating cancers of the prostate, breast, cervix, uterus, vagina, head and neck, soft tissues, brain, and eye. With the availability of both high dose rate (HDR) and low dose rate (LDR) brachytherapy technology and expertise, virtually any area of the body can be implanted if appropriate.

UROLOGY

New England

Althausen, Alex F MD [U] - **Spec Exp:** Urologic Cancer; **Hospital:** Mass Genl Hosp; **Address:** One Hawthorne Pl, Ste 109, Boston, MA 02114-2333; **Phone:** 617-523-5250; **Board Cert:** Urology 76; **Med School:** Tufts Univ 66; **Resid:** Surgery, Albany Med Ctr 68; Urology, Mass Genl Hosp 74; **Fac Appt:** Assoc Prof S, Harvard Med Sch

Heney, Niall M MD [U] - **Spec Exp:** Urologic Cancer; **Hospital:** Mass Genl Hosp; **Address:** Mass Genl Hosp, Dept Urol, 15 Parkman St, WACC 528, Boston, MA 02114; **Phone:** 617-726-3011; **Board Cert:** Urology 77; **Med School:** Ireland 65; **Resid:** Urology, Reg Hosp 72; Urology, Mass Genl Hosp 76; **Fac Appt:** Prof Med, Harvard Med Sch

Libertino, John A MD [U] - **Spec Exp:** Kidney Reconstruction; Prostate Cancer; Adrenal Disorders; **Hospital:** Lahey Clin; **Address:** Lahey Clinic, Dept Urology, 41 Mall Rd, Burlington, MA 01805; **Phone:** 781-744-2511; **Board Cert:** Urology 73; **Med School:** Georgetown Univ 65; **Resid:** Urology, Univ Rochester-Strong Meml Hosp; Urology, Yale-New Haven Hosp 70; **Fellow:** Surgery, Yale-New Haven Hosp; **Fac Appt:** Assoc Clin Prof S, Harvard Med Sch

Loughlin, Kevin R MD [U] - **Spec Exp:** Incontinence; Infertility-Male; Genitourinary Cancer; **Hospital:** Brigham & Women's Hosp (page 87); **Address:** Brigham & Women's Hosp, Div Urology, 45 Francis St, ASBII-3, Boston, MA 02115; **Phone:** 617-732-6325; **Board Cert:** Urology 04; **Med School:** NY Med Coll 75; **Resid:** Pediatrics, NY Hosp-Cornell Univ 78; Surgery, Bellevue Hosp Ctr-NYU 79; **Fellow:** Urology, Brigham & Women's Hosp 83; Urologic Oncology, Meml Sloan Kettering Cancer Ctr; **Fac Appt:** Prof S, Harvard Med Sch

McDougal, William S MD [U] - **Spec Exp:** Urinary Reconstruction; Urologic Cancer; Prostate Cancer; **Hospital:** Mass Genl Hosp; **Address:** Mass Genl Hosp, 55 Fruit St, Bldg GRB - rm 1102, Boston, MA 02114; **Phone:** 617-726-3010; **Board Cert:** Surgery 75; Urology 04; **Med School:** Cornell Univ-Weill Med Coll 68; **Resid:** Surgery, Univ Hosps Cleveland 75; **Fellow:** Physiology, Yale Med Sch 72; **Fac Appt:** Prof U, Harvard Med Sch

McGovern, Francis MD [U] - **Spec Exp:** Prostate Cancer; **Hospital:** Mass Genl Hosp; **Address:** One Hawthorne Pl, Ste 109, Boston, MA 02114; **Phone:** 617-523-5250; **Board Cert:** Urology 99; **Med School:** Case West Res Univ 83; **Resid:** Urology, Mass Genl Hosp 89

Richie, Jerome MD [U] - **Spec Exp:** Prostate Cancer; Testicular Cancer; Kidney Cancer; **Hospital:** Brigham & Women's Hosp (page 87); **Address:** Brigham & Women's Hosp, 45 Francis St, Ste A5B2-3, Boston, MA 02115; **Phone:** 617-732-6325; **Board Cert:** Urology 92; **Med School:** Univ Tex Med Br, Galveston 69; **Resid:** Surgery, UCLA Med Ctr 71; Urology, UCLA Med Ctr 75; **Fac Appt:** Prof U, Harvard Med Sch

Mid Atlantic

Bander, Neil MD [U] - **Spec Exp:** Prostate Cancer; Clinical Trials; **Hospital:** NY-Presby Hosp - NY Weill Cornell Med Ctr (page 103); **Address:** 525 E 68th St, rm E-300, Box 23, New York, NY 10021-4870; **Phone:** 212-746-5460; **Board Cert:** Urology 83; **Med School:** Univ Conn 74; **Resid:** Urology, Bellevue Hosp 77; Urology, U Conn 80; **Fellow:** Urologic Oncology, Meml Sloan Kettering Cancer Ctr 83; **Fac Appt:** Prof U, Cornell Univ-Weill Med Coll

Benson, Mitchell C MD [U] - **Spec Exp:** Prostate Cancer; Bladder Cancer; Kidney Cancer; **Hospital:** NY-Presby Hosp - Columbia Presby Med Ctr (page 103); **Address:** NY Columbia Presbyterian Hospital, Dept Urology, 161 Ft Washington Ave Fl 11 - rm 1153, New York, NY 10032-3713; **Phone:** 212-305-5201; **Board Cert:** Urology 84; **Med School:** Columbia P&S 77; **Resid:** Surgery, Mount Sinai Med Ctr 79; Urology, Columbia-Presby Hosp 82; **Fellow:** Oncology, Johns Hopkins Hosp 84; **Fac Appt:** Prof U, Columbia P&S

Burnett II, Arthur L MD [U] - **Spec Exp:** Prostate Cancer; Erectile Dysfunction; **Hospital:** Johns Hopkins Hosp - Baltimore (page 97); **Address:** 600 N Wolfe St, Marburg Bldg, Ste 407, Baltimore, MD 21287; **Phone:** 410-614-3986; **Board Cert:** Urology 98; **Med School:** Johns Hopkins Univ 88; **Resid:** Urology, Johns Hopkins Hosp 94; Surgery, Johns Hopkins Hosp 90; **Fac Appt:** Prof U, Johns Hopkins Univ

Carter, H. Ballentine MD [U] - **Spec Exp:** Prostate Cancer; **Hospital:** Johns Hopkins Hosp - Baltimore (page 97); **Address:** Brady Urological Inst, Johns Hopkins Hosp, 600 N Wolfe St, Baltimore, MD 21287-2101; **Phone:** 410-955-6100; **Board Cert:** Urology 99; **Med School:** Med Univ SC 81; **Resid:** Surgery, New York Hosp 83; Urology, New York Hosp 87; **Fellow:** Research, Johns Hopkins Hosp 89; **Fac Appt:** Prof U, Johns Hopkins Univ

Droller, Michael J MD [U] - **Spec Exp:** Urologic Cancer; Bladder/Prostate Cancer; Kidney Cancer; **Hospital:** Mount Sinai Med Ctr (page 101); **Address:** 5 E 98th St Fl 6th, Box 1272, New York, NY 10029-6501; **Phone:** 212-241-3868; **Board Cert:** Urology 01; **Med School:** Harvard Med Sch 68; **Resid:** Surgery, Peter Bent Brigham Hosp 70; Urology, Stanford Univ Med Ctr 76; **Fellow:** Immunology, Univ Stockholm 77; **Fac Appt:** Prof U, Mount Sinai Sch Med

Gomella, Leonard G MD [U] - **Spec Exp:** Urologic Cancer; Laparoscopic Surgery; **Hospital:** Thomas Jefferson Univ Hosp (page 110); **Address:** Thomas Jefferson University, 1015 Walnut St Fl 11 - Ste 1112, Philadelphia, PA 19107-5001; **Phone:** 215-955-1000; **Board Cert:** Urology 98; **Med School:** Univ KY Coll Med 80; **Resid:** Surgery, Univ Kentucky Medical Ctr 82; Urology, Univ Kentucky Medical Ctr 86; **Fellow:** Urologic Oncology, Natl Cancer Inst 88; **Fac Appt:** Assoc Prof U, Jefferson Med Coll

Grasso, Michael MD [U] - **Spec Exp:** Urologic Cancer; Laparoscopic Surgery; Kidney Stones; **Hospital:** St Vincent Cath Med Ctrs - Manhattan (page 108); **Address:** 170 W 12th St, Ste 205, Dept. of Urology - Cronin 205, New York, NY 10011; **Phone:** 212-604-1270; **Board Cert:** Urology 02; **Med School:** Jefferson Med Coll 86; **Resid:** Surgery, Jefferson Univ Hosp 88; Urology, Jefferson Univ Hosp 92; **Fac Appt:** Prof U, NY Med Coll

Greenberg, Richard E MD [U] - **Spec Exp:** Prostate Cancer; Bladder Cancer; Kidney Cancer; **Hospital:** Fox Chase Cancer Ctr (page 95); **Address:** Fox Chase Cancer Center,Div of Urology Dept Surgery, 333 Cottman Ave, Ste H3 - rm 116, Philadelphia, PA 19111; **Phone:** 215-728-5341; **Board Cert:** Urology 05; **Med School:** Cornell Univ-Weill Med Coll 76; **Resid:** Surgery, New York Hosp 79; Urology, New York Hosp 83; **Fac Appt:** Prof U, Temple Univ

Herr, Harry W MD [U] - **Spec Exp:** Bladder Cancer; Urologic Tumors; Testicular Cancer; **Hospital:** Meml Sloan Kettering Cancer Ctr (page 100); **Address:** Meml Sloan Kettering Canc Ctr, Dept Urology, 353 E 68th St, New York, NY 10021; **Phone:** 646-422-4411; **Board Cert:** Urology 76; **Med School:** UCSF 69; **Resid:** Urology, UC Irvine Med Ctr 74; **Fellow:** Urology, Meml Sloan Kettering Cancer Ctr 76; **Fac Appt:** Assoc Prof S, Cornell Univ-Weill Med Coll

Huben, Robert P MD [U] - **Spec Exp:** Prostate Cancer; Kidney Cancer; Urologic Cancer; **Hospital:** Roswell Park Cancer Inst (page 107); **Address:** Roswell Park Cancer Inst, Elm & Carlton Sts, Buffalo, NY 14263-0001; **Phone:** 716-845-3159; **Board Cert:** Urology 83; **Med School:** Cornell Univ-Weill Med Coll 76; **Resid:** Urology, East Virginia Med Ctr 81; **Fellow:** Urologic Oncology, Roswell Park Meml Inst 82

Jarow, Jonathan MD [U] - **Spec Exp:** Infertility-Male; Prostate Cancer; Erectile Dysfunction; **Hospital:** Johns Hopkins Hosp - Baltimore (page 97); **Address:** Johns Hopkins Outpatient Ctr, 601 N Caroline St, Fl 4, Baltimore, MD 21287; **Phone:** 410-955-3617; **Board Cert:** Urology 99; **Med School:** Northwestern Univ 80; **Resid:** Surgery, Johns Hopkins Hosp 82; Urology, Johns Hopkins Hosp 86; **Fellow:** Andrology, Baylor Univ; **Fac Appt:** Assoc Prof U, Johns Hopkins Univ

Kaplan, Steven MD [U] - **Spec Exp:** Urodynamics; Voiding Dysfunction; Incontinence after Prostate Cancer; **Hospital:** NY-Presby Hosp - Columbia Presby Med Ctr (page 103); **Address:** 161 Fort Washington Ave Fl 11 - Ste 1174, New York, NY 10032; **Phone:** 212-305-0140; **Board Cert:** Urology 01; **Med School:** Mount Sinai Sch Med 82; **Resid:** Surgery, Mount Sinai Hosp 84; Urology, Columbia Presby Med Ctr 88; **Fellow:** Urology, Columbia Presby Med Ctr 90; **Fac Appt:** Prof U, Columbia P&S

Kirschenbaum, Alexander M MD [U] - **Spec Exp:** Prostate Cancer; Bladder Surgery; **Hospital:** Mount Sinai Med Ctr (page 101); **Address:** 58A E 79th St, New York, NY 10021; **Phone:** 646-422-0926; **Board Cert:** Urology 97; **Med School:** Mount Sinai Sch Med 80; **Resid:** Surgery, Mount Sinai Hosp 82; Urology, Mount Sinai Hosp 85; **Fellow:** Urologic Oncology, Mount Sinai Hosp 87; **Fac Appt:** Assoc Prof U, Mount Sinai Sch Med

Lanteri, Vincent J MD [U] - **Spec Exp:** Prostate Cancer/Robotic Surgery; Urologic Cancer; Minimally Invasive Urologic Surgery; **Hospital:** Hackensack Univ Med Ctr (page 96); **Address:** 5 Summit Ave Fl 2, Hackensack, NJ 07601; **Phone:** 201-487-8866; **Board Cert:** Urology 82; **Med School:** Mexico 74; **Resid:** Surgery, UMDNJ Med Ctr 77; Urology, UMDNJ Med Ctr 80; **Fellow:** Urologic Oncology, Roswell Park Cancer Inst 81

Lepor, Herbert MD [U] - **Spec Exp:** Prostate Cancer; **Hospital:** NYU Med Ctr (page 104); **Address:** 150 E 32nd St, Fl 2, New York, NY 10016; **Phone:** 646-825-6327; **Board Cert:** Urology 97; **Med School:** Johns Hopkins Univ 75; **Resid:** Urology, Johns Hopkins Hosp 86; **Fac Appt:** Prof U, NYU Sch Med

Lowe, Franklin MD [U] - **Spec Exp:** Prostate Disease; Complementary Medicine; Prostate Cancer; **Hospital:** St Luke's - Roosevelt Hosp Ctr - Roosevelt Div (page 93); **Address:** 425 W 59th St, Ste 3A, New York, NY 10019; **Phone:** 212-523-7790; **Board Cert:** Urology 97; **Med School:** Columbia P&S 79; **Resid:** Surgery, Johns Hopkins Hosp 81; Urology, Johns Hopkins Hosp 84; **Fac Appt:** Clin Prof U, Columbia P&S

Macchia, Richard MD [U] - **Spec Exp:** Prostate Disease; Prostate Cancer; Voiding Dysfunction; **Hospital:** SUNY Downstate Med Ctr; **Address:** SUNY Downstate Med School, Dept Urology, 445 Lenox Rd, Box 79, Brooklyn, NY 11203-2098; **Phone:** 718-270-2554; **Board Cert:** Urology 77; **Med School:** NY Med Coll 69; **Resid:** Surgery, St Vincent's Hosp 71; Urology, SUNY Downstate Med Ctr 74; **Fellow:** Urologic Oncology, Meml Sloan Kettering Cancer Ctr 76; **Fac Appt:** Prof U, SUNY Downstate

Malkowicz, Bruce MD [U] - **Spec Exp:** Urologic Cancer; **Hospital:** Hosp Univ Penn - UPHS (page 113); **Address:** Hosp Univ Penn, Dept Urology, 3400 Spruce St, 9 Penn Tower, Philadelphia, PA 19104; **Phone:** 215-662-2891; **Board Cert:** Urology 00; **Med School:** Univ Pennsylvania 81; **Resid:** Surgery, Hosp Univ Penn 83; Urology, Hosp Univ Penn 87; **Fellow:** Urologic Oncology, USC Med Ctr 98; Urologic Oncology, Hosp Univ Penn/Wistar Inst 90; **Fac Appt:** Assoc Prof U, Univ Pennsylvania

Mostwin, Jacek Lech MD/PhD **[U]** - **Spec Exp:** Prostate Cancer; **Hospital:** Johns Hopkins Hosp - Baltimore (page 97); **Address:** Johns Hopkins Hosp, 600 N Wolfe St, Marburg-401C, Baltimore, MD 21287; **Phone:** 410-955-4461; **Board Cert:** Urology 97; **Med School:** Univ MD Sch Med 75; **Resid:** Urology, Johns Hopkins Hosp. 83; Surgery, U Mich. 78; **Fac Appt:** Prof U, Johns Hopkins Univ

Naslund, Michael MD **[U]** - **Spec Exp:** Prostate Cancer; Prostate Disease; **Hospital:** Univ of MD Med Sys; **Address:** Maryland Prostate Ctr, 419 W Redwood St, Ste 320, Baltimore, MD 21201; **Phone:** 410-328-0800; **Board Cert:** Urology 00; **Med School:** Johns Hopkins Univ 81; **Resid:** Urology, Johns Hopkins Hosp 87; Surgery, Johns Hopkins Hosp 83; **Fac Appt:** Assoc Prof S, Univ MD Sch Med

Nelson, Joel Byron MD **[U]** - **Spec Exp:** Prostate Cancer; **Hospital:** UPMC Shadyside (page 114); **Address:** UPMC Shadyside Med Ctr, 5200 Centre Ave, Ste 209, Pittsburgh, PA 15232; **Phone:** 412-605-3013; **Board Cert:** Urology 98; **Med School:** Northwestern Univ 88; **Resid:** Surgery, Northwestern MemL Hosp 90; Urology, Northwestern Meml Hosp 94; **Fellow:** Urology, Johns Hopkins Hosp; **Fac Appt:** Prof U, Univ Pittsburgh

Sawczuk, Ihor S MD **[U]** - **Spec Exp:** Kidney Cancer; Bladder Cancer; Prostate Cancer; **Hospital:** Hackensack Univ Med Ctr (page 96); **Address:** Hackensack Univ Med Ctr, 360 Essex St, Hackensack, NJ 07601; **Phone:** 201-336-8090; **Board Cert:** Urology 96; **Med School:** Med Coll PA Hahnemann 79; **Resid:** Surgery, St Vincent's Hosp & Med Ctr 81; Urology, Columbia-Presby Med Ctr 84; **Fellow:** Urologic Oncology, Columbia-Presby Med Ctr 86; **Fac Appt:** Prof U, Columbia P&S

Scardino, Peter T MD **[U]** - **Spec Exp:** Prostate Cancer; **Hospital:** Meml Sloan Kettering Cancer Ctr (page 100); **Address:** 1275 York Ave, Box 27, New York, NY 10021; **Phone:** 646-422-4329; **Board Cert:** Urology 81; **Med School:** Duke Univ 71; **Resid:** Surgery, Mass Genl Hosp 73; Urology, UCLA Med Ctr 79; **Fellow:** Urology, Natl Cancer Inst 76; **Fac Appt:** Prof U, Cornell Univ-Weill Med Coll

Schlegel, Peter MD **[U]** - **Spec Exp:** Prostate Cancer; Infertility-Male; Fertility Preservation-Male; **Hospital:** NY-Presby Hosp - NY Weill Cornell Med Ctr (page 103); **Address:** 525 E 68th St, Starr 900, New York, NY 10021-4870; **Phone:** 212-746-5491; **Board Cert:** Urology 01; **Med School:** Univ Mass Sch Med 83; **Resid:** Surgery, Johns Hopkins Hosp 85; Urology, Johns Hopkins Hosp 89; **Fellow:** Medical Oncology, Johns Hopkins Hosp 87; Male Reproduction, New York Hosp-Cornell Med Ctr 91; **Fac Appt:** Clin Prof U, Cornell Univ-Weill Med Coll

Sheinfeld, Joel MD **[U]** - **Spec Exp:** Testicular Cancer; Bladder Cancer; Fertility Preservation/Testicular Cancer; **Hospital:** Meml Sloan Kettering Cancer Ctr (page 100); **Address:** Meml Sloan Kettering Cancer Ctr-Kimmel Ctr for Prostate & Urologic Cancers, 1275 York Ave, New York, NY 10021-6007; **Phone:** 646-422-4311; **Board Cert:** Urology 00; **Med School:** Univ Fla Coll Med 81; **Resid:** Urology, Strong Meml Hosp 86; **Fellow:** Urologic Oncology, Meml Sloan Kettering Cancer Ctr 89; **Fac Appt:** Assoc Prof U, Cornell Univ-Weill Med Coll

Taneja, Samir S MD **[U]** - **Spec Exp:** Kidney Cancer-Laparoscopic Surgery; Prostate Cancer; Urologic Cancer-Laparoscopic Surgery; **Hospital:** NYU Med Ctr (page 104); **Address:** 150 E 32nd St, Ste 200, New York, NY 10016; **Phone:** 646-825-6321; **Board Cert:** Urology 99; **Med School:** Northwestern Univ 90; **Resid:** Urology, UCLA Med Ctr 96; **Fac Appt:** Assoc Prof U, NYU Sch Med

Uzzo, Robert MD **[U]** - **Spec Exp:** Kidney Cancer; Prostate & Testicular Cancer; Bladder Cancer; **Hospital:** Fox Chase Cancer Ctr (page 95); **Address:** 333 Cottman Ave, Philadelphia, PA 19111; **Phone:** 215-728-3501; **Board Cert:** Urology 01; **Med School:** Cornell Univ-Weill Med Coll 91; **Resid:** Surgery, New York Hosp-Cornell Med Ctr 93; Urology, New York Hosp-Cornell Med Ctr 97; **Fellow:** Urologic Oncology, Cleveland Clinic 99; Renal Transplant, Cleveland Clinic 00; **Fac Appt:** Assoc Prof S, Temple Univ

Van Arsdalen, Keith N MD [U] - **Spec Exp:** Infertility-Male; Varicocele Microsurgery; Urologic Cancer; **Hospital:** Hosp Univ Penn - UPHS (page 113); **Address:** Hosp Univ Penn, Div Urol, 3400 Spruce St, 9 Penn Tower, Philadelphia, PA 19104; **Phone:** 215-662-2891; **Board Cert:** Urology 84; **Med School:** Med Coll VA 77; **Resid:** Surgery, Univ Maryland Hosp 79; Urology, Med Coll Virginia 82; **Fellow:** Urodynamics, Hosp Univ Penn 83; **Fac Appt:** Prof U, Univ Pennsylvania

Vaughan, Edwin D MD [U] - **Spec Exp:** Urologic Cancer; Adrenal Disorders; Prostate Disease; **Hospital:** NY-Presby Hosp - NY Weill Cornell Med Ctr (page 103); **Address:** New York Presby Hosp, Dept Urology, 525 E 68th St, Starr 900, Box 94, New York, NY 10021-4870; **Phone:** 212-746-5480; **Board Cert:** Urology 86; **Med School:** Univ VA Sch Med 65; **Resid:** Surgery, Vanderbilt Univ Med Ctr 67; Urology, Univ Virginia Hosp 71; **Fellow:** Internal Medicine, Columbia Univ 73; **Fac Appt:** Prof U, Cornell Univ-Weill Med Coll

von Eschenbach, Andrew C MD [U] - **Spec Exp:** Prostate Cancer; Urologic Cancer; **Hospital:** Natl Inst of Hlth - Clin Ctr; **Address:** Natl Cancer Inst, 31 Center Drive Bldg 31 - rm 11A48, MC 2590, Bethesda, MD 20892-2590; **Phone:** 301-496-5615; **Board Cert:** Urology 78; **Med School:** Georgetown Univ 67; **Resid:** Surgery, Penn Hosp 72; Transplant Surgery, Penn Hosp 75; **Fellow:** Urologic Oncology, Univ Texas-MD Anderson Hosp 77

Waldbaum, Robert MD [U] - **Spec Exp:** Prostate Cancer; Prostate Disease; Urologic Cancer; **Hospital:** N Shore Univ Hosp at Manhasset; **Address:** 535 Plandome Rd, Ste 3, Manhasset, NY 11030-1961; **Phone:** 516-627-6188; **Board Cert:** Urology 73; **Med School:** Columbia P&S 62; **Resid:** Surgery, Columbia Presby Med Ctr 66; Urology, New York Hosp-Cornell 70; **Fac Appt:** Clin Prof U, Cornell Univ-Weill Med Coll

Walsh, Patrick MD [U] - **Spec Exp:** Prostate Cancer; Urologic Cancer; **Hospital:** Johns Hopkins Hosp - Baltimore (page 97); **Address:** Brady Urological Inst, 600 N Wolfe St, Marburg 134, Baltimore, MD 21287-2101; **Phone:** 410-955-6100; **Board Cert:** Urology 75; **Med School:** Case West Res Univ 64; **Resid:** Surgery, Peter Bent Brigham Hosp/Childrens Hosp 67; Urology, UCLA Med Ctr 71; **Fellow:** Endocrinology, Harbor Genl Hosp 70; **Fac Appt:** Prof U, Johns Hopkins Univ

Wein, Alan J MD [U] - **Spec Exp:** Neuro-Urology; Prostate Cancer; Incontinence; **Hospital:** Hosp Univ Penn - UPHS (page 113); **Address:** Univ Penn Hlth System, Div Urology, 3400 Spruce St, 9 Penn Tower, Philadelphia, PA 19104-4283; **Phone:** 215-662-2891; **Board Cert:** Urology 95; **Med School:** Univ Pennsylvania 66; **Resid:** Surgery, Hosp Univ Penn 68; Urology, Hosp Univ Penn 72; **Fellow:** Urology, Hosp Univ Penn 69; **Fac Appt:** Prof U, Univ Pennsylvania

Weiss, Robert E MD [U] - **Spec Exp:** Bladder Cancer; Kidney Cancer; Testicular Cancer; **Hospital:** Robert Wood Johnson Univ Hosp - New Brunswick (page 106); **Address:** 1 Robert Wood Johnson Pl Ste MB588, New Brunswick, NJ 08901-1928; **Phone:** 732-235-7775; **Board Cert:** Urology 03; **Med School:** NYU Sch Med 85; **Resid:** Surgery, Mount Sinai Med Ctr 87; Urology, Mount Sinai Med Ctr 91; **Fellow:** Meml Sloan Kettering Cancer Ctr 94; **Fac Appt:** Assoc Prof U, UMDNJ-RW Johnson Med Sch

Yu, George W MD [U] - **Spec Exp:** Urologic Cancer; Nutrition & Disease Prevention/Control; Nutrition & Cancer Remission; **Hospital:** G Washington Univ Hosp; **Address:** 116 Defense Hwy, Ste 200, Annapolis, MD 21401; **Phone:** 410-897-0540; **Board Cert:** Urology 83; **Med School:** Tufts Univ 73; **Resid:** Surgery, Brigham & Women's Hosp 76; Urology, Johns Hopkins Hosp 81; **Fac Appt:** Prof U, Geo Wash Univ

Southeast

Beall, Michael E MD [U] - **Spec Exp:** Prostate & Urologic Cancer; Testicular Cancer; Vasectomy Reversal; **Hospital:** Inova Fairfax Hosp; **Address:** 8503 Arlington Blvd, Ste 310, Fairfax, VA 22030; **Phone:** 703-208-4200; **Board Cert:** Urology 79; **Med School:** Geo Wash Univ 72; **Resid:** Surgery, Geo Wash Univ Hosp 74; Urology, Geo Wash Univ Hosp 77; **Fac Appt:** Assoc Clin Prof U, Geo Wash Univ

Cookson, Michael MD [U] - **Spec Exp:** Bladder Cancer; Testicular Cancer; Prostate Cancer; **Hospital:** Vanderbilt Univ Med Ctr (page 116); **Address:** Vanderbilt U Sch Med, Urol Surg A1302 MCN, Nashville, TN 37232-2765; **Phone:** 615-343-1317; **Board Cert:** Urology 98; **Med School:** Univ Okla Coll Med 88; **Resid:** Urology, U Tex San Antonio 94; **Fellow:** Urologic Oncology, Meml Sloan-Kettering Cancer Ctr 96; **Fac Appt:** Asst Prof U, Vanderbilt Univ

Hall, Marshall Craig MD [U] - **Spec Exp:** Urologic Cancer; Bladder Cancer; **Hospital:** Wake Forest Univ Baptist Med Ctr (page 117); **Address:** Wake Forest U Bapt Med Ctr, Med Ctr Blvd, Reynolds Tower, Winston-Salem, NC 27157; **Phone:** 336-716-4131; **Board Cert:** Urology 97; **Med School:** Univ Louisville Sch Med 87; **Resid:** Surgery, Vanderbilt Univ Med Ctr 89; Urology, Vanderbilt Univ Med Ctr 93; **Fellow:** Urologic Oncology, U Tex MD Anderson Canc Ctr 95; **Fac Appt:** Assoc Prof U, Wake Forest Univ

Harty, James MD [U] - **Spec Exp:** Urologic Cancer; **Hospital:** Norton Hosp; **Address:** 210 E Gray St, Ste 1000, Louisville, KY 40202; **Phone:** 502-629-5904; **Board Cert:** Urology 79; **Med School:** Ireland 69; **Resid:** Surgery, Johns Hopkins Hosp 73; Urology, Johns Hopkins Hosp 77; **Fac Appt:** Prof S, Univ Louisville Sch Med

Jordan, Gerald H MD [U] - **Spec Exp:** Incontinence; Urethral Reconstruction; Prostate Cancer; **Hospital:** Sentara Norfolk Genl Hosp; **Address:** 400 W Brambleton Ave, Ste 100, Norfolk, VA 23510-1196; **Phone:** 757-457-5100; **Board Cert:** Urology 84; **Med School:** Univ Tex, San Antonio 77; **Resid:** Urology, Naval Reg Med Ctr 78; **Fellow:** Reconstructive Surgery, Eastern Va Med Sch 84; **Fac Appt:** Prof U, Eastern VA Med Sch

Kim, Edward D MD [U] - **Spec Exp:** Infertility-Male; Prostate Cancer; Bladder Cancer; **Hospital:** Univ of Tennesee Mem Hosp; **Address:** 1928 Alcoa Hwy Bldg B - Ste 127, Knoxville, TN 37920; **Phone:** 865-544-9254; **Board Cert:** Urology 98; **Med School:** Northwestern Univ 89; **Resid:** Urology, Northwestern Meml Hosp 95; **Fellow:** Baylor Coll Med 96; **Fac Appt:** Assoc Prof U, Univ Tenn Coll Med, Memphis

Lockhart, Jorge L MD [U] - **Spec Exp:** Voiding Dysfunction; Urologic Cancer; **Hospital:** H Lee Moffitt Cancer Ctr & Research Inst; **Address:** H Lee Moffitt Cancer Ctr, Dept Urology, 12902 Magnolia Drive, Tampa, FL 33612; **Phone:** 813-979-3980 x2226; **Board Cert:** Urology 80; **Med School:** Uruguay 73; **Resid:** Urology, Duke Univ Med Ctr 77; **Fellow:** Urodynamics, Duke Univ Med Ctr 78; **Fac Appt:** Prof S, Univ S Fla Coll Med

Marshall, Fray F MD [U] - **Spec Exp:** Urologic Cancer; Prostate Cancer; Kidney Cancer; **Hospital:** Emory Univ Hosp; **Address:** Emory Clinic, Dept Urology, 1365 Clifton Rd NE Bldg B - Ste 1405, Atlanta, GA 30322; **Phone:** 404-778-4898; **Board Cert:** Urology 77; **Med School:** Univ VA Sch Med 69; **Resid:** Surgery, Univ Mich Hosps 72; Urology, Mass Genl Hosp 75; **Fac Appt:** Prof U, Emory Univ

McCullough, David L MD [U] - **Spec Exp:** Genitourinary Cancer; Kidney Stones; **Hospital:** Wake Forest Univ Baptist Med Ctr (page 117); **Address:** Wake Forest University Physicians, Dept Urology, Medical Center Blvd, Winston-Salem, NC 27157; **Phone:** 336-716-4131; **Board Cert:** Urology 95; **Med School:** Wake Forest Univ 64; **Resid:** Urology, Mass Genl Hosp 72; Surgery, Univ Hosp-Case Western Res Univ 66; **Fac Appt:** Prof U, Wake Forest Univ

Moul, Judd W MD [U] - **Spec Exp:** Prostate Cancer; Testicular Cancer; Urologic Cancer; Duke Univ Med Ctr (page 94); **Address:** Duke Univ Med Ctr, Div Urologic Surgery, Box 3707, NC 27710; **Phone:** 919-684-2446; **Board Cert:** Urology 99; **Med School:** Jefferson Med Coll 82; Urology, Walter Reed Army Med Ctr 87; **Fellow:** Urologic Oncology, Duke Univ Med Ctr 89; **Fac App** Prof S, Duke Univ

Pow-Sang, Julio MD [U] - **Spec Exp:** Prostate Cancer; **Hospital:** H Lee Moffitt Cancer Ctr & Research Inst; **Address:** 12902 Magnolia Drive, Tampa, FL 33612-9416; **Phone:** 813-972-8418; **Board Cert:** Urology 99; **Med School:** Mexico 78; **Resid:** Surgery, Univ Miami Sch Med 83; Urology, Univ Miami Sch Med 86; **Fellow:** Urologic Oncology, Univ Fla Coll Med 87; **Fac Appt:** Prof S, Univ S Fla Coll Med

Robertson, Cary N MD [U] - **Spec Exp:** Prostate Cancer; Urologic Cancer; **Hospital:** Duke Univ Med Ctr (page 94); **Address:** Duke Univ Med Ctr, Trent Drive, Box 3833, Durham, NC 27710; **Phone:** 919-681-6768; **Board Cert:** Urology 97; **Med School:** Tulane Univ 77; **Resid:** Urology, Duke Univ Med Ctr 85; **Fellow:** Urologic Oncology, Natl Inst Hlth 87; **Fac Appt:** Assoc Prof U, Duke Univ

Rowland, Randall MD [U] - **Spec Exp:** Urologic Cancer; **Hospital:** Univ Kentucky Med Ctr; **Address:** University of Kentucky Med Ctr, Div Urology, 800 Rose St, rm MS283, Lexington, KY 40536-0298; **Phone:** 859-323-6677; **Board Cert:** Urology 80; **Med School:** Northwestern Univ 72; **Resid:** Urology, Northwestern Meml Hosp 78; **Fac Appt:** Prof U, Univ KY Coll Med

Sanders, William H MD [U] - **Spec Exp:** Prostate Cancer; Kidney Stones; Kidney Cancer; **Hospital:** St Joseph's Hosp - Atlanta; **Address:** 5673 Peachtree Dunwoody Rd, Ste 910, Atlanta, GA 30342-1767; **Phone:** 404-255-3822; **Board Cert:** Urology 96; **Med School:** Emory Univ 88; **Resid:** Urology, Yale Sch of Med 93

Schellhammer, Paul MD [U] - **Spec Exp:** Prostate Cancer; Urologic Cancer; **Hospital:** Sentara Norfolk Genl Hosp; **Address:** 6333 Center Drive, Norfolk, VA 23502; **Phone:** 757-457-5170; **Board Cert:** Urology 99; **Med School:** Cornell Univ-Weill Med Coll 66; **Resid:** Surgery, Univ Hosps 68; Urology, Med Coll Va Hosp 73; **Fellow:** Urology, Memorial Hosp 74; **Fac Appt:** Prof U, Eastern VA Med Sch

Smith, Joseph A MD [U] - **Spec Exp:** Prostate Cancer/Robotic Surgery; Bladder Cancer; **Hospital:** Vanderbilt Univ Med Ctr (page 116); **Address:** Vanderbilt Univ Med Ctr, Dept Urol Surgery, A-1302 MCN, Nashville, TN 37232-2765; **Phone:** 615-343-0234; **Board Cert:** Urology 00; **Med School:** Univ Tenn Coll Med, Memphis 74; **Resid:** Surgery, Parkland Meml Hosp 76; Urology, Univ Utah 79; **Fellow:** Urologic Oncology, Meml Sloan Kettering Cancer Ctr 80; **Fac Appt:** Prof U, Vanderbilt Univ

Teigland, Chris Michael MD [U] - **Spec Exp:** Urologic Cancer; Prostate Cancer; Kidney Cancer; **Hospital:** Carolinas Med Ctr; **Address:** Mckay Urology, 1416 E Morehead St, Ste 101, Charlotte, NC 28204-2925; **Phone:** 704-355-8686; **Board Cert:** Urology 99; **Med School:** Duke Univ 80; **Resid:** Surgery, Univ Utah Affil Hosps 82; Urology, Univ Texas SW Med Ctr 87; **Fac Appt:** Assoc Clin Prof S, Univ NC Sch Med

Wajsman, Zev Lew MD [U] - **Spec Exp:** Urologic Cancer; **Hospital:** North Florida Regl Med Ctr; **Address:** Urology Assocs, 6440 W Newberry Rd, Ste 100, Gainesville, FL 32605; **Phone:** 352-333-5400; **Med School:** Israel 65; **Resid:** Surgery, Central Emek Hosp 70; Urology, Central Emek Hosp 73; **Fellow:** Urology, Rosewell Park Meml Inst 75

D **[U]** - **Spec Exp:** Urologic Cancer & Surgery; Prostate Cancer; **Hospital:** ge 85); **Address:** 4960 Children's Pl, Box 8242, St Louis, MO 63110; **Phone:** rt: Urology 03; **Med School:** Jefferson Med Coll 78; **Resid:** Surgery, U Hosp 80; Urology, Brigham-Womens Hosp-Harvard 83; **Fellow:** Urologic ac Appt: Prof U, Washington Univ, St Louis

Bahnson, Robert MD [U] - **Spec Exp:** Prostate Cancer; Bladder Cancer; Continent Urinary Diversions; **Hospital:** Ohio St Univ Med Ctr (page 105); **Address:** 456 West 10th Avenue, Div of Urology 4960 UHC, Columbus, OH 43210-1228; **Phone:** 614-293-8155; **Board Cert:** Urology 97; **Med School:** Tufts Univ 79; **Resid:** Surgery, Northwestern Univ 81; Urology, Northwestern Univ 85; **Fellow:** Urology, Northwestern Univ 84; Research, Univ Pittsburgh 91; **Fac Appt:** Prof U, Ohio State Univ

Brendler, Charles B MD [U] - **Spec Exp:** Prostate Cancer; **Hospital:** Univ of Chicago Hosps; **Address:** Univ Chicago, Sect Urology, 5841 S Maryland Ave, rm J-653, MC 6038, Chicago, IL 60637; **Phone:** 773-702-1860; **Board Cert:** Urology 81; **Med School:** Univ VA Sch Med 74; **Resid:** Surgery, Duke Univ Med Ctr 76; Urology, Duke Univ Med Ctr 79; **Fellow:** Urologic Oncology, Univ Hosp Wales 80; Johns Hopkins Hosp 82; **Fac Appt:** Prof U, Univ Chicago-Pritzker Sch Med

Bruskewitz, Reginald C MD [U] - **Spec Exp:** Urologic Cancer; Prostate Disease; **Hospital:** Univ WI Hosp & Clins; **Address:** 600 Highland Ave, rm G-5329, Madison, WI 53792; **Phone:** 608-263-4757; **Board Cert:** Urology 81; **Med School:** Univ Wisc 73; **Resid:** Urology, Univ Wisc 78; **Fellow:** Urodynamics, UCLA Med Ctr 79; **Fac Appt:** Assoc Prof S, Univ Wisc

Campbell, Steven C MD/PhD [U] - **Spec Exp:** Kidney Cancer; Prostate Cancer; Bladder Cancer; **Hospital:** Loyola Univ Med Ctr (page 98); **Address:** Loyola University Medical Ctr, 2160 S First Ave Bldg 54 - rm 248, Maywood, IL 60153; **Phone:** 708-216-5098; **Board Cert:** Urology 99; **Med School:** Univ Chicago-Pritzker Sch Med 89; **Resid:** Urology, Cleveland Clinic 95; **Fellow:** Urology, Meml Sloan Kettering Cancer Ctr 96; **Fac Appt:** Assoc Prof U, Loyola Univ-Stritch Sch Med

Catalona, William J MD [U] - **Spec Exp:** Urologic Cancer; Prostate Cancer; Prostate Surgery; **Hospital:** Northwestern Meml Hosp; **Address:** Northwestern Meml Hosp, Dept Urology, 675 N St Clair St, Galter 20-150, Chicago, IL 60611; **Phone:** 312-695-6126; **Board Cert:** Urology 78; **Med School:** Yale Univ 68; **Resid:** Surgery, UCSF Med Ctr 70; Urology, Johns Hopkins Hosp 76; **Fellow:** Surgical Oncology, Natl Cancer Inst 72; **Fac Appt:** Prof U, Washington Univ, St Louis

Chodak, Gerald MD [U] - **Spec Exp:** Prostate Cancer; Prostate Disease; **Hospital:** Weiss Meml Hosp; **Address:** 4646 N Marine Drive, Ste A5500, Chicago, IL 60640-5759; **Phone:** 773-564-5006; **Board Cert:** Urology 84; **Med School:** SUNY Buffalo 75; **Resid:** Surgery, UCLA Med Ctr 77; Urology, Brigham & Womens Hosp 79; **Fellow:** Univ Chicago 81; Research, Harvard Chldns Hosp 82; **Fac Appt:** Prof S, Univ Chicago-Pritzker Sch Med

Coplen, Douglas E MD [U] - **Spec Exp:** Pediatric & Fetal Urology; Urologic Cancer-Pediatric; Testicular Cancer-Pediatric; **Hospital:** St Louis Chldns Hosp; **Address:** Washington Univ Sch Medicine, Dept Urology, 660 S Euclid Ave, Box 8242, St Louis, MO 63110; **Phone:** 314-454-6034; **Board Cert:** Urology 96; **Med School:** Indiana Univ 85; **Resid:** Urology, Barnes Jewish Hosp 92; **Fellow:** Pediatric Urology, Children's Hosp 94; **Fac Appt:** Asst Prof S, Washington Univ, St Louis

Donovan Jr, James F MD [U] - **Spec Exp:** Prostate & Urologic Cancer; Prostate Ca▓
Surgery; Laparoscopic Urologic Surgery; **Hospital:** Univ Hosp - Cincinnati; **Address:** Univer▓
Cincinnat Medical Ctr, Medical Arts Bldg, 222 Piedmont Ave, Ste 7000, Cincinnati, OH 45219;▓
513-475-8787; **Board Cert:** Surgery 97; Urology 99; **Med School:** Northwestern Univ 78; **Resid:▓**
Surgery, Northwestern Meml Hosp 82; Urology, Northwestern Meml Hosp 86; **Fellow:** Baylor Coll Me▓
Fac Appt: Prof U, Univ Cincinnati

Flanigan, Robert C MD [U] - **Spec Exp:** Prostate Cancer; Bladder Cancer; Kidney Cancer. Kidney
Transplant; **Hospital:** Loyola Univ Med Ctr (page 98); **Address:** Loyola Univ Med-Fahey Bldg 54, 2160
S First Ave, rm 267, Maywood, IL 60153; **Phone:** 708-216-5100; **Board Cert:** Surgery 98; Urology 01;
Med School: Case West Res Univ 72; **Resid:** Surgery, Case West Univ Med Ctr 78; Urology, Case
West Univ Med Ctr 78; **Fac Appt:** Prof U, Loyola Univ-Stritch Sch Med

Foster, Richard S MD [U] - **Spec Exp:** Testicular Cancer; **Hospital:** Indiana Univ Hosp (page 90);
Address: 535 Barnhill Drive, Ste 420, Indianapolis, IN 46202; **Phone:** 317-274-3458; **Board Cert:**
Urology 98; **Med School:** Indiana Univ 80; **Resid:** Urology, Indiana Univ Hosp 86; **Fac Appt:** Prof U,
Indiana Univ

Gill, Inderbir Singh MD [U] - **Spec Exp:** Prostate Cancer-Laparoscopic Surgery; Kidney Cancer;
Urologic Cancer-Laparoscopic Surgery; **Hospital:** Cleveland Clin Fdn (page 92); **Address:** Cleveland
Clinic Urological Inst, 9500 Euclid Ave, Ste A100, Cleveland, OH 44195; **Phone:** 216-445-1530; **Board
Cert:** Urology 97; **Med School:** India 80; **Resid:** Surgery, Dayanand Med Coll & Hosp; Urology, Univ
Kentucky Hosp 93; **Fellow:** Cleveland Clinic

Gluckman, Gordon MD [U] - **Spec Exp:** Prostate Cancer; Kidney Cancer; Minimally Invasive
Urologic Surgery; **Hospital:** Adv Luth Genl Hosp; **Address:** Parkside Center, 1875 Dempster St, Ste
506, Park Ridge, IL 60068; **Phone:** 847-823-4700; **Board Cert:** Urology 97; **Med School:** Northwestern
Univ 89; **Resid:** Surgery, UCSF Med Ctr 91; Urology, UCSF Med Ctr 95

Kibel, Adam S MD [U] - **Spec Exp:** Bladder Cancer; Testucular Cancer; Penile Cancer; **Hospital:**
Barnes-Jewish Hosp (page 85); **Address:** Washington University School of Medicine, Dept Urologic
Surgery, 660 S Euclid Ave, Box 8242, St Louis, MO 63110; **Phone:** 314-362-8200; **Board Cert:** Urology
01; **Med School:** Cornell Univ-Weill Med Coll 91; **Resid:** Urology, Brigham & Women's Hosp 96; **Fellow:**
Urologic Oncology, Johns Hopkins Med Ctr 99; **Fac Appt:** Assoc Prof U, Washington Univ, St Louis

Klein, Eric A MD [U] - **Spec Exp:** Prostate Cancer; Testicular Cancer; Urologic Cancer; **Hospital:**
Cleveland Clin Fdn (page 92); **Address:** Cleveland Clinic Fdn, Dept Urol, Sect Urol-Onc, 9500 Euclid
Ave, Fl A100, Cleveland, OH 44195-0001; **Phone:** 216-444-5591; **Board Cert:** Urology 99; **Med
School:** Univ Pittsburgh 81; **Resid:** Urology, Cleveland Clinic Fdn 86; **Fellow:** Urologic Oncology, Meml
Sloan Kettering Canc Ctr 89; **Fac Appt:** Assoc Prof S, Ohio State Univ

Koeneman, Kenneth MD [U] - **Spec Exp:** Robotic Prostatectomy; Prostate Cancer; Urological
Cancer; **Hospital:** Fairview-Univ Med Ctr - Univ Campus; **Address:** MN Hosp Dept of Urology, rm D598,
Box 394, Minneapolis, MN 55455; **Phone:** 612-625-0964; **Board Cert:** Urology 02; **Med School:** Univ
IL Coll Med 92; **Resid:** Urology, Loyola Univ Med Ctr 98; **Fellow:** Urologic Oncology, Univ VA 00; **Fac
Appt:** Assoc Prof U, Univ Minn

Kozlowski, James M MD [U] - **Spec Exp:** Prostate Cancer; Continent Urinary Diversions;
Laparoscopic Surgery; **Hospital:** Northwestern Meml Hosp; **Address:** 675 N St Clair St Bldg Galter Fl
20 - Ste 150, Chicago, IL 60611; **Phone:** 312-695-8146; **Board Cert:** Surgery 93; Urology 83; **Med
School:** Northwestern Univ 75; **Resid:** Surgery, Northwestern Univ-McGaw 79; Urology, Northwestern
Univ-McGaw 81; **Fellow:** Research, NCI-Frederick Cancer Rsch 84; **Fac Appt:** Assoc Prof U,
Northwestern Univ

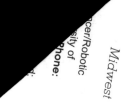

Spec Exp: Prostate Cancer; Erectile Dysfunction; Prostate Disease; Hosp; **Address:** 675 N St Clair St, Galter 20-150, Chicago, IL 60611- **Board Cert:** Urology 00; **Med School:** Northwestern Univ 83; **Resid:** Hosp 85; Urology, Northwestern Meml Hosp 88; **Fellow:** Research, Fac **Appt:** Assoc Prof U, Northwestern Univ

Spec Exp: Prostate Cancer/Robotic Surgery; Transplant-Kidney; Urologic ord Hosp; **Address:** Henry Ford Hosp - Vattikuti Urology Inst, 2799 W Grand Bvd, Detroit, MI 48202; **Phone:** 313-916-2062; **Board Cert:** Urology 82; **Med School:** India 69; **Resid:** Urology, Bryn Mawr Hosp 74; Urology, Johns Hopkins Hosp 80; **Fellow:** Transplant Surgery, Johns Hopkins Univ 77; **Fac Appt:** Prof S, Univ Mass Sch Med

Montie, James MD [U] - **Spec Exp:** Bladder Cancer; Prostate Cancer; Genitourinary Cancer; **Hospital:** Univ Michigan Hlth Sys; **Address:** 1500 E Medical Ctr Dr, Dept Urology, Taubman Hlth Care Ctr, rm 3876, Box 0330, Ann Arbor, MI 48109-0330; **Phone:** 734-647-8903; **Board Cert:** Urology 78; **Med School:** Univ Mich Med Sch 71; **Resid:** Urology, Cleveland Clinic Fdn 76; **Fellow:** Urologic Oncology, Meml Sloan-Kettering Cancer Ctr 79; **Fac Appt:** Prof U, Univ Mich Med Sch

Myers, Robert P MD [U] - **Spec Exp:** Prostate Cancer; **Hospital:** Mayo Med Ctr & Clin - Rochester; **Address:** Mayo Clinic, Dept Urology, 200 First St SW, Rochester, MN 55905; **Phone:** 507-284-3077; **Board Cert:** Urology 76; **Med School:** Columbia P&S 67; **Resid:** Urology, Mayo Clinic 72; **Fac Appt:** Prof U, Mayo Med Sch

Novick, Andrew MD [U] - **Spec Exp:** Transplant-Kidney; Kidney Cancer; Urologic Cancer; **Hospital:** Cleveland Clin Fdn (page 92); **Address:** Cleveland Clinic-Urological Inst, 9500 Euclid Ave, Desk A100, Cleveland, OH 44195; **Phone:** 216-444-5600; **Board Cert:** Urology 96; **Med School:** McGill Univ 72; **Resid:** Surgery, Royal Victoria Hosp 74; Urology, Cleveland Clinic 77

O'Donnell, Michael A MD [U] - **Spec Exp:** Bladder Cancer; Immunotherapy; Urologic Cancer; **Hospital:** Univ Iowa Hosp & Clinics; **Address:** Univ Iowa Hosp & Clins, Dept Urology, 200 Hawkins Drive, Iowa City, IA 52242; **Phone:** 319-384-6040; **Board Cert:** Urology 95; **Med School:** Duke Univ 84; **Resid:** Surgery, Brigham & Womens Hosp 87; Urology, Brigham & Womens Hosp 91; **Fellow:** Urology, Brigham & Womens Hosp 93; **Fac Appt:** Assoc Prof U, Univ Iowa Coll Med

Resnick, Martin MD [U] - **Spec Exp:** Prostate Cancer; Urologic Cancer; Kidney Stones; **Hospital:** Univ Hosps of Cleveland; **Address:** 11100 Euclid Ave, Cleveland, OH 44106-5046; **Phone:** 216-844-3011; **Board Cert:** Urology 98; **Med School:** Wake Forest Univ 69; **Resid:** Surgery, Univ Hosps 71; Urology, Northwestern Univ Med Ctr 75; **Fac Appt:** Prof U, Case West Res Univ

See, William MD [U] - **Spec Exp:** Prostate Cancer; Bladder Cancer; Testicular Cancer; **Hospital:** Froedtert Meml Lutheran Hosp; **Address:** Med Coll of Wisc, Dept Urol, 9200 W Wisconsin Ave, Milwaukee, WI 53226; **Phone:** 414-456-6950; **Board Cert:** Urology 00; **Med School:** Univ Chicago-Pritzker Sch Med 82; **Resid:** Urology, Univ Wash 88; **Fellow:** Research, Natl Kidney Fdn/Univ Wash 86; Research, Amer Fdn for Urol Dis/Univ Iowa 90; **Fac Appt:** Prof U, Med Coll Wisc

Steinberg, Gary D MD [U] - **Spec Exp:** Bladder Cancer; Kidney Cancer; Prostate Cancer; **Hospital:** Univ of Chicago Hosps; **Address:** 5841 S Maryland Ave, MC 6038, Chicago, IL 60637; **Phone:** 773-702-3080; **Board Cert:** Urology 03; **Med School:** Univ Chicago-Pritzker Sch Med 85; **Resid:** Surgery, Johns Hopkins Hosp 87; Urology, Brady Urol Inst/Johns Hopkins 91; **Fellow:** Oncology, Johns Hopkins Hosp 89; **Fac Appt:** Assoc Prof U, Univ Chicago-Pritzker Sch Med

Thomas Jr, Anthony J MD [U] - **Spec Exp:** Infertility-Male; Vasectomy Reversal; Fertility Preservation; **Hospital:** Cleveland Clin Fdn (page 92); **Address:** Cleveland Clinic-Urological Inst, 9500 Euclid Ave, Desk A100, Cleveland, OH 44195; **Phone:** 216-444-5600; **Board Cert:** Urology 78; **Med School:** Univ Cincinnati 69; **Resid:** Surgery, Wayne State Univ Affil Hosp 71; Urology, Wayne State Univ Affil Hosp 76

Totonchi, Emil F MD [U] - **Spec Exp:** Prostate Cancer & Disease; Urologic Cancer; Erectile Dysfunction; **Hospital:** Adv Illinois Masonic Med Ctr; **Address:** 860 N Clark St, Chicago, IL 60610-3218; **Phone:** 312-944-2848; **Board Cert:** Urology 84; **Med School:** Iraq 68; **Resid:** Surgery 77; Urology, Cook County Hosp 82; **Fellow:** Surgical Oncology, Cook County Hosp-Univ Illinois 78

Williams, Richard D MD [U] - **Spec Exp:** Kidney Cancer; Bladder Cancer; Prostate Cancer; **Hospital:** Univ Iowa Hosp & Clinics; **Address:** Univ Iowa Hosp, Dept Urology, 200 Hawkins Dr, rm 3251 RCP, Iowa City, IA 52242-1089; **Phone:** 319-356-0760; **Board Cert:** Urology 79; **Med School:** Univ Kans 70; **Resid:** Surgery, Univ Minn Hosp 72; Urology, Univ Minn Hosp 76; **Fellow:** Urologic Oncology, Univ Minn Hosp 79; **Fac Appt:** Prof U, Univ Iowa Coll Med

Wood, David P MD [U] - **Spec Exp:** Genitourinary Cancer; Bladder Cancer; Prostate Cancer; **Hospital:** Univ Michigan Hlth Sys; **Address:** University of Michigan, Dept Urology, 3875 Taubman Cancer Ctr, 1500 E Medical Center Drive, Ann Arbor, MI 48109-0330; **Phone:** 734-763-9269; **Board Cert:** Urology 02; **Med School:** Univ Mich Med Sch 83; **Resid:** Urology, Cleveland Clinic 88; **Fellow:** Urologic Oncology, Meml Sloan-Kettering Cancer Ctr 91; **Fac Appt:** Prof U, Univ Mich Med Sch

Great Plains and Mountains

Crawford, E David MD [U] - **Spec Exp:** Prostate Cancer; Testicular Cancer; Bladder Cancer; **Hospital:** Univ Colorado Hosp; **Address:** Anschutz Cancer Pavillion, 1665 N Ursula St, Box 6510, MS F-710, Aurora, CO 80010; **Phone:** 720-848-0195; **Board Cert:** Urology 80; **Med School:** Univ Cincinnati 73; **Resid:** Urology, Good Samaritan Hosp 77; **Fellow:** UCLA Med Ctr 78; **Fac Appt:** Prof RadRO, Univ Colorado

Davis, Bradley E MD [U] - **Spec Exp:** Urologic Cancer; Bladder Cancer; Reconstructive Surgery; **Hospital:** Overland Pk Regl Med Ctr; **Address:** Urologic Surgical Associates, 10550 Quivira Rd, Ste 105, Overland Park, KS 66215; **Phone:** 913-438-3833; **Board Cert:** Urology 96; **Med School:** Univ Kans 86; **Resid:** Urology, Univ Kansas Med Ctr 91; **Fellow:** Urologic Oncology, Meml Sloan-Kettering Cancer Ctr 93; **Fac Appt:** Asst Clin Prof U, Univ Kans

Lugg, James A MD [U] - **Spec Exp:** Prostate Cancer; Laparoscopic Surgery; Incontinence; **Hospital:** United Med. Ctr.; **Address:** 2301 House Ave, Ste 500, Cheyenne, WY 82001; **Phone:** 307-635-4131; **Board Cert:** Urology 98; **Med School:** Northwestern Univ 90; **Resid:** Urology, UCLA Med Ctr; **Fac Appt:** Asst Prof U, Univ Colorado

Middleton, Richard MD [U] - **Spec Exp:** Urologic Cancer; Reconstructive Urologic Surgery; Infertility; **Hospital:** Univ Utah Hosps and Clins; **Address:** University of Utah Med Ctr, 50 N Med Dr., Salt Lake City, UT 84132-1001; **Phone:** 801-581-4703; **Board Cert:** Urology 70; **Med School:** Cornell Univ-Weill Med Coll 58; **Resid:** Surgery, New York Hosp-Cornell Med Ctr 61; Urology, New York Hosp-Cornell Med Ctr 67; **Fac Appt:** Prof U, Univ Utah

Southwest

Babaian, Richard MD [U] - **Spec Exp:** Prostate Cancer; **Hospital:** UT MD Anderson Cancer Ctr, The (page 115); **Address:** MD Anderson Cancer Ctr, 1515 Holcombe Blvd, Unit 446, Houston, TX 77030; **Phone:** 713-792-3250; **Board Cert:** Urology 80; **Med School:** Georgetown Univ 72; **Resid:** Surgery, Univ Wisconsin 74; Urology, Univ NC Hosp 77; **Fellow:** Urologic Oncology, MD Anderson Cancer Ctr 79; Immunology, Univ NC Hosps 78; **Fac Appt:** Prof U, Univ Tex, Houston

Bardot, Stephen F MD [U] - **Spec Exp:** Urologic Cancer; Prostate Cancer; **Hospital:** Ochsner Fdn Hosp; **Address:** Ochsner Clinic, 1514 Jefferson Hwy Fl 4, New Orleans, LA 70121-2483; **Phone:** 504-842-4083; **Board Cert:** Urology 93; **Med School:** Univ Kans 85; **Resid:** Surgery, St Luke's Hosp 87; Urology, Kansas City Univ Med Ctr 90; **Fellow:** Urologic Oncology, Cleveland Clinic 91

Basler, Joseph W MD [U] - **Spec Exp:** Prostate Cancer; Urologic Cancer; Kidney Stones; **Hospital:** Audie L Murphy Meml Vets Hosp; **Address:** 7703 Floyd Curl Dr, MC-7845, San Antonio, TX 78229-3900; **Phone:** 210-567-5640; **Board Cert:** Urology 92; **Med School:** Univ MO-Columbia Sch Med 84; **Resid:** Surgery, Univ Missouri 86; Urology, Barnes Hosp/Wash Univ 90; **Fac Appt:** Assoc Prof S, Univ Tex, San Antonio

Greene, Graham MD [U] - **Spec Exp:** Urologic Cancer; **Hospital:** UAMS Med Ctr; **Address:** 4301 W Markham, Slot 774, Little Rock, AR 72205; **Phone:** 501-296-1545; **Board Cert:** Urology 99; **Med School:** Dalhousie Univ 94; **Resid:** Urology, Victoria Genl 94; **Fellow:** Medical Oncology, M.D. Anderson Cancer Ctr 97; **Fac Appt:** Assoc Prof U, Univ Ark

Kadmon, Dov MD [U] - **Spec Exp:** Prostate Cancer; **Hospital:** St Luke's Episcopal Hosp - Houston; **Address:** Baylor College of Medicine, 6560 Fannin St, Ste 2100, Houston, TX 77030; **Phone:** 713-798-7893; **Board Cert:** Urology 84; **Med School:** Israel 70; **Resid:** Surgery, Barnes Jewish Hosp 77; Urology, Barnes Jewish Hosp 80; **Fellow:** Urology, Barnes Jewish Hosp 82; **Fac Appt:** Prof U, Baylor Coll Med

Lerner, Seth P MD [U] - **Spec Exp:** Bladder Cancer; Testicular Cancer; Urinary Tract Reconstruction; **Hospital:** St Luke's Episcopal Hosp - Houston; **Address:** 6560 Fannin St, Ste 2100, Houston, TX 77030; **Phone:** 713-798-6841; **Board Cert:** Urology 94; **Med School:** Baylor Coll Med 84; **Resid:** Surgery, Virginia Mason Hosp 86; Urology, Baylor Coll Med 90; **Fellow:** Urologic Oncology, LAC-USC Med Ctr 92; **Fac Appt:** Assoc Prof U, Baylor Coll Med

McConnell, John Dowling MD [U] - **Spec Exp:** Prostate Cancer; **Hospital:** Zale Lipshy Univ Hosp - Dallas; **Address:** Univ Texas SW Med Ctr, 5323 Harry Hines Blvd, B11.300, Dallas, TX 75390-9131; **Phone:** 214-648-5630; **Board Cert:** Urology 96; **Med School:** Loyola Univ-Stritch Sch Med 78; **Resid:** Surgery, Univ Tex Hlth Sci Ctr-Parkland 80; Urology, Univ Tex Hlth Sci Ctr-Parkland 84; **Fac Appt:** Prof U, Univ Tex SW, Dallas

Miles, Brian J MD [U] - **Spec Exp:** Prostate Cancer; Urologic Cancer; Gene Therapy; **Hospital:** Methodist Hosp - Houston; **Address:** Dept Urology, Scurlock Tower, 6560 Fannin St, Ste 2100, Houston, TX 77030-2769; **Phone:** 713-798-4001; **Board Cert:** Urology 84; **Med School:** Univ Mich Med Sch 74; **Resid:** Urology, Walter Reed Army Med Ctr 82; **Fac Appt:** Prof U, Baylor Coll Med

Pisters, Louis L MD [U] - **Spec Exp:** Prostate Cancer; Bladder Cancer; Genitourinary Cancer; **Hospital:** UT MD Anderson Cancer Ctr, The (page 115); **Address:** MD Anderson Cancer Ctr, 1515 Holcombe Blvd, Box 446, Houston, TX 77030; **Phone:** 713-792-3250; **Board Cert:** Urology 95; **Med School:** Univ Western Ontario 86; **Resid:** Urology, Shands Hosp/UNIV Florida 91; **Fellow:** Urologic Oncology, MD Anderson Cancer Ctr 93; **Fac Appt:** Assoc Prof U, Univ Tex, Houston

Sagalowsky, Arthur I MD [U] - **Spec Exp:** Urologic Cancer; Transplant-Kidney; **Hospital:** Zale Lipshy Univ Hosp - Dallas; **Address:** UT SW Med Ctr, Dept Urology, 5323 Harry Hines Blvd, J8.114, Dallas, TX 75390-9110; **Phone:** 214-648-3976; **Board Cert:** Urology 80; **Med School:** Indiana Univ 73; **Resid:** Surgery, Indiana Univ Hosps 75; Urology, Indiana Univ Hosps 78; **Fellow:** Clinical Pharmacology, Univ Tex SW Med Ctr 80; **Fac Appt:** Prof U, Univ Tex SW, Dallas

Slawin, Kevin Mark MD [U] - **Spec Exp:** Prostate Cancer & Disease; Prostate Cancer/Robotic Surgery; **Hospital:** Methodist Hosp - Houston; **Address:** 6560 Fannin St, Ste 2100, Houston, TX 77030; **Phone:** 713-798-8670; **Board Cert:** Urology 96; **Med School:** Columbia P&S 86; **Resid:** Surgery, Mt Sinai Med Ctr 88; Urology, Columbia-Presby Hosp 92; **Fellow:** Urologic Oncology, Am Fdn Urol Dis/Baylor Coll Med 94; **Fac Appt:** Prof U, Baylor Coll Med

Swanson, David A MD [U] - **Spec Exp:** Genitourinary Cancer; Kidney Cancer; Prostate Cancer; **Hospital:** UT MD Anderson Cancer Ctr, The (page 115); **Address:** UT MD Anderson Canc Ctr, Dept Urol, 1515 Holcombe Blvd , Unit 446, Houston, TX 77030-4095; **Phone:** 713-792-3250; **Board Cert:** Urology 77; **Med School:** Univ Pennsylvania 67; **Resid:** Surgery, Harbor Genl Hosp 69; Urology, UC Davis 75; **Fellow:** Urologic Oncology, Univ Tex-MD Anderson Hosp 78; **Fac Appt:** Prof U, Univ Tex, Houston

Thompson Jr, Ian M MD [U] - **Spec Exp:** Prostate Cancer; Prostate Surgery; **Hospital:** UTSA - Univ Hosp; **Address:** Univ Tex Hlth Scis Ctr, Dept Urol, 7703 Floyd Curl Drive, rm 216L, MC 7845, San Antonio, TX 78229-3900; **Phone:** 210-567-5643; **Board Cert:** Urology 97; **Med School:** Tulane Univ 80; **Resid:** Urology, Brooke Army Med Ctr 85; **Fellow:** Medical Oncology, Meml Sloan-Kettering Canc Ctr 88; **Fac Appt:** Prof S, Univ Tex, San Antonio

West Coast and Pacific

Belldegrun, Arie S MD [U] - **Spec Exp:** Urologic Cancer; Gene Therapy; **Hospital:** UCLA Med Ctr (page 111); **Address:** UCLA -D Geffen Sch Medicine, 10833 LeConte Ave, Rm 66-118, Los Angeles, CA 90095; **Phone:** 310-206-1434; **Board Cert:** Urology 99; **Med School:** Israel 74; **Resid:** Urology, Brigham and Women's Hosp 85; **Fellow:** Urologic Oncology, Natl Cancer Inst, NIH 88; **Fac Appt:** Prof U, UCLA

Boyd, Stuart D MD [U] - **Spec Exp:** Incontinence; Erectile Dysfunction; Urologic Cancer; **Hospital:** USC Norris Canc Comp Ctr; **Address:** 1441 Eastlake Ave, Ste 7416, Los Angeles, CA 90033-4525; **Phone:** 323-865-3704; **Board Cert:** Urology 84; **Med School:** UCLA 75; **Resid:** Urology, UCLA Med Ctr 82; **Fac Appt:** Prof U, USC Sch Med

Brawer, Michael K MD [U] - **Spec Exp:** Prostate Cancer; **Hospital:** NW Hosp; **Address:** NW Prostate Institute, 1570 N 115th St, Ste 15, Seattle, WA 98133; **Phone:** 206-368-6591; **Board Cert:** Urology 98; **Med School:** UCLA 80; **Resid:** Surgery, Stanford Univ 82; **Fellow:** Urology, Stanford Univ 86

Carroll, Peter R MD [U] - **Spec Exp:** Testicular Cancer; Prostate Cancer; Bladder & Pelvic Reconstruction; **Hospital:** UCSF - Mt Zion Med Ctr; **Address:** UCSF Comprehensive Cancer Ctr, 1600 Divisadero St Fl 3, San Francisco, CA 94143-1695; **Phone:** 415-353-7171; **Board Cert:** Urology 98; **Med School:** Georgetown Univ 79; **Resid:** Surgery, UCSF Med Ctr 84; **Fellow:** Urology, Mem Sloan Kettering Cancer Ctr 86; **Fac Appt:** Prof U, UCSF

Danoff, Dudley S MD [U] - **Spec Exp:** Prostate Cancer; Bladder Cancer; Erectile Dysfunction; **Hospital:** Cedars-Sinai Med Ctr (page 88); **Address:** 8631 W 3rd St, Ste 915-E, Los Angeles, CA 90048-5901; **Phone:** 310-854-9898; **Board Cert:** Urology 74; **Med School:** Yale Univ 63; **Resid:** Urology, Yale-New Haven Hosp 65; Urology, Columbia-Presby Med Ctr 69

de Kernion, Jean B MD [U] - **Spec Exp:** Urologic Cancer; Kidney Cancer; Prostate Surgery; **Hospital:** UCLA Med Ctr (page 111); **Address:** UCLA Med Ctr, Dept Urol, 10833 Le Conte Ave, Box 951738, Los Angeles, CA 90095; **Phone:** 310-206-6453; **Board Cert:** Surgery 73; Urology 75; **Med School:** Louisiana State Univ 65; **Resid:** Surgery, Univ Hosps-Case West Res 67; Urology, Univ Hosps-Case West Res 73; **Fellow:** Urologic Oncology, Natl Cancer Inst 69; **Fac Appt:** Prof U, UCLA

Ellis, William J MD [U] - **Spec Exp:** Prostate Cancer; Kidney Cancer; Prostate Disease; **Hospital:** Univ Wash Med Ctr; **Address:** Univ Wash Med Ctr, Dept Urology, Box 356510, Seattle, WA 98195; **Phone:** 206-764-2265; **Board Cert:** Urology 01; **Med School:** Johns Hopkins Univ 85; **Resid:** Surgery, Northwestern Meml Hosp 87; Urology, Northwestern Meml Hosp 91; **Fac Appt:** Assoc Prof U, Univ Wash

Gill, Harcharan Singh MD [U] - **Spec Exp:** Urologic Cancer; Prostate Cancer & Disease; **Hospital:** Stanford Univ Med Ctr; **Address:** 875 Blake Wilbur Drive, Stanford, CA 94305; **Phone:** 650-725-5544; **Board Cert:** Urology 95; **Med School:** Kenya 77; **Resid:** Urology, Inst of Urol; Urology, Univ Penn 91; **Fellow:** Urology, Univ Penn 86; **Fac Appt:** Prof U, Stanford Univ

Holden, Stuart MD [U] - **Spec Exp:** Kidney Cancer; **Hospital:** Cedars-Sinai Med Ctr (page 88); **Address:** 8631 W 3rd St, Ste 915E, Los Angeles, CA 90048; **Phone:** 310-854-9898; **Board Cert:** Urology 77; **Med School:** Cornell Univ-Weill Med Coll 68; **Resid:** Surgery, NY Hosp-Cornell 70; Urology, Emory Univ Hosp 75; **Fellow:** Urology, Meml Sloan Kettering Cancer Ctr 78

Huffman, Jeffry Lee MD [U] - **Spec Exp:** Kidney Stones; Kidney Cancer; Bladder/Prostate Cancer; **Hospital:** USC Univ Hosp - R K Eamer Med Plz; **Address:** USC Care Med Grp, 1510 San Pablo St, Ste 649, Los Angeles, CA 90033; **Phone:** 323-442-6284; **Board Cert:** Urology 95; **Med School:** Loyola Univ-Stritch Sch Med 78; **Resid:** Surgery, St Francis Hosp 80; Urology, Univ Chicago Hosps 83; **Fellow:** Urologic Oncology, Meml Sloan Kettering Cancer Ctr 85; **Fac Appt:** Prof U, USC Sch Med

Kawachi, Mark H MD [U] - **Spec Exp:** Prostate Cancer/Robotic Surgery; Prostate Cancer/Brachytherapy; Minimally Invasive Prostate Surgery; **Hospital:** City of Hope Natl Med Ctr & Beckman Rsch (page 89); **Address:** City of Hope National Medical Ctr, Div Urologic Oncology, 1500 Duarte Rd, Duarte, CA 91010; **Phone:** 626-359-8111 x62655; **Board Cert:** Urology 04; **Med School:** USC Sch Med 79; **Resid:** Urology, USC Med Ctr 84

Lange, Paul MD [U] - **Spec Exp:** Prostate Cancer; **Hospital:** Univ Wash Med Ctr; **Address:** Univ Wash Med Ctr, Dept Urology, Box 356510, Seattle, WA 98195; **Phone:** 206-543-3918; **Board Cert:** Urology 78; **Med School:** Washington Univ, St Louis 67; **Resid:** Surgery, Duke Univ Med Ctr 72; Urology, Univ Minn Med Ctr 75; **Fellow:** Immunology, Univ Minn 73; Research, NIH 70; **Fac Appt:** Prof U, Univ Wash

Lieskovsky, Gary MD [U] - **Spec Exp:** Prostate Cancer; **Hospital:** USC Norris Canc Comp Ctr; **Address:** 1441 Eastlake Ave, Ste 7416, Los Angeles, CA 90089-0112; **Phone:** 323-865-3702; **Board Cert:** Urology 80; **Med School:** Canada 73; **Resid:** Urology, Univ Alberta Hosp 78; **Fellow:** Urology, UCLA Med Ctr 80; **Fac Appt:** Prof U, USC Sch Med

Presti Jr, Joseph C MD [U] - **Spec Exp:** Prostate Cancer; Bladder Cancer; Kidney Cancer; **Hospital:** Stanford Univ Med Ctr; **Address:** Stanford Univ Sch of Med-Dept of Urology, 875 Blake Wilbur Dr. MC 5821, Stanford, CA 94305; **Phone:** 650-725-5544; **Board Cert:** Urology 02; **Med School:** UC Irvine 84; **Resid:** Surgery, UC San Francisco 86; Urology, UC San Francisco 89; **Fellow:** Urologic Oncology, Meml Sloan-Kettering 92; **Fac Appt:** Assoc Prof U, Stanford Univ

Schmidt, Joseph MD **[U]** - **Spec Exp:** Prostate Cancer; Clinical Trials/Prostate Cancer; **Hospital:** UCSD Med Ctr; **Address:** 200 W Arbor Drive, San Diego, CA 92103-8897; **Phone:** 619-543-5904; **Board Cert:** Urology 71; **Med School:** Univ IL Coll Med 61; **Resid:** Surgery, Rush-Presby-St Lukes Hosp 63; Urology, Johns Hopkins Hosp 67; **Fellow:** Urology, Johns Hopkins Sch Med 67; **Fac Appt:** Prof U, UCSD

Skinner, Donald G MD **[U]** - **Spec Exp:** Bladder Cancer; Testicular Cancer; Prostate Cancer; **Hospital:** USC Norris Canc Comp Ctr; **Address:** 1441 Eastlake Ave, Ste 7416, Los Angeles, CA 90033; **Phone:** 323-865-3707; **Board Cert:** Urology 74; **Med School:** Yale Univ 64; **Resid:** Surgery, Mass Genl Hosp 66; Urology, Mass Genl Hosp 71; **Fac Appt:** Prof U, USC Sch Med

Skinner, Eila C MD **[U]** - **Spec Exp:** Urologic Cancer; Genitourinary Disorders-Geriatric; **Hospital:** USC Norris Canc Comp Ctr; **Address:** USC-Keck Sch Med, Dept Urology, 1441 Eastlake Ave, Ste 7416, Los Angeles, CA 90089; **Phone:** 323-865-3700; **Board Cert:** Urology 01; **Med School:** USC Sch Med 83; **Resid:** Urology, LAC-USC Med Ctr 88; **Fellow:** Urologic Oncology, LAC-USC Med Ctr 90; **Fac Appt:** Assoc Prof U, USC Sch Med

Smith, Robert B MD **[U]** - **Spec Exp:** Urologic Cancer; **Hospital:** UCLA Med Ctr (page 111); **Address:** UCLA Med Ctr, Clark Urology Ctr, 10833 Le Conte Ave, rm 66-118 CHS, Los Angeles, CA 90095; **Phone:** 310-825-9273; **Board Cert:** Urology 72; **Med School:** UCLA 63; **Resid:** Surgery, UCLA Med Ctr 65; Urology, UCLA Med Ctr 69; **Fac Appt:** Prof S, UCLA

Stein, John P MD **[U]** - **Spec Exp:** Bladder Cancer; Prostate Cancer; Testicular Cancer; **Hospital:** USC Norris Canc Comp Ctr; **Address:** 1441 Eastlake Ave, Ste 7416, Los Angeles, CA 90089; **Phone:** 323-865-3709; **Board Cert:** Urology 99; **Med School:** Loyola Univ-Stritch Sch Med 89; **Resid:** Surgery, LAC-USC Med Ctr 91; Urology, LAC-USC Med Ctr 93; **Fellow:** Urologic Oncology, LAC-USC Med Ctr 97; **Fac Appt:** Assoc Prof U, USC Sch Med

Tomera, Kevin M MD **[U]** - **Spec Exp:** Urologic Cancer; Voiding Dysfunction; **Hospital:** Alaska Regl Hosp; **Address:** 1200 Airport Heights Drive, Ste 101, Anchorage, AK 99508-2944; **Phone:** 907-276-2803; **Board Cert:** Urology 95; **Med School:** Northwestern Univ 78; **Resid:** Urology, Mayo Clinic 83

Wilson, Timothy G MD **[U]** - **Spec Exp:** Prostate Cancer/Robotic Surgery; Minimally Invasive Urologic Surgery; Urinary Reconstruction; **Hospital:** City of Hope Natl Med Ctr & Beckman Rsch (page 89); **Address:** City of Hope National Medical Ctr, Div Urologic Oncology, 1500 Duarte Rd, Duarte, CA 91010-3012; **Phone:** 626-256-4673 x62655; **Board Cert:** Urology 01; **Med School:** Oregon Hlth Sci Univ 84; **Resid:** Urology, USC Med Ctr 90; **Fellow:** Urologic Oncology, City Hosp Natl Med Ctr 91; **Fac Appt:** Assoc Clin Prof U, USC Sch Med

OTHER SPECIALISTS

ALLERGY & IMMUNOLOGY

*A*n allergist-immunologist is trained in evaluation, physical and laboratory diagnosis and management of disorders involving the immune system. Selected examples of such conditions include asthma, anaphylaxis, rhinitis, eczema and adverse reactions to drugs, foods, and insect stings as well as immune deficiency diseases (both acquired and congenital), defects in host defense and problems related to autoimmune disease, organ transplantation or malignancies of the immune system. As our understanding of the immune system develops, the scope of this specialty is widening.

Training programs are available at some medical centers to provide individuals with expertise in both allergy/immunology and adult rheumatology, or in both

539

allergy/immunology and pediatric pulmonology. Such individuals are candidates for dual certification.

Training required: Two years in allergy/immunology OR prior certification in internal medicine or pediatrics plus additional training and examination

CARDIOLOGY

(a subspecialty of INTERNAL MEDICINE)

Cardiovascular Disease: A cardiologist specializes in diseases of the heart, lungs and blood vessels and manages complex cardiac conditions such a heart attacks and life-threatening, abnormal heartbeat rhythms.

Cardiac Electrophysiology: A field of special interest within the subspecialty of cardiovascular disease which involves intricate technical procedures to evaluate heart rhythms and determine appropriate treatment for them.

Interventional Cardiology: An area of medicine within the subspecialty of cardiology which uses specialized imaging and other diagnostic techniques to evaluate blood flow and pressure in the coronary arteries and chambers of the heart, and uses technical procedures and medications to treat abnormalities that impair the function of the heart.

Training required: Three years in internal medicine plus additional training and examination for certification in cardiovascular disease, clinical electrophysiology or interventional cardiology

CLINICAL GENETICS

A specialist trained in diagnostic and therapeutic procedures for patients with genetically linked diseases. This specialist uses modern cytogenetic, radiologic and biochemical testing to assist in specialized genetic counseling, implements needed therapeutic interventions and provides prevention through prenatal diagnosis.

A clinical geneticist demonstrates competence in providing comprehensive diagnostic, management and counseling services for genetic disorders.

A medical geneticist plans and coordinates large scale screening programs for inborn errors of metabolism, hemoglobinopathies, chromosome abnormalities and neural tube defects.

Training required: Two or four years

INFECTIOUS DISEASE

(a subspecialty of INTERNAL MEDICINE)

An internist who deals with infectious diseases of all types and in all organs. Conditions requiring selective use of antibodies call for this special skill. This physician often diagnoses and treats AIDS patients and patients with fevers which have not been explained. Infectious disease specialists may also have expertise in preventive medicine and conditions associated with travel.

Training required: Three years in internal medicine plus additional training and examination for certification in infectious disease

INTERNAL MEDICINE

A personal physician who provides long-term, comprehensive care in the office and the hospital, managing both common and complex illness of adolescents, adults and the elderly. Internists are trained in the diagnosis and treatment of cancer, infections and diseases

PHYSICIAN LISTINGS:

INFECTIOUS DISEASES

Mid Atlantic	549
Great Plains & Mountains	549
West Coast & Pacific	549

INTERNAL MEDICINE

Mid Atlantic	550
Southeast	550
Midwest	550
Southwest	550

affecting the heart, blood, kidneys, joints and digestive, respiratory and vascular systems. They are also trained in the essentials of primary care internal medicine which incorporates an understanding of disease prevention, wellness, substance abuse, mental health and effective treatment of common problems of the eyes, ears, skin, nervous system and reproductive organs.

Note: *Internal Medicine normally includes many primary care physicians. However, for the purpose of this directory, no primary care physicians are included.*

Training required: *Three years*

PHYSICAL MEDICINE & REHABILITATION

Physical medicine and rehabilitation, also referred to as rehabilitation medicine, is the medical specialty concerned with diagnosing, evaluating and treating patients with physical disabilities. These disabilities may arise from conditions affecting the musculoskeletal system such as neck and back pain, sports injuries, or other painful conditions affecting the limbs, for example carpal tunnel syndrome. Alternatively, the disabilities may result from neurological trauma or disease such as spinal cord injury, head injury or stroke.

A physician certified in physical medicine and rehabilitation is often called a physiatrist. The primary goal of the physiatrist is to achieve maximal restoration of physical, psychological, social and vocational function through comprehensive rehabilitation. Pain management is often an important part of the role of the physiatrist. For diagnosis and evaluation, a physiatrist may include the techniques of electromyography to supplement the standard history, physical, X-ray and laboratory examinations. The physiatrist has expertise in the appropriate use of therapeutic exercise, prosthetics (artificial limbs), orthotics and mechanical and electrical devices.

Training required: *Four years plus one year clinical practice*

542

PREVENTIVE MEDICINE

A preventive medicine specialist focuses on the health of individuals and defined populations in order to protect, promote and maintain health and well-being and prevent disease, disability and premature death. A preventive medicine physician may be a specialist in general preventive medicine, public health, occupational medicine, or aerospace medicine. This specialist works with large population groups as well as with individual patients to promote health and understand the risks of disease, injury, disability and death, seeking to modify and eliminate these risks.

Training required: *Three years*

543

CANCER RISK ASSESSMENT
FOX CHASE CANCER CENTER

333 Cottman Avenue
Philadelphia, Pennsylvania 19111-2497
Phone: 1-888-FOX CHASE • Fax: 215-728-2702 • www.fccc.edu

Unique programs for healthy people provide screening, education and early detection for people with a personal or family history of certain cancers or other special risk factors. The staff includes medical oncologists, gynecologists, gastroenterologists, a dermatologist, radiation oncologists, nurses and nurse practitioners, genetic counselors, radiologists, pathologists and health educators trained in cancer prevention. Participants may also have the opportunity for genetic testing and counseling when appropriate and the option of enrolling in available prevention trials.

Fox Chase opened the region's first risk-assessment program in 1991. A memorial to Margaret M. Dyson, who died of ovarian cancer in 1990, the Margaret Dyson Family Risk Assessment Program was developed by Mary B. Daly, M.D., Ph.D., of Fox Chase and established with funds from the National Cancer Institute and the Dyson Foundation. The program became a model for additional Fox Chase risk-assessment programs focused on other cancers.

- **Margaret Dyson Family Risk Assessment Program:**
  1-800-325-4145
  For women with a family history of breast and/or ovarian cancer
- **Familial Melanoma Risk Assessment Program:**
  215-214-1448
  For people with a family history of melanoma, a potentially fatal form of skin cancer
- **Gastrointestinal Tumor Risk Assessment Program:**
  215-728-7041
  For people with increased risk of gastrointestinal cancers, including a family or personal history of colorectal polyps or inflammatory bowel disease
- **Prostate Cancer Risk Assessment Program:**
  215-728-2406
  For men with increased risk of prostate cancer, including family history or being African American

CANCER PREVENTION

Our Research Institute for Cancer Prevention, the first comprehensive program of its kind in the nation, opened in 2000, culminating a decade of leadership in cancer prevention research. The five-story Prevention Pavilion provides 120,000 square feet of space to house both research and clinical programs dedicated to preventing specific types of cancer. The research covers a broad spectrum from basic laboratory studies to clinical prevention trials and behavioral studies.

Fox Chase started its chemoprevention program in 1991—a laboratory program to develop and test natural or synthetic substances to prevent cancer. Director Margie L. Clapper, Ph.D., is now collaborating with colleagues in preclinical studies of various agents aimed at preventing colitis-associated colorectal cancer.

In addition, Fox Chase's behavioral research program conducts a wide range of studies to make cancer prevention and control programs more effective.

NYU MEDICAL CENTER
550 1st Avenue (at 31st Street)
New York, NY 10016
Physician Referral:
1-888-7-NYU-MED
www.nyumc.org

SCHOOL OF MEDICINE

NEW YORK UNIVERSITY

NYU CANCER INSTITUTE
at the NYU Clinical Cancer Center
160 East 34th Street
New York, NY 1001
1-212-731-6000
www.nyuci.org

CLINICAL GENETICS

The Clinical Genetics Program at NYU Medical Center offers a comprehensive program of genetic evaluation, counseling, and testing, supported by vital, ongoing research efforts and active treatment protocols. Our integrated team approach includes centralized, easy access to medical geneticists and genetic counselors. We are nationally known for groundbreaking work identifying genetic markers for breast, colorectal, ovarian, and prostate cancer, and assessing cancer risks.

BREAST AND OVARIAN CANCER - a leading participant in the New York Breast Cancer Study and the National Ovarian Cancer Early Detection Program; latest blood test can help identify early indications of ovarian cancer.

COLORECTAL CANCER - diagnostic evaluations followed by tests for identifying high-risk individuals.

PROSTATE CANCER - the latest research and ongoing protocols.

EARLY DETECTION - in the absence of a targeted test, we provide screening tests to identify high-risk patients in need of follow-up care.

COUNSELING - personalized, confidential insight into matters related to prevention, surveillance, and early diagnosis and treatment in a non-judgmental atmosphere.

Specialists at the NCI-designated NYU Cancer Institute seek to enhance and coordinate the extensive resources of NYU Medical Center to optimize research, treatment, and the ultimate control of cancer.

Our new NYU Clinical Cancer Center is located at 160 East 34th Street. This state-of-the-art 13-level, 85,000-square-foot building serves as "home base" for patients, by providing the latest cancer prevention, screening, diagnostic treatment, genetic counseling, and support services in one central location. The NYU Clinical Cancer Center stands to dramatically improve the lives of people with cancer. As part of NYU Medical Center, patients can access a variety of other non-cancer services throughout the institution.

PHYSICIAN REFERRAL
1-888-7-NYU-MED
(1-888-769-8633)
www.nyumc.org
www.nyuci.org

ALLERGY & IMMUNOLOGY
West Coast and Pacific

Cowan, Morton J MD [A&I] - **Spec Exp:** Immunodeficiency Disorders; Stem Cell Transplant-Fetal; Bone Marrow Transplant-Pediatric; **Hospital:** UCSF Med Ctr; **Address:** UCSF Med Ctr, Peds BMT Program, 505 Parnassus Ave, rm M659, San Francisco, CA 94143-1278; **Phone:** 415-476-2188; **Board Cert:** Pediatrics 81; Allergy & Immunology 83; **Med School:** Univ Pennsylvania 70; **Resid:** Surgery, Duke Univ Med Ctr 72; Pediatrics, UCSF Med Ctr 77; **Fellow:** Research, Natl Inst Hlth 75; Immunology, UCSF Med Ctr; **Fac Appt:** Prof Ped, UCSF

CARDIOVASCULAR DISEASE
Mid Atlantic

Steingart, Richard MD [Cv] - **Spec Exp:** Heart Failure; Nuclear Cardiology; Heart Disease in Cancer Patients; **Hospital:** Meml Sloan Kettering Cancer Ctr (page 100); **Address:** Memorial Sloan-Kettering Cancer Ctr - Cardiology, 1275 York Ave, New York, NY 10021; **Phone:** 212-639-8488; **Board Cert:** Internal Medicine 77; Cardiovascular Disease 79; **Med School:** Mount Sinai Sch Med 74; **Resid:** Internal Medicine, Yale-New Haven Hosp 77; **Fellow:** Cardiovascular Disease, Mt Sinai Med Ctr 79; **Fac Appt:** Prof Med, Cornell Univ-Weill Med Coll

CLINICAL GENETICS
Mid Atlantic

Ostrer, Harry MD [CG] - **Spec Exp:** Genetic Disorders; Hereditary Cancer; **Hospital:** NYU Med Ctr (page 104); **Address:** NYU Medical Ctr, 550 1st Ave, rm MSB136, New York, NY 10016; **Phone:** 212-263-5746; **Board Cert:** Clinical Genetics 84; Pediatrics 85; Clinical Cytogenetics 90; Clinical Molecular Genetics 04; **Med School:** Columbia P&S 76; **Resid:** Pediatrics, Johns Hopkins Hosp 78; Clinical Genetics, Natl Inst Health 81; **Fellow:** Molecular Genetics, Johns Hopkins Hosp 83; **Fac Appt:** Prof Ped, NYU Sch Med

Shapiro, Lawrence R MD [CG] - **Spec Exp:** Dysmorphology; Prenatal Diagnosis; Hereditary Cancer; **Hospital:** Westchester Med Ctr; **Address:** Regional Med Genetics Ctr, 19 Bradhurst Ave, Ste 1600, Hawthorne, NY 10532-2140; **Phone:** 914-593-8900; **Board Cert:** Pediatrics 67; Clinical Genetics 82; Clinical Cytogenetics 82; **Med School:** NYU Sch Med 62; **Resid:** Pediatrics, Chldns Hosp 64; Pediatrics, Bellevue Hosp 65; **Fellow:** Clinical Genetics, NYU Med Ctr; Clinical Genetics, Mount Sinai Med Ctr 68; **Fac Appt:** Prof Ped, NY Med Coll

Southeast

Sutphen, Rebecca MD [CG] - **Spec Exp:** Genetic Disorders; **Hospital:** All Children's Hosp; **Address:** All Children's Hosp, 880 6th St S, Ste 240, Saint Petersburg, FL 33701; **Phone:** 727-892-8491; **Board Cert:** Pediatrics 01; Clinical Cytogenetics 96; Clinical Molecular Genetics 96; Clinical Genetics 96; **Med School:** Temple Univ 90; **Resid:** Pediatrics, All Children's Hosp 93; **Fellow:** Clinical Genetics, Univ S Fla Coll Med 95; **Fac Appt:** Assoc Prof CG, Univ S Fla Coll Med

Midwest

Rubinstein, Wendy S MD/PhD **[CG]** - **Spec Exp:** Breast Cancer; Colon Cancer; Pancreatic Cancer; **Hospital:** Evanston Hosp; **Address:** Ctr for Medical Genetics, 1000 Central St, Ste 620, Evanston, IL 60201; **Phone:** 847-570-1029; **Board Cert:** Internal Medicine 03; Clinical Genetics 96; Clinical Molecular Genetics 96; **Med School:** Mount Sinai Sch Med 89; **Resid:** Internal Medicine, Strong Meml Hosp 92; **Fellow:** Clinical Genetics, Univ Pittsburgh 96; Clinical Molecular Genetics, Univ Pittsburgh 96; **Fac Appt:** Asst Prof Med, Northwestern Univ

Whelan, Alison MD **[CG]** - **Spec Exp:** Gynecologic Cancer Risk Assessment; Colon & Rectal Cancer Risk Assessment; **Hospital:** Barnes-Jewish Hosp (page 85); **Address:** Washington Univ Sch Med, 660 S Euclid Ave, Campus Box 8073, St Louis, MO 63110; **Phone:** 314-454-6093; **Board Cert:** Clinical Genetics 96; **Med School:** Washington Univ, St Louis 86; **Resid:** Internal Medicine, Barnes Hosp 89; Pediatrics, Wash Univ Sch Med 94; **Fellow:** Research, Wash Univ Sch Med 91; Clinical Genetics, Wash Univ Sch Med 94; **Fac Appt:** Assoc Prof Med, Washington Univ, St Louis

Southwest

Mulvihill, John J MD **[CG]** - **Spec Exp:** Cancer Treatment & Genetic Disorders; Neurofibromatosis; Fertility/Pregnancy after Cancer Therapy; **Hospital:** Chldns Hosp OU Med Ctr; **Address:** Chldns Hosp, 940 NE 13th St, rm 2B2418, Oklahoma City, OK 73104; **Phone:** 405-271-8685; **Board Cert:** Pediatrics 75; Clinical Genetics 82; **Med School:** Univ Wash 69; **Resid:** Pediatrics, Johns Hopkins Hosp 74; **Fellow:** Research, NCI-Natl Inst Hlth 72; **Fac Appt:** Prof CG, Univ Okla Coll Med

West Coast and Pacific

Grody, Wayne W MD/PhD **[CG]** - **Spec Exp:** Genetic Disorders; Hereditary Cancer; **Hospital:** UCLA Med Ctr (page 111); **Address:** UCLA School of Medicine, Los Angeles, CA 90095-1732; **Phone:** 310-825-5648; **Board Cert:** Clinical Genetics 90; Anatomic & Clinical Pathology 87; Clinical Biochemical Genetics 90; Molecular Genetic Pathology 01; **Med School:** Baylor Coll Med 77; **Resid:** Pathology, UCLA Med Ctr 86; **Fellow:** Clinical Genetics, UCLA Med Ctr 87; **Fac Appt:** Prof CG, UCLA

Weitzel, Jeffrey N MD **[CG]** - **Spec Exp:** Breast Cancer; Ovarian Cancer; Hereditary Cancer; **Hospital:** City of Hope Natl Med Ctr & Beckman Rsch (page 89); **Address:** City of Hope Cancer Ctr, 1500 E Duarte Rd, Duarte, CA 91010; **Phone:** 626-359-8111 x64324; **Board Cert:** Internal Medicine 86; Medical Oncology 89; Clinical Genetics 96; **Med School:** Univ Minn 83; **Resid:** Internal Medicine, Univ Minn Hosps 86; Hematology, Hammersmith Hosp 87; **Fellow:** Hematology and Oncology, Tufts -New England Med Ctr 92; Clinical Genetics, Tufts-New England Med Ctr 96; **Fac Appt:** Assoc Clin Prof Med, USC Sch Med

INFECTIOUS DISEASE

Mid Atlantic

Polsky, Bruce MD [Inf] - **Spec Exp:** AIDS/HIV; Viral Infections; Infectious Complications of Cancer; **Hospital:** St Luke's - Roosevelt Hosp Ctr - Roosevelt Div (page 93); **Address:** 1111 Amsterdam Ave, New York, NY 10025; **Phone:** 212-523-2525; **Board Cert:** Internal Medicine 83; Infectious Disease 86; **Med School:** Wayne State Univ 80; **Resid:** Internal Medicine, Montefiore Hosp 83; **Fellow:** Infectious Disease, Meml Sloan Kettering Cancer Ctr 86; **Fac Appt:** Prof Med, Columbia P&S

Sepkowitz, Kent MD [Inf] - **Spec Exp:** Tuberculosis; Infections in Cancer Patients; Fungal Infections; **Hospital:** Meml Sloan Kettering Cancer Ctr (page 100); **Address:** 1275 York Ave, New York, NY 10021-0033; **Phone:** 212-639-2441; **Board Cert:** Internal Medicine 83; Infectious Disease 00; **Med School:** Univ Okla Coll Med 80; **Resid:** Internal Medicine, Roosevelt Hosp 84; **Fellow:** Infectious Disease, Meml Sloan Kettering Cancer Ctr 91; **Fac Appt:** Prof Med, Cornell Univ-Weill Med Coll

Great Plains and Mountains

Freifeld, Alison G MD [Inf] - **Spec Exp:** Infectious Disease during Chemotherapy; Infections in Cancer Patients; **Hospital:** Nebraska Med Ctr; **Address:** University of Nebraska, 985400 Nebraska Medical Center, Omaha, NE 68198-5400; **Phone:** 402-559-8650; **Board Cert:** Internal Medicine 85; Infectious Disease 88; **Med School:** Johns Hopkins Univ 82; **Resid:** Internal Medicine, Johns Hopkins Univ Med Ctr 85

West Coast and Pacific

Palefsky, Joel M MD [Inf] - **Spec Exp:** AIDS Related Cancers; **Hospital:** UCSF - Mt Zion Med Ctr; **Address:** UCSF Med Ctr, Infectious Disease, 505 Parnassus Ave, rm M1203, San Francisco, CA 94143; **Phone:** 415-476-1574; **Board Cert:** Internal Medicine 84; Infectious Disease 88; **Med School:** McGill Univ 80; **Resid:** Internal Medicine, Royal Victoria Hosp 84; **Fellow:** Infectious Disease, Stanford Univ 89

INTERNAL MEDICINE

Mid Atlantic

Rivlin, Richard S MD [IM] - **Spec Exp:** Cancer Prevention & Nutrition; Nutrition & Disease Prevention/Control; Endocrinology & Thyroid Disease; **Hospital:** NY-Presby Hosp - NY Weill Cornell Med Ctr (page 103); **Address:** Strang Cancer Prevention Center, c/o Rockefeller University, 1230 York Ave, Box 231, New York, NY 10021; **Phone:** 212-734-1436; **Board Cert:** Internal Medicine 69; **Med School:** Harvard Med Sch 59; **Resid:** Internal Medicine, Bellevue Hosp 60; Internal Medicine, Johns Hopkins Hosp 61; **Fellow:** Endocrinology, Diabetes & Metabolism, Natl Inst Hlth 63; Biochemistry, Johns Hopkins Hosp 66; **Fac Appt:** Prof Med, Cornell Univ-Weill Med Coll

Southeast

Heimburger, Douglas C MD [IM] - **Spec Exp:** Nutriton & Disease Prevention/Control; Nutrition & Cancer Prevention; **Hospital:** Univ of Ala Hosp at Birmingham; **Address:** University of Alabama, Dept Nutrition Science & Medicine, 1675 University Blvd, Webb 222, Birmingham, AL 35294-3360; **Phone:** 205-934-7058; **Board Cert:** Internal Medicine 81; **Med School:** Vanderbilt Univ 78; **Resid:** Internal Medicine, Washington Univ Hosps 81; **Fellow:** Nutrition, Univ Alabama Med Ctr 82; **Fac Appt:** Prof Med, Univ Ala

Jensen, Gordon L MD/PhD [IM] - **Spec Exp:** Nutrition in Chronic Disease; Nutrition in Cancer Patients; **Hospital:** Vanderbilt Univ Med Ctr (page 116); **Address:** Vanderbilt Ctr for Human Nutrition, 514 Medical Arts Bldg, 1211 21st Ave, Ste South, Nashville, TN 37212-2713; **Phone:** 615-936-1288; **Board Cert:** Internal Medicine 87; **Med School:** Cornell Univ-Weill Med Coll 84; **Resid:** Internal Medicine, New England Deaconess Hosp 87; **Fellow:** Nutrition, New England Deaconess Hosp 88; **Fac Appt:** Prof Med, Vanderbilt Univ

Vance, Mary Lee MD [IM] - **Spec Exp:** Pituitary Disorders; Adrenal Tumors; **Hospital:** Univ Virginia Med Ctr; **Address:** UVA Health System, 5840 Hospital Drive, Box 800601, Charlottesville, VA 22908-0601; **Phone:** 434-924-2284; **Board Cert:** Internal Medicine 80; **Med School:** Louisiana State Univ 77; **Resid:** Internal Medicine, Baylor Univ Med Ctr 80; **Fellow:** Endocrinology, Univ Virginia Med Ctr 83; **Fac Appt:** Prof Med, Univ VA Sch Med

Midwest

Remick, Scot Clifton MD [IM] - **Spec Exp:** AIDS Related Cancers; Clinical Trials; Drug Development; **Hospital:** Univ Hosps of Cleveland; **Address:** U Hosp Cleveland- Div Hemat Oncol, 11100 Euclid Ave BHC-6, Cleveland, OH 44106; **Phone:** 216-844-3951; **Board Cert:** Internal Medicine 85; Medical Oncology 87; **Med School:** NY Med Coll 82; **Resid:** Internal Medicine, Johns Hopkins 85; **Fellow:** Medical Oncology, U Wisc Clin Cancer Ctr 88; **Fac Appt:** Prof Med, Case West Res Univ

Southwest

Witte, Marlys H MD [IM] - **Spec Exp:** Lymphedema; **Hospital:** Univ Med Ctr - Tucson; **Address:** Univ Arizona Hlth Scis Ctr, 1501 N Campbell Ave, rm 4406, PO Box 245063, Tucson, AZ 85724-5063; **Phone:** 520-626-6118; **Board Cert:** Internal Medicine 67; **Med School:** NYU Sch Med 60; **Resid:** Internal Medicine, Bellevue Hosp 63; **Fellow:** Internal Medicine, NYU Med Ctr 66; **Fac Appt:** Prof S, Univ Ariz Coll Med

PHYSICAL MEDICINE & REHABILITATION

Mid Atlantic

Cheville, Andrea MD **[PMR]** - **Spec Exp:** Lymphedema; Cancer Rehabilitation; Acupuncture; **Hospital:** Hosp Univ Penn - UPHS (page 113); **Address:** Hosp Univ Penn, 3400 Spruce St, 5 W Gates, Philadelphia, PA 19104; **Phone:** 215-349-8769; **Board Cert:** Physical Medicine & Rehabilitation 98; **Med School:** Harvard Med Sch 93; **Resid:** Physical Medicine & Rehabilitation, UMDNJ Med Ctr 97; **Fellow:** Pain & Palliative Care, Meml Sloan Kettering Cancer Ctr 99; **Fac Appt:** Asst Prof PMR, Univ Pennsylvania

Francis, Kathleen MD **[PMR]** - **Spec Exp:** Lymphedema; Amyotrophic Lateral Sclerosis (ALS); Neurodegenerative Disease; **Address:** 200 S Orange Ave, Livingston, NJ 07039; **Phone:** 973-322-7366; **Board Cert:** Physical Medicine & Rehabilitation 04; **Med School:** UMDNJ-NJ Med Sch, Newark 89; **Resid:** Physical Medicine & Rehabilitation, UMDNJ-Kessler Inst Rehab 93; **Fac Appt:** Asst Clin Prof PMR, UMDNJ-NJ Med Sch, Newark

Levinson, Stephen F MD/PhD **[PMR]** - **Spec Exp:** Cancer Rehabilitation; Lymphedema; Spinal Cord Injury; **Hospital:** Univ of Rochester Strong Meml Hosp; **Address:** Strong Meml Hosp, Dept Phys Med & Rehab, 601 Elmwood Ave, Box 664, Rochester, NY 14642; **Phone:** 585-275-3271; **Board Cert:** Physical Medicine & Rehabilitation 87; Spinal Cord Injury Medicine 99; **Med School:** Indiana Univ 83; **Resid:** Physical Medicine & Rehabilitation, Stanford Univ Hosp 86; **Fac Appt:** Assoc Prof PMR, Univ Rochester

Schwartz, L Matthew MD **[PMR]** - **Spec Exp:** Lymphedema Rehabilitation; Head & Neck Cancer Rehabilitation; Pain-Cancer; **Hospital:** Hosp Univ Penn - UPHS (page 113); **Address:** Hosp Univ Penn, Dept Phys Med & Rehab, 3400 Spruce St, 5 West Gates, Philadelphia, PA 19104; **Phone:** 215-662-3259; **Board Cert:** Physical Medicine & Rehabilitation 92; Pain Medicine 03; **Med School:** UMDNJ-NJ Med Sch, Newark 87; **Resid:** Physical Medicine & Rehabilitation, Hosp Univ Penn 89; Physical Medicine & Rehabilitation, Thomas Jefferson Univ Hosp 91; **Fac Appt:** Clin Prof PMR, Univ Pennsylvania

Southeast

King, Richard W MD **[PMR]** - **Spec Exp:** Cancer Rehabilitation; Lymphedema; Soft Tissue Radiation Necrosis; **Hospital:** WellStar Windy Hill Hosp; **Address:** HyOx Medical Treatment Ctr, 2550 Windy Hill Rd, Ste 110, Marietta, GA 30067; **Phone:** 678-303-3200; **Board Cert:** Physical Medicine & Rehabilitation 88; Undersea & Hyperbaric Medicine 02; **Med School:** Emory Univ 79; **Resid:** Physical Medicine & Rehabilitation, Emory Univ Hosp 87

Stewart, Paula JB MD **[PMR]** - **Spec Exp:** Lymphedema; Brain Tumors; Spinal Cord Tumors; **Hospital:** Healthsouth Lakeshore Rehab Hosp; **Address:** Healttsouth Lakeshore Rehab Hosp, 3900 Ridgeway Drive, Birmingham, AL 35209; **Phone:** 205-868-2347; **Board Cert:** Physical Medicine & Rehabilitation 96; Spinal Cord Injury Medicine 00; **Med School:** Univ Minn 87; **Resid:** Physical Medicine & Rehabilitation, Mayo Clinic 91

Midwest

DePompolo, Robert W MD **[PMR]** - **Spec Exp:** Cancer Rehabilitation; Lymphedema; **Hospital:** St Mary's Hosp - Rochester; **Address:** Mayo Clinic, Dept Phys Med & Rehab, 200 1st St SW, Rochester, MN 55905; **Phone:** 507-255-8972; **Board Cert:** Physical Medicine & Rehabilitation 81; **Med School:** Wayne State Univ 77; **Resid:** Physical Medicine & Rehabilitation, Univ Minnesota 80

Feldman, Joseph MD **[PMR]** - **Spec Exp:** Lymphedema; Pain-Back; Electromyography; **Hospital:** Evanston Hosp; **Address:** 2650 Ridge Ave, Evanston, IL 60201-1718; **Phone:** 847-570-2066; **Board Cert:** Physical Medicine & Rehabilitation 71; **Med School:** Univ IL Coll Med 65; **Resid:** Physical Medicine & Rehabilitation, Univ of Ilinois 69; **Fac Appt:** Asst Prof PMR, Northwestern Univ

Gamble, Gail L MD **[PMR]** - **Spec Exp:** Lymphedema; Head & Neck Cancer; Metastatic Bone Disease; **Hospital:** Mayo Med Ctr & Clin - Rochester; **Address:** Mayo Clinic, Dept Phys Med & Rehab, 200 1st St SW, Rochester, MN 55905; **Phone:** 507-284-2608; **Board Cert:** Physical Medicine & Rehabilitation 85; **Med School:** Mayo Med Sch 79; **Resid:** Physical Medicine & Rehabilitation, Mayo Med Sch 83

PREVENTIVE MEDICINE
Mid Atlantic

Lane, Dorothy S MD **[PrM]** - **Spec Exp:** Women's Health; Cancer Screening; Health Promotion & Disease Prevention; **Hospital:** Stony Brook Univ Hosp; **Address:** Stony Brook Univ Sch Med, HSC 4, rm 179, Stony Brook, NY 11794-8437; **Phone:** 631-444-2094; **Board Cert:** Public Health & General Preventive Medicine 70; Family Medicine 00; **Med School:** Columbia P&S 65; **Resid:** Internal Medicine, Beth Israel Med Ctr 66; Public Health & General Preventive Medicine, NY Hlth Dept 68; **Fac Appt:** Prof PrM, SUNY Stony Brook

Weiss, Stanley H MD **[PrM]** - **Spec Exp:** Cancer Epidemiology & Control; AIDS/HIV/Infectious Disease; Bioterrorism Preparedness; **Hospital:** UMDNJ-Univ Hosp-Newark; **Address:** NJ Medical School, 30 Bergen St, ADMC, Ste 1614, Newark, NJ 07107-3000; **Phone:** 973-972-7716; **Board Cert:** Internal Medicine 81; Medical Oncology 85; **Med School:** Harvard Med Sch 78; **Resid:** Internal Medicine, Montefiore Med Ctr 81; **Fellow:** Medical Oncology, National Cancer Inst 85; Epidemiology, National Cancer Inst 87; **Fac Appt:** Assoc Prof PrM, UMDNJ-NJ Med Sch, Newark

Midwest

Wallace, Robert B MD **[PrM]** - **Spec Exp:** Epidemiology of Aging; Cancer Epidemiology & Control; Disability Prevention; **Hospital:** Univ Iowa Hosp & Clinics; **Address:** University of Iowa, Dept Epidemiology, 200 Hawkins Drive, rm C-21N GH, Iowa City, IA 52242; **Phone:** 319-384-5005; **Board Cert:** Public Health & General Preventive Medicine 74; **Med School:** Northwestern Univ 67; **Resid:** Internal Medicine, NY-Cornell Med Ctr 69; **Fac Appt:** Prof PrM, Univ Iowa Coll Med

SECTION IV

APPENDICES

APPENDIX A

AMERICAN BOARD OF MEDICAL SPECIALTIES

THE STATEMENT OF PURPOSE INCLUDED IN THE ARTICLES OF INCORPORATION IS:

- *To improve the standards of medical care.*

- *To act as spokesman for all approved specialty boards, as a group.*

- *To resolve problems encountered among and between specialty boards.*

- *To deal with the applications for approval of proposed new specialty boards, new types of certification, modification of existing types of certification, and related matters.*

- *To endeavor to avoid duplication of effort by specialty boards.*

- *To establish and maintain standards of organization and operation of specialty boards.*

Following is a list of the addresses of the various medical specialty boards approved by the ABMS. Note that there are 24 board organizations for 25 medical specialties. Psychiatry and Neurology share the same board.

To find out if a physician is certified, consumers can call the individual boards which may charge a fee for the information, or they can contact the ABMS at (866) 275-2267 (no fee) or www.abms.org.

BOARD SPECIALTIES

◼ **American Board of Allergy and Immunology**
510 Walnut Street, Suite 1701
Philadelphia, PA 19106-3699
(215) 592-9466
General Certification in Allergy and Immunology; with Added Qualification in Diagnostic Laboratory Immunology. Certifications awarded since 1989 are valid for 10 years. For those certified prior to 1989 there is no recertification requirement.

◼ **American Board of Anesthesiology**
4101 Lake Boone Trail
Suite 510
Raleigh, NC 27607-7506
(919) 881-2570
General Certification in Anesthesiology; with Special and Added Qualifications in Critical Care Medicine and Pain Management. Certifications awarded since 2000 are valid for 10 years.

◼ **American Board of Colon and Rectal Surgery**
20600 Eureka Road, Suite 600
Taylor, MI 48180
(734) 282-9400
General Certification is in Colon and Rectal Surgery. Certifications awarded since 1991 are valid for 8 years.

◼ **American Board of Dermatology**
Henry Ford Hospital
One Ford Place
Detroit, MI 48202
(313) 874-1088
General Certification in Dermatology; with Special Qualifications in Dermatopathology, Dermatological Immunology/Diagnostic and Laboratory Immunology. Certifications awarded since 1991 are valid for 10 years. For those certified prior to 1991, there is no recertification requirement.

◼ **American Board of Emergency Medicine**
3000 Coolidge Road
East Lansing, MI 48823
(517) 332-4800
General Certification in Emergency Medicine; with Special and Added Qualifications in Pediatric Emergency Medicine and Sports Medicine. Certifications are valid for a 10-year period.

■ **American Board of Family Practice**
2228 Young Drive
Lexington, KY 40505
(859) 269-5626
General Certification in Family Practice; with Added Qualifications in Geriatric Medicine and Sports Medicine. Certifications are valid for a 7-year period.

■ **American Board of Internal Medicine**
510 Walnut Street, Suite 1700
Philadelphia, PA 19106-3699
(215) 446-3500, (800) 441-ABIM
General Certification in Internal Medicine; with Special Qualifications in Cardiovascular Disease, Critical Care Medicine, Endocrinology, Diabetes and Metabolism, Gastroenterology, Hematology, Infectious Disease, Medical Oncology, Nephrology, Pulmonary Disease, and Rheumatology; and Added Qualifications in Adolescent Medicine, Cardiac Electrophysiology, Diagnostic Laboratory Immunology, Geriatric Medicine and Sports Medicine. Certifications awarded since 1990 are valid for 10 years. For those certified prior to 1990 there is no recertification requirement.

■ **American Board of Medical Genetics**
9650 Rockville Pike
Bethesda, MD 20814
(301) 571-1825
General Certification in Clinical Genetics, Medical Genetics, Clinical Biochemical Genetics, Clinical Cytogenetics, Clinical Biochemical/Molecular Genetics and Clinical Molecular Genetics. Certifications are valid for a 10-year period.

■ **American Board of Neurological Surgery**
Smith Tower, Suite 2139
6550 Fannin Street
Houston, TX 77030-2701
(713) 790-6015
General Certification in Neurological Surgery. Certifications awarded since 1999 are valid for 10 years.

■ **American Board of Nuclear Medicine**
900 Veteran Avenue, Room 13-152
Los Angeles, CA 90024-1786
(310) 825-6787
General Certification in Nuclear Medicine. Certifications awarded since 1992 are valid for 10 years. For those certified prior to 1992, there is no recertification requirement.

557

APPENDIX A

■ **American Board of Obstetrics and Gynecology**
2915 Vine Street, Suite 300
Dallas, TX 75204
(214) 871-1619
General Certification in Obstetrics and Gynecology; with Special Qualifications in Gynecologic Oncology, Maternal and Fetal Medicine, Reproductive Endocrinology and Added Qualification in Critical Care. Certifications awarded since 1986 are valid for 10 years. For those certified prior to 1986, there is no recertification requirement.

■ **American Board of Ophthalmology**
111 Presidential Boulevard, Suite 241
Bala Cynwyd, PA 19004
(610) 664-1175
Certifications awarded since 1992 are valid for 10 years. For those certified prior to 1992, there is no recertification requirement.

■ **American Board of Orthopaedic Surgery**
400 Silver Cedar Court
Chapel Hill, NC 27514
(919) 929-7103
General Certification in Orthopaedic Surgery; with Added Qualification in Hand Surgery. Certifications awarded since 1986 are valid for 10 years. For those certified prior to 1986, there is no recertification requirement.

■ **American Board of Otolaryngology**
3050 Post Oak Boulevard, Suite 1700
Houston, TX 77056
(713) 850-0399
General Certification in Otolaryngology; with Added Qualification in Otology/Neurotology and Pediatric Otolaryngology. Presently, there is no recertification requirement.

■ **American Board of Pathology**
P.O. Box 25915
Tampa, FL 33622-5915
(813) 286-2444
General Certification in Anatomic and Clinical Pathology, Anatomic Pathology and Clinical Pathology; with Special Qualifications in Blood Banking/Transfusion Medicine, Chemical Pathology, Dermatopathology, Forensic Pathology, Hematology, Immunopathology, Medical Microbiology, Neuropathology and Pediatric Pathology and Added Qualification in Cytopathology. Certifications awarded since 1997 are valid for 10 years.

■ **American Board of Pediatrics**
111 Silver Cedar Court
Chapel Hill, NC 27514-1651
(919) 929-0461
General Certification in Pediatrics; with Special Qualifications in Adolescent Medicine, Allergy &
Immunology, Pediatric Cardiology, Pediatric Critical Care Medicine, Pediatric Emergency
Medicine, Pediatric Endocrinology, Pediatric Gastroenterology, Pediatric Hematology-Oncology,
Pediatric Infectious Diseases, Pediatric Nephrology, Pediatric Pulmonology, Neonatal-Perinatal
Medicine and Pediatric Rheumatology. Added Qualifications in Diagnostic Laboratory
Immunology, Medical Toxicology and Sports Medicine. Certifications valid for 7 years.

■ **American Board of Physical Medicine and Rehabilitation**
3015 Allegro Park Lane, S.W.
Rochester, MN 55902-4139
(507) 282-1776
General Certification in Physical Medicine and Rehabilitation; with Special Qualifications in Spinal
Cord Injury Medicine. Certifications awarded since 1993 are valid for 10 years.

■ **American Board of Plastic Surgery**
Seven Penn Center, Suite 400
1635 Market Street
Philadelphia, PA 19103-2204
(215) 587-9322
General Certification in Plastic Surgery; with Added Qualification in Hand Surgery. Certifications
are valid for a 10-year period.

■ **American Board of Preventive Medicine**
330 South Wells Street, Suite 1018
Chicago, IL 60606
(312) 939-2276
General Certification in Aerospace Medicine, Occupational Medicine and Public Health and General
Preventive Medicine; with Added Qualification in Underseas Medicine and Medical Toxicology. In
the subspecialty of Underseas Medicine and Medical Toxicology certifications are valid for a 10-
year period.

■ **American Board of Psychiatry & Neurology**
500 Lake Cook Road, Suite 335
Deerfield, IL 60015
(847) 945-7900
General Certification in Psychiatry, Neurology and Neurology with Special Qualification in Child
Neurology; with Special Qualification in Child and Adolescent Psychiatry and Added Qualification
in Addiction Psychiatry, Clinical Neurophysiology, Forensic Psychiatry and Geriatric Psychiatry.
Certifications are valid for a 10-year period.

APPENDIX A

■ **American Board of Radiology**
5441 E. Williams Boulevard, Suite 200
Tucson, AZ 85711
(520) 790-2900
General Certification in Diagnostic Radiology or Radiation Oncology; with Special Competency in Nuclear Radiology and Added Qualifications in Neuroradiology, Pediatric Radiology and Vascular and Interventional Radiology. Radiation Physics is a non-clinical certification. Certificates are valid for a 10-year period.

■ **American Board of Surgery**
1617 John F. Kennedy Boulevard, Suite 860
Philadelphia, PA 19103-1847
(215) 568-4000
General Certification in Surgery; with Special Qualifications in Pediatric Surgery and General Vascular Surgery and Added Qualifications in Surgery of the Hand, Surgical Critical Care and General Vascular Surgery. Certifications are valid for a 10-year period.

■ **American Board of Thoracic Surgery**
One Rotary Center, Suite 803
Evanston, IL 60201
(847) 475-1520
General Certification in Thoracic Surgery. Certifications awarded since 1976 are valid for 10 years. For those certified prior to 1976, there is no recertification requirement.

■ **American Board of Urology**
2216 Ivy Road, Suite 210
Charlottesville, VA 22903
(434) 979-0059
General Certification in Urology. Certifications awarded as of 1985 are valid for 10 years. For those certified prior to 1985, there is no recertification requirement.

Appendix B

Osteopathic Boards

American Osteopathic Association
142 E Ontario Street
Chicago, IL 60611
(800) 621-1773

GENERAL CERTIFICATION

■ **American Osteopathic Board of Anesthesiology**
General certification in Anesthesiology; with Added Qualification in Pain Management. Certifications awarded since 2004 are valid for 10 years. For those certified prior to 2004 there is no recertification requirement.

■ **American Osteopathic Board of Dermatology**
Dermatology
General certification in Dermatology. Certifications awarded since 2004 are valid for 10 years. For those certified prior to 2004 there is no recertification requirement.

■ **American Osteopathic Board of Emergency Medicine**
General certification in Emergency Medicine. Certifications awarded since 1994 are valid for 10 years. For those certified prior to 1994 there is no recertification requirement.

■ **American Osteopathic Board of Family Physicians**
General certification in Family Practice. Certifications awarded since March 1, 1997 are valid for 8 years. For those certified prior to 1997 there is no recertification requirement.

■ **American Osteopathic Board of Internal Medicine**
General certification in Internal Medicine; with Special and Added Qualifications in Allergy/Immunology, Cardiology, Endocrinology, Gastroenterology, Hematology, Infectious Disease, Neprhology, Oncology, Pulmonary Disease, Rheumatology, Addiction Medicine, Clinical Cardiac Electrophysiology, Geriatric Medicine, Interventional Cardiology and Sports Medicine. Certifications awarded since 1993 are valid for 10 years. For those certified prior to 1993 there is no recertification requirement.

■ **American Osteopathic Board of Neurology and Psychiatry**
General certification in Neurology and Psychiatry. Certifications awarded since 1996 are valid for 10 years. For those certified prior to 1996 there is no recertification requirement.

- **American Osteopathic Board of Neuromusculoskeletal Medicine (Formerly American Osteopathic Board of Special Proficiency in Osteopathic Manipulative Medicine)**

  General certification in Neuromusculoskeletal Medicine. Certifications awarded since 1995 are valid for 10 years. For those certified prior to 1995 there is no recertification requirement.

- **American Osteopathic Board of Nuclear Medicine**

  General certification in Nuclear Medicine. Certifications awarded since 1995 are valid for 10 years. For those certified prior to 1995 there is no recertification requirement.

- **American Osteopathic Board of Obstetrics and Gynecology**

  General certification in Obstetrics and Gynecology with Special Qualifications in Gynecologic Oncology; Maternal and Fetal Medicine and Reproductive Endocrinology. Certifications awarded since June, 2002 are valid for 6 years. For those certified prior to June, 2002 there is no recertification requirement.

- **American Osteopathic Board of Ophthalmology and Otolaryngology/Head and Neck Surgery**

  General certification in Ophthalmology, Otolaryngolgy, Facial Plastic Surgery and Otolaryngology/Facial Plastic Surgery. Certifications awarded in Ophthalmology since 2000 are valid for 10 years. For those certified prior to 2000 there is no recertification requirement. Certifications awarded in Otolaryngology and/or Otolaryngology/Facial Plastic Surgery since 2002 are valid for 10 years. For those certified prior to 2002 there is no recertification requirement.

- **American Osteopathic Board of Orthopaedic Surgery**

  General certification in Orthopaedic Surgery with Added Qualifications in Hand Surgery. Certifications awarded since 1994 are valid for 10 years. For those certified prior to 1994 there is no recertification requirement.

- **American Osteopathic Board of Pathology**

  General certification in Laboratory Medicine, Anatomic Pathology and Anatomic Pathology and Laboratory Medicine. Certifications awarded since 1995 are valid for 10 years. For those certified prior to 1995 there is no recertification requirement.

- **American Osteopathic Board of Pediatrics**

  General certification in Pediatrics with Special Qualifications in Neonatology, Pediatric Allergy/Immunology and Pediatric Endocrinology. Certifications awarded since 1995 are valid for 7 years. For those certified prior to 1995 there is no recertification requirement.

■ **American Osteopathic Board of Physical Medicine & Rehabilitation Medicine**

General certification in Physical Medicine and Rehabilitation. Certifications awarded since 2004 are valid for 10 years. For those certified prior to 2004 there is no recertification requirement.

■ **American Osteopathic Board of Preventive Medicine**

General certification in Preventive Medicine/Aerospace Medicine, Preventive Medicine/Occupational-Environmental Medicine and Preventive Medicine/Public Health. Certifications awarded since 1994 are valid for 10 years. For those certified prior to 1994 there is no recertification requirement.

■ **American Osteopathic Board of Proctology**

General certification in Proctology. Certifications awarded since 2004 are valid for 10 years. For those certified prior to 2004 there is no recertification requirement.

■ **American Osteopathic Board of Radiology**

General certification in Diagnostic Radiology and Radiation Oncology with Special Qualifications in Body Imaging, Neuroradiology, Pediatric Radiology and Vascular and Interventional Radiology. Certifications awarded since 2004 are valid for 10 years. For those certified prior to 2004 there is no recertification requirement.

■ **American Osteopathic Board of Surgery**

General certification in Surgery, Neurological Surgery, Plastic and Reconstructive Surgery, Thoracic Cardiovascular Surgery, Urological Surgery and General Vascular Surgery with Added Qualifications in Surgical Critical Care. Certifications awarded since 1997 are valid for 10 years. For those certified prior to 1997 there is no recertification requirement.

Consumers may call the American Osteopathic Association at (800) 621-1773 or visit the website, www.osteopathic.org, for general certification information.

APPENDIX C

Hospital Listings

Following is an alphabetical listing of hospitals noted in doctors' entries. The abbreviations as they appear in the listings are in italics below. Due to the many mergers taking place in the hospital industry these days, the names on this list may have changed subsequent to publication of this guide.

Abbott - Northwestern Hospital
Abbott - Northwestern Hosp
800 E 28th St
Minneapolis, MN 55407
Midwest
(612) 863-4000

Advocate Christ Medical Center
Adv Christ Med Ctr
4440 W 95th St
Oak Lawn, IL 60453
Midwest
(708) 425-8000

Advocate Illinois Masonic Medical Center
Adv Illinois Masonic Med Ctr
836 W Wellington Ave
Chicago, IL 60657-5147
Midwest
(773) 975-1600

Advocate Lutheran General Hospital
Adv Luth Genl Hosp
1775 West Dempster St
Park Ridge, IL 60068
Midwest
(847) 723-2210

Alaska Regional Hospital
Alaska Regl Hosp
2801 DeBarr Rd
Anchorage, AK 99508
West Coast and Pacific
(907) 276-1131

Albany Medical Center
Albany Med Ctr
43 New Scotland Ave
Albany, NY 12208
Mid Atlantic
(518) 262-3125

Alfred I duPont Hospital for Children
Alfred I duPont Hosp for Children
1600 Rockland Rd
Wilmington, DE 19803
Mid Atlantic
(302) 651-4000

All Children's Hospital
All Children's Hosp
801 Sixth Street South
St. Petersburg, FL 33701
Southeast
(727) 767-7451

Institutions in bold are profiled in this edition of the Castle Connolly Guide.

Allegheny General Hospital
Allegheny General Hosp
320 E. North Avenue
Pittsburgh, PA 15212
Mid Atlantic
(412) 359-3131

Alta Bates Summit Medical Center -
Ashby Campus
*Alta Bates Summit Med Ctr - Ashby
Campus*
2450 Ashby Avenue
Berkeley, CA 94705
West Coast and Pacific
(510) 204-4444

Arkansas Children's Hospital
Arkansas Chldns Hosp
800 Marshall St
Little Rock, AR 72202
Southwest
(501) 364-1100

Armed Forces Institute of Pathology
Armed Forces Inst of Path
6825 16th St NW, Bldg 54
Washington, DC 20306-6000
Mid Atlantic
(202) 782-2100

**Arthur G. James Cancer Hospital &
Research Institute**
*Arthur G James Cancer Hosp &
Research Inst*
300 West 10th Avenue
Columbus, OH 43210
Midwest
(614) 293-3300

Audie L Murphy Memorial Veterans
Hospital
Audie L Murphy Meml Vets Hosp
7400 Merton Minter Blvd
San Antonio, TX 78229
Southwest
(210) 617-5300

Aultman Hospital
Aultman Hosp
2600 6th St SW
Canton, OH 44710-1799
Midwest
(330) 452-9911

Banner Desert Medical Center
Banner Desert Med Ctr
1400 S Dobson Rd
Mesa, AZ 85202
Southwest
(480) 512-3000

Baptist Hospital
Baptist Hosp
2000 Church St
Nashville, TN 37236
Southeast
(615) 284-5555

Baptist Hospital of Miami
Baptist Hosp of Miami
8900 N Kendall Dr
Miami, FL 33176
Southeast
(786) 596-1960

Baptist Medical Center - Jacksonville
Baptist Medical Center - Jacksonville
800 Prudential Drive
Jacksonville, FL 32207
Southeast
(904) 202-2000

Institutions in bold are profiled in this edition of the Castle Connolly Guide.

Barnes-Jewish Hospital
Barnes-Jewish Hosp
One Barnes-Jewish Hospital Plaza
St. Louis, MO 63110
Midwest
(314) 362-5000

Bascom Palmer Eye Institute
Bascom Palmer Eye Inst.
900 NW 17 St
Miami, FL 33136
Southeast
(305) 326-6000

Baylor University Medical Center
Baylor Univ Medical Ctr
3500 Gaston Avenue
Dallas, TX 75246
Southwest
(214) 820-0111

Ben Taub General Hospital
Ben Taub General Hosp
1504 Taub Loop
Houston, TX 77001
Southwest
(713) 873-2000

Beth Israel Deaconess Medical Center -
Boston
Beth Israel Deaconess Med Ctr - Boston
330 Brookline Ave
Boston, MA 02215
New England
(617) 667-7000

Beth Israel Medical Center - Milton &
Caroll Petrie Division
Beth Israel Med Ctr - Petrie Division
First Avenue @ 16th Street
New York, NY 10003
Mid Atlantic
(212) 420-2000

Boston Medical Center
Boston Med Ctr
1 Boston Medical Center Pl
Boston, MA 02118
New England
(617) 638-8000

Brigham & Women's Hospital
Brigham & Women's Hosp
75 Francis St
Boston, MA 02115
New England
(617) 732-5500

Bryn Mawr Hospital
Bryn Mawr Hosp
130 S Bryn Mawr Ave
Bryn Mawr, PA 19010-3143
Mid Atlantic
(610) 526-3000

California Pacific Medical Center - Pacific
Campus
CA Pacific Med Ctr - Pacific Campus
2333 Buchanan St
San Francisco, CA 94115
West Coast and Pacific
(415) 600-6000

Institutions in bold are profiled in this edition of the Castle Connolly Guide.

APPENDIX C

Carolinas Medical Center
Carolinas Med Ctr
1000 Blythe Blvd
Charlotte, NC 28203-5871
Southeast
(704) 355-2000

Cedars Medical Center - Miami
Cedars Med Ctr - Miami
1400 NW 12 Ave
Miami, FL 33136
Southeast
(305) 325-5511

Cedars-Sinai Medical Center
Cedars-Sinai Med Ctr
8700 Beverly Boulevard
Los Angeles, CA 90048
West Coast and Pacific
(310) 423-3277

Centennial Medical Center
Centennial Med Ctr
2300 Patterson Street
Nashville, TN 37203
Southeast
(615) 342-1000

Children's Healthcare of Atlanta -
Egleston
Chldns Hlthcare Atlanta - Egleston
1405 Clifton Rd NE
Atlanta, GA 30322
Southeast
(404) 325-6000

Children's Hospital - Boston
Children's Hospital - Boston
300 Longwood Avenue
Boston, MA 02115
New England
(617) 355-6000

Children's Hospital - Denver, The
Chldn's Hosp - Denver, The
1056 E 19th Ave
Denver, CO 80218-1088
Great Plains and Mountains
(303) 861-8888

Children's Hospital - Los Angeles
Chldns Hosp - Los Angeles
4650 Sunset Blvd
Los Angeles, CA 90027
West Coast and Pacific
(323) 660-2450

Children's Hospital - New Orleans
Children's Hospital - New Orleans
200 Henry Clay Ave
New Orleans, LA 70118
Southwest
(504) 899-9511

Children's Hospital - Omaha
Children's Hosp - Omaha
8200 Dodge St
Omaha, NE 68114
Great Plains and Mountains
(402) 955-5400

Children's Hospital and Clinics -
Minneapolis
Chldns Hosp and Clinics - Minneapolis
2525 Chicago Ave S
Minneapolis, MN 55404
Midwest
(612) 813-6111

Children's Hospital and Health Center
Children's Hosp and Hlth Ctr - San Diego
3020 Childrens Way
San Diego, CA 92123
West Coast and Pacific
(858) 576-1700

Institutions in bold are profiled in this edition of the Castle Connolly Guide.

568

Children's Hospital and Regional Medical
Center - Seattle
Chldns Hosp and Regl Med Ctr - Seattle
4800 Sand Point Way NE
Seattle, WA 98145
West Coast and Pacific
(206) 987-2000

Children's Hospital at OU Medical Center
Chldns Hosp OU Med Ctr
940 Northeast 13th St
Oklahoma City, OK 73104
Southwest
(405) 271-5437

Children's Hospital Medical Center -
Akron
Children's Hosp & Med Ctr- Akron
One Perkins Square
Akron, OH 44308
Midwest
(330) 379-8200

Children's Hospital of Alabama -
Birmingham
Children's Hospital - Birmingham
1600 7th Ave South
Birmingham, AL 35233
Southeast
(205) 939-9100

Children's Hospital of Philadelphia, The
Chldns Hosp of Philadelphia, The
34th St & Civic Center Blvd
Philadelphia, PA 19104
Mid Atlantic
(215) 590-1000

**Children's Hospital of Pittsburgh -
UPMC**
Chldns Hosp of Pittsburgh - UPMC
3705 Fifth Avenue
Pittsburgh, PA 15213
Mid Atlantic
(412) 692-5325

Children's Hospital of Wisconsin
Chldns Hosp - Wisconsin
9000 W Wisconsin Ave
Milwaukee, WI 53201
Midwest
(414) 266-2000

Children's Medical Center of Dallas
Chldns Med Ctr of Dallas
1935 Motor St
Dallas, TX 75235
Southwest
(214) 456-7000

Children's Memorial Hospital
Children's Mem Hosp
2300 Children's Plaza
Chicago, IL 60614
Midwest
(773) 880-4000

Children's Mercy Hospitals & Clinics
Chldns Mercy Hosps & Clinics
2401 Gilham Rd
Kansas City, MO 64108
Midwest
(816) 234-3000

Children's National Medical Center - DC
Chldns Natl Med Ctr
111 Michigan Ave NW
Washington, DC 20010
Mid Atlantic
(202) 884-5000

Institutions in bold are profiled in this edition of the Castle Connolly Guide.

Christiana Care Health Services
Christiana Care Hlth Svs
501 W 14th St
Wilmington, DE 19899-1038
Mid Atlantic
(302) 428-2229

Christiana Hospital
Christiana Hospital
4755 Ogletown-Stanton Rd
Newark, DE 19718-0001
Mid Atlantic
(302) 733-1000

Cincinnati Children's Hospital Medical Center
Cincinnati Chldns Hosp Med Ctr
3333 Burnet Ave
Cincinnati, OH 45229-3039
Midwest
(800) 344-2462

**City of Hope National Medical Center
& Beckman Research**
City of Hope Natl Med Ctr & Beckman Rsch
1500 E Duarte Rd
Duarte, CA 91010
West Coast and Pacific
(626) 359-8111

Cleveland Clinic Florida - Naples
Cleveland Clin - Naples
6101 Pine Ridge Rd
Naples, FL 34119
Southeast
(239) 348-4000

Cleveland Clinic Florida - Weston
Cleveland Clin - Weston
2950 Cleveland Clinic Blvd
Weston, FL 33331
Southeast
(954) 659-5000

Cleveland Clinic Foundation
Cleveland Clin Fdn
9500 Euclid Avenue
Cleveland, OH 44195
Midwest
(800) 223-2273

Community Memorial Hospital - Toms River
Comm Mem Hosp - Toms River
99 Route 37 W
Toms River, NJ 08753
Mid Atlantic
(908) 240-8000

Concord Hospital
Concord Hospital
250 Pleasant St
Concord, NH 03301-2598
New England
(603) 225-2711

Connecticut Children's Medical Center
CT Chldns Med Ctr
282 Washington St
Hartford, CT 06106
New England
(860) 545-9000

Cooper University Hospital
Cooper Univ Hosp
1 Cooper Plaza
Camden, NJ 08103-1489
Mid Atlantic
(856) 342-2000

Institutions in bold are profiled in this edition of the Castle Connolly Guide.

Dana-Farber Cancer Institute
Dana-Farber Cancer Inst
44 Binney St
Boston, MA 02115
New England
(617) 632-3000

Dartmouth - Hitchcock Medical Center
Dartmouth - Hitchcock Med Ctr
1 Medical Center Dr
Lebanon, NH 03756-0002
New England
(603) 650-5000

Doctors Medical Center
Doctors Med Ctr
2000 Vale Rd
San Pablo, CA 94806
West Coast and Pacific
(510) 970-5000

Doctors' Hospital
Doctors' Hosp
5000 University Dr
Coral Gables, FL 33146
Southeast
(305) 666-2111

Doernbecher Children's Hospital/Oregon
Health Science University
Doernbecher Chldns Hosp/OHSU
3181 SW Sam Jackson Park Rd
Portland, OR 97201-3098
West Coast and Pacific
(503) 494-8811

Duke University Medical Center
Duke Univ Med Ctr
DUMC, Box 3708
Durham, NC 27710
Southeast
(919) 684-8111

Emory University Hospital
Emory Univ Hosp
1364 Clifton Rd NE
Atlanta, GA 30322
Southeast
(404) 712-2000

Englewood Hospital & Medical Center
Englewood Hosp & Med Ctr
350 Engle Street
Englewood, NJ 07631
Mid Atlantic
(201) 894-3000

Evanston Hospital
Evanston Hosp
2650 Ridge Ave
Evanston, IL 60201
Midwest
(847) 570-2000

Fairview-University Medical Center -
University Campus
Fairview-Univ Med Ctr - Univ Campus
420 Delaware St SE
Minneapolis, MN 55455
Midwest
(612) 273-3000

Fletcher Allen Health Care - Medical
Center Campus
FAHC - Med Ctr Campus
111 Colchester Ave (Burgess 1)
Burlington, VT 05401
New England
(802) 847-0000

Institutions in bold are profiled in this edition of the Castle Connolly Guide.

Fletcher Allen Health Care - UHC Campus
FAHC - UHC Campus
1 S Prospect St
Burlington, VT 05401
New England
(802) 847-0000

Four Winds Hospital
Four Winds Hosp
800 Cross River Road
Katonah, NY 10536
Mid Atlantic
(914) 763-8151

Fox Chase Cancer Center
Fox Chase Cancer Ctr
333 Cottman Avenue
Philadelphia, PA 19111
Mid Atlantic
(215) 728-6900

Franklin Square Hospital
Franklin Sqaure Hosp
9000 Franklin Square Drive
Baltimore, MD 21237
Mid Atlantic
(410) 682-7000

Froedtert Memorial Lutheran Hospital
Froedtert Meml Lutheran Hosp
9200 W Wisconsin Ave
Milwaukee, WI 53226
Midwest
(414) 805-6644

George Washington University Hospital
G Washington Univ Hosp
901 23rd St NW
Washington, DC 20037
Mid Atlantic
(202) 715-4000

Georgetown University Hospital
Georgetown Univ Hosp
3800 Reservoir Rd NW
Washington, DC 20007
Mid Atlantic
(202) 444-2000

Good Samaritan Hospital - San Jose
Good Samaritan Hosp - San Jose
2425 Samaritan Drive
San Jose, CA 95124
West Coast and Pacific
(408) 559-2011

Greenwich Hospital
Greenwich Hosp
Five Perryridge Road
Greenwich, CT 06830
New England
(203) 863-3000

H Lee Moffitt Cancer Center & Research
Institute
H Lee Moffitt Cancer Ctr & Research Inst
12902 Magnolia Drive
Tampa, FL 33612-9497
Southeast
(813) 972-4673

Hackensack University Medical Center
Hackensack Univ Med Ctr
30 Prospect Avenue
Hackensack, NJ 07601
Mid Atlantic
(201) 996-2000

Hahnemann University Hospital
Hahnemann Univ Hosp
Broad & Vine St
Philadelphia, PA 19102
Mid Atlantic
(215) 762-7000

Institutions in bold are profiled in this edition of the Castle Connolly Guide.

Harper University Hospital
Harper Univ Hosp
3990 John R St
Detroit, MI 48201-2097
Midwest
(313) 745-8040

Harrison Memorial Hospital
Harrison Meml Hosp
2520 Cherry Ave
Bremerton, WA 98310-4270
West Coast and Pacific
(360) 377-3911

Hartford Hospital
Hartford Hosp
80 Seymour St, Box 5037
Hartford, CT 06102-5037
New England
(860) 545-5000

Healthsouth Lakeshore Rehabilitation
Hospital
Healthsouth Lakeshore Rehab Hosp
3900 Ridgeway Dr
Birmingham, AL 35209
Southeast
(205) 868-2000

Henry Ford Hospital
Henry Ford Hosp
2799 W Grand Blvd
Detroit, MI 48202
Midwest
(313) 916-2600

Hinsdale Hospital
Hinsdale Hosp
120 N Oak St
Hinsdale, IL 60521
Midwest
(630) 856-9000

Hospital for Joint Diseases
Hosp For Joint Diseases
301 East 17th Street
New York, NY 10003
Mid Atlantic
(212) 598-6000

Hospital for Special Surgery
Hosp For Special Surgery
535 East 70th Street
New York, NY 10021
Mid Atlantic
(212) 606-1000

**Hospital of the University of
Pennsylvania - UPHS**
Hosp Univ Penn - UPHS
3400 Spruce Street
Philadelphia, PA 19104
Mid Atlantic
(215) 662-4000

Howard University Hospital
Howard Univ Hosp
2041 Georgia Ave NW
Washington, DC 20060
Mid Atlantic
(202) 865-6100

Indiana University Hospital
Indiana Univ Hosp
550 N University Blvd
Indianapolis, IN 46202
Midwest
(317) 274-5555

Inova Fairfax Hospital
Inova Fairfax Hosp
3300 Gallows Road
Falls Church, VA 22042
Southeast
(703) 698-1110

Institutions in bold are profiled in this edition of the Castle Connolly Guide.

APPENDIX C

Jackson Memorial Hospital
Jackson Meml Hosp
1611 NW 12th Ave
Miami, FL 33136
Southeast
(305) 585-1111

Johns Hopkins Hospital - Baltimore, The
Johns Hopkins Hosp - Baltimore
600 N Wolfe St
Baltimore, MD 21287
Mid Atlantic
(410) 955-5000

Kaiser Permanente Santa Clara Medical Center
Kaiser Permanente Santa Clara Med Ctr
900 Kiley Blvd
Santa Clara, CA 95051
West Coast and Pacific
(408) 236-6400

Kapiolani Medical Center for Women & Children
Kapiolani Med Ctr for Women & Chldn
1319 Punahou St
Honolulu, HI 96826
West Coast and Pacific
(808) 983-6000

Kootenai Medical Center
Kootenai Med Ctr
2003 Lincoln Way
Coeur d'Alene, ID 83814-2677
Great Plains and Mountains
(208) 666-2000

Kosair Children's Hospital
Kosair Chldn's Hosp
231 E Chestnut St
Louisville, KY 40202
Southeast
(502) 629-6000

LAC & USC Medical Center
LAC & USC Med Ctr
1200 N State St
Los Angeles, CA 90033-4525
West Coast and Pacific
(323) 226-2622

LAC - Harbor - UCLA Medical Center
LAC - Harbor - UCLA Med Ctr
1000 W Carson St
Torrance, CA 90509-2059
West Coast and Pacific
(310) 222-2345

Lahey Clinic
Lahey Clin
41 Mall Road
Burlington, MA 01805
New England
(781) 744-5100

Lake Forest Hospital
Lake Forest Hosp
660 N Westmoreland Road
Lake Forest, IL 60045
Midwest
(847) 234-5600

Lakeland Regional Medical Center
Lakeland Regl Med Ctr
1324 Lakeland Hills Blvd
Lakeland, FL 33805
Southeast
(863) 687-1100

Institutions in bold are profiled in this edition of the Castle Connolly Guide.

Lankenau Hospital
Lankenau Hosp
100 Lancaster Ave
Wynnewood, PA 19096-3498
Mid Atlantic
(610) 645-2000

LDS Hospital
LDS Hosp
8th Ave & C St
Salt Lake City, UT 84143
Great Plains and Mountains
(801) 408-1100

Le Bonheur Children's Medical Center
Le Bonheur Chldns Med Ctr
50 N Dunlap
Memphis, TN 38103-2893
Southeast
(901) 572-3000

Lenox Hill Hospital
Lenox Hill Hosp
100 East 77th Street
New York, NY 10021
Mid Atlantic
(212) 434-2000

Lindy Boggs Medical Center
L Boggs Med Ctr
301 N Jefferson Davis Pkwy
New Orleans, LA 70119
Southwest
(504) 483-5000

Loma Linda University Medical Center
Loma Linda Univ Med Ctr
11234 Anderson St
Loma Linda, CA 92354
West Coast and Pacific
(909) 558-4000

Long Beach Memorial Medical Center
Long Beach Meml Med Ctr
2801 Atlantic Ave
Long Beach, CA 90801
West Coast and Pacific
(562) 933-2000

Long Island College Hospital
Long Island Coll Hosp
339 Hicks Street
Brooklyn, NY 11201
Mid Atlantic
(718) 780-1000

Long Island Jewish Medical Center
Long Island Jewish Med Ctr
270-05 76th Avenue
New Hyde Park, NY 11040
Mid Atlantic
(516) 470-7000

Louis A Weiss Memorial Hospital
Weiss Meml Hosp
4646 N Marine Dr
Chicago, IL 60640
Midwest
(773) 878-8700

Louisiana State University Hospital
Louisiana State Univ Hosp
1501 Kings Highway P.O. Box 33932
Shreveport, LA 71130
Southwest
(318) 675-4239

Loyola University Medical Center
Loyola Univ Med Ctr
2160 S 1st Ave
Maywood, IL 60153
Midwest
(708) 216-9000

Institutions in bold are profiled in this edition of the Castle Connolly Guide.

575

Lucile Packard Children's
Hospital/Stanford University Medical
Center
*Lucile Packard Chldns Hosp/Stanford
Univ Med Ctr*
725 Welch Rd
Palo Alto, CA 94304
West Coast and Pacific
(650) 497-8000

Magee-Womens Hospital - UPMC
Magee-Womens Hosp - UPMC
300 Halket Street
Pittsburgh, PA 15213
Mid Atlantic
(412) 641-1000

Maimonides Medical Center
Maimonides Med Ctr
4802 Tenth Avenue
Brooklyn, NY 11219
Mid Atlantic
(718) 283-6000

Maine Medical Center
Maine Med Ctr
22 Bramhall St
Portland, ME 04102
New England
(207) 871-0111

Marin General Hospital
Marin Genl Hosp
250 Bon Air Rd
Greenbrae, CA 94904
West Coast and Pacific
(415) 925-7000

Massachusetts General Hospital
Mass Genl Hosp
55 Fruit St
Boston, MA 02114
New England
(617) 726-2000

Mayo Clinic - Jacksonville, FL
Mayo - Jacksonville
4500 San Pablo Road
Jacksonville, FL 32224
Southeast
(904) 953-2000

Mayo Clinic - Rochester, MN
Mayo Med Ctr & Clin - Rochester
200 First St SW
Rochester, MN 55905
Midwest
(507) 284-2511

Mayo Clinic - Scottsdale
Mayo Clin Hosp - Scottsdale
13400 E Shea Blvd
Scottsdale, AZ 85259
Southwest
(480) 301-8000

McLaren Regional Medical Center
McLaren Reg Med Ctr
401 S. Ballenger Highway
Flint, MI 48532
Midwest
(810) 342-2000

Medical City Dallas Hospital
Med City Dallas Hosp
7777 Forest Ln
Dallas, TX 75230-2594
Southwest
(972) 566-7000

Institutions in bold are profiled in this edition of the Castle Connolly Guide.

Medical College of Virginia Hospitals
Med Coll of VA Hosp
401 N 12th St, Box 980510
Richmond, VA 23219
Southeast
(804) 828-9000

Medical University of South Carolina
Medical Center
MUSC Med Ctr
169 Ashley Ave
Charleston, SC 29425
Southeast
(843) 792-2300

Memorial Medical Center - Baptist
Campus
Meml Med Ctr - Baptist Campus
2700 Napoleon Ave
New Orleans, LA 70115
Southwest
(504) 899-9311

Memorial Medical Center - Savannah
Meml Med Ctr - Savannah
4700 Waters Ave
Savannah, GA 31404
Southeast
(912) 350-8000

Memorial Regional Hospital - Hollywood
Meml Regl Hosp - Hollywood
3501 Johnson Street
Hollywood, FL 33021
Southeast
(954) 987-2000

**Memorial Sloan-Kettering Cancer
Center**
Meml Sloan Kettering Cancer Ctr
1275 York Avenue
New York, NY 10021
Mid Atlantic
(212) 639-2000

Mercy Hospital - Miami, FL
Mercy Hosp - Miami
3663 S Miami Ave
Miami, FL 33133
Southeast
(305) 854-4400

Mercy Medical Center - Cedar Rapids
Mercy Med Ctr - Cedar Rapids
701 10th St SE
Cedar Rapids, IA 52403
Midwest
(319) 398-6217

Methodist Healthcare - University
Hospital
Meth Healthcare Central - Univ Hosp
1265 Union Ave
Memphis, TN 38104
Southeast
(901) 726-7000

Methodist Hospital - Houston
Methodist Hosp - Houston
6565 Fannin St, D200
Houston, TX 77030
Southwest
(713) 790-3311

Institutions in bold are profiled in this edition of the Castle Connolly Guide.

Methodist Hospital - Indianapolis
Methodist Hosp - Indianapolis
1701 N Senate Blvd
Indianapolis, IN 46202
Midwest
(317) 962-2000

Metropolitan Methodist Hospital
Metro Methodist Hosp
1310 McCullough Ave
San Antonio, TX 78209
Southwest
(210) 208-2200

Miami Children's Hospital
Miami Children's Hosp
3100 SW 62nd Ave
Miami, FL 33155
Southeast
(305) 666-6511

Montefiore Medical Center
Montefiore Med Ctr
111 East 210 Street
Bronx, NY 10467
Mid Atlantic
(718) 920-4321

Montefiore Medical Center - Weiler-
Einstein Division
Montefiore Med Ctr - Weiler-Einstein Div
1825 Eastchester Road
Bronx, NY 10461
Mid Atlantic
(718) 904-2000

Moses H Cone Memorial Hospital
Moses H Cone Mem Hosp
1200 N. Elm Street
Greenboro, NC 27401
Southeast
(336) 832-7000

Mount Sinai Medical Center
Mount Sinai Med Ctr
One Gustave L. Levy Pl
New York, NY 10029
Mid Atlantic
(212) 241-6500

Mount Sinai Medical Center - Miami
Mount Sinai Med Ctr - Miami
4300 Alton Rd
Miami Beach, FL 33140
Southeast
(305) 674-2121

National Institutes of Health - Clinical
Center
Natl Inst of Hlth - Clin Ctr
6100 Executive Blvd, rm 3C01, MS 7511
Bethesda, MD 20892-7511
Mid Atlantic
(301) 496-4000

Nebraska Medical Center
Nebraska Med Ctr
987400 Nebraska Med Ctr
Omaha, NE 68198-7400
Great Plains and Mountains
(402) 552-2000

Nebraska Methodist Hospital
Nebraska Meth Hosp
8303 Dodge St
Omaha, NE 68114
Great Plains and Mountains
(402) 354-4000

New York Eye & Ear Infirmary
New York Eye & Ear Infirm
310 East 14th Street
New York, NY 10003
Mid Atlantic
(212) 979-4000

Institutions in bold are profiled in this edition of the Castle Connolly Guide.

NewYork-Presbyterian Hospital -
Columbia Presbyterian Medical Center
NY-Presby Hosp - Columbia Presby Med
Ctr
622 W 168th St
New York, NY 10032
Mid Atlantic
(212) 305-2500

NewYork-Presbyterian Hospital - New
York Weill Cornell Medical Center
NY-Presby Hosp - NY Weill Cornell Med
Ctr
525 E 68th St
New York, NY 10021
Mid Atlantic
(212) 746-5454

North Florida Regional Medical Center
North Florida Regl Med Ctr
6500 Newberry Rd
Gainesville, FL 32605
Southeast
(352) 333-4000

North Shore University Hospital at
Manhasset
N Shore Univ Hosp at Manhasset
300 Community Dr
Manhasset, NY 11030
Mid Atlantic
(516) 562-0100

Northwest Hospital
NW Hosp
1550 N 115th St
Seattle, WA 98133-0806
West Coast and Pacific
(206) 364-0500

Northwestern Memorial Hospital
Northwestern Meml Hosp
251 E Huron St
Chicago, IL 60611
Midwest
(312) 926-2000

Norton Hospital
Norton Hosp
200 E Chestnut St
Louisville, KY 40202
Southeast
(502) 629-8000

NYU Medical Center
NYU Med Ctr
550 First Avenue
New York, NY 10016
Mid Atlantic
(212) 263-7300

Ochsner Foundation Hospital
Ochsner Fdn Hosp
1516 Jefferson Hwy
New Orleans, LA 70121
Southwest
(504) 842-3000

Ohio State University Medical Center
Ohio St Univ Med Ctr
410 W 10th Avenue
Columbus, OH 43210
Midwest
(614) 293-8000

Olathe Medical Center
Olathe Med Ctr
20333 W 151st St
Olathe, KS 66061-5352
Great Plains and Mountains
(913) 791-4200

Institutions in bold are profiled in this edition of the Castle Connolly Guide.

APPENDIX C

Oregon Health & Science University
OR Hlth & Sci Univ
3181 SW Sam Jackson Park Rd
Portland, OR 97239-3098
West Coast and Pacific
(503) 494-8311

Orlando Regional Medical Center
Orlando Regl Med Ctr
1414 Kuhl Ave
Orlando, FL 32806
Southeast
(407) 841-5111

Orthopaedic Hospital
Orthopaedic Hosp
2400 South Flower Street
Los Angeles, CA 90007
West Coast and Pacific
(213) 742-1000

OU Medical Center
OU Med Ctr
1200 Everett Dr
Oklahoma City, OK 73104-5098
Southwest
(405) 271-4700

Our Lady of Mercy Medical Center
Our Lady of Mercy Med Ctr
600 E 233rd St
Bronx, NY 10466
Mid Atlantic
(718) 920-9000

Overlake Hospital Medical Center
Overlake Hosp Med Ctr
1035 116th Ave NE
Bellevue, WA 98004-4687
West Coast and Pacific
(425) 688-5000

Overland Park Regional Medical Center
Overland Pk Regl Med Ctr
10500 Quivira Rd
Overland Park, KS 66215
Great Plains and Mountains
(913) 541-5000

Pennsylvania Hospital
Pennsylvania Hosp
800 Spruce Street
Philadelphia, PA 19107
Mid Atlantic
(215) 829-3000

Pitt County Memorial Hospital - Univ
Health System East Carolina
Pitt Cty Mem Hosp - Univ Med Ctr East Carolina
2100 Stantonsburg Rd
Greenville, NC 27835-6028
Southeast
(252) 847-4100

Presbyterian - St Luke's Medical Center
Presby - St Luke's Med Ctr
1719 E 19th Ave
Denver, CO 80218
Great Plains and Mountains
(303) 839-6000

Presbyterian Hospital - Albuquerque
Presbyterian Hospital - Albuquerque
1100 Central Ave SE
Albuquerque, NM 87106
Southwest
(505) 841-1234

Institutions in bold are profiled in this edition of the Castle Connolly Guide.

Presbyterian Hospital of Dallas
Presby Hosp of Dallas
8200 Walnut Hill Ln
Dallas, TX 75231
Southwest
(214) 345-6789

Primary Children's Medical Center
Primary Children's Med Ctr
100 N Medical Drive
Salt Lake City, UT 84113-1100
Great Plains and Mountains
(801) 588-2000

Providence Hospital - Southfield
Providence Hosp - Southfield
16001 W Nine Mile Rd
Southfield, MI 48075
Midwest
(248) 424-3000

Providence Portland Medical Center
Providence Portland Med Ctr
4805 NE Glisan
Portland, OR 97213-2967
West Coast and Pacific
(503) 215-1111

Providence Saint Joseph Medical Center
Providence St Joseph Med Ctr
501 S Buena Vista St
Burbank, CA 91505
West Coast and Pacific
(818) 843-5111

Queen's Medical Center - Honolulu
Queen's Med Ctr - Honolulu
1301 Punchbowl Street
Honolulu, HI 96813
West Coast and Pacific
(808) 538-9011

Rainbow Babies & Children's Hospital
Rainbow Babies & Chldns Hosp
11100 Euclid Ave
Cleveland, OH 44106
Midwest
(216) 844-1000

Rapid City Regional Hospital
Rapid City Reg Hosp
353 Fairmount Blvd
Rapid City, SD 57701
Great Plains and Mountains
(605) 719-1000

Rhode Island Hospital
Rhode Island Hosp
593 Eddy Street
Providence, RI 02903
New England
(401) 444-4000

Riley Children's Hospital
Riley Chldns Hosp
702 Barnhill Drive
Indianapolis, IN 46202
Midwest
(317) 274-5000

**Robert Wood Johnson University
Hospital - New Brunswick**
***Robert Wood Johnson Univ Hosp - New
Brunswick***
1 Robert Wood Johnson Pl
New Brunswick, NJ 08901
Mid Atlantic
(732) 828-3000

Institutions in bold are profiled in this edition of the Castle Connolly Guide.

Rochester Methodist Hospital
Rochester Meth Hosp
201 W Center St
Rochester, MN 55905-3003
Midwest
(507) 284-2511

Roswell Park Cancer Institute
Roswell Park Cancer Inst
Elm and Carlton Streets
Buffalo, NY 14263
Mid Atlantic
(716) 845-5770

Rush University Medical Center
Rush Univ Med Ctr
1653 W Congress Pkwy
Chicago, IL 60612-3833
Midwest
(312) 942-5000

Sacred Heart Medical Center
Sacred Heart Med Ctr
1255 Hilyard St
Eugene, OR 97440-3700
West Coast and Pacific
(541) 686-7300

Saint John's Health Center
St John's Hlth Ctr, Santa Monica
1328 22nd St
Santa Monica, CA 90404
West Coast and Pacific
(310) 829-5511

Saint Vincent Catholic Medical Centers
- St Vincent's Manhattan
St Vincent Cath Med Ctrs - Manhattan
170 West 12th Street
New York, NY 10011
Mid Atlantic
(212) 604-7000

Salt Lake Regional Medical Center
Salt Lake Regional Med Ctr
1050 E South Temple
Salt Lake City, UT 84102
Great Plains and Mountains
(801) 350-4111

San Francisco General Hospital
San Francisco Genl Hosp
1001 Potrero Avenue
San Francisco, CA 94110
West Coast and Pacific
(415) 206-8000

Santa Clara Valley Medical Center
Santa Clara Vly Med Ctr
751 S Bascom Ave
San Jose, CA 95128
West Coast and Pacific
(408) 885-5000

Santa Rosa Children's Hospital
Santa Rosa Children's Hosp
519 W Houston St
San Antonio, TX 78207
Southwest
(512) 228-2011

Sarasota Memorial Hospital
Sarasota Meml Hosp
1700 S Tamiami Trail
Sarasota, FL 34239
Southeast
(941) 917-9000

Schneider Children's Hospital
Schneider Chldn's Hosp
269-01 76th Ave
New Hyde Park, NY 11040
Mid Atlantic
(718) 470-3000

Institutions in bold are profiled in this edition of the Castle Connolly Guide.

Scott & White Memorial Hospital
Scott & White Mem Hosp
2401 South 31st Street
Temple, TX 76508-0001
Southwest
(254) 724-2111

Scottsdale Healthcare - Osborn
Scottsdale Hlthcare - Osborn
7400 E Osborn Rd
Scottsdale, AZ 85251-6403
Southwest
(480) 675-4000

Scottsdale Healthcare - Shea
Scottsdale Hlthcare - Shea
9000 E Shea Blvd
Scottsdale, AZ 85258-4514
Southwest
(602) 860-3000

Scripps Green Hospital
Scripps Green Hosp
10666 N Torrey Pines Rd
La Jolla, CA 92037
West Coast and Pacific
(858) 455-9100

Scripps Memorial Hospital - La Jolla
Scripps Meml Hosp - La Jolla
9888 Genesee Ave
La Jolla, CA 92037
West Coast and Pacific
(858) 457-4123

Sentara Norfolk General Hospital
Sentara Norfolk Genl Hosp
600 Gresham Dr
Norfolk, VA 23507
Southeast
(757) 668-3000

Shands Healthcare at University of Florida
Shands Hlthcre at Univ of FL
1600 SW Archer Rd
Gainesville, FL 32610
Southeast
(352) 265-0111

Shands Jacksonville
Shands Jacksonville
655 W 8th St
Jacksonville, FL 32209
Southeast
(904) 244-0411

Sibley Memorial Hospital
Sibley Mem Hosp
5255 Loughboro Road NorthWest
Washington, DC 20016
Mid Atlantic
(202) 537-4000

Southwest Texas Methodist Hospital
SW TX Meth Hosp
7700 Floyd Curl Dr
San Antonio, TX 78229
Southwest
(210) 575-4000

Sparrow Hospital
Sparrow Hosp
1215 E Michigan Ave, MS 0
Lansing, MI 48912
Midwest
(517) 364-1000

Spectrum Health - Blodgett Campus
Spectrum Hlth Blodgett Campus
1840 Wealthy St SE
Grand Rapids, MI 49506
Midwest
(616) 774-7444

Institutions in bold are profiled in this edition of the Castle Connolly Guide.

APPENDIX C

St Anthony Hospital
St Anthony Hosp
1000 N Lee St
Oklahoma City, OK 73102
Southwest
(405) 272-7000

St Anthony's Hospital - St Petersburg
St Anthony's Hosp - St Petersburg
1200 7th Avenue North
St Petersburg, FL 33705
Southeast
(727) 893-6814

St Barnabas Medical Center
St Barnabas Med Ctr
94 Old Short Hills Rd
Livingston, NJ 07039-5672
Mid Atlantic
(973) 322-5000

St Elizabeth's Medical Center
St Elizabeth's Med Ctr
736 Cambridge St
Brighton, MA 02135
New England
(617) 789-3000

St Joseph Hospital
St Joseph Hosp - Bellingham
2901 Squalicum Pkwy
Bellingham, WA 98225-1898
West Coast and Pacific
(360) 734-5400

St Joseph's Hospital & Medical Center -
Phoenix
St Joseph's Hosp & Med Ctr - Phoenix
350 W Thomas Rd
Phoenix, AZ 85013-4496
Southwest
(602) 406-3000

St Joseph's Hospital - Atlanta
St Joseph's Hosp - Atlanta
5665 Peachtree Dunwoody Road
NorthEast
Atlanta, GA 30342
Southeast
(404) 851-7001

St Joseph's Hospital - Tampa
St Joseph's Hosp - Tampa
3001 W Martin Luther King Jr Blvd
Tampa, FL 33607
Southeast
(813) 870-4000

St Jude Children's Research Hospital
St Jude Children's Research Hosp
332 N Lauderdale St
Memphis, TN 38105
Southeast
(901) 495-3300

St Louis Children's Hospital
St Louis Chldns Hosp
One Children's Pl
St Louis, MO 63110
Midwest
(314) 454-6000

St Louis University Hospital
St Louis Univ Hosp
3635 Vista at Grand Blvd
St Louis, MO 63110
Midwest
(314) 577-8000

Institutions in bold are profiled in this edition of the Castle Connolly Guide.

584

St Luke's - Roosevelt Hospital Center - Roosevelt Division
St Luke's - Roosevelt Hosp Ctr - Roosevelt Div
1000 Tenth Avenue
New York, NY 10019
Mid Atlantic
(212) 523-4000

St Luke's Episcopal Hospital - Houston
St Luke's Episcopal Hosp - Houston
6720 Bertner Avenue
Houston, TX 77030
Southwest
(832) 355-1000

St Luke's Hospital - Chesterfield, MO
St Luke's Hosp - Chesterfield, MO
232 S Woods Mill Rd
Chesterfield, MO 63017
Midwest
(314) 434-1500

St Luke's Hospital - Jacksonville
St Luke's Hosp - Jacksonville
4201 Belfort Rd
Jacksonville, FL 32216
Southeast
(904) 296-3700

St Mary's Hospital - Huntington, WV
St Mary's Hosp - Huntington, WV
2900 1st Ave
Huntington, WV 25702-1272
Mid Atlantic
(304) 526-1234

St Mary's Hospital - Rochester, MN (Mayo Clinic)
St Mary's Hosp - Rochester
1216 2nd St SW
Rochester, MN 55902
Midwest
(507) 255-5123

St Mary's Medical Center - West Palm Beach
St Mary's Med Ctr - W Palm Bch
901 45th St
West Palm Beach, FL 33407
Southeast
(561) 844-6300

St Patrick Hospital & Health Sciences Center
St Patrick Hospital - Missoula
500 W Broadway
Missoula, MT 59802
Great Plains and Mountains
(406) 543-7271

St Paul University Hospital
St Paul Univ Hosp
5909 Harry Hines Boulevard
Dallas, TX 75235
Southwest
(214) 879-1000

St Thomas Hospital - Nashville
St Thomas Hosp - Nashville
4220 Harding Road
Nashville, TN 37205
Southeast
(615) 222-2111

Institutions in bold are profiled in this edition of the Castle Connolly Guide.

APPENDIX C

St Vincent Carmel Hospital
St Vincent Carmel Hosp
13500 N Meridian St
Carmel, IN 46032-1496
Midwest
(317) 573-7000

St Vincent Hospital - Santa Fe
St Vincent Hosp - Santa Fe
455 St Michaels Dr
Santa Fe, NM 87504-2107
Southwest
(505) 983-3361

St Vincent's Medical Center - Jacksonville
St Vincent's Med Ctr - Jacksonville
1800 Barrs St
Jacksonville, FL 32204
Southeast
(904) 308-7300

St Vincent's Medical Center - Los Angeles
St Vincent's Med Ctr - Los Angeles
2131 W 3rd St
Los Angeles, CA 90057
West Coast and Pacific
(213) 484-7111

St. Luke's Regional Medical Center
St. Luke's Reg Med Ctr - Boise
190 E Bannock St
Boise, ID 83712
Great Plains and Mountains
(208) 381-2222

Stanford University Medical Center
Stanford Univ Med Ctr
300 Pasteur Dr
Stanford, CA 94305
West Coast and Pacific
(650) 723-4000

Stony Brook University Hospital
Stony Brook Univ Hosp
Nicolls Rd
Stony Brook, NY 11794
Mid Atlantic
(631) 689-8333

Suburban Hospital Healthcare Systems
Suburban Hosp - Bethesda
8600 Old Georgetown Road
Bethesda, MD 20814
Mid Atlantic
(301) 896-3100

SUNY Downstate Medical Center
SUNY Downstate Med Ctr
450 Clarkson Ave
Brooklyn, NY 11203
Mid Atlantic
(718) 270-1000

Swedish Medical Center - Seattle
Swedish Med Ctr - Seattle
747 Broadway
Seattle, WA 98122
West Coast and Pacific
(206) 386-6000

Swedish Medical Center Providence
Campus
Swedish Med Ctr Providence Campus
500 17th Ave
Seattle, WA 98122
West Coast and Pacific
(206) 320-2000

Tacoma General Hospital
Tacoma Genl Hosp
315 S Martin Luther King Jr Way
Tacoma, WA 98405
West Coast and Pacific
(253) 403-1000

Institutions in bold are profiled in this edition of the Castle Connolly Guide.

586

Tampa General Hospital
Tampa Genl Hosp
PO BOX 1289
Tampa, FL 33601
Southeast
(813) 844-7000

Temple University Hospital
Temple Univ Hosp
3401 N Broad St
Philadelphia, PA 19140-5189
Mid Atlantic
(215) 707-2000

Texas Children's Hospital - Houston
Texas Chldns Hosp - Houston
6621 Fannin
Houston, TX 77030
Southwest
(832) 824-1000

The University of Kansas Hospital
Univ of Kansas Hosp
3901 Rainbow Blvd
Kansas City, KS 66160
Great Plains and Mountains
(913) 588-5000

Thomas Jefferson University Hospital
Thomas Jefferson Univ Hosp
111 S 11th St
Philadelphia, PA 19107
Mid Atlantic
(215) 955-6000

Tufts - New England Medical Center
Tufts-New England Med Ctr
750 Washington Street
Boston, MA 02111-1533
New England
(617) 636-5000

Tulane University Hospital & Clinic
Tulane Univ Med Ctr Hosp & Clin
1415 Tulane Ave
New Orleans, LA 70112
Southwest
(504) 588-5263

UCLA Medical Center
UCLA Med Ctr
10833 Le Conte Avenue
Los Angeles, CA 90095
West Coast and Pacific
(310) 825-9111

UCSD Medical Center
UCSD Med Ctr
200 W Arbor Dr
San Diego, CA 92103
West Coast and Pacific
(619) 543-6222

UCSF - Mount Zion Medical Center
UCSF - Mt Zion Med Ctr
1600 Divisadero St
San Francisco, CA 94115
West Coast and Pacific
(415) 567-6600

UCSF Medical Center
UCSF Med Ctr
500 Parnassus Ave
San Francisco, CA 94143
West Coast and Pacific
(415) 476-1000

UMass Memorial Medical Center
UMass Memorial Med Ctr
55 Lake Ave N
Worcester, MA 01655
New England
(508) 334-1000

Institutions in bold are profiled in this edition of the Castle Connolly Guide.

APPENDIX C

UMDNJ-University Hospital-Newark
UMDNJ-Univ Hosp-Newark
150 Bergen St
Newark, NJ 07103-2406
Mid Atlantic
(973) 972-4300

Union Memorial Hospital - Baltimore
Union Meml Hosp - Baltimore
201 E University Pkwy
Baltimore, MD 21218
Mid Atlantic
(410) 554-2000

United Medical Center
United Med. Ctr.
214 E 23rd St
Cheyenne, WY 82001
Great Plains and Mountains
(307) 634-2273

University Hospital & Clinics- Mississippi
Univ Hosps & Clins - Jackson
2500 N State St
Jackson, MS 39216
Southeast
(601) 984-1000

University Hospital - Cincinnati
Univ Hosp - Cincinnati
234 Goodman St
Cincinnati, OH 45219
Midwest
(513) 584-1000

University Hospital - SUNY Upstate
Medical University
Univ. Hosp.- SUNY Upstate
750 E Adams Street
Syracuse, NY 13210
Mid Atlantic
(315) 464-5540

University Hospital and Medical Center -
Tamarac
University Hosp and Med Ctr -Tamarac
7201 N University Drive
Tamarac, FL 33321
Southeast
(954) 721-2200

University Hospitals of Cleveland
Univ Hosps of Cleveland
11100 Euclid Ave
Cleveland, OH 44106
Midwest
(216) 844-1000

University Medical Center Health System
Univ Med Ctr - Lubbock
PO Box 5980
Lubbock, TX 79408
Southwest
(806) 775-8200

University Medical Center of Southern
Nevada - Las Vegas
Univ Med Ctr - Las Vegas
1800 W Charleston Blvd
Las Vegas, NV 89102
West Coast and Pacific
(702) 383-2000

University Medical Center- Tucson
Univ Med Ctr - Tucson
1501 N Campbell Ave
Tucson, AZ 85724-5128
Southwest
(520) 694-0111

Institutions in bold are profiled in this edition of the Castle Connolly Guide.

University New Mexico Health & Science
Center
Univ NM Hlth & Sci Ctr
2211 Lomas Blvd NE
Albuquerque, NM 87106
Southwest
(505) 272-2111

University of Alabama Hospital at
Birmingham
Univ of Ala Hosp at Birmingham
619 South 19th Street
Birmingham, AL 35249-6544
Southeast
(205) 934-4011

University of Arkansas for Medical
Sciences Medical Center
UAMS Med Ctr
4301 W Markham St
Little Rock, AR 72205
Southwest
(501) 686-7000

University of California - Davis Medical
Center
UC Davis Med Ctr
2315 Stockton Blvd
Sacramento, CA 95817
West Coast and Pacific
(916) 734-2011

University of California - Irvine Medical
Center
UC Irvine Med Ctr
101 The City Dr
Orange, CA 92868
West Coast and Pacific
(714) 456-6011

University of Chicago Hospitals
Univ of Chicago Hosps
5841 S Maryland Ave, MC-1114
Chicago, IL 60637
Midwest
(773) 702-1000

University of Colorado Hospital
Univ Colorado Hosp
4200 E 9th Ave
Denver, CO 80262
Great Plains and Mountains
(303) 372-0000

University of Illinois Medical Center at
Chicago
Univ of IL Med Ctr at Chicago
1740 W Taylor St
Chicago, IL 60612
Midwest
(312) 996-7000

University of Iowa Hospitals and Clinics
Univ Iowa Hosp & Clinics
200 Hawkins Drive
Iowa City, IA 52242
Midwest
(319) 356-1616

University of Kentucky Medical Center
Univ Kentucky Med Ctr
800 Rose Street
Lexington, KY 40536
Southeast
(859) 323-5445

University of Louisville Hospital
Univ of Louisville Hosp
530 S Jackson St
Louisville, KY 40202
Southeast
(502) 562-3000

Institutions in bold are profiled in this edition of the Castle Connolly Guide.

589

APPENDIX C

University of Maryland Medical System
Univ of MD Med Sys
22 S Greene St
Baltimore, MD 21201
Mid Atlantic
(410) 328-8667

University of Miami Hosp &
Clinics/Sylvester Comprehensive Cancer
Cntr
Univ of Miami Hosp & Clins/Sylvester
Comp Canc Ctr
1475 NW 12th Ave
Miami, FL 33136
Southeast
(305) 243-1000

University of Michigan Health System
Univ Michigan Hlth Sys
1500 E Medical Center Dr
Ann Arbor, MI 48109
Midwest
(734) 936-4000

University of Missouri Hospitals & Clinics
Univ of Missouri Hosp & Clins
1 Hospital Dr
Columbia, MO 65212
Midwest
(573) 882-4141

University of North Carolina Hospitals
Univ NC Hosps
101 Manning Drive, Box 7600
Chapel Hill, NC 27514-4335
Southeast
(919) 966-4131

University of Pennsylvania Medical
Center - Philadelphia
Univ Penn Med Ctr - Presbyterian
51 N 39th St
Philadelphia, PA 19104
Mid Atlantic
(215) 662-8000

University of Rochester Strong Memorial
Hospital
Univ of Rochester Strong Meml Hosp
601 Elmwood Ave
Rochester, NY 14642
Mid Atlantic
(585) 275-2121

University of South Florida - Tampa
Univ of S FL - Tampa
4202 E Fowler Ave
Tampa, FL 33620
Southeast
(813) 974-2011

University of Tennesee Memorial Hospital
Univ of Tennesee Mem Hosp
1924 Alcoa Hwy
Knoxville, TN 37920
Southeast
(865) 544-9000

University of Texas MD Anderson
Cancer Center, The
UT MD Anderson Cancer Ctr, The
1515 Holcombe Blvd
Houston, TX 77030-4095
Southwest
(713) 792-2121

Institutions in bold are profiled in this edition of the Castle Connolly Guide.

University of Texas Medical Branch
Hospital at Galveston
UT Med Br Hosp at Galveston
301 University Blvd
Galveston, TX 77555
Southwest
(409) 772-1011

University of Texas San Antonio -
University Hospital
UTSA - Univ Hosp
4502 Medical Dr
San Antonio, TX 78229
Southwest
(210) 358-4000

University of Texas Southwestern Medical
Center at Dallas, The
UTSW Med Ctr - Dallas
5323 Harry Hines Blvd
Dallas, TX 75390
Southwest
(214) 648-3111

University of Utah Hospitals and Clinics
Univ Utah Hosps and Clins
50 N Medical Dr
Salt Lake City, UT 84132-0001
Great Plains and Mountains
(801) 581-2121

University of Virginia Medical Center
Univ Virginia Med Ctr
Lee Street
Charlottesville, VA 22908-0001
Southeast
(434) 924-0211

University of Washington Medical Center
Univ Wash Med Ctr
1959 NE Pacific St, Box 356355
Seattle, WA 98195
West Coast and Pacific
(206) 598-3300

University of Wisconsin Hospital &
Clinics
Univ WI Hosp & Clins
600 Highland Avenue
Madison, WI 53792
Midwest
(608) 263-6400

UPMC Presbyterian
UPMC Presby, Pittsburgh
200 Lothrop St
Pittsburgh, PA 15213
Mid Atlantic
(412) 647-2345

UPMC Shadyside
UPMC Shadyside
5230 Centre Ave
Pittsburgh, PA 15232-1381
Mid Atlantic
(412) 623-2121

USC Norris Cancer Comprehensive Center
and Hospital
USC Norris Canc Comp Ctr
1441 Eastlake Ave
Los Angeles, CA 90033
West Coast and Pacific
(323) 865-3000

Institutions in bold are profiled in this edition of the Castle Connolly Guide.

591

USC University Hospital - Richard K.
Eamer Medical Plaza
USC Univ Hosp - R K Eamer Med Plz
1500 San Pablo St
Los Angeles, CA 90033
West Coast and Pacific
(323) 442-8444

VA Medical Center - Atlanta
VA Med Ctr - Atlanta
1670 Clairmont Rd
Decatur, GA 30003
Southeast
(404) 321-6111

VA Medical Center - Portland
VA Medical Center - Portland
3710 SW US Veteran Hospital Rd
Portland, OR 97207
West Coast and Pacific
(503) 220-8262

VA Medical Center - West Los Angeles
VA Med Ctr - W Los Angeles
11301 Wilshire Blvd
Los Angeles, CA 90073
West Coast and Pacific
(310) 478-3711

Vanderbilt University Medical Center
Vanderbilt Univ Med Ctr
1313 21st Avenue South, Suite 405
Nashville, TN 37232-4335
Southeast
(615) 936-0301

Veterans Affairs Medical Center - Denver
VA Med Ctr
1055 Clermont Street
Denver, CO 80220
Great Plains and Mountains
(303) 399-8020

Veterans Affairs Medical Center - Tucson
VA Medical Center - Tucson
3601 S 6th Avenue
Tucson, AZ 85723
Southwest
(520) 792-1450

Virginia Hospital Center - Arlington
Virginia Hosp Ctr - Arlington
1701 N George Mason Dr
Arlington, VA 22205-3698
Southeast
(703) 558-5000

Virginia Mason Medical Center
Virginia Mason Med Ctr
1100 Ninth Ave, Box 900
Seattle, WA 98111
West Coast and Pacific
(206) 223-6600

**Wake Forest University Baptist Medical
Center**
Wake Forest Univ Baptist Med Ctr
Medical Center Blvd
Winston-Salem, NC 27157-1015
Southeast
(336) 716-2011

WakeMed Cary Hospital
WakeMed Cary
1900 Kildaire Farm Rd
Cary, NC 27511-6616
Southeast
(919) 350-2300

Washington Hospital Center
Washington Hosp Ctr
110 Irving St NW
Washington, DC 20010
Mid Atlantic
(202) 877-7000

Institutions in bold are profiled in this edition of the Castle Connolly Guide.

WellStar Kennestone Hospital
WellStar Kennestone Hosp
677 Church Street
Marietta, GA 30060
Southeast
(770) 793-5000

WellStar Windy Hill Hospital
WellStar Windy Hill Hosp
2540 Windy Hill Road
Marietta, GA 30067
Southeast
(770) 644-1000

West Virginia University Hospital - Ruby
Memorial
WV Univ Hosp - Ruby Memorial
1 Medical Center Drive
Morgantown, WV 26506
Mid Atlantic
(304) 598-4000

Westchester Medical Center
Westchester Med Ctr
95 Grasslands Road
Valhalla, NY 10595
Mid Atlantic
(914) 493-7000

William Beaumont Hospital
William Beaumont Hosp
3601 W 13 Mile Rd
Royal Oak, MI 48073
Midwest
(248) 551-5000

Wills Eye Hospital
Wills Eye Hosp
840 Walnut St
Philadelphia, PA 19107-5598
Mid Atlantic
(215) 928-3000

Wolfson Children's Hospital
Wolfson Chldns Hosp
800 Prudential Dr
Jacksonville, FL 32207
Southeast
(904) 202-8000

Women's and Children's Hospital of
Buffalo, The
Women's & Chldn's Hosp of Buffalo, The
219 Bryant St
Buffalo, NY 14222
Mid Atlantic
(716) 878-7000

Yale - New Haven Hospital
Yale - New Haven Hosp
20 York St
New Haven, CT 06510
New England
(203) 688-4242

Zale Lipshy University Hospital - Dallas
Zale Lipshy Univ Hosp - Dallas
5151 Harry Hines Blvd
Dallas, TX 75235
Southwest
(214) 590-3101

Institutions in bold are profiled in this edition of the Castle Connolly Guide.

APPENDIX D
MEDICAL SCHOOLS

The following is a list of U.S. and Canadian medical schools and the abbreviations used for each in the doctor listings. The abbreviations as they appear in the listings are in italics below.

ALABAMA

University of Alabama School of Medicine
University of Alabama at Birmingham
Univ Ala

University of South Alabama
College of Medicine
Univ S Ala Coll Med

ARIZONA

Arizona College of Osteopathic Medicine,
Midwestern University
Ariz Coll Osteo Med

University of Arizona College of
Medicine/Arizona Health Sciences Center
Univ Ariz Coll Med

ARKANSAS

University of Arkansas
College of Medicine
Univ Ark

CALIFORNIA

Charles Drew University
of Medicine and Science
Charles Drew Univ Med & Sci

Loma Linda University
School of Medicine
Loma Linda Univ

Stanford University School of Medicine
Stanford Univ

University of California Davis
School of Medicine
UC Davis

University of California Irvine
College of Medicine
UC Irvine

University of California Los Angeles
UCLA School of Medicine
UCLA

University of California San Diego
School of Medicine
UCSD

University of California San Francisco
School of Medicine
UCSF

University of Southern California
School of Medicine
USC Sch Med

Western University
College of Osteopathic Medicine
Western Univ Coll Osteo Med

COLORADO

University of Colorado
School of Medicine
Univ Colorado

CONNECTICUT

Southeastern University
College of Osteopathic Medicine
Southeastern Univ Coll Osteo Med

University of Connecticut
School of Medicine
Univ Conn

Yale University School of Medicine
Yale Univ

DISTRICT OF COLUMBIA

George Washington University
School of Medicine and Health Science
Geo Wash Univ

Georgetown University
School of Medicine
Georgetown Univ

Howard University College of Medicine
Howard Univ

FLORIDA

Nova Southeastern University,
College of Osteopathic Medicine
Nova SE Univ Coll Osteo Med

University of Florida College of Medicine
Univ Fla Coll Med

University of Miami School of Medicine
Univ Miami Sch Med

University of South Florida
College of Medicine
Univ S Fla Coll Med

GEORGIA

Emory University School of Medicine
Emory Univ

Medical College of Georgia
School of Medicine
Med Coll GA

Mercer University School of Medicine
Mercer Univ Sch Med

Morehouse School of Medicine
Morehouse Sch Med

HAWAII

University of Hawaii John A. Burns
School of Medicine
Univ Hawaii JA Burns Sch Med

ILLINOIS

Chicago College of Osteopathic Medicine,
Midwestern University
Chicago Coll Osteo Med

Loyola University of Chicago -
Stritch School of Medicine
Loyola Univ-Stritch Sch Med

Northwestern University Medical School
Northwestern Univ

Rush Medical College of Rush University
Rush Med Coll

Southern Illinois University
School of Medicine
Southern IL Univ

University of Chicago (Div Bio Sci)
Pritzker School of Medicine
Univ Chicago-Pritzker Sch Med

University of Health Sciences
Chicago Medical School
Univ Hlth Sci/Chicago Med Sch

University of Illinois College of Medicine
Univ IL Coll Med

INDIANA

Indiana University School of Medicine
Indiana Univ

IOWA

University of Iowa College of Medicine
Univ Iowa Coll Med

University of Osteopathic Medicine and
Health Sciences, Desmoine
Univ Osteo Med & Hlth Sci, Des Moines

KANSAS

Karl Menninger School of Psychiatry
Karl Menninger Sch Psych

University of Kansas Medical Center
School of Medicine
Univ Kans

KENTUCKY

University of Kentucky
College of Medicine
Univ KY Coll Med

University of Louisville
School of Medicine
Univ Louisville Sch Med

LOUISIANA

Louisiana State University
School of Medicine
Louisiana State Univ

Tulane University School of Medicine
Tulane Univ

MAINE

University of New England
College of Osteopathic Medicine
Univ New Eng Coll Osteo Med

MARYLAND

F. Edward A. Hebert School of Medicine
Uniformed Services University of Health
Sciences
Uniformed Srvs Univ, Betheseda

Johns Hopkins University
School of Medicine
Johns Hopkins Univ

University of Maryland
School of Medicine
Univ MD Sch Med

MASSACHUSETTS

Boston University School of Medicine
Boston Univ

Harvard Medical School
Harvard Med Sch

Middlesex University School of Medicine
Middlesex Univ

Tufts University School of Medicine
Tufts Univ

University of Massachusetts
Medical School
Univ Mass Sch Med

MICHIGAN

Michigan State University
College of Human Medicine
Mich State Univ

Michigan State University
College of Osteopathic Medicine
Mich State Univ Coll Osteo Med

University of Michigan Medical School
Univ Mich Med Sch

Wayne State University
School of Medicine
Wayne State Univ

MINNESOTA

Mayo Medical School
Mayo Med Sch

University of Minnesota Duluth
School of Medicine
Univ Minn-Duluth Sch Med

University of Minnesota Medical School
Univ Minn

MISSISSIPPI

University of Mississippi
School of Medicine
Univ Miss

MISSOURI

Kirksville College of Osteopathic
Medicine
Kirksville Coll Osteo Med

Saint Louis University
School of Medicine
St Louis Univ

University of Health Sciences/College of
Osteopathic Medicine
Univ Hlth Sci, Coll Osteo Med

University of Missouri Columbia
School of Medicine
Univ MO-Columbia Sch Med

University of Missouri Kansas City
School of Medicine
Univ MO-Kansas City

Washington University
School of Medicine
Wash Univ, St. Louis

NEBRASKA

Creighton University School of Medicine
Creighton Univ

University of Nebraska
College of Medicine
Univ Nebr Coll Med

NEVADA

University of Nevada School of Medicine
Univ Nevada

NEW HAMPSHIRE

Dartmouth Medical School
Dartmouth Med Sch

NEW JERSEY

Rutgers University
Rutgers Univ

Seton Hall University
School of Graduate Medical Eduction
Seton Hall Univ Sch Grad Med Ed

University of Medicine and Dentistry
of New Jersey, Newark
UMDNJ-NJ Med Sch, Newark

University of Medicine and Dentistry of New
Jersey, Robert Wood Johnson Medical School
UMDNJ-RW Johnson Med Sch

University of Medicine and Dentistry of
New Jersey/School of Osteopathic Medicine
UMDNJ Sch of Osteo Med

NEW MEXICO

University of New Mexico
School of Medicine
Univ New Mexico

NEW YORK

Albany Medical College
Albany Med Coll

Albert Einstein
College of Medicine of Yeshiva University
Albert Einstein Coll Med

Columbia University
College of Physicians and Surgeons
Columbia P&S

Cornell University-Weill Medical College
Cornell Univ-Weill Med Coll

Mount Sinai School of Medicine
Mount Sinai Sch Med

New York
College of Osteopathic Medicine
NY Coll Osteo Med

New York Medical College
NY Med Coll

New York University School of Medicine
NYU Sch Med

Robert Wood Johnson Medical School
Robert W Johnson Med Sch

State University of New York at Buffalo
School of Medicine & Biomedical Sciences
SUNY Buffalo

State University of New York
Health Science Center at Brooklyn
SUNY Downstate

State University of New York
Health Science Center at Brooklyn
SUNY Hlth Sci Ctr

State University of New York
Health Science Center at Syracuse
SUNY Upstate Med Univ

State University of New York at Stony Brook
Health Sciences Center
SUNY Stony Brook

University of Rochester
School of Medicine and Dentistry
Univ Rochester

NORTH CAROLINA

Bowman Gray School of Medicine
Bowman Gray

Duke University School of Medicine
Duke Univ

**East Carolina University
School of Medicine**
E Carolina Univ

**University of North Carolina at Chapel Hill
School of Medicine**
Univ NC Sch Med

Wake Forest University
Wake Forest Univ

NORTH DAKOTA

**University of North Dakota
School of Medicine**
Univ ND Sch Med

OHIO

**Case Western Reserve University
School of Medicine**
Case West Res Univ

Cleveland Clinic Medical School
Cleveland Clinic Med Sch

Medical College of Ohio
Med Coll OH

**Northeastern Ohio University
College of Medicine**
NE Ohio Univ

**Ohio State University
College of Medicine**
Ohio State Univ

**Ohio University,
College of Osteopathic Medicine**
Ohio Univ, Coll Osteo Med

**University of Cincinnati
College of Medicine**
Univ Cincinnati

**Wright State University
School of Medicine**
Wright State Univ

OKLAHOMA

**Oklahoma State University
College of Osteopathic Medicine**
Okla State Univ, Coll Osteo Med

**University of Oklahoma
College of Medicine**
Univ Okla Coll Med

OREGON

**Oregon Health Science University
School of Medicine**
Oregon Hlth Sci Univ

PENNSYLVANIA

Drexel University College of Medicine
Drexel Univ Coll Med

**Hahnemann University
School of Medicine**
Hahnemann Univ

**Jefferson Medical College
of Thomas Jefferson University**
Jefferson Med Coll

Lake Erie College of Osteopathic Medicine
Lk Erie Coll Osteo Med

Medical College of Pennsylvania
Med Coll PA Hahnermann

Pennsylvania State University
College of Medicine
Penn State Univ-Hershey Med Ctr

Philadelphia
College of Osteopathic Medicine
Philadelphia Coll Osteo Med

Temple University School of Medicine
Temple Univ

Thomas Jefferson University
Thomas Jefferson Univ

University of Pennsylvania
School of Medicine
Univ Pennsylvania

University of Pittsburgh
School of Medicine
Univ Pittsburgh

RHODE ISLAND

Brown University Program in Medicine
Brown Univ

SOUTH CAROLINA

Medical University of South Carolina
College of Medicine
Med Univ SC

University of South Carolina
School of Medicine
Univ SC Sch Med

SOUTH DAKOTA

University of South Dakota
School of Medicine
Univ SD Sch Med

TENNESSEE

East Tennessee State University
James H. Quillen College of Medicine
E Tenn State Univ

Meharry Medical College School of
Medicine
Meharry Med Coll

University of Tennessee
College of Medicine, Memphis
Univ Tenn Coll Med, Memphis

University of Tennessee
College of Medicine, Chattanooga
Univ Tenn Coll Med, Chattanooga

Vanderbilt University School of Medicine
Vanderbilt Univ

TEXAS

Baylor College of Medicine
Baylor Coll Med

Texas A&M University Health Science
Center College of Medicine
Texas A&M Univ

Texas Tech University Health Science
Center School of Medicine
Texas Tech Univ

University of North Texas Health Science
Center/College of Osteopathic Medicine
Univ N Tex Hlth Sci Ctr, Coll Osteo Med

University of Texas
Medical School at Galveston
Univ Texas Med Br, Galveston

University of Texas
Medical School at Houston
Univ Texas, Houston

University of Texas
Medical School, Southwest
U Texas SW, Dallas

University of Texas
Medical School at San Antonio
Univ Tex, San Antonio

UTAH

Oral Roberts School of Medicine
Oral Roberts Sch Med

University of Utah School of Medicine
Univ Utah

VERMONT

University of Vermont College of Medicine
Univ VT Coll Med

VIRGINIA

Eastern Virginia Medical School of the
Medical College of Hampton Roads
Eastern VA Med Sch

Virginia Commonwealth University Medical
College of Virginia School of Medicine
Med Coll VA

University of Virginia School of Medicine
Univ VA Sch Med

Virginia Commonwealth University
VA Commonwealth Univ

WASHINGTON

University of Washington
School of Medicine
Univ Wash

WEST VIRGINIA

Marshall University School of Medicine
Marshall Univ

Robert C. Byrd Health Sciences Center of
West Virginia University School of
Medicine
W VA Univ

West Virginia School
of Osteopathic Medicine
W VA Sch Osteo Med

WISCONSIN

Medical College of Wisconsin
Med Coll Wisc

University of Wisconsin School of
Medicine
Univ Wisc

APPENDIX E

SELECTED CANCER RESOURCES

While the following resources have been checked
for accuracy as of June 2005, we cannot guarantee
the complete content of each source.

GENERAL RESOURCES

AMERICAN CANCER SOCIETY
A site with many resources on types
of cancer, treatments, coping,
support, clinical research data,
volunteering and current news
articles. It also has a database that, by
entering a zip code, one may locate
local resources, activities and news.

National Office
1599 Clifton Road, NE
Atlanta, GA 30329
800-ACS-2345
www.cancer.org

AMERICAN INSTITUTE FOR CANCER RESEARCH
Discusses current research findings on
diet, nutrition and cancer prevention
and provides an online Cancer
Resource Book.

1759 R Street, NW
Washington, DC 20009
800-843-8114
www.aicr.org

ANNIE APPLESEED PROJECT
Provides information, education,
advocacy and awareness for people
with cancer, family and friends
interested in alternative medical
treatments.

7319 Serrano Terrace
Delray Beach, FL 33446-2215
annfonfa@aol.com
www.annieappleseedproject.org

ASSOCIATION OF CANCER ONLINE RESOURCES (ACOR)
Maintains many support groups and
cancer-specific information, treatment
options, clinical trial findings and a
large collection of cancer-related
online communities.

173 Duane Street, Suite 3A
New York, NY 10013-3334
212-226-5525
www.acor.org

CANCERBACUP
Europe-based organization with over
4,500 of pages of online cancer
information, practical advice and
support for cancer patients and their
families.

www.cancerbacup.org.uk

CANCER CARE

Provides free resources and support to cancer patients, caregivers and families with all cancers through counseling, education, information, referrals and direct financial assistance.

National Office
275 7th Ave
New York, NY 10001
800-813-HOPE or 212-302-2400
www.cancercare.org

CANCEREDUCATION.COM

Provides cancer-specific information and educational programming for patients, their families and physicians.

750 Lexington Avenue
26th Floor
New York, NY 10022
212-531-5960
webmaster@cancereducation.com
www.cancereducation.com

CANCERFACTS.COM

Resources for cancer patients, their families and caregivers, including personalized cancer information and a profiler to learn about current treatment options.

NexCura, Inc.
1725 Westlake Avenue North
Suite 300
Seattle, WA 98109
206-270-0225
answers@support.nextura.com
www.cancerfacts.com

CANCERNETWORK.COM

Provides research findings and information on complications, cancers, therapies and insurance and payment issues.

CMP Healthcare Media
Oncology Publishing Group
600 Community Drive
Manhasset, NY 11030
516-562-5000
info@cancernetwork.com
www.cancernetwork.com

CANCER RESEARCH & PREVENTION FOUNDATION OF AMERICA

Scientific research and cancer education with a focus on cancers that can be prevented through lifestyle changes or early detection followed by prompt treatment. Includes breast, cervical, colorectal, lung, prostate, skin, oral and testicular cancers.

1600 Duke Street
Suite 500
Alexandria, VA 22314
800-227-2732
www.preventcancer.org

CANCERSOURCE.COM

Information, articles, advice, interactive tools and community resources for patients, physicians, children, women and nurses.

263 Summer Street
Boston, MA 02210
866-234-5025
www.cancersource.com

CANCER TRACK

Comprehensive source for links to news, research, medications, treatments, support groups, regulatory agencies and online references.

www.cancertrack.com

HEALTH FINDER

A service of the Department of Health and Human Services, Health Finder has many resources ranging from topics specifically related to cancer to broader health topics such as locating public clinics, nursing homes, health fraud advice, medical privacy and links to universities, medical dictionaries and journals. It also has a guide that presents information and resources to help patients and families get better quality healthcare.

www.healthfinder.gov

CANCER NEWS

News and information on cancer diagnosis, treatment and prevention.

www.cancernews.com

NATIONAL COMPREHENSIVE CANCER NETWORK

Outlines cancer treatment guidelines and offers cancer patients and their families information to help work with their physicians to make more informed decisions about care and treatments.

National Comprehensive Cancer Network
500 Old York Road, Suite 250
Jenkintown, PA 19046
215-690-0300

TREATMENT GUIDELINES FOR PATIENTS:
888-909-NCCN

www.nccn.org/

ONCOLINK

Information on specific types of cancer, updates on cancer treatments and news about research advances.

OncoLink
Abramson Cancer Center of the University of Pennsylvania
3400 Spruce Street - 2 Donner
Philadelphia, PA 19104-4283
www.oncolink.com/

ONCOLOGY NURSING SOCIETY (ONS)

Resources on prevention, detection, diagnosis, treatment and survivorship.

Oncology Nursing Society
125 Enterprise Drive
RIDC Park West
Pittsburgh, PA 15275-1214
866-257-4ONS
customer.service@ons.org
www.ons.org/patientEd/

ONCOLOGY TOOLS

Information related to cancers and approved cancer drug therapies organized by disease category.

www.fda.gov/cder/cancer/

PEOPLE LIVING WITH CANCER

A website by the American Society of Clinical Oncology for patients that provides oncologist-approved information on more than 50 types of cancer and their treatments, clinical trials, coping, and side effects. It includes a "Find an Oncologist" database, live chats, message boards, a drug database and links to patient support organizations.

American Society of Clinical Oncology
1900 Duke Street, Suite 200
Alexandria, Virginia 22314
703-797-1914
contactus@plwc.org
www.peoplelivingwithcancer.org

605

SPECIAL POPULATIONS NETWORKS FOR CANCER AWARENESS, RESEARCH AND TRAINING
Resources and programs for minority communities.

http://crchd.nci.nih.gov/spn/current
_network/current_initiatives.html

YOUR DISEASE RISK
Provides education on cancers and focuses on prevention as the primary approach to controlling cancer and other chronic diseases.

Harvard Center for Cancer
Prevention
677 Huntington Ave, Landmark 3 East
Boston, MA 02115
617-998-1034
www.yourdiseaserisk.harvard.edu

WOMEN

BREASTCANCER.ORG
Offers information on breast cancer prevention, symptoms, treatment, research, recovery and support.

www.breastcancer.org

ENTRE MUJERES
Un guia sobre la recuperación física y emocional después de la mastectomía.

www.cancerlinks.com/Mujeres/
mujeres_index.html

LOOK GOOD...FEEL BETTER
Provides resources and links for women who are undergoing cancer treatment including cosmetics advice and support.

www.lookgoodfeelbetter.org

NATIONAL WOMEN'S HEALTH RESOURCE CENTER
Women's health site that includes information on various cancers.

NWHRC
157 Broad Street
Suite 315
Red Bank, NJ 07701
www.healthywomen.org (Note: Click on "Health Center" and select the appropriate topic.)

NCI WOMEN OF COLOR
Provides basic data on how cancer affects women in minority populations.

http://cancercontrol.cancer.gov/
womenofcolor

WOMEN'S CANCER CENTER
Many resources for women with various kinds of cancer.

www.womenscancercenter.com

YWCA
"ENCOREplus", a program available at some YWCA locations that focuses on cancer prevention, nutrition and rehabilitation.

YWCA USA
1015 18th Street, NW
Suite 1100
Washington, DC 20036
800-YWCA-US1
info@ywca.org
www.ywca.org(Note: click on the "I need help" link.)

CHILDREN AND YOUNG ADULTS

BRAVE KIDS

Provides online resources for children with chronic or life-threatening illnesses and disabilities and their families and local resources searchable by zip code.

Brave Kids: West Coast
1223 Wilshire Boulevard
#1411
Santa Monica, CA 90403
800-568-1008
Brave Kids: East Coast
1208 Lake Cove Court
Ponte Vedra Beach, FL 32082
904-827-9571
info@bravekids.org
www.bravekids.org/

CANDLELIGHTERS CHILDHOOD CANCER FOUNDATION

Offers support, education and advocacy for families of children with cancer, survivors of childhood cancer and the professionals who care for them.

National Office
P.O. Box 498
Kensington, MD 20895-0498
800-366-CCCF or 301-962-3520
staff@candlelighters.org
www.candlelighters.org

CHILDREN'S ONCOLOGY GROUP

Offers educational and support resources.

PO Box 60012
Arcadia, CA 91066-6012
626-447-0064 (COG, Research Operations Center)
www.childrensoncologygroup.org

CURESEARCH

Provides educational resources about cancer diagnoses and the different phases of treatment. (In partnership with the National Childhood Cancer Foundation.)

CureSearch Headquarters
4600 East West Highway, #600
Bethesda, MD 20814-3457
800-458-6223
www.curesearch.org/

KIDSHEALTH.ORG

Site designed for parents, kids and teens that discusses many health topics including cancer.

www.kidshealth.org

NATIONAL CHILDHOOD CANCER FOUNDATION

Provides educational resources about cancer diagnoses and the different phases of treatment. (In partnership with CureSearch.)

440 E Huntington Drive, Suite 300
Arcadia, CA 91066-6012
800-458-NCCF
www.nccf.org

PEDIATRIC ONCOLOGY RESOURCE CENTER

A site with resources, internet links, and references for parents, friends and families of children who have or had childhood cancer.

www.acor.org/ped-onc

TEENS LIVING WITH CANCER

A website for teenagers with cancer with information on treatments, combating fear, testimonials from other teens who have or had cancer and support chat rooms.

Melissa's Living Legacy Foundation
245 Citation Drive
Henrietta, NY 14467
Phone: 585-334-0858

607

info@teenslivingwithcancer.org
teenslivingwithcancer.org

YOUNG ADULT CANCER RESOURCE SITE
An online support and resources for 15-45 year-olds who have or may be developing cancer.

wableyer.oncologymail.com

SPECIFIC CANCERS

RARE CANCER ALLIANCE
Provides support and other resources for adults and children with rare cancers.

www.rare-cancer.org
Note: You are encouraged to explore the other websites listed in this appendix, as many also include information on rare cancers.

TREATMENT

AMERICAN SOCIETY FOR THERAPEUTIC RADIOLOGY AND ONCOLOGY
Provides downloadable brochures and publications on treatment options for several specific cancers.

ASTRO Headquarters
12500 Fair Lakes Circle
Suite 375
Fairfax, VA 22033
800-962-7876
www.astro.org/patient/
treatment_information

BLOOD AND MARROW TRANSPLANT INFORMATION NETWORK
Provides information about blood and marrow transplants, support groups, a list of transplant centers and testimonials from survivors.

www.bmtinfonet.org

CANCERSYMPTOMS.ORG
Provides information and resources for learning about and managing symptoms often associated with cancer treatment.

www.cancersymptoms.org

SURVIVORS

CANCER SURVIVORS NETWORK
Provides a forum for cancer survivors to share their stories, join chats, post messages on discussion boards and create your own webpage about your experiences.

www.acscsn.org

CANCERVIVE
Provides support, public education and advocacy to those who have had cancer.

11636 Chayote Street
Los Angeles, CA 90049
800-4TO-CURE or 310-203-9232
cancervivr@aol.com
cancervive.org

LANCE ARMSTRONG FOUNDATION
LAF provides advocacy, education, support and research for both cancer survivors and people who currently have cancer.

www.laf.org

NATIONAL COALITION FOR CANCER SURVIVORSHIP (NCCS)
Provides education, advocacy and support to those affected by cancer and cancer survivors. Specifically address quality of care and minority issues.

1010 Wayne Avenue
Suite 770
Silver Spring, MD 20910
877-622-7937
info@canceradvocacy.org
www.canceradvocacy.org

OUTLOOK – LIFE BEYOND CHILDHOOD CANCER

Addresses the needs and provides information to help give survivors and their families the tools to help them become their own advocate and is a forum for support.

www.outlook-life.org

SUPPORT

FERTILE HOPE

Provides reproductive information and support to cancer patients whose medical treatments present the risk of infertility.

www.fertilehope.org
Note: You are encouraged to explore the other websites listed in this appendix, as many also include resources for support including education materials, chat rooms, community groups and clinical advice.

CLINICAL TRIALS

NATIONAL CANCER INSTITUTE (NCI)

A branch of the US National Institutes of Health, NCI provides information about cancer, clinical trials, statistics, and research. (For more information about NCI, see separate listing below.)

www.cancer.gov/clinicaltrials

AMERICAN CANCER SOCIETY

Free clinical trial matching and referral service.

clinicaltrials.cancer.org/

CENTERWATCH

Provides information and resources used by patients, pharmaceutical, biotechnology and medical device companies, CROs and research centers involved in clinical research around the world. The web site provides an extensive list of IRB approved clinical trials being conducted internationally and also lists promising therapies newly approved by the Food and Drug Administration. CenterWatch also offers reports on specific illnesses, clinical trial information and therapies that patients and advocates can buy.
Thomson CenterWatch
22 Thomson Place, 47F1
Boston, MA 02210-1212
617-856-5900
www.centerwatch.com

NATIONAL COMPREHENSIVE CANCER NETWORK (NCCN)

An alliance of 19 of the world's leading cancer centers, NCCN is a source of information to help patients and health professionals make informed decisions about cancer care. Through the collective expertise of its member institutions, the NCCN develops, updates, and disseminates a complete library of clinical practice guidelines.

National Comprehensive Cancer Network
500 Old York Road, Suite 250
Jenkintown, PA 19046
215-690-0300
Fax: 215-690-0280
Treatment Guidelines for Patients:
888-909-NCCN
www.nccn.org/

609

NATIONAL COALITION FOR CANCER SURVIVORSHIP (NCCS)

Provides education, advocacy and support to those affected by cancer and cancer survivors. Specifically address quality of care and minority issues.

1010 Wayne Avenue
Suite 770
Silver Spring, MD 20910
877-622-7937
info@canceradvocacy.org
www.canceradvocacy.org

OUTLOOK – LIFE BEYOND CHILDHOOD CANCER

Addresses the needs and provides information to help give survivors and their families the tools to help them become their own advocate and is a forum for support.

www.outlook-life.org

SUPPORT

FERTILE HOPE

Provides reproductive information and support to cancer patients whose medical treatments present the risk of infertility.

www.fertilehope.org

Note: You are encouraged to explore the other websites listed in this appendix, as many also include resources for support including education materials, chat rooms, community groups and clinical advice.

CLINICAL TRIALS

NATIONAL CANCER INSTITUTE (NCI)

A branch of the US National Institutes of Health, NCI provides information about cancer, clinical trials, statistics, and research. (For more information about NCI, see separate listing below.)

www.cancer.gov/clinicaltrials

AMERICAN CANCER SOCIETY

Free clinical trial matching and referral service.

www.clinicaltrials.cancer.org/

CENTERWATCH

Provides information and resources used by patients, pharmaceutical, biotechnology and medical device companies, CROs and research centers involved in clinical research around the world. The web site provides an extensive list of IRB approved clinical trials being conducted internationally and also lists promising therapies newly approved by the Food and Drug Administration. CenterWatch also offers reports on specific illnesses, clinical trial information and therapies that patients and advocates can buy.

Thomson CenterWatch
22 Thomson Place, 47F1
Boston, MA 02210-1212
617-856-5900
www.centerwatch.com

NATIONAL COMPREHENSIVE CANCER NETWORK (NCCN)

An alliance of 19 of the world's leading cancer centers, NCCN is a source of information to help patients and health professionals make informed decisions about cancer care. Through the collective expertise of its member institutions, the NCCN develops, updates, and disseminates a complete library of clinical practice guidelines.

National Comprehensive Cancer Network
500 Old York Road, Suite 250
Jenkintown, PA 19046
215-690-0300
Fax: 215-690-0280
Treatment Guidelines for Patients:
888-909-NCCN
www.nccn.org/

COALITION OF NATIONAL CANCER COOPERATIVE GROUPS (CNCC)

A network of cancer clinical trials specialists including cooperative groups, cancer centers, academic medical centers, community hospitals, physician practices, and patient advocate groups, CNCC aims at improving the clinical trials experience for patients and physicians, regulatory requirements, and providing professional support services. It offers a variety of programs and information for physicians, patient advocate groups, and patients designed to increase awareness of, and participation in, cancer clinical trials.

1818 Market Street, #1100
Philadelphia, PA 19103
877-520-4457
www.cancertrialshelp.org

NATIONAL CANCER INSTITUTE (NCI)

The National Cancer Institute's (NCI's) Cancer Information Service (CIS) is a national information and education network. The CIS is a free public service of the NCI, the Nation's primary agency for cancer research. The CIS provides current cancer information to patients, their families, the public, and health professionals. The CIS provides personalized, confidential responses to specific questions about cancer.

Cancer Information Service (CIS)
Building 31, Room 10A07
Bethesda, MD 20892
email: cancernet@icicb.nci.nih.gov
1-800-4-CANCER (1-800-422-6237)
www.cis.nci.nih.gov
www.cancer.gov

NCI-DESIGNATED CANCER CENTERS

Cancer centers listed by state.

www3.cancer.gov/cancercenters
NCI Dictionary of Cancer Terms

www.cancer.gov/dictionary

SECTION V

INDICES

SUBJECT INDEX

SPECIAL EXPERTISE INDEX

This index lists the areas which the physicians listed in the Guide have identified as their "special expertise." These are not medical specialities. They are specific elements of disease, procedures, techniques and treatments for which these physicians are best known and are referred patients.

SPECIAL EXPERTISE INDEX

SPECIAL EXPERTISE INDEX

Special Expertise	Spec	Name	Pg	Special Expertise	Spec	Name	Pg
Brain Tumors	RadRO	Pezner, R (CA)	449	Brain Tumors-Pediatric	NS	Fuchs, H (NC)	265
Brain Tumors	NS	Apuzzo, M (CA)	271	Brain Tumors-Pediatric	NS	Goodrich, J (NY)	261
Brain Tumors	N	Levin, V (TX)	283	Breast Augmentation	PlS	Cram, A (IA)	414
Brain Tumors	RadRO	Pollack, J (NY)	438	Breast Cancer	S	Pockaj, B (AZ)	493
Brain Tumors	NRad	Atlas, S (CA)	456	Breast Cancer	DR	Monsees, B (MO)	454
Brain Tumors	NS	Bilsky, M (NY)	260	Breast Cancer	Hem	Wisch, N (NY)	200
Brain Tumors	NS	Origitano, T (IL)	268	Breast Cancer	Onc	Cohen, S (NY)	213
Brain Tumors	NS	Boop, F (TN)	264	Breast Cancer	DR	Dershaw, D (NY)	452
Brain Tumors	NS	Greene Jr, C (CA)	272	Breast Cancer	S	McMasters, K (KY)	484
Brain Tumors	N	Cloughesy, T (CA)	283	Breast Cancer	Onc	Offit, K (NY)	220
Brain Tumors	NS	Laws Jr., E (VA)	265	Breast Cancer	RadRO	Rosenman, J (NC)	441
Brain Tumors	NS	Dacey Jr, R (MO)	266	Breast Cancer	RadRO	Hancock, S (CA)	449
Brain Tumors	NS	Ellenbogen, R (WA)	271	Breast Cancer	S	Byrd, D (WA)	494
Brain Tumors	NS	Albright, A (PA)	260	Breast Cancer	NuM	Podoloff, D (TX)	460
Brain Tumors	RadRO	Herman, T (TX)	447	Breast Cancer	RadRO	Myerson, R (MO)	445
Brain Tumors	PMR	Stewart, P (AL)	551	Breast Cancer	DR	Helvie, M (MI)	454
Brain Tumors	PHO	Gold, S (NC)	388	Breast Cancer	Onc	Livingston, R (WA)	249
Brain Tumors	NS	O'Rourke, D (PA)	263	Breast Cancer	Onc	Rosen, S (IL)	238
Brain Tumors	NS	Link, M (MN)	267	Breast Cancer	S	Urist, M (AL)	485
Brain Tumors	PHO	Manera, R (IL)	392	Breast Cancer	DR	Mitnick, J (NY)	453
Brain Tumors	NS	Goumnerova, L (MA)	259	Breast Cancer	RadRO	Berson, A (NY)	435
Brain Tumors	RadRO	Machtay, M (PA)	437	Breast Cancer	Onc	Loprinzi, C (MN)	236
Brain Tumors	PHO	Kadota, R (CA)	398	Breast Cancer	Onc	Fracasso, P (MO)	234
Brain Tumors	NS	Warnick, R (OH)	269	Breast Cancer	Path	Schnitt, S (MA)	362
Brain Tumors	NS	Raffel, C (MN)	268	Breast Cancer	Onc	Johnson, D (TN)	227
Brain Tumors	PHO	Arndt, C (MN)	390	Breast Cancer	S	Krag, D (VT)	474
Brain Tumors	NS	Heros, R (FL)	265	Breast Cancer	Path	Young, R (MA)	362
Brain Tumors	RadRO	Sandler, H (MI)	445	Breast Cancer	DR	Orel, S (PA)	453
Brain Tumors	RadRO	Loeffler, J (MA)	433	Breast Cancer	RadRO	Lee, C (MN)	443
Brain Tumors	NS	Bakay, R (IL)	266	Breast Cancer	Onc	Chabner, B (MA)	208
Brain Tumors	PHO	Israel, M (NH)	381	Breast Cancer	S	Ross, M (TX)	493
Brain Tumors	Path	Bollen, A (CA)	371	Breast Cancer	Onc	Perry, M (MO)	237
Brain Tumors	N	Posner, J (NY)	281	Breast Cancer	Onc	Rosen, P (CA)	251
Brain Tumors	PHO	Halpern, S (NJ)	384	Breast Cancer	Path	Dubeau, L (CA)	372
Brain Tumors	PHO	Garvin, J (NY)	383	Breast Cancer	RadRO	Juillard, G (CA)	449
Brain Tumors	NS	DiGiacinto, G (NY)	261	Breast Cancer	RadRO	Rose, C (CA)	450
Brain Tumors	NS	Camins, M (NY)	261	Breast Cancer	DR	Mendelson, E (IL)	454
Brain Tumors	Onc	Prados, M (CA)	251	Breast Cancer	Onc	Brescia, F (SC)	225
Brain Tumors	N	Greenberg, H (MI)	282	Breast Cancer	Onc	Hoffman, P (IL)	235
Brain Tumors	NS	Chandler, W (MI)	266	Breast Cancer	S	Goodnight, J (CA)	495
Brain Tumors	NS	Al-Mefty, O (AR)	269	Breast Cancer	S	Johnson, D (CA)	495
Brain Tumors	NS	Adler Jr, J (CA)	270	Breast Cancer	RadRO	Underhill, K (NH)	434
Brain Tumors	PHO	Horn, B (CA)	398	Breast Cancer	RadRO	Prosnitz, L (NC)	441
Brain Tumors	NS	Ruge, J (IL)	268	Breast Cancer	Onc	Vaughan, W (AL)	230
Brain Tumors	NS	Pollack, I (PA)	263	Breast Cancer	Onc	Canellos, G (MA)	208
Brain Tumors	NS	Cosgrove, G (MA)	259	Breast Cancer	RadRO	Pistenmaa, D (TX)	448
Brain Tumors	N	Yung, W (TX)	283	Breast Cancer	Onc	Von Roenn, J (IL)	239
Brain Tumors	NS	Loftus, C (PA)	262	Breast Cancer	Onc	Lynch Jr, J (FL)	228
Brain Tumors	RadRO	Curran Jr, W (PA)	435	Breast Cancer	S	Hoffman, J (PA)	478
Brain Tumors	NS	Bauer, J (IL)	266	Breast Cancer	Onc	Grossbard, M (NY)	216
Brain Tumors	NS	Levy, R (IL)	267	Breast Cancer	Onc	Weber, J (CA)	252
Brain Tumors	PHO	Goldman, S (IL)	391	Breast Cancer	Path	Cote, R (CA)	371
Brain Tumors	RadRO	Shaw, E (NC)	441	Breast Cancer	S	August, D (NJ)	475
Brain Tumors	PHO	Luchtman-Jones, L (MO)	392	Breast Cancer	S	Wagman, L (CA)	496
Brain Tumors & Disorders	NS	Ott, K (CA)	272	Breast Cancer	S	Grant, C (MN)	487
Brain Tumors-Adult & Pediatric	RadRO	Suh, J (OH)	445	Breast Cancer	S	Feig, B (TX)	491
Brain Tumors-Adult & Pediatric	NS	Kondziolka, D (PA)	262	Breast Cancer	RadRO	Rotman, M (NY)	438
Brain Tumors-Pediatric	RadRO	Merchant, T (TN)	440	Breast Cancer	RadRO	Schiff, P (NY)	438
Brain Tumors-Pediatric	N	Janss, A (GA)	281	Breast Cancer	Hem	Walters, T (ID)	204
Brain Tumors-Pediatric	NS	Carmel, P (NJ)	261	Breast Cancer	Onc	Ross, M (VA)	228
Brain Tumors-Pediatric	NS	Tomita, T (IL)	269	Breast Cancer	Onc	Doroshow, J (MD)	214
Brain Tumors-Pediatric	NS	Scott, R (MA)	260	Breast Cancer	Path	Ross, J (NY)	364
Brain Tumors-Pediatric	ChiN	Mandelbaum, D (RI)	284	Breast Cancer	Onc	Chitambar, C (WI)	233
Brain Tumors-Pediatric	NS	Wisoff, J (NY)	264	Breast Cancer	Path	Mies, C (PA)	364

621

SPECIAL EXPERTISE INDEX

Special Expertise	Spec	Name	Pg	Special Expertise	Spec	Name	Pg
Breast Cancer	Onc	Hutchins, L (AR)	244	Breast Cancer	S	Alfonso, A (NY)	475
Breast Cancer	S	Klimberg, V (AR)	492	Breast Cancer	Onc	Budd, G (OH)	232
Breast Cancer	Onc	Ganz, P (CA)	249	Breast Cancer	Onc	Jones, S (TX)	245
Breast Cancer	Onc	Chap, L (CA)	248	Breast Cancer	Onc	Garber, J (MA)	209
Breast Cancer	CG	Weitzel, J (CA)	548	Breast Cancer	Onc	Winer, E (MA)	211
Breast Cancer	Onc	Anderson, J (MI)	231	Breast Cancer	Onc	Ingle, J (MN)	236
Breast Cancer	S	Ames, F (TX)	491	Breast Cancer	Onc	Hortobagyi, G (TX)	244
Breast Cancer	Onc	Overmoyer, B (OH)	237	Breast Cancer	Onc	Shapiro, C (OH)	239
Breast Cancer	S	Skinner, K (NY)	481	Breast Cancer	Onc	Robert, N (VA)	228
Breast Cancer	Onc	Smith, T (VA)	230	Breast Cancer	RadRO	McNeese, M (TX)	448
Breast Cancer	S	Osteen, R (MA)	474	Breast Cancer	Onc	Weber, B (PA)	223
Breast Cancer	RadRO	Herman, T (TX)	447	Breast Cancer	Onc	Salem, P (TX)	247
Breast Cancer	Onc	Sledge Jr, G (IN)	239	Breast Cancer	RadRO	Strom, E (TX)	448
Breast Cancer	RadRO	Recht, A (MA)	434	Breast Cancer	RadRO	Kuske, R (AZ)	447
Breast Cancer	S	Smith, B (MA)	474	Breast Cancer	RadRO	Berg, C (MD)	434
Breast Cancer	S	Borgen, P (NY)	476	Breast Cancer	RadRO	Wazer, D (RI)	434
Breast Cancer	S	O'Hea, B (NY)	479	Breast Cancer	RadRO	Vicini, F (MI)	446
Breast Cancer	Path	Page, D (TN)	367	Breast Cancer	Onc	Buzdar, A (TX)	243
Breast Cancer	Onc	Osborne, C (TX)	246	Breast Cancer	RadRO	Taylor, M (MO)	445
Breast Cancer	Onc	Yee, D (MN)	240	Breast Cancer	S	Goulet Jr, R (IN)	487
Breast Cancer	S	Gabram, S (IL)	487	Breast Cancer	S	Robinson, D (FL)	485
Breast Cancer	Onc	Moore, A (NY)	219	Breast Cancer	S	Frazier, T (PA)	477
Breast Cancer	Onc	Horton, J (FL)	227	Breast Cancer	Path	Patchefsky, A (PA)	364
Breast Cancer	S	Roses, D (NY)	480	Breast Cancer	S	Eisenberg, B (NH)	473
Breast Cancer	Onc	Muggia, F (NY)	220	Breast Cancer	Onc	Daly, M (PA)	214
Breast Cancer	S	Witt, T (IL)	490	Breast Cancer	Path	Hoda, S (NY)	362
Breast Cancer	DR	Evers, K (PA)	453	Breast Cancer	Onc	Mintzer, D (PA)	219
Breast Cancer	S	Sener, S (IL)	489	Breast Cancer	Onc	Fox, K (PA)	215
Breast Cancer	Onc	Carpenter Jr, J (AL)	225	Breast Cancer	Onc	Seewaldt, V (NC)	229
Breast Cancer	Onc	Piel, I (IL)	237	Breast Cancer	S	Israel, P (GA)	483
Breast Cancer	RadRO	Halpern, H (IL)	443	Breast Cancer	S	Hunt, K (TX)	492
Breast Cancer	S	Singletary, S (TX)	493	Breast Cancer	S	Mamounas, E (OH)	488
Breast Cancer	Path	Thor, A (OK)	371	Breast Cancer	Onc	Lyman, G (NY)	218
Breast Cancer	RadRO	Hellman, S (IL)	443	Breast Cancer	RadRO	Mendenhall, N (FL)	440
Breast Cancer	S	Kern, K (CT)	473	Breast Cancer	RadRO	Buchholz, T (TX)	447
Breast Cancer	RadRO	Halle, J (NC)	439	Breast Cancer	Onc	Stockdale, F (CA)	251
Breast Cancer	Onc	Graham, M (NC)	226	Breast Cancer	Onc	Albain, K (IL)	231
Breast Cancer	Onc	Chlebowski, R (CA)	248	Breast Cancer	S	Bass, B (MD)	476
Breast Cancer	Onc	Dickler, M (NY)	214	Breast Cancer	S	Ponn, T (CT)	474
Breast Cancer	CG	Rubinstein, W (IL)	548	Breast Cancer	GO	Kelley II, J (PA)	293
Breast Cancer	S	Hughes, K (MA)	473	Breast Cancer	Onc	Muss, H (VT)	210
Breast Cancer	Onc	Disis, M (WA)	248	Breast Cancer	S	Herrmann, V (GA)	483
Breast Cancer	RadRO	Solin, L (PA)	438	Breast Cancer	S	Beauchamp, R (TN)	482
Breast Cancer	Onc	Silverman, P (OH)	239	Breast Cancer	RadRO	Goodman, R (NJ)	436
Breast Cancer	S	Eberlein, T (MO)	487	Breast Cancer	Onc	Hartmann, L (MN)	235
Breast Cancer	Path	Sanchez, M (NJ)	364	Breast Cancer	RadRO	Ferree, C (NC)	439
Breast Cancer	S	Leffall Jr, L (DC)	478	Breast Cancer	Path	Tomaszewski, J (PA)	365
Breast Cancer	Onc	Urba, W (OR)	252	Breast Cancer	Onc	Valero, V (TX)	247
Breast Cancer	Onc	Glick, J (PA)	216	Breast Cancer	S	Wood, W (GA)	485
Breast Cancer	Onc	Gradishar, W (IL)	235	Breast Cancer	Onc	Fleming, G (IL)	234
Breast Cancer	Onc	Kosova, L (IL)	236	Breast Cancer	S	Crowe Jr, J (OH)	486
Breast Cancer	Onc	Nissenblatt, M (NJ)	220	Breast Cancer	S	Chang, A (MI)	486
Breast Cancer	Onc	Cobleigh, M (IL)	233	Breast Cancer	RadRO	Pierce, L (MI)	445
Breast Cancer	RadRO	Haffty, B (CT)	433	Breast Cancer	Onc	Come, S (MA)	209
Breast Cancer	Onc	Bitran, J (IL)	232	Breast Cancer	S	Schwartz, G (PA)	480
Breast Cancer	Onc	Hudis, C (NY)	217	Breast Cancer	S	Edge, S (NY)	476
Breast Cancer	S	Anderson, B (WA)	494	Breast Cancer	S	Iglehart, J (MA)	473
Breast Cancer	RadRO	Lewin, A (FL)	440	Breast Cancer	Onc	Shulman, L (MA)	211
Breast Cancer	Onc	Schwartz, M (FL)	229	Breast Cancer	S	Farrar, W (OH)	487
Breast Cancer	Onc	Jahanzeb, M (MN)	236	Breast Cancer	S	Nelson, E (UT)	490
Breast Cancer	S	Niederhuber, J (WI)	488	Breast Cancer	S	Newman, L (MI)	488
Breast Cancer	Onc	Dreicer, R (OH)	234	Breast Cancer	Onc	Goldstein, L (PA)	216
Breast Cancer	Path	Masood, S (FL)	366	Breast Cancer	DR	Conant, E (PA)	452
Breast Cancer	Hem	Abramson, N (FL)	200	Breast Cancer	Onc	Grana, G (NJ)	216

SPECIAL EXPERTISE INDEX

SPECIAL EXPERTISE INDEX

SPECIAL EXPERTISE INDEX

SPECIAL EXPERTISE INDEX

SPECIAL EXPERTISE INDEX

SPECIAL EXPERTISE INDEX

SPECIAL EXPERTISE INDEX

SPECIAL EXPERTISE INDEX

SPECIAL EXPERTISE INDEX

638

SPECIAL EXPERTISE INDEX

Special Expertise	Spec	Name	Pg	Special Expertise	Spec	Name	Pg
Lymphoma	Path	Warnke, R (CA)	373	Lymphoma	Hem	Zalusky, R (NY)	200
Lymphoma	Onc	Czuczman, M (NY)	214	Lymphoma	Onc	Offit, K (NY)	220
Lymphoma	Hem	Forman, S (CA)	206	Lymphoma	Hem	Kempin, S (NY)	198
Lymphoma	RadRO	Cox, J (TX)	447	Lymphoma	Path	Braylan, R (FL)	366
Lymphoma	Onc	Armitage, J (NE)	241	Lymphoma	Onc	Rosen, S (IL)	238
Lymphoma	Path	Weiss, L (CA)	373	Lymphoma	Onc	Horning, S (CA)	249
Lymphoma	Onc	Fisher, R (NY)	215	Lymphoma	Onc	Beatty, P (MT)	241
Lymphoma	Onc	Canellos, G (MA)	208	Lymphoma	Onc	Yunus, F (TN)	231
Lymphoma	RadRO	Glatstein, E (PA)	436	Lymphoma	Onc	Bernstein, Z (NY)	212
Lymphoma	Hem	Gregory, S (IL)	202	Lymphoma	RadRO	Constine III, L (NY)	435
Lymphoma	Hem	Gaynor, E (IL)	202	Lymphoma	RadRO	Russell, K (WA)	450
Lymphoma	NuM	Dillehay, G (IL)	460	Lymphoma	PHO	Pui, C (TN)	389
Lymphoma	Onc	Williams, M (VA)	231	Lymphoma	PHO	Goldman, S (TX)	395
Lymphoma	Onc	Hurd, D (NC)	227	Lymphoma	RadRO	Lin, H (MO)	444
Lymphoma	Onc	Colon-Otero, G (FL)	225	Lymphoma	RadRO	Tripuraneni, P (CA)	451
Lymphoma	Onc	De Vita Jr, V (CT)	209	Lymphoma	PHO	Cairo, M (NY)	383
Lymphoma	Onc	Rosen, P (CA)	251	Lymphoma	RadRO	Macklis, R (OH)	444
Lymphoma	Onc	Grossbard, M (NY)	216	Lymphoma	Onc	Mitchell, B (NC)	228
Lymphoma	Onc	Press, O (WA)	251	Lymphoma	PHO	Weinstein, H (MA)	382
Lymphoma	D	McDonald, C (RI)	137	Lymphoma	Path	Knowles, D (NY)	363
Lymphoma	Onc	Bierman, P (NE)	241	Lymphoma	Path	Frizzera, G (NY)	362
Lymphoma	Onc	Nadler, L (MA)	210	Lymphoma	RadRO	Lee, C (MN)	443
Lymphoma	Hem	Lill, M (CA)	206	Lymphoma	NuM	Silberstein, E (OH)	460
Lymphoma	Onc	Zelenetz, A (NY)	224	Lymphoma	Onc	Dakhil, S (KS)	241
Lymphoma	Hem	Vose, J (NE)	204	Lymphoma	Path	Kurtin, P (MN)	368
Lymphoma	Path	Swerdlow, S (PA)	365	Lymphoma	PHO	Manera, R (IL)	392
Lymphoma	Path	Jaffe, E (MD)	363	Lymphoma	PHO	Andrews, R (WA)	396
Lymphoma	Path	Harris, N (MA)	361	Lymphoma & Multiple Myeloma	Onc	Nissenblatt, M (NJ)	220
Lymphoma	Hem	van Besien, K (IL)	204	Lymphoma, Cutaneous B Cell (CBCL)	RadRO	Wilson, L (CT)	434
Lymphoma	Onc	Lynch Jr, J (FL)	228	Lymphoma, Cutaneous T Cell (CTCL)	RadRO	Wilson, L (CT)	434
Lymphoma	Onc	Schwartz, B (MN)	238	Lymphoma, Non-Hodgkin's	PHO	Sandlund Jr, J (TN)	389
Lymphoma	Onc	Smith, M (PA)	222	Lymphoma, Non-Hodgkin's	PHO	Murphy, S (TX)	395
Lymphoma	Hem	Mears, J (NY)	198	Lymphoma, Non-Hodgkin's	NuM	Wiseman, G (MN)	460
Lymphoma	Hem	Rai, K (NY)	199	Lymphoma, Non-Hodgkin's	Hem	Winter, J (IL)	204
Lymphoma	Onc	O'Brien, S (TX)	246	Lymphoma, Non-Hodgkin's	Hem	Gordon, L (IL)	202
Lymphoma	RadRO	Rabinovitch, R (CO)	446	Lymphoma, Non-Hodgkin's	Hem	Stiff, P (IL)	203
Lymphoma	Hem	Saven, A (CA)	207	Lymphoma, Non-Hodgkin's	Onc	Gerson, S (OH)	234
Lymphoma	Onc	Kaplan, L (CA)	249	Lymphoma, Non-Hodgkin's	Onc	Glick, J (PA)	216
Lymphoma	Onc	Chao, N (NC)	225	Lymphoma-Ocular (eye)	Oph	Gigantelli, J (NE)	313
Lymphoma	Onc	Schiffer, C (MI)	238				
Lymphoma	Onc	Bunn Jr, P (CO)	241	**M**			
Lymphoma	RadRO	Roberts, K (CT)	434				
Lymphoma	Hem	Baron, J (IL)	201	Macular Disease/Degeneration	Oph	Grossniklaus, H (GA)	311
Lymphoma	Path	Grogan, T (AZ)	370	Macular Disease/Degeneration	Oph	Sternberg Jr, P (TN)	312
Lymphoma	RadRO	Goodman, R (NJ)	436	Macular Disease/Degeneration	Oph	Finger, P (NY)	311
Lymphoma	RadRO	Ferree, C (NC)	439	Mammography	DR	Evers, K (PA)	453
Lymphoma	Path	Banks, P (NC)	366	Mammography	DR	Helvie, M (MI)	454
Lymphoma	Onc	Gockerman, J (NC)	226	Mammography	DR	Monsees, B (MO)	454
Lymphoma	Onc	Shulman, L (MA)	211	Mammography	DR	Otto, P (TX)	455
Lymphoma	Onc	Moore, J (NC)	228	Mammography	DR	Huynh, P (TX)	455
Lymphoma	PHO	Reaman, G (DC)	386	Mammography	DR	Mitnick, J (NY)	453
Lymphoma	Hem	Cooper, B (TX)	205	Mediastinal & Thoracic Cancers	TS	Vallieres, E (WA)	512
Lymphoma	Onc	Kosova, L (IL)	236	Mediastinal Cancer	Path	Koss, M (CA)	372
Lymphoma	Path	McCurley, T (TN)	366	Mediastinal Cancer	Path	Moran, C (TX)	370
Lymphoma	Path	Kinney, M (TX)	370	Mediastinal Cancer	Path	Suster, S (OH)	368
Lymphoma	RadRO	Mittal, B (IL)	444	Mediastinal Masses	TS	Kiernan, P (VA)	508
Lymphoma	Hem	Tallman, M (IL)	204	Mediastinal Tumors	TS	Keenan, R (PA)	506
Lymphoma	Onc	Golomb, H (IL)	235	Mediastinal Tumors	TS	Detterbeck, F (NC)	508
Lymphoma	Hem	Strauss, J (TX)	205	Mediastinal Tumors	TS	Kaiser, L (PA)	506
Lymphoma	Onc	Nichols, C (OR)	250	Mediastinal Tumors	Onc	Kris, M (NY)	218
Lymphoma	Onc	Piel, I (IL)	237	Medulloblastoma	NS	Raffel, C (MN)	268
Lymphoma	Hem	Savage, D (NY)	199	Melanoma	S	Kavanah, M (MA)	473
Lymphoma	Path	Nathwani, B (CA)	372	Melanoma	D	Bystryn, J (NY)	138
Lymphoma	Onc	Jillella, A (PA)	217	Melanoma	S	Kaufman, H (NY)	478

SPECIAL EXPERTISE INDEX

Special Expertise	Spec	Name	Pg	Special Expertise	Spec	Name	Pg
Metastatic Bone Disease	PMR	Gamble, G (MN)	552	Multiple Myeloma	RadRO	Meredith, R (AL)	441
Metastatic Cancer	Onc	Holland, J (NY)	217	Multiple Myeloma	PHO	Corey, S (TX)	395
Metastatic Disease Management	S	Dooley, W (OK)	491	Multiple Myeloma	Hem	Singhal, S (IL)	203
Microsurgery	PlS	Caffee, H (FL)	413	Multiple Myeloma	Onc	Yunus, F (TN)	231
Microsurgery	PlS	Brandt, K (MO)	414	Multiple Myeloma	Hem	Fonseca, R (AZ)	205
Microsurgery	PlS	Fix, R (AL)	413	Multiple Myeloma	Hem	Roodman, G (PA)	199
Microsurgery	PlS	Mathes, S (CA)	415	Multiple Myeloma	Onc	Kwak, L (TX)	245
Microsurgery	PlS	Wilkins, E (MI)	414	Multiple Myeloma	Hem	Coutre, S (CA)	206
Microsurgery	NS	Camins, M (NY)	261	Multiple Myeloma	Onc	Czuczman, M (NY)	214
Microvascular Reconstruction	Oto	Burkey, B (TN)	338	Multiple Myeloma	Hem	Savage, D (NY)	199
Microvascular Reconstruction	Oto	Urken, M (NY)	337	Multiple Myeloma	Onc	Coleman, M (NY)	213
Middle Ear Disorders	Oto	Miyamoto, R (IN)	341	Multiple Myeloma	Onc	Straus, D (NY)	222
Minimally Invasive Cancer Surgery	S	Tuttle, T (MN)	490	Multiple Myeloma	NuM	Wiseman, G (MN)	460
Minimally Invasive Neurosurgery	NS	Cohen, A (OH)	266	Multiple Myeloma	Onc	Williams, M (VA)	231
Minimally Invasive Prostate Surgery	U	Kawachi, M (CA)	536	Multiple Myeloma	Hem	Linker, C (CA)	207
Minimally Invasive Surgery	S	Schneider, P (CA)	496	Multiple Myeloma	RadRO	Yahalom, J (NY)	439
Minimally Invasive Surgery	CRS	Beck, D (LA)	130	Multiple Myeloma	Hem	Raphael, B (NY)	199
Minimally Invasive Surgery	GO	Poliakoff, S (FL)	296	Multiple Myeloma	OrS	Biermann, J (MI)	323
Minimally Invasive Thoracic Surgery	TS	Maddaus, M (MN)	509	Multiple Myeloma	Hem	Larson, R (IL)	202
Minimally Invasive Thoracic Surgery	TS	Friedberg, J (PA)	506	Multiple Myeloma	Onc	Schiffer, C (MI)	238
Minimally Invasive Urologic Surgery	U	Lanteri, V (NJ)	525	Multiple Myeloma	Onc	Ball, E (CA)	248
Minimally Invasive Urologic Surgery	U	Gluckman, G (IL)	531	Multiple Myeloma	Hem	Barlogie, B (AR)	204
Minimally Invasive Urologic Surgery	U	Wilson, T (CA)	537	Multiple Myeloma	Hem	Linenberger, M (WA)	206
Mitral Valve Repair	TS	Harrison, L (LA)	511	Multiple Myeloma	Onc	Smith, M (PA)	222
Mohs' Surgery	D	Orengo, I (TX)	143	Multiple Myeloma	Hem	Lyons, R (TX)	205
Mohs' Surgery	D	Hruza, G (MO)	141	Multiple Myeloma	Onc	Wingard, J (FL)	231
Mohs' Surgery	D	Leshin, B (NC)	141	Multiple Myeloma	Onc	Stadtmauer, E (PA)	222
Mohs' Surgery	D	Johnson, T (MI)	142	Multiple Sclerosis Imaging	NRad	Provenzale, J (NC)	456
Mohs' Surgery	D	Greenway, H (CA)	144	Musculoskeletal Tumors	OrS	Luck Jr, J (CA)	324
Mohs' Surgery	D	Wheeland, R (AZ)	143	Musculoskeletal Tumors	OrS	Benevenia, J (NJ)	324
Mohs' Surgery	D	Amonette, R (TN)	140	Musculoskeletal Tumors	OrS	Gebhardt, M (MA)	321
Mohs' Surgery	D	Otley, C (MN)	142	Musculoskeletal Tumors	OrS	Scully, S (FL)	322
Mohs' Surgery	D	Braun III, M (DC)	138	Musculoskeletal Tumors-	OrS	Neff, J (NE)	324
Mohs' Surgery	D	Brodland, D (PA)	138	Musculoskeletal Tissue Banking	OrS	Joyce, M (OH)	324
Mohs' Surgery	D	Leffell, D (CT)	137	Mycosis Fungoides	D	Rook, A (PA)	140
Mohs' Surgery	D	Bennett, R (CA)	143	Myelodysplasia, Leukemia, & Lymphoma	Hem	Zuckerman, K (FL)	201
Mohs' Surgery	D	Zitelli, J (PA)	140	Myelodysplastic Syndromes	Hem	List, A (FL)	201
Mohs' Surgery	D	Glogau, R (CA)	144	Myelodysplastic Syndromes	Onc	Gabrilove, J (NY)	215
Mohs' Surgery	D	Neuburg, M (WI)	142	Myelodysplastic Syndromes	Hem	Nand, S (IL)	203
Mohs' Surgery	D	Dzubow, L (PA)	138	Myelodysplastic Syndromes	Hem	Greer, J (TN)	200
Mohs' Surgery	D	Maloney, M (MA)	137	Myelodysplastic Syndromes	Onc	Petersdorf, S (WA)	250
Mohs' Surgery	D	Flowers, F (FL)	140	Myelodysplastic Syndromes	Hem	Pecora, A (NJ)	199
Mohs' Surgery	D	Robins, P (NY)	139	Myelodysplastic Syndromes	Onc	Powell, B (NC)	228
Mohs' Surgery	D	Green, H (FL)	141	Myeloproliferative Disorders	Hem	Nand, S (IL)	203
Mohs' Surgery	D	Taylor, R (TX)	143	Myeloproliferative Disorders	Hem	Baron, J (IL)	201
Mohs' Surgery	D	Bailin, P (OH)	141	Myeloproliferative Disorders	Hem	Spivak, J (MD)	200
Mohs' Surgery	D	Hanke, C (IN)	141	Myeloproliferative Disorders	Hem	Zuckerman, K (FL)	201
Mohs' Surgery	D	Geronemus, R (NY)	138	Myeloproliferative Disorders	Hem	Fruchtman, S (NY)	198
Movement Disorders	NS	Germano, I (NY)	261	Myeloproliferative Disorders	Hem	Solberg, L (FL)	201
Movement Disorders	NS	Kelly, P (NY)	262				
Movement Disorders	NS	Kondziolka, D (PA)	262	**N**			
Movement Disorders	NS	Lunsford, L (PA)	263				
MRI	NRad	Atlas, S (CA)	456	Nasal & Eyelid Reconstruction	PlS	Miller, T (CA)	415
MRI	DR	Weinreb, J (CT)	452	Nasal & Sinus Cancer	Oto	Carrau, R (PA)	333
Mucositis	RadRO	Martenson Jr, J (MN)	444	Nasal & Sinus Disorders	Oto	Stringer, S (MS)	339
Multiple Myeloma	Onc	Anderson, K (MA)	208	Nasal & Sinus Disorders	Oto	Siegel, G (IL)	342
Multiple Myeloma	Hem	Gertz, M (MN)	202	Nasal & Sinus Surgery	Oto	Krespi, Y (NY)	336
Multiple Myeloma	Hem	Greipp, P (MN)	202	Nasal Reconstruction	PlS	Walton Jr, R (IL)	414
Multiple Myeloma	Onc	Hussein, M (OH)	235	Nasal Surgery	PlS	Rohrich, R (TX)	415
Multiple Myeloma	Hem	Damon, L (CA)	206	Neonatal Surgery	PS	Jackson, R (AR)	404
Multiple Myeloma	Onc	Vescio, R (CA)	252	Neonatal Surgery	PS	Ginsburg, H (NY)	402
Multiple Myeloma	Onc	Bensinger, W (WA)	248	Neonatal Surgery	PS	Weinberger, M (FL)	403
Multiple Myeloma	Onc	Chanan-Khan, A (NY)	213	Neonatal Surgery	PS	Stolar, C (NY)	402
Multiple Myeloma	Hem	Djulbegovic, B (FL)	200	Neonatal Surgery-Gastrointestinal	PS	Sawin, R (WA)	404

SPECIAL EXPERTISE INDEX

644

645

SPECIAL EXPERTISE INDEX

SPECIAL EXPERTISE INDEX

648

SPECIAL EXPERTISE INDEX

653

SPECIAL EXPERTISE INDEX

ALPHABETICAL LISTING OF DOCTORS

Name	Specialty	Page
A		
Abbitt, P (FL)	DR	454
Abbruzzese, J (TX)	Onc	243
Abcarian, H (IL)	CRS	128
Abella, E (AZ)	PHO	394
Abeloff, M (MD)	Onc	211
Abrams, D (CA)	Onc	247
Abrams, R (IL)	RadRO	442
Abramson, A (NY)	Oto	333
Abramson, D (NY)	Oph	311
Abramson, N (FL)	Hem	200
Abromowitch, M (NE)	PHO	393
Ackerman, A (NY)	D	138
Acquadro, M (MA)	PM	353
Adler Jr, J (CA)	NS	270
Agarwala, S (PA)	Onc	211
Ahlgren, J (DC)	Onc	211
Ahmann, F (AZ)	Onc	243
Aiken, J (WI)	PS	403
Aisner, J (NJ)	Onc	211
Akerley, W (UT)	Onc	241
Al-Mefty, O (AR)	NS	269
Alavi, A (PA)	NuM	459
Alazraki, N (GA)	NuM	459
Albain, K (IL)	Onc	231
Albert, D (WI)	Oph	312
Alberts, D (AZ)	Onc	243
Alberts, W (FL)	Pul	424
Albright, A (PA)	NS	260
Albritton, K (MA)	PHO	381
Alexander, F (OH)	PS	403
Alfonso, A (NY)	S	475
Algazy, K (PA)	Onc	212
Alleyn, J (FL)	GO	294
Allred, D (TX)	Path	369
Althausen, A (MA)	U	523
Altman, A (CT)	PHO	381
Altorki, N (NY)	TS	505
Alvarez, R (AL)	GO	294
Ambinder, R (MD)	Onc	212
Ames, F (TX)	S	491
Amin, M (GA)	Path	365
Amonette, R (TN)	D	140
Andersen, J (CA)	PlS	415
Anderson, B (WA)	S	494
Anderson, J (MI)	Onc	231
Anderson, K (MA)	Onc	208
Anderson, R (UT)	Oph	313
Andrews, D (PA)	NS	260
Andrews, R (WA)	PHO	396
Andriole, G (MO)	U	530
Ang, K (TX)	RadRO	446
Anscher, M (NC)	RadRO	439

Name	Specialty	Page
Anthony, L (LA)	Onc	243
Antin, J (MA)	Onc	208
Antman, K (MD)	Onc	212
Antonia, S (FL)	Onc	224
Appelbaum, F (WA)	Onc	248
Apuzzo, M (CA)	NS	271
Aranha, G (IL)	S	486
Arber, D (CA)	Path	371
Arceci, R (MD)	PHO	382
Ariyan, S (CT)	PlS	411
Armitage, J (NE)	Onc	241
Arndt, C (MN)	PHO	390
Arriaga, M (PA)	Oto	333
Arteaga, C (TN)	Onc	224
Arts, H (MI)	Oto	339
Arun, B (TX)	Onc	243
Athanasian, E (NY)	HS	325
Atkins, M (MA)	Onc	208
Atlas, S (CA)	NRad	456
Augsburger, J (OH)	Oph	312
August, D (NJ)	S	475
Austin, J (NY)	DR	452
Awasthi, D (LA)	NS	270
Axelrod, D (NY)	S	475
B		
Babaian, R (TX)	U	534
Badie, B (WI)	NS	266
Bahnson, R (OH)	U	530
Bailey, H (TX)	CRS	130
Bailin, P (OH)	D	141
Bains, M (NY)	TS	505
Bakay, R (IL)	NS	266
Baker, L (MI)	Onc	231
Balch, C (VA)	S	482
Balducci, L (FL)	Onc	224
Ball, E (CA)	Onc	248
Balla, A (IL)	Path	367
Ballantyne, G (NJ)	S	475
Bander, N (NY)	U	523
Banks, P (NC)	Path	366
Barakat, R (NY)	GO	292
Barbosa, J (FL)	PHO	387
Bardot, S (LA)	U	534
Barkin, J (FL)	Ge	158
Barlogie, B (AR)	Hem	204
Barnes, W (DC)	GO	292
Barnett, G (OH)	NS	266
Baron, J (IL)	Hem	201
Barredo, J (SC)	PHO	387
Barter, J (MD)	GO	292
Bartlett, D (PA)	S	476
Bartlett, S (PA)	PlS	411

ALPHABETICAL LISTING OF DOCTORS

Name	Specialty	Page	Name	Specialty	Page
Basch, S (NY)	Psyc	419	Boland, C (TX)	Ge	159
Bashevkin, M (NY)	Onc	212	Boldt, D (TX)	Hem	204
Basler, J (TX)	U	534	Bollen, A (CA)	Path	371
Bass, B (MD)	S	476	Bolwell, B (OH)	Onc	232
Bassett, L (CA)	DR	455	Boniuk, M (TX)	Oph	313
Bastian, B (CA)	D	143	Bonomi, P (IL)	Onc	232
Batzdorf, U (CA)	NS	271	Boop, F (TN)	NS	264
Bauer, J (IL)	NS	266	Borden, E (OH)	Onc	232
Beall, M (VA)	U	528	Borgen, P (NY)	S	476
Beart Jr, R (CA)	CRS	130	Borges, L (MA)	NS	259
Beatty, P (MT)	Onc	241	Bosl, G (NY)	Onc	212
Beauchamp, R (TN)	S	482	Bostwick, D (VA)	Path	366
Beck, D (LA)	CRS	130	Bouwman, D (MI)	S	486
Becker, J (MA)	S	473	Bowen, G (UT)	D	142
Beecham, J (NH)	GO	291	Boxrud, C (CA)	Oph	314
Behm, F (TN)	Path	366	Boyce Jr, H (FL)	Ge	158
Behrns, K (NC)	S	482	Boyd, S (CA)	U	535
Belani, C (PA)	Onc	212	Brackmann, D (CA)	Oto	345
Belinson, J (OH)	GO	297	Bradford, C (MI)	Oto	340
Bell, D (MA)	Path	361	Brandt, K (MO)	PlS	414
Belldegrun, A (CA)	U	535	Braun III, M (DC)	D	138
Benedetti, C (OH)	PM	354	Braverman, I (CT)	D	137
Benevenia, J (NJ)	OrS	321	Brawer, M (WA)	U	535
Benjamin, R (TX)	Onc	243	Brawley, O (GA)	Onc	224
Bennett, R (CA)	D	143	Braylan, R (FL)	Path	366
Bensinger, W (WA)	Onc	248	Brecher, M (NY)	PHO	382
Benson, M (NY)	U	524	Breitbart, W (NY)	Psyc	419
Benson III, A (IL)	Onc	231	Breitfeld, P (NC)	PHO	387
Bentz, B (UT)	Oto	343	Brem, H (MD)	NS	260
Benz Jr., E (MA)	Hem	197	Brem, S (FL)	NS	264
Berchuck, A (NC)	GO	295	Brems, J (IL)	S	486
Berek, J (CA)	GO	301	Brendler, C (IL)	U	530
Berg, C (MD)	RadRO	434	Brennan, M (NY)	S	476
Berg, D (WA)	D	143	Brenner, M (TX)	Hem	204
Berg, S (TX)	PHO	394	Bresalier, R (TX)	Ge	160
Berg, W (MD)	DR	452	Brescia, F (SC)	Onc	225
Berger, M (CA)	NS	271	Brewer, M (AZ)	GO	300
Berke, G (CA)	Oto	345	Bricker, L (MI)	Onc	232
Berlin, J (TN)	Onc	224	Bristow, R (MD)	GO	292
Berman, M (CA)	GO	301	Brizel, D (NC)	RadRO	439
Bernard, S (NC)	Onc	224	Brockstein, B (IL)	Onc	232
Bernstein, Z (NY)	Onc	212	Brodeur, G (PA)	PHO	382
Berson, A (NY)	RadRO	435	Brodland, D (PA)	D	138
Bertolone, S (KY)	PHO	387	Brown, K (MI)	Ge	159
Bhan, A (MA)	Path	361	Bruce, J (NY)	NS	260
Bierman, P (NE)	Onc	241	Bruera, E (TX)	Onc	243
Biermann, J (MI)	OrS	323	Brufsky, A (PA)	Onc	212
Bilchik, A (CA)	S	494	Bruggers, C (UT)	PHO	394
Bilsky, M (NY)	NS	260	Bruner, J (TX)	Path	369
Bitran, J (IL)	Onc	232	Brunicardi, F (TX)	S	491
Black, K (CA)	NS	271	Brunt, L (MO)	S	486
Black, P (MA)	NS	259	Bruskewitz, R (WI)	U	530
Blair, N (IL)	Oph	312	Buchholz, T (TX)	RadRO	447
Bland, K (AL)	S	482	Buckner, J (MN)	Onc	232
Blaney, S (TX)	PHO	394	Bucky, L (PA)	PlS	411
Blanke, C (OR)	Onc	248	Budd, G (OH)	Onc	232
Blasko, J (WA)	RadRO	448	Bukowski, R (OH)	Hem	201
Bleday, R (MA)	CRS	125	Bull, D (UT)	TS	510
Bleyer, W (TX)	PHO	395	Bumpous, J (KY)	Oto	337
Blumenthal, D (UT)	N	283	Bunn Jr, P (CO)	Onc	241
Bockenstedt, P (MI)	Hem	201	Burger, P (MD)	Path	362
Boggan, J (CA)	NS	271	Burkey, B (TN)	Oto	338
Bojrab, D (MI)	Oto	340	Burnett II, A (MD)	U	524

Name	Specialty	Page	Name	Specialty	Page
Burris III, H (TN)	Onc	225	Char, D (CA)	Oph	314
Burstein, H (MA)	Onc	208	Charboneau, J (MN)	RadRO	442
Burt, R (UT)	Ge	159	Chari, R (TN)	S	482
Burt, R (IL)	Onc	233	Chen, A (MD)	PHO	383
Bussel, J (NY)	PHO	382	Cheng, E (MN)	OrS	323
Butler, D (TX)	D	142	Cheson, B (DC)	Hem	198
Buzdar, A (TX)	Onc	243	Cheville, A (PA)	PMR	551
Byrd, D (WA)	S	494	Chitambar, C (WI)	Onc	233
Bystryn, J (NY)	D	138	Chlebowski, R (CA)	Onc	248
			Cho, H (NY)	Oto	334
			Cho, K (MI)	Path	367
C			Chodak, G (IL)	U	530
			Choi, N (MA)	RadRO	433
Cady, B (RI)	S	473	Choti, M (MD)	S	476
Caffee, H (FL)	PlS	413	Chowdhury, K (CO)	Oto	343
Cagle, P (TX)	Path	369	Choy, H (TX)	RadRO	447
Cain, J (OR)	GO	301	Chu, E (CT)	Onc	208
Cairo, M (NY)	PHO	383	Cioffi, W (RI)	S	473
Calvo, B (NC)	S	482	Civin, C (MD)	PHO	383
Cameron, J (MD)	S	476	Clamon, G (IA)	Onc	233
Camins, M (NY)	NS	261	Clark, J (IL)	Onc	233
Camitta, B (WI)	PHO	390	Clark, O (CA)	S	494
Campbell, B (WI)	Oto	340	Clarke-Pearson, D (NC)	GO	295
Campbell, S (IL)	U	530	Clayman, G (TX)	Oto	343
Cance, W (FL)	S	482	Cleary, J (WI)	Onc	233
Canellos, G (MA)	Onc	208	Clinton, S (OH)	Onc	233
Caputo, T (NY)	GO	292	Clohisy, D (MN)	OrS	323
Carbone, D (TN)	Onc	225	Close, L (NY)	Oto	334
Cardenosa, G (NC)	DR	454	Cloughesy, T (CA)	N	283
Carey, L (FL)	S	482	Clutter, W (MO)	EDM	148
Carey, L (NC)	Onc	225	Cobleigh, M (IL)	Onc	233
Carlson, J (PA)	GO	292	Cobos, E (TX)	Hem	205
Carlson, R (CA)	Onc	248	Coccia, P (NE)	PHO	394
Carmel, P (NJ)	NS	261	Cochran, A (CA)	Path	371
Carpenter Jr, J (AL)	Onc	225	Cockerham, K (CA)	Oph	314
Carrau, R (PA)	Oto	333	Cohen, A (OH)	NS	266
Carroll, P (CA)	U	535	Cohen, A (KY)	CRS	127
Carroll, W (NY)	PHO	383	Cohen, B (OH)	ChiN	284
Carson, B (MD)	NS	261	Cohen, C (NY)	GO	293
Carter, H (MD)	U	524	Cohen, J (OR)	Oto	345
Cascino, T (MN)	N	282	Cohen, M (IA)	Path	367
Cassisi, N (FL)	Oto	338	Cohen, N (NY)	Oto	334
Castle, V (MI)	PHO	390	Cohen, P (DC)	Onc	213
Castleberry Jr, R (AL)	PHO	387	Cohen, R (PA)	Onc	213
Catalano, P (MA)	Oto	333	Cohen, S (NY)	Onc	213
Catalona, W (IL)	U	530	Cohn, S (IL)	PHO	390
Chabner, B (MA)	Onc	208	Coia, L (NJ)	RadRO	435
Chabot, J (NY)	S	476	Coit, D (NY)	S	476
Chait, A (WA)	EDM	148	Coker, N (TX)	Oto	344
Chakravarthy, A (TN)	RadRO	439	Colby, T (AZ)	Path	369
Chalas, E (NY)	GO	292	Coldwell, D (MS)	VIR	457
Chalian, A (PA)	Oto	333	Coleman, J (IN)	PlS	414
Champlin, R (TX)	Hem	205	Coleman, M (NY)	Onc	213
Chanan-Khan, A (NY)	Onc	213	Coleman, R (NC)	NuM	459
Chandler, W (MI)	NS	266	Coller, J (MA)	CRS	125
Chandrasoma, P (CA)	Path	371	Collins, E (NH)	PlS	411
Chang, A (MI)	S	486	Colombani, P (MD)	PS	402
Chang, H (CA)	S	494	Colon-Otero, G (FL)	Onc	225
Chao, N (NC)	Onc	225	Come, S (MA)	Onc	209
Chap, L (CA)	Onc	248	Comis, R (PA)	Onc	213
Chapman, P (NY)	Onc	213	Conant, E (PA)	DR	452
Chapman, P (MA)	NS	259	Conant, M (CA)	D	143
Chapman, R (MI)	Onc	233	Connolly, J (MA)	Path	361
Chapman, W (MO)	S	486			

ALPHABETICAL LISTING OF DOCTORS

Name	Specialty	Page	Name	Specialty	Page
Eberlein, T (MO)	S	487	Finan, M (LA)	GO	300
Eckardt, J (CA)	OrS	324	Fine, H (MD)	Onc	215
Edelson, R (CT)	D	137	Finger, P (NY)	Oph	311
Edelstein, B (NY)	DR	453	Finklestein, J (CA)	PHO	397
Edge, S (NY)	S	476	Finlay, J (CA)	PHO	397
Edington, H (PA)	S	477	Fiorica, J (FL)	GO	295
Edney, J (NE)	S	490	Fisher, M (NY)	D	138
Edwards, M (AR)	S	491	Fisher, P (CA)	N	283
Egan, T (NC)	TS	508	Fisher, R (NY)	Onc	215
Eichler, C (FL)	D	140	Fisher, W (TX)	S	492
Eifel, P (TX)	RadRO	447	Fishman, D (NY)	GO	293
Eilber, F (CA)	S	494	Fishman, E (MD)	DR	453
Einhorn, L (IN)	Onc	234	Fishman, S (CA)	PM	354
Eisele, D (CA)	Oto	346	Fitzgerald, P (CA)	EDM	149
Eisenberg, B (NH)	S	473	Fitzgibbon, D (WA)	PM	355
Eisenberg, H (MD)	NS	261	Fix, R (AL)	PlS	413
Eisenberger, M (MD)	Onc	214	Flamm, E (NY)	NS	261
Eisenstat, T (NJ)	CRS	126	Flanigan, R (IL)	U	531
Ellenbogen, R (WA)	NS	271	Fleischer, D (AZ)	Ge	160
Ellenhorn, J (CA)	S	495	Fleming, G (IL)	Onc	234
Ellis, W (WA)	U	536	Fleshman, J (MO)	CRS	128
Ellison, E (OH)	S	487	Fletcher, C (MA)	Path	361
Elmets, C (AL)	D	140	Flickinger, J (PA)	RadRO	436
Emami, B (IL)	RadRO	442	Flomenberg, N (PA)	Onc	215
Emanuel, P (AL)	Hem	200	Flowers, F (FL)	D	140
Emerson, S (PA)	Hem	198	Flynn, M (KY)	S	483
Emond, J (NY)	S	477	Flynn, P (MN)	Hem	201
Eng, C (OH)	Onc	234	Foley, E (VA)	CRS	127
Eng, K (NY)	S	477	Foley, K (NY)	PM	353
Enker, W (NY)	S	477	Follen-Mitchell, M (TX)	GO	300
Ennis, R (NY)	RadRO	435	Fong, Y (NY)	S	477
Epstein, J (MD)	Path	362	Fonseca, R (AZ)	Hem	205
Esserman, L (CA)	S	495	Forastiere, A (MD)	Onc	215
Essner, R (CA)	S	495	Forman, J (MI)	RadRO	442
Estabrook, A (NY)	S	477	Forman, S (CA)	Hem	206
Ettinger, D (MD)	Onc	215	Forman, W (NM)	Onc	244
Euhus, D (TX)	S	491	Formenti, S (NY)	RadRO	436
Evans, D (TX)	S	491	Forscher, C (CA)	Onc	249
Evers, K (PA)	DR	453	Fossella, F (TX)	Onc	244
Ewend, M (NC)	NS	264	Foster, R (IN)	U	531
			Foucar, M (NM)	Path	370
			Fowler, J (OH)	GO	297
F			Fowler Jr, W (NC)	GO	295
			Fox, K (PA)	Onc	215
Faber, L (IL)	TS	509	Fracasso, P (MO)	Onc	234
Fabian, C (KS)	Onc	242	Fraker, D (PA)	S	477
Falletta, J (NC)	PHO	388	Francis, K (NJ)	PMR	551
Fallon, R (IN)	PHO	391	Frangoul, H (TN)	PHO	388
Fann, J (WA)	Psyc	420	Frantz, C (DE)	PHO	383
Fanucchi, M (GA)	Onc	226	Frassica, F (MD)	OrS	321
Farrar, W (OH)	S	487	Frazier, T (PA)	S	477
Fay, J (TX)	Onc	244	Freedman, R (TX)	GO	300
Fee Jr, W (CA)	Oto	346	Freifeld, A (NE)	Inf	549
Feig, B (TX)	S	491	Friebert, S (OH)	PHO	391
Feig, S (CA)	PHO	397	Friedberg, J (PA)	TS	506
Feinstein, D (CA)	Hem	206	Friedlaender, G (CT)	OrS	321
Feldman, J (IL)	PMR	552	Friedman, A (NC)	NS	264
Felix, C (PA)	Onc	215	Friedman, D (WA)	PHO	397
Fenske, N (FL)	D	140	Friedman, H (NC)	PHO	388
Ferguson, M (IL)	TS	509	Frim, D (IL)	NS	267
Ferrara, J (MI)	PHO	391	Frizzera, G (NY)	Path	362
Ferraz, F (VA)	NS	264	Fromm, G (TX)	GO	300
Ferree, C (NC)	RadRO	439	Fruchtman, S (NY)	Hem	198
Fields, K (FL)	Hem	200			

ALPHABETICAL LISTING OF DOCTORS

Name	Specialty	Page	Name	Specialty	Page
Fry, R (PA)	CRS	126	Goldberg, M (PA)	TS	506
Fuchs, C (MA)	Onc	209	Goldberg, M (IL)	Ge	159
Fuchs, H (NC)	NS	265	Goldberg, R (NC)	Onc	226
Fuller, A (MA)	GO	291	Goldblum, J (OH)	Path	368
Fung, J (OH)	S	487	Goldman, A (FL)	Pul	424
Funk, G (IA)	Oto	340	Goldman, S (TX)	PHO	395
Futran, N (WA)	Oto	346	Goldman, S (IL)	PHO	391
			Goldsmith, S (NY)	NuM	459
			Goldstein, L (PA)	Onc	216
G			Golomb, H (IL)	Onc	235
			Golub, R (FL)	CRS	127
Gabram, S (IL)	S	487	Gomella, L (PA)	U	524
Gabrilove, J (NY)	Onc	215	Goodman, A (MA)	GO	291
Gaffney, D (UT)	RadRO	446	Goodman, R (NJ)	RadRO	436
Gagel, R (TX)	EDM	148	Goodnight, J (CA)	S	495
Galandiuk, S (KY)	CRS	127	Goodrich, J (NY)	NS	261
Galask, R (IA)	ObG	303	Goodwin, S (CA)	VIR	458
Gamble, G (MN)	PMR	552	Goodwin, W (FL)	Oto	338
Gandara, D (CA)	Onc	249	Gordon, L (IL)	Hem	202
Ganz, P (CA)	Onc	249	Gordon, M (NY)	D	138
Garber, J (MA)	Onc	209	Gorfine, S (NY)	CRS	126
Garnick, M (MA)	Onc	209	Goulet Jr, R (IN)	S	487
Garver Jr, R (AL)	Pul	424	Goumnerova, L (MA)	NS	259
Garvin, J (NY)	PHO	383	Gradishar, W (IL)	Onc	235
Gaynor, E (IL)	Hem	202	Grado, G (AZ)	RadRO	447
Gebhardt, M (MA)	OrS	321	Graham, M (NC)	Onc	226
Geller, K (CA)	Oto	346	Graham, M (AZ)	PHO	395
Gelmann, E (DC)	Onc	216	Graham-Pole, J (FL)	PHO	388
Georgiade, G (NC)	PlS	413	Grana, G (NJ)	Onc	216
Germano, I (NY)	NS	261	Grandis, J (PA)	Oto	334
Geronemus, R (NY)	D	138	Granstein, R (NY)	D	139
Gershenson, D (TX)	GO	300	Grant, C (MN)	S	487
Gerson, S (OH)	Onc	234	Grant, M (TX)	S	492
Gertz, M (MN)	Hem	202	Grasso, M (NY)	U	524
Geschwind, J (MD)	VIR	457	Greco, F (TN)	Onc	226
Gewirtz, A (PA)	Hem	198	Green, D (NY)	PHO	384
Geyer, J (WA)	PHO	397	Green, H (FL)	D	141
Gharagozloo, F (DC)	TS	506	Green, M (SC)	Onc	226
Giannotta, S (CA)	NS	271	Greenberg, D (MA)	Psyc	419
Gibbs, J (NY)	S	477	Greenberg, H (MI)	N	282
Gigantelli, J (NE)	Oph	313	Greenberg, R (PA)	U	524
Gilbert, M (TX)	N	283	Greenberger, J (PA)	RadRO	436
Gilchrest, B (MA)	D	137	Greene, G (AR)	U	534
Gill, H (CA)	U	536	Greene Jr, C (CA)	NS	272
Gill, I (OH)	U	531	Greenson, J (MI)	Path	368
Ginsburg, E (MA)	RE	305	Greenway, H (CA)	D	144
Ginsburg, H (NY)	PS	402	Greer, B (WA)	GO	301
Giuliano, A (CA)	S	495	Greer, J (TN)	Hem	200
Glader, B (CA)	PHO	397	Gregory, S (IL)	Hem	202
Glassburn, J (PA)	RadRO	436	Greipp, P (MN)	Hem	202
Glatstein, E (PA)	RadRO	436	Grem, J (NE)	Onc	242
Glick, J (PA)	Onc	216	Grier, H (MA)	PHO	381
Glisson, B (TX)	Onc	244	Grigsby, P (MO)	RadRO	442
Glode, L (CO)	Onc	242	Grody, W (CA)	CG	548
Glogau, R (CA)	D	144	Grogan, T (AZ)	Path	370
Gluckman, G (IL)	U	531	Groopman, J (MA)	Hem	197
Gluckman, J (OH)	Oto	340	Grosfeld, J (IN)	PS	403
Gockerman, J (NC)	Onc	226	Grosh, W (VA)	Onc	226
Godder, K (OR)	PHO	397	Grossbard, M (NY)	Onc	216
Godwin, J (IL)	Hem	202	Grossniklaus, H (GA)	Oph	311
Goff, B (WA)	GO	301	Grubb Jr, R (MO)	NS	267
Goffinet, D (CA)	RadRO	449	Gruber, S (MI)	Onc	235
Goggins, M (MD)	Ge	157	Grunberg, S (VT)	Onc	209
Gold, S (NC)	PHO	388			

Name	Specialty	Page
Grupp, S (PA)	PHO	384
Guillem, J (NY)	CRS	126
Gunderson, L (AZ)	RadRO	447
Gupta, P (PA)	Path	362
Gutierrez, F (IL)	NS	267
Gutin, P (NY)	NS	262

H

Name	Specialty	Page
Haase, G (CO)	PS	404
Habermann, T (MN)	Hem	202
Haffty, B (CT)	RadRO	433
Haik, B (TN)	Oph	312
Hait, W (NJ)	Onc	216
Halberg, F (CA)	RadRO	449
Hall, M (NC)	U	528
Halle, J (NC)	RadRO	439
Haller, D (PA)	Onc	216
Hallisey, M (CT)	VIR	457
Halpern, A (NY)	D	139
Halpern, H (IL)	RadRO	443
Halpern, S (NJ)	PHO	384
Haluszka, O (PA)	Ge	157
Hamaker, R (IN)	Oto	340
Hamilton, S (TX)	Path	370
Hammar, S (WA)	Path	372
Hancock, S (CA)	RadRO	449
Hande, K (TN)	Onc	227
Hanke, C (IN)	D	141
Hankinson, H (NM)	NS	270
Hanks, J (VA)	S	483
Hann, L (NY)	DR	453
Hanna, E (TX)	Oto	344
Har-El, G (NY)	Oto	334
Haraf, D (IL)	RadRO	443
Harbour, J (MO)	Oph	313
Harkema, J (MI)	S	487
Harper, D (NH)	ObG	303
Harris, J (MA)	RadRO	433
Harris, M (NJ)	PHO	384
Harris, N (MA)	Path	361
Harrison, L (NY)	RadRO	436
Harrison, L (LA)	TS	511
Harsh IV, G (CA)	NS	272
Hartmann, L (MN)	Onc	235
Harty, J (KY)	U	528
Haskal, Z (NY)	VIR	457
Hassenbusch, S (TX)	NS	270
Haughey, B (MO)	Oto	340
Hawkins, D (WA)	PHO	397
Hayani, A (IL)	PHO	391
Hayashi, R (MO)	PHO	391
Hayes, D (MI)	Onc	235
Healey, J (NY)	OrS	321
Heber, D (CA)	EDM	149
Heimburger, D (AL)	IM	550
Heinrich, M (OR)	Hem	206
Heitmiller, R (MD)	TS	506
Hekmatpanah, J (IL)	NS	267
Hellman, S (IL)	RadRO	443
Helman, L (MD)	PHO	384
Helvie, M (MI)	DR	454
Hemming, A (FL)	S	483

Name	Specialty	Page
Hendrickson, M (CA)	Path	372
Heney, N (MA)	U	523
Herbst, A (IL)	GO	297
Herbst, R (TX)	Onc	244
Herman, T (TX)	RadRO	447
Heros, R (FL)	NS	265
Herr, H (NY)	U	524
Herrmann, V (GA)	S	483
Hesdorffer, C (NY)	Onc	216
Hester Jr, T (GA)	PlS	413
Hetherington, M (MO)	PHO	391
Hicks Jr, W (NY)	Oto	335
Hiesiger, E (NY)	N	281
Hilden, J (OH)	PHO	392
Himelstein, B (WI)	PHO	392
Hinder, R (FL)	S	483
Hinkle, A (NY)	PHO	384
Hirsch, B (PA)	Oto	335
Hochster, H (NY)	Onc	217
Hoda, S (NY)	Path	362
Hoffman, A (CA)	EDM	149
Hoffman, H (IA)	Oto	340
Hoffman, J (PA)	S	478
Hoffman, L (NY)	PlS	412
Hoffman, P (IL)	Onc	235
Holden, S (CA)	U	536
Holland, J (NY)	Onc	217
Holland, J (NY)	Psyc	419
Holliday, M (MD)	Oto	335
Holmes, E (CA)	TS	511
Holt, P (NY)	Ge	157
Homans, A (VT)	PHO	381
Hong, W (TX)	Onc	244
Hoppe, R (CA)	RadRO	449
Hoque, L (HI)	S	495
Horn, B (CA)	PHO	398
Horn, T (AR)	D	143
Horning, S (CA)	Onc	249
Horowitz, I (GA)	GO	295
Hortobagyi, G (TX)	Onc	244
Horton, J (FL)	Onc	227
Horwitz, E (TN)	PHO	388
Horwitz, E (PA)	RadRO	436
Hoskins, W (GA)	GO	295
Houghton, A (NY)	Onc	217
Howe, J (IA)	S	487
Hricak, H (NY)	DR	453
Hruban, R (MD)	Path	363
Hruza, G (MO)	D	141
Huben, R (NY)	U	525
Huber Jr, P (TX)	CRS	130
Hudes, G (PA)	Onc	217
Hudis, C (NY)	Onc	217
Hudson, M (TN)	PHO	388
Huffman, J (CA)	U	536
Hug, E (NH)	RadRO	433
Hughes, K (MA)	S	473
Hunt, K (TX)	S	492
Hurd, D (NC)	Onc	227
Hurley, J (NY)	EDM	147
Hussain, M (MI)	Onc	235
Hussein, M (OH)	Onc	235
Hutchins, L (AR)	Onc	244

ALPHABETICAL LISTING OF DOCTORS

ALPHABETICAL LISTING OF DOCTORS

Name	Specialty	Page	Name	Specialty	Page
Knudson, M (CA)	S	496	Larson, D (CA)	RadRO	449
Kobrine, A (DC)	NS	262	Larson, R (IL)	Hem	202
Koch, W (MD)	Oto	335	Larson, S (NY)	NuM	459
Kodner, I (MO)	CRS	128	Laterra, J (MD)	N	281
Koeller, K (DC)	NRad	456	Lauer, S (GA)	PHO	389
Koeneman, K (MN)	U	531	Laughlin, M (OH)	Hem	203
Kohler, M (SC)	GO	296	Lavertu, P (OH)	Oto	341
Komaki, R (TX)	RadRO	447	Lavery, I (OH)	CRS	128
Kondziolka, D (PA)	NS	262	Lavyne, M (NY)	NS	262
Konski, A (PA)	RadRO	437	Lawrence, T (MI)	RadRO	443
Kopans, D (MA)	DR	452	Laws Jr., E (VA)	NS	265
Kopel, S (NY)	Hem	198	Lawson, D (GA)	Onc	227
Korones, D (NY)	PHO	385	Lawson, W (NY)	Oto	336
Kosova, L (IL)	Onc	236	Lazarus, H (OH)	Hem	203
Koss, M (CA)	Path	372	Le Boit, P (CA)	Path	372
Koulos, J (NY)	GO	293	Lebwohl, M (NY)	D	139
Kovnar, E (WI)	ChiN	284	Lederberg, M (NY)	Psyc	420
Kozlowski, J (IL)	U	531	Lee, C (MN)	RadRO	443
Krag, D (VT)	S	474	Lee, J (TX)	S	492
Kramer, E (NY)	NuM	459	Lee, K (PA)	S	478
Kranzler, L (IL)	NS	267	Lee, W (NC)	RadRO	440
Krasna, M (MD)	TS	507	Leffall Jr, L (DC)	S	478
Kraus, D (NY)	Oto	335	Leffell, D (CT)	D	137
Kraybill Jr, W (NY)	S	478	Legha, S (TX)	Onc	245
Kreissman, S (NC)	PHO	388	Leibel, S (CA)	RadRO	449
Kreitzer, J (NY)	PM	353	Leight, G (NC)	S	483
Krellenstein, D (NY)	TS	507	Leitch, A (TX)	S	492
Krespi, Y (NY)	Oto	336	Lema, M (NY)	PM	353
Kretschmar, C (MA)	PHO	382	Lentz, S (NC)	GO	296
Kris, M (NY)	Onc	218	Leonetti, J (IL)	Oto	341
Krouse, R (AZ)	S	492	Lepanto, P (WV)	RadRO	437
Kuettel, M (NY)	RadRO	437	Lepor, H (NY)	U	525
Kuhn, J (TX)	S	492	Lerner, S (TX)	U	534
Kun, L (TN)	RadRO	440	Leshin, B (NC)	D	141
Kung, F (CA)	PHO	398	Leslie, K (AZ)	Path	370
Kunkel, E (PA)	Psyc	419	Lesser, G (NC)	Onc	227
Kurman, R (MD)	Path	363	Lessin, S (PA)	D	139
Kurtin, P (MN)	Path	368	Levenback, C (TX)	GO	300
Kurtzberg, J (NC)	PHO	389	Levetown, M (TX)	Ped	405
Kushner, B (NY)	PHO	385	Levin, B (TX)	Ge	160
Kuske, R (AZ)	RadRO	447	Levin, V (TX)	N	283
Kvols, L (FL)	Onc	227	Levine, A (CA)	Hem	206
Kwak, L (TX)	Onc	245	Levine, E (NC)	S	484
Kwon, T (NY)	GO	293	Levine, E (NY)	Onc	218
			Levine, P (VA)	Oto	338
L			Levinson, S (NY)	PMR	551
			Levy, R (IL)	NS	267
La Quaglia, M (NY)	PS	402	Lewin, A (FL)	RadRO	440
Lackman, R (PA)	OrS	322	Li, B (LA)	S	493
Ladenson, P (MD)	EDM	147	Li Volsi, V (PA)	Path	363
Lagasse, L (CA)	GO	301	Liau, L (CA)	NS	272
Lage, J (SC)	Path	366	Libby, D (NY)	Pul	423
Landreneau, R (PA)	TS	507	Libertino, J (MA)	U	523
Lane, D (NY)	PrM	552	Libutti, S (MD)	S	478
Lane, J (NY)	OrS	322	Licciardi, F (NY)	RE	305
Lang Jr, F (TX)	NS	270	Liddle, R (NC)	Ge	158
Lange, B (PA)	PHO	385	Lieberman, R (MD)	Onc	218
Lange, P (WA)	U	536	Lieskovsky, G (CA)	U	536
Langer, C (PA)	Onc	218	Lightdale, C (NY)	Ge	157
Lanteri, V (NJ)	U	525	Lilenbaum, R (FL)	Hem	201
Lanza, D (FL)	Oto	338	Lill, M (CA)	Hem	206
Lanzkowsky, P (NY)	PHO	385	Lillehei, K (CO)	NS	269
Larach, S (FL)	CRS	128	Lillemoe, K (IN)	S	488

665

ALPHABETICAL LISTING OF DOCTORS

Name	Specialty	Page	Name	Specialty	Page
Lim, H (MI)	D	142	Mamelak, A (CA)	NS	272
Lin, H (MO)	RadRO	444	Mamounas, E (OH)	S	488
Linenberger, M (WA)	Hem	206	Manco-Johnson, M (CO)	PHO	394
Link, M (MN)	NS	267	Mandelbaum, D (RI)	ChiN	284
Link, M (CA)	PHO	398	Manera, R (IL)	PHO	392
Linker, C (CA)	Hem	207	Marcus Jr, R (GA)	RadRO	440
Linstrom, C (NY)	Oto	336	Marentette, L (MI)	Oto	341
Lippman, M (MI)	Onc	236	Margolin, K (CA)	Onc	250
Lippman, S (TX)	Onc	245	Marina, N (CA)	PHO	398
Lipshutz, W (PA)	Ge	157	Maris, J (PA)	PHO	385
Lipton, J (NY)	PHO	385	Mark, E (MA)	Path	361
List, A (FL)	Hem	201	Markman, M (TX)	Onc	245
Litzow, M (MN)	Hem	203	Markowitz, S (OH)	Onc	237
Livingston, P (NY)	Onc	218	Marks, K (OH)	OrS	323
Livingston, R (WA)	Onc	249	Marks, L (NC)	RadRO	440
Ljung, B (CA)	Path	372	Marks, S (PA)	Onc	219
Lockhart, J (FL)	U	528	Marsh Jr, J (PA)	S	479
Loeffler, J (MA)	RadRO	433	Marshall, F (GA)	U	528
Loehrer, P (IN)	Onc	236	Marshall, J (DC)	Onc	219
Loftus, C (PA)	NS	262	Martenson Jr, J (MN)	RadRO	444
Logothetis, C (TX)	Onc	245	Martuza, R (MA)	NS	259
Logrono, R (TX)	Path	370	Mason, J (MA)	Ge	157
Long, D (MD)	NS	263	Masood, S (FL)	Path	366
Longo, W (CT)	CRS	125	Masters, G (DE)	Onc	219
Look, K (IN)	GO	298	Mathes, S (CA)	PlS	415
Loprinzi, C (MN)	Onc	236	Mathisen, D (MA)	TS	505
Loree, T (NY)	PlS	412	Matthay, K (CA)	PHO	398
Lossos, I (FL)	Onc	227	Matthay, R (CT)	Pul	423
Lotze, M (PA)	S	479	Mattox, D (GA)	Oto	338
Loughlin, K (MA)	U	523	Mauro, M (NC)	VIR	457
Lowe, F (NY)	U	525	Maxwell, G (TN)	PlS	413
Lowe, L (MI)	D	142	May Jr, J (MA)	PlS	411
Lowe, N (CA)	D	144	Mayberg, M (WA)	NS	272
Luchtman-Jones, L (MO)	PHO	392	Mayer, R (MA)	Onc	210
Luck Jr, J (CA)	OrS	324	Maziarz, R (OR)	Hem	207
Lueder, G (MO)	Oph	313	McCaffrey, T (FL)	Oto	338
Lugg, J (WY)	U	533	McCarthy, S (CT)	DR	452
Lunsford, L (PA)	NS	263	McConnell, J (TX)	U	534
Lurain, J (IL)	GO	298	McCormick, B (NY)	RadRO	437
Lyckholm, L (VA)	Onc	228	McCormick, P (NY)	NS	263
Lydiatt, D (NE)	Oto	343	McCormick, S (NY)	Path	363
Lydiatt, W (NE)	Oto	343	McCraw, J (MS)	PlS	413
Lyerly, H (NC)	S	484	McCullough, D (NC)	U	528
Lyman, G (NY)	Onc	218	McCurley, T (TN)	Path	366
Lynch, T (MA)	Onc	210	McDonald, C (RI)	D	137
Lynch Jr, J (FL)	Onc	228	McDonald, D (MO)	OrS	323
Lyons, R (TX)	Hem	205	McDougal, W (MA)	U	523
			McGill, T (MA)	PO	401
			McGlave, P (MN)	Hem	203
M			McGovern, F (MA)	U	523
			McGrath, P (KY)	S	484
Macchia, R (NY)	U	525	McGuire III, W (MD)	Onc	219
Macdonald, J (NY)	Onc	219	McGuirt, W (NC)	Oto	338
Macdonald, R (IL)	NS	267	McKenna, W (PA)	RadRO	437
Machtay, M (PA)	RadRO	437	McKenna Jr, R (CA)	TS	511
Maciejewski, J (OH)	Hem	203	McLennan, G (IA)	Pul	424
MacKeigan, J (MI)	CRS	129	McMasters, K (KY)	S	484
Macklis, R (OH)	RadRO	444	McMenomey, S (OR)	Oto	346
Maddaus, M (MN)	TS	509	McNeese, M (TX)	RadRO	448
Madoff, R (MN)	CRS	129	McVary, K (IL)	U	532
Malawer, M (DC)	OrS	322	Meacham, L (GA)	PEn	400
Malik, G (MI)	NS	268	Mears, J (NY)	Hem	198
Malkowicz, B (PA)	U	525	Medbery, C (OK)	RadRO	448
Maloney, M (MA)	D	137			

Name	Specialty	Page
Medich, D (PA)	CRS	126
Medina, J (OK)	Oto	344
Meehan, K (NH)	Hem	197
Meek, R (DE)	PHO	385
Mehta, M (WI)	RadRO	444
Melamed, J (NY)	Path	364
Melmed, S (CA)	EDM	149
Melvin, W (OH)	S	488
Mendelson, E (IL)	DR	454
Mendenhall, N (FL)	RadRO	440
Mendenhall, W (FL)	RadRO	440
Menon, M (MI)	U	532
Merchant, T (TN)	RadRO	440
Meredith, R (AL)	RadRO	441
Meropol, N (PA)	Onc	219
Meyers, B (MO)	TS	510
Meyers, P (NY)	PHO	386
Meyskens, F (CA)	Onc	250
Michalski, J (MO)	RadRO	444
Michelassi, F (NY)	S	479
Middleton, R (UT)	U	533
Mieler, W (TX)	Oph	313
Mies, C (PA)	Path	364
Mihm Jr., M (MA)	D	137
Mikkelsen, T (MI)	NS	268
Miles, B (TX)	U	534
Miller, J (GA)	TS	508
Miller, K (MA)	Hem	197
Miller, S (MD)	D	139
Miller, T (AZ)	Onc	246
Miller, T (CA)	PlS	415
Millikan, R (TX)	Onc	246
Millis, J (IL)	S	488
Mills, S (VA)	Path	367
Milsom, J (NY)	CRS	126
Minsky, B (NY)	RadRO	437
Mintzer, D (PA)	Onc	219
Mitchell, B (NC)	Onc	228
Mitnick, J (NY)	DR	453
Mittal, B (IL)	RadRO	444
Miyamoto, R (IN)	Oto	341
Moley, J (MO)	S	488
Monsees, B (MO)	DR	454
Montgomery, E (MD)	Path	364
Montie, J (MI)	U	532
Moore, A (NY)	Onc	219
Moore, D (IN)	GO	298
Moore, J (NC)	Onc	228
Moran, C (TX)	Path	370
Morgan, E (IL)	PHO	392
Morgan, L (FL)	ObG	303
Morgan, M (PA)	GO	294
Morgan III, W (TN)	PS	403
Morrison, G (FL)	NS	265
Morrow, C (CA)	GO	302
Morrow, M (PA)	S	479
Mortimer, J (CA)	Onc	250
Morton, D (CA)	TS	512
Moscow, J (KY)	PHO	389
Mostwin, J (MD)	U	526
Motzer, R (NY)	Onc	220
Moul, J (NC)	U	529
Movsas, B (MI)	RadRO	444

Name	Specialty	Page
Muggia, F (NY)	Onc	220
Mulvihill, J (OK)	CG	548
Mulvihill, S (UT)	S	490
Mundt, A (IL)	RadRO	444
Muntz, H (WA)	GO	302
Murphree, A (CA)	Oph	314
Murphy, S (TX)	PHO	395
Murphy, W (FL)	Path	367
Murray, T (FL)	Oph	312
Murtagh, F (FL)	NRad	456
Muss, H (VT)	Onc	210
Mutch, D (MO)	GO	298
Myers, E (PA)	Oto	336
Myers, J (MN)	Path	368
Myers, J (TX)	Oto	344
Myers, R (MN)	U	532
Myerson, R (MO)	RadRO	445

N

Name	Specialty	Page
Nachman, J (IL)	PHO	392
Nadler, L (MA)	Onc	210
Nand, S (IL)	Hem	203
Nascimento, A (MN)	Path	368
Naslund, M (MD)	U	526
Natale, R (CA)	Onc	250
Nathanson, S (MI)	S	488
Nathwani, B (CA)	Path	372
Nava-Villarreal, H (NY)	S	479
Neff, J (NE)	OrS	324
Neglia, J (MN)	PHO	392
Negrin, R (CA)	Hem	207
Neifeld, J (VA)	S	484
Nelson, E (UT)	S	490
Nelson, H (MN)	CRS	129
Nelson, J (PA)	U	526
Nemunaitis, J (TX)	Onc	246
Nesbitt, J (TN)	TS	508
Netterville, J (TN)	Oto	339
Neuburg, M (WI)	D	142
Neumann, D (OH)	NuM	460
Neuwelt, E (OR)	NS	272
Newman, L (MI)	S	488
Newton, H (OH)	N	282
Nichols, C (OR)	Onc	250
Nicholson, H (OR)	PHO	398
Nicosia, S (FL)	Path	367
Niederhuber, J (WI)	S	488
Nigra, T (DC)	D	139
Niloff, J (MA)	GO	291
Nimer, S (NY)	Hem	199
Ninan, M (TN)	TS	508
Nissenblatt, M (NJ)	Onc	220
Nivatvongs, S (MN)	CRS	129
Nogueras, J (FL)	CRS	128
Noller, K (MA)	ObG	303
Noone, R (PA)	PlS	412
Nori, D (NY)	RadRO	437
Norton, J (CA)	S	496
Norton, L (NY)	Onc	220
Novick, A (OH)	U	532
Noyes, N (NY)	RE	305
Numann, P (NY)	S	479

ALPHABETICAL LISTING OF DOCTORS

Name	Specialty	Page	Name	Specialty	Page
Nuss, D (LA)	Oto	344	Patrizio, P (CT)	RE	305
			Patt, R (TX)	PM	354
			Patt, Y (NM)	Onc	246
O			Patterson, G (MO)	TS	510
			Patterson, J (OR)	Pul	424
O'Brien, J (CA)	Oph	314	Patz, E (NC)	DR	454
O'Brien, S (TX)	Onc	246	Payne, R (NC)	PM	354
O'Day, S (CA)	Onc	250	Peabody, T (IL)	OrS	324
O'Donnell, M (IA)	U	532	Pearlman, N (CO)	S	490
O'Hea, B (NY)	S	479	Pecora, A (NJ)	Hem	199
O'Leary, M (MN)	PHO	393	Pegram, M (CA)	Onc	250
O'Malley Jr, B (PA)	Oto	336	Pellegrini, C (WA)	S	496
O'Reilly, E (NY)	Onc	220	Pelzer, H (IL)	Oto	341
O'Reilly, R (NY)	PHO	386	Pemberton, J (MN)	CRS	129
O'Rourke, D (PA)	NS	263	Penalver, M (FL)	GO	296
O'Shaughnessy, J (TX)	Onc	246	Pendergrass, T (WA)	PHO	399
Odom, L (CO)	PHO	394	Pensak, M (OH)	Oto	341
Odze, R (MA)	Path	361	Perez, E (FL)	Onc	228
Oeffinger, K (TX)	Ped	405	Perlman, E (IL)	Path	368
Offit, K (NY)	Onc	220	Perry, M (MO)	Onc	237
Olopade, O (IL)	Onc	237	Persky, M (NY)	Oto	336
Olsen, E (NC)	D	141	Peschel, R (CT)	RadRO	433
Olsen, K (MN)	Oto	341	Peters, G (AL)	Oto	339
Onders, R (OH)	S	488	Petersdorf, S (WA)	Onc	250
Opelka, F (MA)	CRS	125	Peterson, B (MN)	Onc	237
Orel, S (PA)	DR	453	Petrelli, N (DE)	S	479
Orengo, I (TX)	D	143	Petruzzelli, G (IL)	Oto	342
Orenstein, J (DC)	Path	364	Petrylak, D (NY)	Onc	221
Origitano, T (IL)	NS	268	Pezner, R (CA)	RadRO	449
Orringer, M (MI)	TS	510	Pfister, D (NY)	Onc	221
Osborne, C (TX)	Onc	246	Phillips, P (PA)	ChiN	284
Osborne, M (NY)	S	479	Phillips, T (CA)	RadRO	450
Osteen, R (MA)	S	474	Picus, J (MO)	Onc	237
Oster, M (NY)	Onc	220	Piel, I (IL)	Onc	237
Ostrer, H (NY)	CG	547	Pienta, K (MI)	Onc	237
Otley, C (MN)	D	142	Piepmeier, J (CT)	NS	260
Ott, K (CA)	NS	272	Pierce, L (MI)	RadRO	445
Otto, P (TX)	DR	455	Pierson III, R (MD)	TS	507
Otto, R (TX)	Oto	344	Piest, K (TX)	Oph	314
Overmoyer, B (OH)	Onc	237	Pinson, C (TN)	S	484
Ozols, R (PA)	Onc	220	Pinto, H (CA)	Onc	251
			Pisano, E (NC)	DR	454
P			Pistenmaa, D (TX)	RadRO	448
			Pisters, K (TX)	Onc	246
Packer, R (DC)	ChiN	284	Pisters, L (TX)	U	534
Page, D (TN)	Path	367	Pisters, P (TX)	S	493
Paidas, C (FL)	PS	403	Pitman, K (MS)	Oto	339
Pairolero, P (MN)	TS	510	Pitts, L (CA)	NS	272
Palefsky, J (CA)	Inf	549	Pochapin, M (NY)	Ge	157
Panicek, D (NY)	DR	453	Pockaj, B (AZ)	S	493
Papadopoulos, N (TX)	Onc	246	Podoloff, D (TX)	NuM	460
Papel, I (MD)	Oto	336	Podratz, K (MN)	GO	298
Pappas, T (NC)	S	484	Poliakoff, S (FL)	GO	296
Parent, A (MS)	NS	265	Polk Jr, H (KY)	S	484
Parham, G (AL)	GO	296	Pollack, A (PA)	RadRO	438
Park, T (MO)	NS	268	Pollack, I (PA)	NS	263
Parker, R (NY)	PHO	386	Pollack, J (NY)	RadRO	438
Partridge, E (AL)	GO	296	Pollock, R (TX)	S	493
Pasmantier, M (NY)	Onc	221	Polsky, B (NY)	Inf	549
Pass, H (MI)	TS	510	Ponn, T (CT)	S	474
Pass, H (MI)	S	489	Portenoy, R (NY)	PM	353
Patchefsky, A (PA)	Path	364	Porter, D (PA)	Hem	199
Patchell, R (KY)	N	281	Posner, J (NY)	N	281

ALPHABETICAL LISTING OF DOCTORS

Name	Specialty	Page	Name	Specialty	Page
S			Schusterman, M (TX)	PlS	415
			Schwartz, B (MN)	Onc	238
Saclarides, T (IL)	CRS	129	Schwartz, C (MD)	PHO	386
Safai, B (NY)	D	140	Schwartz, G (PA)	S	480
Sagalowsky, A (TX)	U	535	Schwartz, L (PA)	PMR	551
Sagar, S (OH)	N	282	Schwartz, M (FL)	Onc	229
Sagel, S (MO)	DR	455	Schwartz, P (CT)	GO	291
Saha, S (MI)	S	489	Scott, R (MA)	NS	260
Sahler, O (NY)	Ped	405	Scott-Conner, C (IA)	S	489
Saiki, J (NM)	Onc	247	Scully, S (FL)	OrS	322
Sailer, S (NC)	RadRO	441	Seagren, S (CA)	RadRO	450
Salem, P (TX)	Onc	247	See, W (WI)	U	532
Salem, R (IL)	VIR	458	Seewaldt, V (NC)	Onc	229
Salem, R (CT)	S	474	Seiff, S (CA)	Oph	314
Sallan, S (MA)	Ped	405	Sen, C (NY)	NS	263
Saltz, L (NY)	Onc	221	Senagore, A (OH)	CRS	129
Salvi, S (IL)	PHO	393	Sener, S (IL)	S	489
Samlowski, W (UT)	Onc	242	Senzer, N (TX)	RadRO	448
Sampson, J (NC)	NS	265	Sepkowitz, K (NY)	Inf	549
Samuels, B (ID)	Onc	242	Serody, J (NC)	Onc	229
Sanchez, M (NJ)	Path	364	Sevin, B (FL)	GO	296
Sanders, W (GA)	U	529	Sewell, C (GA)	Path	367
Sandler, A (TN)	Onc	229	Shah, J (NY)	S	480
Sandler, E (FL)	PHO	389	Shaha, A (NY)	S	481
Sandler, H (MI)	RadRO	445	Shahian, D (MA)	TS	505
Sandlund Jr, J (TN)	PHO	389	Shamberger, R (MA)	S	474
Sarr, M (MN)	S	489	Shank, B (CA)	RadRO	450
Sasaki, C (CT)	Oto	333	Shapiro, C (OH)	Onc	239
Savage, D (NY)	Hem	199	Shapiro, L (NY)	CG	547
Saven, A (CA)	Hem	207	Shapiro, S (IN)	NS	269
Sawaya, R (TX)	NS	270	Shapiro, W (AZ)	N	283
Sawczuk, I (NJ)	U	526	Shapshay, S (MA)	Oto	333
Sawin, R (WA)	PS	404	Shaw, E (NC)	RadRO	441
Scarborough, M (FL)	OrS	322	Shea, T (NC)	Onc	229
Scardino, P (NY)	U	526	Sheinfeld, J (NY)	U	526
Schantz, S (NY)	Oto	337	Shellito, P (MA)	CRS	125
Schechter, N (CT)	Ped	405	Sherman, R (CA)	PlS	415
Scheff, A (CA)	NuM	460	Sherman, S (TX)	EDM	148
Scheinberg, D (NY)	Onc	221	Shields, C (PA)	Oph	311
Scheithauer, B (MN)	Path	368	Shields, J (PA)	Oph	311
Schellhammer, P (VA)	U	529	Shields, P (DC)	Onc	222
Schepps, B (RI)	DR	452	Shike, M (NY)	Ge	158
Scher, C (LA)	PHO	396	Shin, D (GA)	Onc	229
Scher, H (NY)	Onc	221	Shina, D (NM)	RadRO	448
Schiff, D (VA)	N	282	Shindo, M (NY)	Oto	337
Schiff, P (NY)	RadRO	438	Shipley, W (MA)	RadRO	434
Schiffer, C (MI)	Onc	238	Shochat, S (TN)	PS	403
Schiller, A (NY)	Path	365	Shrieve, D (UT)	RadRO	446
Schiller, G (CA)	Hem	207	Shulman, L (MA)	Onc	211
Schiller, J (WI)	Onc	238	Shulman, L (IL)	ObG	303
Schink, J (IL)	GO	299	Sibley, R (CA)	Path	373
Schlegel, P (NY)	U	526	Sidransky, D (MD)	Onc	222
Schmidt, J (CA)	U	537	Siegel, B (MO)	NuM	460
Schnabel, F (NY)	S	480	Siegel, G (IL)	Oto	342
Schneider, P (CA)	S	496	Siegel, S (CA)	PHO	399
Schnitt, S (MA)	Path	362	Sigurdson, E (PA)	S	481
Schoetz, D (MA)	CRS	125	Silbergeld, D (WA)	NS	272
Schold Jr, S (FL)	N	282	Silberstein, E (OH)	NuM	460
Schomberg, P (MN)	RadRO	445	Silva, E (TX)	Path	371
Schraut, W (PA)	S	480	Silver, M (IL)	Pul	424
Schuchter, L (PA)	Onc	221	Silverberg, S (MD)	Path	365
Schuller, D (OH)	Oto	342	Silverman, J (PA)	Path	365
Schuster, M (NY)	Hem	199	Silverman, P (OH)	Onc	239

ALPHABETICAL LISTING OF DOCTORS

Name	Specialty	Page	Name	Specialty	Page
Waxman, A (CA)	NuM	461	Wilson, T (CA)	U	537
Waxman, I (IL)	Ge	159	Winawer, S (NY)	Ge	158
Waye, J (NY)	Ge	158	Winer, E (MA)	Onc	211
Wazen, J (NY)	Oto	337	Wingard, J (FL)	Onc	231
Wazer, D (RI)	RadRO	434	Winick, N (TX)	PHO	396
Weber, B (PA)	Onc	223	Winter, J (IL)	Hem	204
Weber, J (CA)	Onc	252	Wisch, N (NY)	Hem	200
Weber, R (TX)	Oto	345	Wiseman, G (MN)	NuM	460
Weber, S (TX)	Oto	345	Wisoff, J (NY)	NS	264
Weichselbaum, R (IL)	RadRO	446	Witt, T (IL)	S	490
Weigel, R (PA)	S	481	Witte, M (AZ)	IM	550
Wein, A (PA)	U	527	Wolf, G (MI)	Oto	343
Weinberger, M (FL)	PS	403	Wolfe, L (MA)	PHO	382
Weinberger, M (NY)	PM	353	Wolff, A (MD)	Onc	224
Weiner, G (IA)	Onc	240	Wolff, B (MN)	CRS	130
Weiner, L (PA)	Onc	223	Woltering, E (LA)	S	494
Weiner, M (NY)	PHO	387	Wong, J (CA)	RadRO	451
Weingeist, T (IA)	Oph	313	Wong, W (NY)	CRS	127
Weinreb, J (CT)	DR	452	Woo, P (NY)	Oto	337
Weinstein, G (PA)	Oto	337	Wood, D (MI)	U	533
Weinstein, H (MA)	PHO	382	Wood, D (WA)	TS	512
Weinstein, S (UT)	PM	354	Wood, G (WI)	D	142
Weisberg, T (ME)	Onc	211	Wood, R (TX)	S	494
Weisenburger, D (NE)	Path	369	Wood, W (GA)	S	485
Weisman, R (CA)	Oto	347	Wood Molo, M (IL)	RE	306
Weiss, G (VA)	Onc	231	Woods, W (GA)	PHO	390
Weiss, L (CA)	Path	373	Worden, F (MI)	Onc	240
Weiss, M (CA)	NS	273	Wright, C (MA)	TS	505
Weiss, R (NJ)	U	527			
Weiss, S (GA)	Path	367			
Weiss, S (NJ)	PrM	552	**Y**		
Weissler, M (NC)	Oto	339			
Weissman, D (WI)	Onc	240	Yahalom, J (NY)	RadRO	439
Weitzel, J (CA)	CG	548	Yang, J (MD)	S	481
Welton, M (CA)	CRS	131	Yang, S (MD)	TS	507
Wexler, L (NY)	PHO	387	Yarbrough, W (TN)	Oto	339
Wexner, S (FL)	CRS	128	Yeager, A (AZ)	PHO	396
Weymuller, E (WA)	Oto	347	Yeatman, T (FL)	S	485
Wharam Jr, M (MD)	RadRO	438	Yee, D (MN)	Onc	240
Wharen Jr, R (FL)	NS	265	Yen, Y (CA)	Onc	252
Wheeland, R (AZ)	D	143	Yetman, R (OH)	PlS	414
Wheeler, T (TX)	Path	371	Young, A (KY)	NS	266
Whelan, A (MO)	CG	548	Young, R (MA)	Path	362
Whelan, R (NY)	CRS	127	Yousem, S (PA)	Path	365
Whitaker, L (PA)	PlS	412	Yu, G (MD)	U	527
White, D (NY)	Pul	423	Yu, J (CA)	NS	273
Whitlock, J (TN)	PHO	390	Yueh, B (WA)	Oto	347
Whyte, R (CA)	TS	512	Yung, W (TX)	N	283
Wicha, M (MI)	Onc	240	Yunus, F (TN)	Onc	231
Wiener, E (PA)	PS	402			
Wiet, R (IL)	Oto	342			
Wilkins, E (MI)	PlS	414	**Z**		
Wilkins, R (CO)	OrS	324			
Wilkinson, R (HI)	PHO	399	Zalusky, R (NY)	Hem	200
Willett, C (NC)	RadRO	442	Zelefsky, M (NY)	RadRO	439
Williams, M (VA)	Onc	231	Zelenetz, A (NY)	Onc	224
Williams, R (IA)	U	533	Zimmerman, D (IL)	PEn	400
Williams, S (IN)	Onc	240	Zinner, M (MA)	S	475
Willis, I (FL)	S	485	Zitelli, J (PA)	D	140
Wilson, J (WI)	RadRO	446	Zorn, G (AL)	TS	509
Wilson, K (OH)	Oto	343	Zuckerman, K (FL)	Hem	201
Wilson, L (CT)	RadRO	434			
Wilson, M (TN)	Oph	312			

CASTLE CONNOLLY ORDER FORM

I want to order the following Castle Connolly Guides
at these discounted prices (15%):

America's Top Doctors, 5th edition # ___ of books at $25.46 $_____

Top Doctors:
New York Metro Area, 9th edition # ___ of books at $21.21 $_____
Chicago Metro Area, 3rd edition # ___ of books at $21.21 $_____

America's Cosmetic Doctors
and Dentists: 2nd edition # ___ of books at $25.46 $_____

Cancer Made Easier: *New York Metro Area* # ___ of books at $16.96 $_____

The Buyer's Guide to Choosing
the Best Healthcare # ___ of books at $11.01 $_____

The ABCs of HMOs: How To
Get The Best From Managed Care # ___ of books at $10.16 $_____

How to Find the Best Doctors:
Florida (pub. date: 2000) # ___ of books at $21.21 $_____

Subtotal $_____

*NY residents, please add 8.25% sales tax $_____
**NJ residents, please add 6% sales tax $_____

Add $4.99 per book for shipping and handling: # ____ of books x $4.99 $_____

TOTAL $_____

Please fill in the following information (please print):

Name: _____

Address: _____

City: _____

State: _____ Zip: _____

Phone (day): _____ (eve): _____

E-mail: _____

___ Check or Money Order enclosed
(payable to Castle Connolly Medical Ltd.)
___ Credit Card: please circle one Amex MC Visa

Card #: _____

Exp. Date: _____ Today's Date: _____

Signature: _____

Mail to: Castle Connolly Medical Ltd. 42 West 24th Street, New York, NY 10010
or fax to: (212) 367-0964
Order online: www.castleconnolly.com

ACKNOWLEDGMENTS

ACKNOWLEDGMENTS The publishers would like to thank the entire staff for their many hours and days of intense and precise work on this guide in order to further its goal of assisting consumers in making the best healthcare choices.

CASTLE CONNOLLY EXECUTIVE MANAGEMENT:

President & CEO	John J. Connolly, Ed.D.
Vice President, Chief Medical & Research Officer	Jean Morgan, M.D.
Vice President, Chief Strategy & Operations Officer	William Liss-Levinson, Ph.D.
Director, Information Technology	Taishi Thompson

We also would like to extend our gratitude to the American Board of Medical Specialties (ABMS) for allowing us to use excerpts, especially the descriptions of medical specialties and subspecialties, from the text of their publication "Which Medical Specialist for You?"

A special thank you to our Senior Advisor, Ina Bendis, M.D., Ph.D. and additional thanks to our layout/editorial staff: Stephenie Galvan; Nicole Haddad; Russell Hodgson and Matt Pretka.

OTHER PUBLICATIONS FROM CASTLE CONNOLLY MEDICAL LTD.:
America's Top Doctors; *Top Doctors: New York Metro Area; Top Doctors: Chicago Metro Area; America's Cosmetic Doctors and Dentists; Cancer Made Easier: New York—Metro Area* and others...

TO ORDER, USE FORM ON PREVIOUS PAGE

CUSTOMER FEEDBACK OFFER

We would appreciate your help improving our guide. If you will take a few minutes to complete this survey, we will give you a *free copy* of a Healthcare Choice Guide.

How did you find out about this book?
❏ From a Friend ❏ TV ❏ Newspaper ❏ Radio
❏ From a Doctor ❏ Bookstore ❏ Other _____

Why did you purchase this book?
❏ Needed a Specialist ❏ As a General Reference Guide
❏ Needed a Primary Care Physician ❏ Other _____

Did you use this book to find any physicians?
❏ No ❏ Yes – If yes, ❏ 1 doctor ❏ 2-3 doctors ❏ 4 or more doctors

Where do you primarily use this book?
❏ Home ❏ Office

Did you use this book as a reference to find a doctor for a friend or relative?
❏ No ❏ Yes – If yes, # of times _____

Did you loan this book to a friend or relative?
❏ No ❏ Yes – If yes, # of times _____

Do you have any suggestions for improving the book? _____

_____

Are there any other books you would like to see us publish? _____

_____

To Thank You for Helping Us...
Please check the *ONE* Healthcare Choice Guide that you wish to receive:

❏ *Board and Care Facilities and Adult Foster Homes*
❏ *Catching Costly Billing Errors*
❏ *Choosing a Chiropractor*
❏ *Choosing a Comprehensive Women's Health Center*
❏ *Choosing a Dentist*
❏ *Choosing a Diagnostic Cardiology Center*
❏ *Choosing a Diagnostic Imaging Center*
❏ *Choosing a Hospital*
❏ *Choosing a Nursing Home*
❏ *Choosing a Primary Care Doctor*
❏ *Choosing a Specialist*

❏ *Choosing a Veterinarian*
❏ *Choosing an Ambulatory Surgery Center*
❏ *Choosing an Assisted Living Facility*
❏ *Choosing Eldercare Advisors*
❏ *Family Caregivers*
❏ *Home Healthcare*
❏ *Home Modification for Elder-Friendly Living*
❏ *Rehabilitation Services*
❏ *Understanding Health Plans*

Name: _____

Address: _____

City: _____ State: _____ Zip Code _____

Mail or fax to:
Castle Connolly Medical Ltd. 42 West 24th Street, New York, NY 10010
Fax: (212) 367-0964 www.castleconnolly.com

DOCTOR-PATIENT ADVISOR

Doctor-Patient Advisor is a Castle Connolly Medical Ltd., service providing one-on-one consultations with a physician or nurse to individuals who have serious or complex medical problems or to anyone who feels he/she needs assistance finding the right physician for any purpose. Each client will receive personalized assistance in identifying the appropriate specialists for his/her condition. The Castle Connolly trained staff will utilize the extensive Castle Connolly Medical Ltd. database of physicians and hospitals, as well as individual searches, to locate the best resources to meet the client's needs. Fee: $275.00. For further information call (212) 367-8400 x 16.

For further information on physicians and hospitals please
visit the Castle Connolly Web site at
www.CastleConnolly.com or at
www.AmericasTopDoctorsforCancer.com